ENCYCLOPEDIA OF
SPORTS MEDICINE

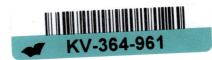

ENCYCLOPEDIA OF
SPORTS
MEDICINE

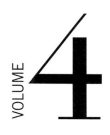

VOLUME 4

EDITOR
LYLE J. MICHELI, M.D.

O'Donnell Family Professor of Orthopaedic Sports Medicine and Director, Division of Sports Medicine, Children's Hospital Boston

Clinical Professor of Orthopaedic Surgery, Harvard Medical School

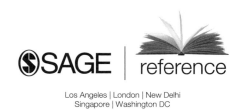

$SAGE | reference

Los Angeles | London | New Delhi
Singapore | Washington DC

For information:

SAGE Publications, Inc.
2455 Teller Road
Thousand Oaks, California 91320
E-mail: order@sagepub.com

SAGE Publications Ltd.
1 Oliver's Yard
55 City Road
London, EC1Y 1SP
United Kingdom

SAGE Publications India Pvt. Ltd.
B 1/I 1 Mohan Cooperative Industrial Area
Mathura Road, New Delhi 110 044
India

SAGE Publications Asia-Pacific Pte. Ltd.
33 Pekin Street #02-01
Far East Square
Singapore 048763

Printed in the United States of America.

Library of Congress Cataloging-in-Publication Data

Encyclopedia of sports medicine / edited by Lyle J. Micheli.
    p. cm.
"A SAGE Reference Publication."
Includes bibliographical references and index.
ISBN 978-1-4129-6115-8 (cloth)
    1. Sports medicine—Encyclopedias. 2. Sports injuries—Encyclopedias. I. Micheli, Lyle J., 1940–[DNLM:
1. Sports Medicine—Encyclopedias—English. 2. Athletic Injuries—Encyclopedias—English.
3. Sports—Encyclopedias—English. QT 13 E5298 2011]

RC1206.E53 2011
617.1′02703—dc22   2010023364

10 11 12 13 14 10 9 8 7 6 5 4 3 2 1

Publisher:	Rolf A. Janke
Acquisitions Editor:	Jim Brace-Thompson
Assistant to the Publisher:	Michele Thompson
Developmental Editor:	Sanford Robinson
Reference Systems Coordinator:	Laura Notton
Reference Systems Manager:	Leticia M. Gutierrez
Production Editor:	Kate Schroeder
Copy Editors:	QuADS Prepress (P) Ltd.
Typesetter:	C&M Digitals (P) Ltd.
Proofreaders:	Kristin Bergstad, Scott Oney, Christina West
Indexer:	Virgil Diodato
Cover Designer:	Gail Buschman

DISCLAIMER: All information contained in the *Encyclopedia of Sports Medicine* is intended only for informational and educational purposes. The information is not intended to diagnose medical problems, prescribe remedies for illness, or treat disease. We recommend that you always seek the advice of a healthcare professional with respect to any medical condition, illness or disease.

Contents

List of Entries

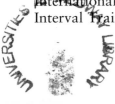

Reader's Guide

The Reader's Guide is designed to assist readers in finding articles on related topics. Headwords are organized into 16 major categories. Note, however, that some topics defy easy categorization and belong to more than one grouping.

Conditioning and Training

Aerobic Endurance
Body Composition (Body Mass Index)
Burnout in Sports
Cardiovascular and Respiratory Anatomy and Physiology: Responses to Exercise
Circuit Training
Conditioning
Core Strength
Cross-Training
Detraining (Reversibility)
Exercise Prescription
Exercise Programs
Fitness Testing
Gender and Age Differences in Response to Training
Home Exercise Equipment
Immune System, Exercise and
Interval Training/Fartlek
Lean Body Weight Assessment
Osteoporosis Prevention Through Exercise
Overtraining
Periodization
Physiological Effects of Exercise on Cardiopulmonary System
Plyometrics
Principles of Training
Resistance Training
Speed, Agility, and Speed Endurance Development
Static Stretching
Strength Training for the Female Athlete
Strength Training for the Young Athlete
Stretching and Warming Up
Target Heart Rate

Temperature and Humidity, Effects on Exercise
Women's Health, Effects of Exercise on

Diagnosis and Treatment of Sports Injuries

Acupuncture
Ankle Support
Arthroscopy
Bracing
Casting and Immobilization
Complementary Treatment
Crutches, How to Use
Dual-Energy X-Ray Absorptiometry (DEXA)
Electrical Stimulation
Electromyography
Extracorporeal Shock Wave Therapy
Fieldside Assessment and Triage
Joint Injection
Joints, Magnetic Resonance Imaging of
Nonsteroidal Anti-Inflammatory Drugs (NSAIDs)
Operating Room Equipment and Environment
Orthotics
Pain Management in Sports Medicine
Pharmacology and Exercise
Physical Examination and History
Preparticipation Cardiovascular Screening
Presports Physical Examination
PRICE/MICE
Taping
Ultrasound

Musculoskeletal Examination Techniques

Musculoskeletal Tests, Ankle
Musculoskeletal Tests, Elbow

Rehabilitation and Physical Therapy

Cryotherapy
Deep Heat: Ultrasound, Diathermy
Electrotherapy
Hydrotherapy and Aquatic Therapy
Principles of Rehabilitation and Physical Therapy
Superficial Heat
Therapeutic Exercise

Special Populations

Pediatric Obesity, Sports, and Exercise
Physically and Mentally Challenged Athletes
Psychology of the Young Athlete
Senior Athletes
Strength Training for the Female Athlete
Strength Training for the Young Athlete
Title IX, Education Amendments of 1972
Transsexual Athletes
Young Athlete
Youth Fitness

Specialties and Occupations in Sports Medicine

Athletic Trainers
Dietitian/Sports Nutritionist
Emergency Medicine and Sports
Exercise Physiologist
Family Doctor
Group Fitness Instructor
Manual Medicine
Orthopedist in Sports Medicine, Role of
Physical and Occupational Therapist
Physiatry and Sports Medicine
Podiatric Sports Medicine
Sport and Exercise Psychology
Sports Biomechanist
Sports Massage Therapist
Team Physician
Sport Psychology

Sport Psychology

Anger and Violence in Sports
Arousal and Athletic Performance
Attention Focus in Sports
Biofeedback
Bulimia Nervosa

Burnout in Sports
Exercise Addiction/Overactivity Disorders
Hypnosis and Sport Performance
Imagery and Visualization
Leadership in Sports
Mental Health Benefits of Sports and Exercise
Motivation
Overtraining
Personality and Exercise
Psychological Aspects of Injury and
    Rehabilitation
Psychological Assessment in Sports
Sport and Exercise Psychology
Sports Socialization
Team and Group Dynamics in Sports

Sports and Society

Air Pollution, Effects on Exercise and Sports
Anger and Violence in Sports
Benefits of Exercise and Sports
Diversity in Sports
Doping and Performance Enhancement: A New
    Definition
Doping and Performance Enhancement:
    Historical Overview
Doping and Performance Enhancement: Olympic
    Games From 2004 to 2008
Epidemiology of Sports Injuries
Legal Aspects of Sports Medicine
Protective Equipment in Sports
Sports Injuries, Overuse
Team and Group Dynamics in Sports
Title IX, Education Amendments of 1972
World Anti-Doping Agency

Sports and Sports Medicine

Air Pollution, Effects on Exercise and Sports
Anatomy and Sports Medicine
Benefits of Exercise and Sports
Circadian Rhythms and Exercise
Diversity in Sports
Emergency Medicine and Sports
Epidemiology of Sports Injuries
Exercise and Disease Prevention
Future Directions in Sports Medicine
History of Sports Medicine
Immune System, Exercise and
Physical Examination and History

S

Sacroiliac Pain

As the link between the spine and the lower extremities, the sacroiliac (SI) joint plays a prominent role in both acute and chronic low back pain. Low back pain is a common problem in both the general population and in athletes. Due to its complex anatomy and biomechanics, the SI joint can be a difficult clinical entity to accurately diagnose and treat. A thorough understanding of its anatomy and functional biomechanics is required to appropriately manage the patient with low back pain due to SI joint dysfunction.

The approach to the athlete with low back pain starts with an accurate and thorough history and physical examination, with special attention to the mechanism of injury and careful palpatory and functional clinical examination techniques. A comprehensive treatment program is required, including functional core and abdominal strengthening, improving lower extremity flexibility, manual medicine, and possibly medications. Other complementary techniques, such as prolotherapy, SI joint injections, and acupuncture may provide benefits but are less well researched.

Anatomy

The region surrounding the SI joint consists of three bony structures: the sacrum, the pelvis, and the lumbar vertebrae. Connecting these structures and providing its movement and function are several muscles, tendons, and ligaments. For example,

the sacrotuberous ligament is a fibrous tissue that connects and stabilizes the sacrum and the ischial tuberosity of the pelvis. Its site of attachment on the ischial tuberosity is shared with the long head of the biceps femoris, one of the three components of the hamstring muscle group. The importance of this anatomical relationship is that tight hamstring muscles will often lead to low back pain due to a strain on the sacrotuberous ligament and into the SI joint. Overlying this ligamentous sling is the thoracolumbar fascia, which is a sheet of connective tissue that provides attachment points for multiple major muscle groups of the spine, abdomen, and upper and lower extremities (Figure 1). The breakdown and degeneration of these soft tissue structures often leads to instability in the region, which in turn promotes chronic pain syndromes.

The adult SI joint is a synovial joint, meaning that it is encased in a joint capsule that helps maintain its balance and integrity. The bony structure is described as an L-shaped articulation with a long (upper) vertical pole and a short (lower) horizontal pole. It has also been described as an S- or a C-shaped articulation. There is much variability in SI joint size, shape, and contour, even within the same person. As the population ages, the SI joint develops different elevations and depressions within the cavity in response to repetitive stresses. Due to its role in the transfer of forces between the torso and the lower extremities, the SI joint endures demanding biomechanical loads during sports activities. As a result of these repetitive forces, the joint capsule thickens, and the underlying bone can be eroded, ultimately resulting in arthritic changes.

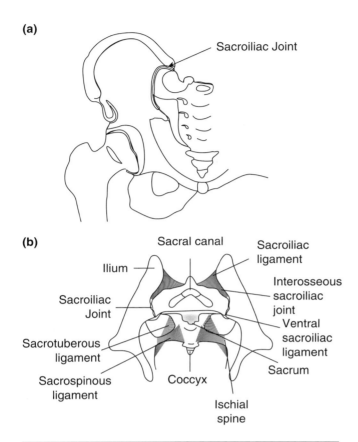

(a)

Sacroiliac Joint

(b)

Sacral canal

Sacroiliac
ligament

Ilium

Interosseous
sacroiliac
joint

Sacroiliac
Joint

Ventral
sacroiliac
ligament

Sacrotuberous
ligament

Sacrum

Sacrospinous
ligament

Coccyx

Ischial
spine

Figure 1   (a) Sacroiliac Joint and (b) Coronal Section
of Sacroiliac Joint and Surroundings,
Showing Ligamentous Attachments

Although it was previously thought that there
is very little motion in the SI joint, most clinicians
now accept that there is motion in it throughout
life. The hormones released during pregnancy and
the increased weight of the baby result in a significant increase in the motion at the SI joint during
pregnancy. This is a common reason for low back
pain during pregnancy. Further studies and observations have demonstrated that asymmetrical patterns of motion at the SI joints also lead to
movement at the pubic symphysis, which is the
point where the two pelvic bones meet in the front.
Pubic symphysis asymmetry can lead to groin and
pelvic pain.

Motion at the SI joint during the normal gait
cycle occurs as combined activities in opposite
directions at the right and left pelvic bones. At heel
strike when stepping forward with the right foot,

the right pelvic bone rotates backward and the left
pelvic bone rotates frontward. While this is happen-
ing, the front surface of the sacrum turns toward
the left, the top surface of the sacrum levels off, and
the spine straightens upward, slightly turning to the
left. Moving toward the right foot midstance, the
right pelvic bone rotates frontward, and the sacrum
rotates right, while the lumbar spine rotates to the
left. The process is repeated in the opposite direction as the left foot approaches heel strike.

Diagnosis

The approach to diagnosis is based on several components, including the subjective complaint of pain,
as well as a functional biomechanical examination
and the clinician's palpatory findings. There are several SI joint screening tests commonly used. When
these tests are used in combination with a thorough
history, careful examination, and appropriate diagnostic imaging, an accurate diagnosis and treatment
regimen can be established.

The differential diagnosis is broad and can include
a number of orthopedic, soft tissue, and visceral
conditions that may refer pain to the low back and
sacral regions. Some important diagnoses to consider are infections and inflammatory conditions
such as arthritis, tumors, fractures, pregnancy, vascular conditions, and hip problems.

When the history and physical examination do
not completely uncover the cause of the low back
pain, one should consider performing standard
radiographs of the lumbosacral spine and pelvis. It
is important to obtain oblique views to fully assess
the SI joint. If the diagnosis remains elusive or the
athlete is not responding to treatment as expected,
a further diagnostic workup may include a bone
scan, computed tomography (CT) scan, or magnetic resonance imaging (MRI) scan. Laboratory
studies may be necessary to rule out infectious or
metabolic conditions.

Treatment

Once the diagnosis has been made, treatment generally includes analgesic and/or anti-inflammatory
medications. Physical therapy targeting core
strengthening and a functional therapeutic exercise program for the lower extremities and pelvis
should be initiated. It is important that the

demands of the athlete's sport be carefully considered in the design of the rehabilitative program. Using sport-specific concepts in the functional treatment program allows one to reintroduce the loads and motions of a sport in a controlled clinical fashion. Hands-on treatments, including massages, Rolfing, and various manipulative approaches, have been used with varying degrees of success. Finally, injection therapy with local anesthetics, cortisone, and/or prolotherapy can be of benefit, especially in refractory cases. It is important to match the diagnosis with the most appropriate treatment protocol.

Per Gunnar Brolinson and Greg Beato

See also Anatomy and Sports Medicine; Back Injuries, Surgery for; Lower Back Injuries and Low Back Pain

Further Readings

Brolinson PG, Gray G. Principle-centered rehabilitation. In: Garrett WE, Kirkendall DT, Squire DH, eds. *Principles and Practice of Primary Care Sports Medicine.* Philadelphia, PA: Lippincott Williams & Wilkins; 2001:645–652.

Brolinson PG, Kozar AJ, Cibor G. Sacroiliac joint dysfunction in athletes. *Curr Sports Med Rep.* 2003;2(1):47–56.

Dreyfuss P, Dryer S, Griffin J, Hoffman J, Walsh N. Positive sacroiliac screening tests in asymptomatic adults. *Spine.* 1994 19(10):1138–1143.

Greenman PE. Clinical aspects of the sacroiliac joint in walking. In: Vleeming A, Mooney V, Dorman T, Stoeckart R, eds. *Movement, Stability and Low Back Pain: The Essential Role of the Pelvis.* New York, NY: Churchill Livingstone; 1997:235–242.

Jacob HA, Kissling RO. The mobility of the sacroiliac joints in healthy volunteers between 20 and 50 years of age. *Clin Biomech.* 1995;10(7):252–361.

Snijders CJ, Vleeming A, Stoeckart R. Transfer of lumbosacral load to iliac bones and legs. II: loading of the sacroiliac joints when lifting in stooped posture. *Clin Biomech.* 1993;8(6):295–301.

Willard FH. The muscular, ligamentous and neural structure of the low back and its relation to back pain. In: Vleeming A, Mooney V, Dorman T, Stoeckart R, eds. *Movement Stability, and Low Back Pain: The Essential Role of the Pelvis.* New York, NY: Churchill Livingstone; 1997:3–35.

Sailing and Yacht Racing, Injuries in

Sailing and yacht racing is a long-standing competitive sport. The America's Cup, first won in 1851, is the oldest active international sports trophy. The few studies that document medical concerns of sailing involve highly experienced sailors. Injuries and illnesses occur with similar frequency to other non-contact sports. These concerns are mostly minor, yet some are life threatening. The tendency for injury increases as the wind velocity rises. Medical concerns differ in dinghy and large-boat sailing. Further differences are seen based on boat class, kind of race, level of experience, and crew position. Disabled sailors have injury patterns similar to those of able-bodied sailors. Yacht racing is generally considered a safe sport; however, sailors, governing bodies, boat designers, and sports medicine personnel need to be aware of the associated risks.

Dinghy

Dinghies range in length from 2 to 6 meters (m) and are typically sailed by one to three people. Racing may include multiple short, back-to-back races or one long course. To keep a boat from turning over and to enhance forward momentum, it is important to keep the hull of the boat relatively flat against the water. This is accomplished by *hiking,* the action of leaning much of one's body weight over the edge of the boat. Hiking is usually from a seated position, with bent or straight knees. Dinghies are often equipped with hiking straps, under which sailors slip their feet and lean out to balance the boat. Hiking causes the most injuries in dinghy sailing. Hiking relies heavily on lower extremity and trunk muscle groups. The forces are translated to the lower back and knee.

Collegiate and Olympic dinghy racers are extremely competitive, and they often round marks close together. Injuries tend to be open wounds, sprains, strains, contusions, or fractures. The most common sites of injury are the lumbar spine, knee, and shoulder. The spine is susceptible to ligamentous, muscle, and disk injuries. Repetitive movements, improper lumbar positions, and weak abdominal muscles contribute to excessive loading.

Poor posture and weak core strength can lead to back and knee pain, body aches, fatigue, reduced strength, and muscle imbalance. Sailors should try to achieve a neutral spine/neck and proper scapula setting, "think tall," and avoid a slumped position. Common knee injuries are ligamentous or meniscal injuries, patellar tendinitis, and patellofemoral pain syndrome. Young women may be at greater risk for knee injuries from hiking due to often internally rotated knees. A proper hiking technique with correct strap placement and foot position limits the torque and imbalanced forces on the knee. Land-based hiking benches are quite useful to work on body positioning and muscle strengthening. The shoulder is at risk for rotator cuff and biceps tendinitis because the sailor is steering, trimming a sail(s), or doing both. In high winds, the loads are larger and necessitate persistent contractions of the shoulder muscles.

Another medical concern of dinghy racing is stress to the cardiovascular system. This system should be assessed when doing a preparticipation evaluation since a sailor's cardiorespiratory demands increase with increasing wind velocities and cardiac output and blood pressure rise significantly during strenuous hiking. Another concern for both genders is that of eating disorders, as some classes have weight limits.

Youth racing is very popular. There are 132,000 registered Optimist boats with sailors between the ages of 8 and 15 years. Most youths are required to wear life jackets when racing, though very few programs mandate children to wear a sports helmet. There is not much written on sailing injuries in this age-group. However, growth spurts are often associated with reduced coordination, which may lead to injuries. This typically occurs for girls between 11 and 13 years and boys between 13 and 15 years.

Large Boat

Large-boat competitions may be held on a single day or multiple days, with one or more races per day, local or offshore, or even around-the-world endurance contests. Radio consult provisions permit racers to discuss medical concerns with other racers or gain medical advice via satellite communication. Seldom is medical evacuation required. Sports medicine concerns in large-boat racing include injury, illness, and, rarely, fatalities.

Many large-boat ocean races have an almost century-long tradition. Two had been relatively free of fatalities until one extreme storm occurred during each of them, resulting in 21 deaths. Man overboard (MOB) and head injuries are the most common causes of death while sailing.

There is a high fatality risk from hypothermia or drowning with MOBs during a storm. Sails need to be expediently doused/changed. Even with a global positioning system (GPS), a boat can get 1 mile (mi; 1 mi = 1.61 kilometers) away in 5 minutes and take 20 minutes to return to the MOB site. The overboard sailor may be at risk for hypothermia, drowning, or near drowning. Even if the sailor is found, it may be technically difficult to retrieve the possibly unconscious sailor.

Head injuries while sailing have caused more than 20 deaths in the past 60 years. A direct blow from a moving boom, spinnaker, or jockey pole is typically responsible and often knocks the athlete overboard. Violent weather puts extra stresses on boat parts, often causing unexpected breakages. Life jackets and harnesses greatly increase survival.

Different crew positions have differing responsibilities and tend to have different patterns of injury. A number of actions in yacht racing are sudden, sporadic, and powerful, such as hoisting a large sail. Others may be repetitive and prolonged, such as long-distance steering. Bowmen, grinders, and helmsmen are particularly at risk for injury.

Many above-deck injuries occur from overuse or direct impacts with boat hardware. Falls on deck or down stairs or hatches or while getting on or off a boat often result in injuries. Below-deck injuries typically result from violent and sudden movements of the boat during rough conditions or from cuts and burns incurred while working in the galley.

A 2006 study of America's Cup sailors by V. J. Neville and colleagues, published in the British *Journal of Sports Medicine,* noted an incidence of 5.7 injuries per 1,000 hours of sailing and off-boat training. Training injuries occurred almost four times more frequently than sailing injuries. Twice as many acute injuries as overuse injuries were seen.

The most common injuries encountered while racing are to the upper extremity (finger, hand, shoulder), head and face, and spine and neck. The types of injury most often seen are abrasions, contusions, burns (thermal, rope, sun), closed fractures, lacerations, ligament sprains, tendinopathies, and head injuries without loss of consciousness. Training injuries include sprains, tendinopathies, and muscle strains.

Illness among racing/training sailors tends to be infrequent and minor. The 2006 study by Neville and colleagues showed a 3.1 incidence of illness per 1,000 sailing and training hours.

Upper respiratory tract infections, seasickness, and gastrointestinal issues are the most common illnesses. Contributing factors are a stressful training routine, close living quarters, rough seas, and contaminated water. Sitting on wet, salty surfaces with infrequent bathing causes dermatologic issues. Insomnia, hypertension, sunburn, headache, and infections are also seen.

Medical Preparation

All yachts should be equipped with a medical kit and a communication system that at least two sailors are trained to use. For long offshore racing, a very high-frequency (VHF), single sideband and a satellite system for voice/e-mail are necessary, in addition to an arrangement with a local hospital or telemedicine company for emergencies. Each yacht should designate a medical officer who has attended a marine medical course. Drills for emergencies such as MOBs should be practiced.

Conclusion

While the incidence of injury and illness remains low in competitive sailing, there is room for prevention. Sports medicine personnel can aid the athlete by advising strength and endurance training, cardiovascular fitness, proper nutrition and hydration, prompt medical attention, and mental and safety preparedness. Further research documenting medical concerns, particularly among young sailors, is needed.

Lizanne Backe Barone

See also Dehydration; Knee Injuries; Lower Back Muscle Strain and Ligament Sprain; Shoulder Injuries; Sunburn and Skin Cancers

Further Readings

Allen JB. Sailing. In: Madden CC, Putukian M, Young CC, McCarty EC, eds. *Netter's Sports Medicine.* Philadelphia, PA: Saunders Elsevier; 2009:627–633.

Allen JB, De Jong MR. Sailing and sports medicine: a literature review. *Br J Sports Med.* 2006;40(7): 587–593.

Gill PG. The Onboard Medical Guide: First Aid and Emergency Medicine Afloat. Camden, ME: International Marine; 1997.

Nathanson AT, Fischer EG, Mello MJ, Baird J. Injury and illness at the Newport-Bermuda Race 1998–2006. *Wilderness Environ Med.* 2008;19(2):129–132.

Neville VJ, Molloy J, Brooks JH, Speedy DB, Atkinson G. Epidemiology of injuries and illnesses in America's Cup yacht racing. *Br J Sports Med.* 2006;40(4): 304–312.

Price CJ, Spalding TJ, McKenzie C. Patterns of illness and injury encountered in amateur ocean yacht racing. *Br J Sports Med.* 2002;36(6):457–462.

Snellenburg K. Dinghy sailing. In: Shamus E, ed. *Sports Injury: Prevention & Rehabilitation.* Columbus, OH: McGraw-Hill; 2001:227–239.

Salt in the Athlete's Diet

Human blood contains sodium chloride (NaCl)—common salt—in solution and, in addition, contains smaller quantities of other ions. Electrolytes such as sodium chloride cannot be stored, nor can they be manufactured in the body. These electrolytes must be obtained from our diet. Sodium and potassium salts are needed in greater quantity than any other electrolyte. Maintaining an equilibrium between the salt loss and dietary intake is vital.

A fluid and electrolyte balance is critical to optimal exercise performance. Many athletes, especially endurance athletes, often do not meet their fluid requirements during exercise. However, successful athletes come close to meeting fluid needs, at the same time accounting for their salt loss. Increasing ambient temperature and humidity can increase the rate of sweating on average to 1 liter (L)/hour. Depending on the individual, exercise type, and exercise intensity, sweat rates can range from extremely low values to more than 3 L/hour. Overhydrating with a low or negligible sodium intake can result in reduced performance and hyponatremia. Adding salt to the sports drink actually promotes better absorption in the gut. Sodium also becomes important in the recovery period.

The minimum amount of urinary sodium lost in a day is between 4 and 6 grams (g). This does not include the amount of salt lost in sweat. A dietary intake of 5 to 10 g of salt/day or 2 to 3 kilograms (kg)/year is necessary to maintain homeostasis.

Athletes have varying degrees of salt concentration in their sweat. Those with high salt concentrations may need more salt than the average sweating athlete.

Salt consists of sodium and chloride ions, which are important for normal physiologic functioning. High sweat rates in athletes result in the loss of both fluids and sodium. Fluid replacement with hypotonic solutions such as water will lead to incomplete rehydration and possible complications such as hyponatremia, decreased performance, and heat-related illnesses. There is significant individual variation in the sodium lost during activity. In some, the losses can be replaced by the normal dietary intake, whereas in others, the losses can be so dramatic that extra salt needs to be added to the diet. There are various methods to raise the sodium intake, such as increased use of table salt on foods, eating salty snacks, adding salt to sports drinks, and the use of salt tablets. The emphasis on fluid replacement is also important, but care must be taken to avoid overhydration. Simple measures such as recording the daily pre- and postexercise body weight aid in making fluid and sodium ingestion decisions.

Sweat has an average sodium concentration of 10 to 100 millimoles (mmol)/L. The sweat rate, the amount of fluid lost in 1 hour, can be as high as 3 L/hour. Insufficient substitution can lead to cramps and, as noted earlier, hyponatremia. This is particularly true in hot, humid weather. Athletes can lose up to 5 g of sodium/hour. This can cause a negative balance in the total exchangeable sodium of 30%.

Researchers at the Cleveland Clinic have developed a formula to estimate an athlete's salt loss:

$$\text{Salt loss} = 0.0263 \times \text{Sweat [Na]} \times \text{Weight loss.}$$

As mentioned earlier, the sweat sodium concentration can range between 10 and 100 mmol/L. For simplification purposes in this example, the sweat concentration is set at 50 mmol/L. For individualized calculations, the specific salt concentration of the athlete's sweat should be used.

Example: If a player loses 10 pounds (lb; 1 lb = 0.45 kg) during practice with a sweat sodium concentration of 50 mmol/L, he or she will have lost $0.0263 \times 50 \times 10 = 13.15$ g of salt.

The use of sports drinks has increased dramatically in recent years. How much do these sport drinks actually help in stabilizing the sodium balance?

Modifying the preceding formula, the sodium salt content of a beverage can be assessed as follows:

$$\text{NaCl (g)} = 0.00252 \times \text{[Na] (milligrams [mg]/vol)} \times \text{vol.}$$

A popular beverage targeting athletes has 110 mg of sodium in 8 ounces (oz; 1 oz = 29.57 milliliters [ml]). If an athlete drinks one 20-oz bottle of it, he or she will have consumed

$$0.00252 \times 110/8 \times 20 = 0.693 \text{ g of salt.}$$

In the example above, the athlete lost 13.15 g of salt. To replace that by just drinking the sports drink (second example), he would have to drink nineteen 20-oz bottles!

An average diet contains between 8 and 10 g of salt. Thus, much of the sodium lost in an event will be replenished by regular dietary intake. If, though, an athlete has a weight loss of 5 lb or more during an athletic event, a salt substitution should be considered. A basic rule would be to supply 1 g of salt and 500 ml (=16 oz of fluid) for each pound of weight loss over 5 lb.

Marc P. Hilgers

See also Dietitian/Sports Nutritionist; Fat in the Athlete's Diet; Nutrition and Hydration; Sports Drinks

Further Readings

Pelly F. The salt story. http://www.coolrunning.com.au/runningguide/wiki/index.php/The_Salt_Story. Accessed June 21, 2010.

Sodium (salt) intake for athletes. http://www.faqs.org/sports-science/Sc-Sp/Sodium-Salt-Intake-for-Athletes.html. Accessed June 21, 2010.

Tamborlane WV, Weiswasser JZ, Held NA, Fung T, eds. *The Yale Guide to Children's Nutrition.* New Haven, CT: Yale University Press.

Volpe SL. A nutritionist's' view: sodium and fluid needs for athletes. *ACSM'S Health Fitness J.* 2007;11(1):33–34.

SCAPHOID FRACTURE

The *scaphoid* is one of the small bones of the wrist. It is the most frequently fractured carpal bone, accounting for 71% of all carpal bone fractures. The incidence of fracture is greater in young and middle-aged men, typically those between 15 and 60 years.

Many cases of painful wrists due to a fractured scaphoid are seen in the emergency department. Early diagnosis is important as 90% of all acute scaphoid fractures heal if treated early. On the other hand, a delay in diagnosis can lead to a variety of adverse outcomes.

Anatomy

The wrist is made up of eight carpal bones, which are arranged in two rows (Figure 1). The scaphoid is the most lateral bone of the proximal row. It articulates with the radius superiorly.

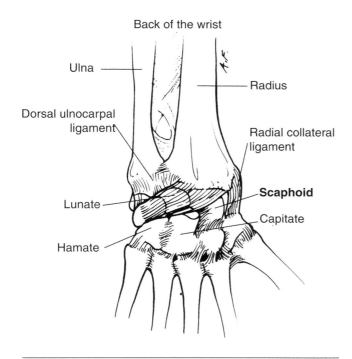

Figure 1 Anatomy of the Wrist

On surface anatomy, it is located below the anatomic snuffbox—a triangular depression lying below the thumb, best visible when the thumb is extended. This boat-shaped bone is key to wrist motion and stability. It can be divided into four distinct parts: the proximal pole, the wrist, the distal body, and the tuberosity. Most scaphoid fractures occur at the waist and the proximal pole.

The scaphoid is supplied by the radial artery near the tubercle and waist. The blood supply to this bone is paradoxical, going from distal to proximal. Thus, fractures in this part heal slowly, and the bone fragments may even fail to fuse.

Causes

Most patients who have broken their scaphoid have done it while participating in sports such as football or basketball; two-wheeled sports such as motocross, bicycle motocross (BMX), and cycling; or in an automobile accident. It usually happens from a fall on an outstretched hand (FOOSH) with the wrist pronated (palm facing backward).

Symptoms

A fracture of the scaphoid almost never shows any obvious deformity of the wrist. Symptoms of a fracture include pain at the base of the thumb and a swelling around the wrist. Loss of the concavity of the anatomic snuffbox is usually seen.

Pain may subside and then return as a deep, dull ache that may worsen when the thumb is moved or the hand grips an object. In some cases, the pain is not severe and may be mistaken for a sprain.

Clinical Evaluation

Physical Examination

The age and sex of the patient are considered together with the mechanism of injury. It is important to compare the injured wrist with the uninjured wrist.

The following observations on performing specific maneuvers suggest a fracture of the scaphoid:

- There is tenderness on palpation at the anatomical snuffbox.
- The scaphoid tubercle is tender. Extend the patient's wrist with one hand, and apply

pressure on the tuberosity at the proximal wrist crease with the other.

- Absence of tenderness on performing the first two examinations makes a scaphoid fracture highly unlikely.
- There is pain on performing the "scaphoid compression test." This test involves longitudinally compressing the patient's thumb along the line of the first metacarpal.
- Pain is felt on pronation followed by ulnar deviation.
- There is reduced range of motion of the hand.

Imaging

There are various imaging options to figure out the fracture in a patient with a suspected scaphoid injury:

- *Radiography:* Anteroposterior, lateral, and oblique radiographic views of the wrist are required. A special radiograph called a scaphoid view is also recorded occasionally. Nondisplaced fractures (fractures in which the bone fragments have not been displaced) are usually not seen on initial radiographs.
- *Bone scintigraphy:* It is a cost-effective and accurate method for assessing occult scaphoid fractures.
- *Magnetic resonance imaging:* It is a highly sensitive, noninvasive modality that can not only detect occult scaphoid fractures but can also access bone healing and evaluate for bone contusions and ligamentous injuries.
- *Ultrasonography:* Ultrasound examination is not appropriate in the initial evaluation of a suspected scaphoid fracture. Nevertheless, it is reliable and accurate in identifying occult scaphoid fractures.

Treatment

Nonsurgical Treatment

Scaphoid fractures are usually not visible on X-rays immediately after an injury. A wrist injury suspected of a scaphoid fracture by examination should be casted, with follow-up examination done in 7 to 14 days. However, it is possible that the fracture line is still not visible; in such cases, an MRI or CT scan may be necessary to confirm the diagnosis.

In a fracture where bone is not displaced (bone fragments are in the right place) and/or fractures that do not extend across the bone's length, simple treatment with cast immobilization may heal the fracture within 9 to 12 weeks; inclusion of the thumb in the cast is usually recommended. Recovery is monitored by examining plain radiographs. If the fracture does not heal, surgery is recommended.

Surgical Treatment

Surgery is indicated in the following situations:

- When the bone is displaced (fragments are not in their anatomical position) and is hence at a higher risk of nonunion (failure of bone to heal)
- When the athlete is anxious to return to play as soon as possible (Surgery allows the patient to get early mobilization and complete functionality in a shorter duration. This reduced time spent in a cast also helps reduce muscle atrophy.)
- When the scaphoid fracture is undiagnosed initially, with nonhealing (nonunion)
- In a nondisplaced fracture when healing does not occur in a timely manner with cast immobilization
- When the fracture is in the middle or proximal part (nearer the forearm), since it may not heal with only the cast because of the reduced blood supply in this part of the bone

Two surgical options are available: (1) open reduction and internal fixation and (2) closed reduction and percutaneous fixation. The former is for displaced fractures, whereas the latter is for fractures that have minimal displacement. In the surgical method, cannulated screws or wires are used to stabilize the fragments. The length of the incision and the area where it is placed depend on the degree of displacement of the fragments and the part of the scaphoid that is fractured. It can be on the front or back of the wrist. The incision is larger when fragments have to be realigned into their anatomical position before they are stabilized with screws. Postoperatively, the hand is placed in a cast and regularly monitored with radiographs to check the progress of the healing process. The bone heals within 8 to 12 weeks.

Even with surgery, this fracture takes time to heal or may not heal properly. If the bone does not heal, a bone graft is added in addition to internal fixation. (The grafts are usually taken from the patient's pelvis.) During this process, the hand is placed in a cast. Bone grafts speed up the healing process, and the cast is usually removed in 3 weeks, allowing rehabilitation exercises of the hand and wrist. Also, in fractures where the blood supply has been severed, special grafts, called vascularized grafts, are used that have their own blood supply.

Complications

The proper treatment of scaphoid fractures is extremely important. If the bone fails to heal, it is called a *nonunion*. One cause of nonunions, as noted earlier, is the poor blood supply to the fractured part, which results in bone death. This is referred to as *avascular necrosis*. Nonunion and avascular necrosis subsequently lead to arthritis of the wrist, resulting in pain and a reduced range of motion; the person experiences difficulties in performing even normal activities such as lifting and gripping.

Rehabilitation

Cast immobilization and functional disuse can lead to swelling (edema) of the injured wrist. Elevation and active motion of the uninjured joints of the hand can help avoid this fluid accumulation. During the healing period, the patient must avoid any strenuous activity with the injured arm, including lifting, pushing, pulling, and throwing. Participation in contact sports must be avoided, and care must be taken to avoid activities that increase the risk of falling onto the hand.

After the cast is removed, active range-of-motion (ROM) exercises for wrist flexion and extension and radial and ulnar deviation are performed to overcome the stiffness. About 2 weeks later, passive range-of-motion (PROM) exercises are started, together with gentle muscle-strengthening exercises. Progressive strengthening over several weeks by means of weight bearing and other activities will help restore complete functionality to the wrist.

Hira Bashir and Fatima tuz Zahra

See also Wrist Dislocation; Wrist Fracture; Wrist Injuries; Wrist Sprain; Wrist Tendinopathy

Further Readings

Bucholz CA, Heckman JD, Court-Brown CM, Tornetta P, Koval KJ. *Rockwood and Green's Fractures in Adults*. Philadelphia, PA: Lippincott Williams & Wilkins; 2006.

Dutton M. *Orthopaedic Examination, Evaluation, and Intervention*. New York, NY: McGraw-Hill; 2004.

Geissler WB, ed. *Wrist Arthroscopy*. Berlin, Germany: Springer; 2005.

SCHEUERMANN KYPHOSIS

When viewed from the side, the human spine has a series of normal curves. The lower back or lumbar spine is curved anteriorly (*lordosis*). The upper back curves outward and is referred to as a *thoracic kyphosis*. This is a C-shaped opening anteriorly. The cervical spine maintains a mild lordosis. When any of these curves are excessive, they can cause pain and cosmetic deformity. The normal thoracic kyphosis is between 20° and 40°. There are several causes of excessive kyphosis. A congenital fusion or abnormality may cause a fixed kyphosis noted early in life. Later in life, osteoporosis may cause an excessive kyphosis, or dowager's hump, due to compression fractures. In the adolescent, there are two causes of noted kyphosis. One is postural, due to slouching and poor spinal extension strength, and is usually correctible with postural strengthening. The second is *Scheuermann kyphosis*.

Scheuermann kyphosis is a developmental fixed deformity of adolescence. By definition, there are at least three consecutive vertebrae involved, with anterior wedging of 5° or more. The prevalence has been estimated to be between 4% and 8% of the population. It is usually recognized during the adolescent growth spurt. When detected with spinal growth remaining, it can be minimized with exercises and bracing. Thus, early recognition is important.

Etiology

There have been a number of theories as to the causes of Scheuermann kyphosis. Genetic factors have been strongly implicated, but there has been no specific genetic marker identified. Some have attributed this to an osteochondrosis, which refers to a loss of blood supply to the growth cartilage rings that are located on the superior and inferior parts of each spinal vertebral body. Repetitive compression of the anterior portion of this ring will inhibit the growth and cause anterior wedging. In keeping with this theory, muscular imbalances with stronger anterior trunk muscles would put excessive pressure on the anterior ring apophysis. Furthermore, it has been noted in industrial workers in excessive forward flexion. There has also been a noted association with elite levels of water skiing in the pre-adolescent and adolescent age-groups. Other possible etiologies include transient osteoporosis and growth hormone imbalance.

With regard to gender, some studies have indicated that there is a male predominance, while others have shown a more equal, 1:1, ratio.

Clinical Presentation

The most common presentation is a cosmetic deformity noted by parents during the adolescent growth period. It is a very gradual development that is usually painless. Parents often consider this to be postural. About 25% of these adolescents have an associated scoliosis of less than 25° to 30°. Scoliosis is a lateral curvature of the spine. Kyphosis is best detected on forward flexion, viewed from the side (see photo, right column). Scoliosis is also seen on this forward flexion test but viewed from behind. Scoliosis will manifest with an asymmetry of the rib humps in flexion. When a kyphosis is detected, one should determine if it is fixed or postural. When the patient extends backward or is prone while suspended on the elbows, the postural kyphosis is corrected, while the Scheuermann kyphosis remains.

One of the significant problems of excessive kyphosis is loss of self-esteem. The kyphosis may cause a cosmetic deformity and make the individual appear heavier. Although the adolescent may complain of pain at the apex of the deformity, it is more common for an adult to complain of pain. It is likely that in the adult, the local degenerative processes of the disk and posterior spinal elements are causing focal irritation. The increased thoracic kyphosis alters the biomechanics of the lumbar

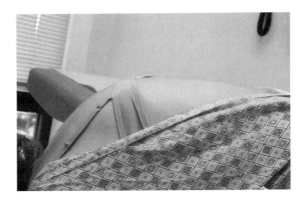

Kyphosis. Patient is in forward flexion, viewed from the side.

Source: Photo courtesy of Pierre A. d'Hemecourt.

spine, with increased lordosis to compensate. This excessive lordosis may cause stress in the posterior elements of the lumbar spine with a spondylolysis (stress fracture). Although quite uncommon, neurologic compression may also occur with peripheral manifestations. These may include pain radiation to the chest wall, to the abdominal wall, or into the legs.

Imaging

The standard evaluation of a suspected kyphosis includes a standing series of the thoracolumbar spine, which involves posteroanterior (PA) and lateral views. The PA view will detect any scoliosis. The lateral view is useful for determining the amount of kyphosis using the Cobb method (Figure see radiograph, next page). This measures the angle from the superiormost vertebrae to the inferiormost vertebrae. To meet the criteria of Scheuermann kyphosis, there must be an overall kyphosis of more than 45°, and at least 5°, with three consecutive wedged vertebrae. A lateral radiograph in extension may be considered if there is a question whether the kyphosis is more postural.

If there is a kyphosis, one must determine bone growth as improvement can only occur in the setting of remaining spinal growth. Therefore, the pelvic portion of the plain PA radiograph will help determine the remaining growth potential by calculating the Risser score of the iliac crest growth cartilage (Figure 1). The iliac apophysis ossification appears laterally to medially. Each 25% is divided into the first four scores. Risser I is the

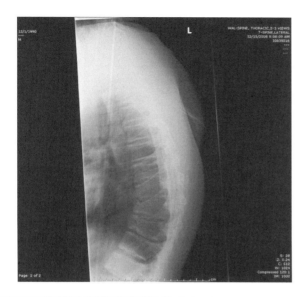

Kyphosis, plain posteroanterior radiograph

Source: Photo courtesy of Pierre A. d'Hemecourt.

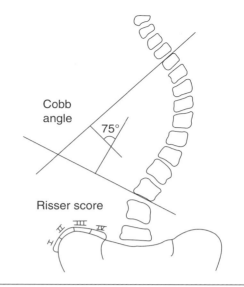

Figure 1   Risser Score

Source: Pierre A. d'Hemecourt.

appearance of the first 25%. Risser II is the first 50%. Spinal growth is most noted up to Risser II. A left hand/wrist radiograph may also be obtained for bone aging.

Further imaging with an MRI scan is useful if there is significant pain. This will demonstrate any significant disk disease as well as spinal cord abnormalities such as a syrinx (cystlike structure).

Treatment

The ideal treatment candidate is the adolescent with significant growth potential and a curve in excess of 45°. Treatment consists of an upper back extension–based strengthening program combined with a core stabilization program. This is an important part of the treatment and is very useful for the postural component. Bracing is also optimal here. Usually, the apex is at T7 or above it and requires a Milwaukee brace. This brace comprises a pelvic girdle, a pad at the curve apex, and a shoulder with a cervical ring fixation. Ideal treatment is at least 18 hours/day for the first year and nighttime wear until skeletal maturity. Radiographs are repeated every 4 to 6 months. This brace is not well tolerated and at times is just used for nighttime wear. When the kyphosis has an apex below T7, a more tolerable thoracolumbarsacral orthosis (TLSO) is used. The TLSO is also continued until skeletal maturity.

Surgical intervention is reserved for those curves in excess of 75°. The Milwaukee brace is ineffective at this degree of curvature. The surgical stabilization usually involves an anterior and posterior approach with fusion with fixation. A posterior-only approach may be followed if there is some flexibility to the curve, but this provides less curve correction than does the combined approach. Complications can include spinal cord injury, nonunion of the fusion, and infection. The results can be very satisfying.

Return-to-Sports Considerations

There is no real restriction to play in most of these athletes unless there has been a surgical fusion with instrumentation. In the latter case, contact sports are a contraindication. In the nonoperatively treated group, sports participation of all kinds is encouraged as long as the principles of sports biomechanics are addressed. In sports that require forward thoracolumbar flexion such as crew and wrestling, the athlete is instructed in upper back extension postures with a good upper back–strengthening program. When bracing is used, the athlete is usually allowed out of the brace for all practice and competition events. This allows better compliance and enhances spinal stabilization.

Pierre A. d'Hemecourt

See also Back Injuries, Surgery for; Lower Back Injuries and Low Back Pain; Musculoskeletal Tests, Spine

Further Readings

Ascani E, Salsano V, Giglio G. The incidence and early detection of spinal deformities. A study based on the screening of 16,104 schoolchildren. *Ital J Orthop Traumatol.* 1977;3(1):111–117.

Bradford DS, Moe JH, Montalvo FJ, Winter RB. Scheuermann kyphosis and roundback deformity. Results of Milwaukee brace treatment. *J Bone Joint Surg Am.* 1974;56(4):740–758.

Lee SS, Lenke LG, Kuklo TR, et al. Comparison of Scheuermann kyphosis correction by posterior-only thoracic pedicle screw fixation versus combined anterior/posterior fusion. *Spine.* 2006;31(20): 2316–2321.

Lowe TG, Line BG. Evidence based medicine: analysis of Scheuermann kyphosis. *Spine.* 2007;32(19 suppl): S115–S119.

Murray PM, Weinstein SL, Spratt KF. The natural history and long-term follow-up of Scheuermann kyphosis. *J Bone Joint Surg Am.* 1993;75(2):236–248.

Shelton YA. Scoliosis and kyphosis in adolescents: diagnosis and management. *Adolesc Med State Art Rev.* 2007;18(1):121–139.

Sorensen KH. *Scheuermann's Juvenile Kyphosis: Clinical Appearances, Radiography, Aetiology, and Prognosis.* Copenhagen, Denmark: Munksgaard; 1964.

SCIATICA

Low back pain affects a significant portion of the population, with epidemiologic studies reporting a lifetime prevalence of 49% to 70%. *Sciatica*, also referred to as *lumbosacral radicular syndrome*, is a type of low back pain that is characterized by pronounced posterior radiating leg pain. The pain follows a distribution served by a lumbar or sacral spinal nerve root and is often accompanied by sensory, motor, or tendon reflex abnormalities. The prevalence of sciatica has been estimated to be around 2% to 10%. This prevalence is likely higher in athletes, especially high-level or elite athletes, due to the increased physical demands placed on the spine during many athletic activities. Clinicians that care for athletes must have a good understanding of the causes, diagnosis, and treatment of sciatica to expedite a safe return to athletic activity.

Anatomy

In the lower back, the lumbar spine is composed of five vertebral bodies. The sacrum, a large triangular bone consisting of five fused vertebrae, connects the lumbar spine and the tailbone or coccyx. The spinal cord traverses through the spinal canal of the vertebrae, and nerves coming off the spinal cord travel through the spinal canal and exit through small openings on the sides of the vertebrae called *foramina* (singular foramen). The sciatic nerve is the largest and longest nerve in the body and originates from a group of nerves in the lower back. It then runs through the buttock and down the lower leg, supplying motor and sensory functions to the thigh, knee, calf, ankle, foot, and toes. Between each of the vertebrae is a vertebral or spinal disk that serves as a shock absorber. Each disk is composed of two parts: (1) an outer tough exterior (annulus fibrosis) that surrounds and contains (2) an inner jelly-like material (nucleus pulposus).

Causes

The leading etiology of sciatica (approximately 90% of cases) is a herniated disk causing nerve root compression. Other etiologies include lumbar stenosis (narrowing of the lumbar spinal canal), facet joint osteoarthritis, spinal cord tumors, and infection. Disk prolapse is more commonly identified as a cause of nerve root compression among younger athletes (20- to 50-year-olds), while osteophytes and degenerative disease are often the culprits in older athletes. The red flags for life-threatening etiologies have been widely recognized, and more aggressive and urgent workup is needed if these are identified (Table 1). Several factors have been shown to increase one's risk for sciatica: age (peak between 45 and 64 years of age), increasing height, mental stress, cigarette smoking, strenuous physical activity, and exposure to vibrations from vehicles.

Clinical Evaluation

History

The first step in managing an athlete with sciatica is to recognize the condition. The physician's

Table 1   Red Flags for Low Back Pain

History or Physical Exam Clue	Possible Diagnostic Etiology
Saddle anesthesia	Cauda equina syndrome
Urinary retention	Cauda equina syndrome
Bowel or bladder incontinence	Cauda equina syndrome
Loss of rectal tone	Cauda equina syndrome
Major motor or sensory loss	Cauda equina syndrome, significant herniated disk
History of cancer	Metastatic disease
Age over 50 years	Neoplasm
Unexplained weight loss	Neoplasm
Nighttime pain	Neoplasm or infection
Fevers	Spinal infection
Recent infection (pyelonephritis, cellulitis, etc.)	Spinal infection
Vertebral tenderness	Spinal infection or fracture
Unrelenting pain	Spinal infection, neoplasm, or fracture
Immunosuppression	Spinal infection
Intravenous drug use	Spinal infection
Fall in osteoporotic patient	Vertebral compression fracture
Trauma (motor vehicle accident, fall from a height, etc.) in young patient	Vertebral fracture

Source: Susan Bettcher and James Borchers.

main diagnostic tool is obtaining a thorough history and performing a comprehensive yet focused physical examination. Patients frequently report a shooting, radiating, or burning leg pain that extends to the ankle and foot, often with athletic activity. Pain commonly travels along the lateral and posterior aspects of the thigh and leg. These symptoms are often accompanied by a component of numbness or a tingling sensation. Sciatica pain attributed to disk herniation can increase with maneuvers such as coughing and with running activities.

Physical Exam

The physical exam should include inspection, palpation, and range-of-motion testing of the lower back and legs, along with documentation of vascular integrity. Emphasis should be placed on neurological testing. A key diagnostic tool to help assess for radiculopathy is the *Lasegue sign,* more commonly referred to as the straight leg raise test. For this maneuver, the clinician elevates the supine patient's extended leg without his or her assistance. The test is positive if sciatica is reproduced between 10° and 60° of elevation. A second maneuver is the crossed straight leg raise test. This test focuses on raising the unaffected leg; a positive result occurs if pain is reproduced in the affected leg. A variation of the above tests, the seated straight leg test, is performed with the patient seated. The leg is extended until there is 90° of flexion at the hip. The test is positive if pain is elicited as the leg is raised. If one or more of these maneuvers are positive and the pain description is consistent with sciatica, a diagnosis of sciatica can be made.

Diagnostic Tests

Performing laboratory or imaging studies is often not necessary when diagnosing sciatica as these tests do not affect the typical treatment course, which is conservative management. However, if any red flags are present, further workup should be initiated at the time of diagnosis. In addition, imaging studies are often indicated if the diagnosis is uncertain or if there is a lack of response to conservative management after 6 to 8 weeks. Imaging can be used to help identify the pain source, such as a herniated disk. This information can be used to determine if surgical intervention is indicated. Disk herniations are frequently seen on computed tomography (CT) scans and more commonly on magnetic resonance imaging (MRI) scans. The findings must be correlated to the distribution of symptoms, and a decision must be made as to whether the pattern makes sense. Imaging studies depend on various factors (availability of testing, patient health, cost, etc.) and the physician's preference.

Treatment

The overall prognosis for sciatica is good as a majority of patients and athletes recover from related disabilities within a couple of weeks to months. However, the symptoms can become chronic, and a minority of athletes can continue to have pain for periods greater than 1 year. The mainstay of the treatment is conservative management, which focuses on pain control. However, if there is a lack of clinical improvement after 6 to 8 weeks, surgical intervention can be considered. The effectiveness of certain conservative measures and the optimal timing of surgery still need to be established.

Nonsurgical Treatment

Conservative management involves one or more of the following: patient education, bed rest, remaining active, use of analgesics such as nonsteroidal anti-inflammatory drugs (NSAIDs), epidural steroid injections, physical therapy, spinal manipulation, acupuncture, traction therapy, and behavioral treatment. While there is no solid evidence for the effectiveness of any of these measures, bed rest is no longer recommended because no significant difference in pain and functional status measures has been seen when compared with staying active. As such, physicians recommend that their athletes with sciatica remain active but avoid activities that aggravate their pain. Formal physical therapy is also recommended by certain providers and may be helpful in individuals with more severe pain and/or disability. For athletes with access to training facilities, a certified athletic trainer can guide the rehabilitation and monitor a graduated return to play. Physicians often prescribe NSAIDs for the initial pain associated with sciatica. Other non-NSAID analgesic pain medications, muscle relaxants, and antidepressants may be used instead of or in addition to NSAIDs. A conservative treatment plan should be made in conjunction with the athlete, keeping in mind the current knowledge of treatment modalities, our understanding of the expected course of sciatica, and the athlete's performance goals.

Surgical Treatment

An immediate neurosurgical referral needs to be made for the cauda equina syndrome, which is characterized by saddle anesthesia, decreased rectal tone, and changes in the urination and bowel functions. Urgent referrals should be made if progressive paresis and/or acute severe paresis are present. Other nonurgent referral indications to neurosurgery, neurology, or orthopedic surgery include severe pain in spite of adequate medication, uncertain diagnosis, and lack of clinical improvement after 6 to 8 weeks. Surgical intervention can be undertaken in cases of refractory sciatica in which there is an identifiable source of pain, such as lumbar disk prolapse. Surgery aims at removing the disk herniation through surgical diskectomy or microdiskectomy. There may be an initial improvement in leg pain and faster recovery in individuals treated with early surgery, but the long-term outcomes of surgery have not been shown to be better than those managed conservatively. As such, providers need to discuss the available evidence and knowledge of treatment modalities and outcomes with their affected athletes so that they can make well-informed decisions.

Susan Bettcher and James Borchers

See also Back Injuries in Sports, Surgery for; Cervical and Thoracic Disk Disease; Lower Back Injuries and Low Back Pain; Musculoskeletal Tests, Spine; Slipped Disk

Further Readings

Frymoyer JW, Cats-Baril WL. An overview of the incidences and costs of low back pain. *Orthop Clin North Am*. 1991;22(2):263–271.

Hagen KB, Jamtvedt G, Hilde G, Winnem MF. The updated Cochrane review of bed rest for low back pain and sciatica. *Spine*. 2005;30(5):542–546.

Koes BW, van Tulder MW, Peul WC. Diagnosis and treatment of sciatica. *BMJ*. 2007;334(7607): 1313–1317.

Luijsterburg PAJ, Verhagen AP, Ostelo RW, et al. Physical therapy plus general practitioners' care versus general practitioners' care alone for sciatica: a randomized clinical trial with a 12-month follow-up. *Eur Spine J*. 2008;17(4):509–517.

Peul WC, van den Hout WB, Brand R, Thomeer RTWM, Koes BW. Prolonged conservative care versus early surgery in patients with sciatica caused by lumbar disc herniation: two year results of a randomized controlled trial. *BMJ*. 2008;336(7657):1355–1358.

SCOLIOSIS

Scoliosis is an abnormal curvature of the spine when viewed from the back. In this position, the spine normally appears as a straight line from the occiput to the pelvis. With scoliosis, this may appear as a single C-shaped curve or a double S-shaped curve. There is often an associated rotational component that presents with a rib hump or lumbar prominence, depending on the location of the curve. The overall prevalence of scoliosis is 2% to 3%. However, severe curves occur in less than 0.1% of the population. The prevalence of minor curves is equal between men and women, but more significant curves demonstrating progression are at least five times more common in women.

Scoliosis curves may be described by the location of the apical vertebra. This is the vertebra that is most deviated from the midline. There are 7 cervical vertebrae, 12 thoracic vertebrae, and 5 lumbar vertebrae. The position of the apical vertebra defines the curve level: cervical from C2 to C6, cervicothoracic from C7 to T1, thoracic from T2 to T11, thoracolumbar from T12 to L1, lumbar from L2 to L4, and lumbosacral from L5 to the sacrum. Single or multiple curves may be seen. The curve is further defined by the direction of the convexity (outer portion of the curve). A curve that is convex to the right is called dextroscoliosis; convexity to the left is levoscoliosis. Curves may be single or multiple.

The objective of scoliosis identification is to prevent the progression, which may be associated with functional deformity, cosmetic deformity, and potentially pain in the adult. The young woman athlete is often seen with this on preparticipation examination.

Classification

Scoliosis may be classified according to the etiology. Curves may be secondary to congenital, neuromuscular, and idiopathic causes. Congenital causes usually reflect bony abnormalities, as a result of which one is born with the spinal vertebrae incompletely separated from an adjacent level or incompletely formed. These curves often present early in life.

Neuromuscular scoliosis refers to curves that are secondary to neurologic and muscular disorders. Spinal cord abnormalities such as a syringomyelia (a cystic-like structure in the cord) and a tethered cord may cause an abnormal curvature. Some inherited muscular and neurologic diseases such as muscular dystrophy may present with a gradually progressive curve. Connective tissue abnormalities such as Marfan syndrome and Ehlers-Danlos syndrome also fall in this category. Certain tumors such as neurofibromatosis and osteoid osteomas also represent neuromuscular causes.

At least 80% of scoliosis cases are classified as *idiopathic*, which means that there is no known cause. Idiopathic scoliosis is further subclassified by the age of onset:

- *Infantile, under the age of 3:* Unlike the older idiopathic forms, this is more prevalent in the male population and has a more positive ability to be corrected on its own.

- *Juvenile, between 3 years and 10 years of age:* This has a much higher risk of progression and must be monitored closely. It also has a significant risk of comorbid spinal cord abnormalities that must be considered.
- *Adolescent idiopathic scoliosis, over the age of 10 years:* This is the most common entity and is most often seen in the young woman athlete.

Numerous hypotheses have been postulated regarding the cause of scoliosis. However, it remains unclear. Chromosome mapping has made specific identifications, but there appears to be an incomplete genetic expression. Other factors that have been considered include abnormalities of growth hormone secretion, melatonin secretion, and skeletal muscle contractile protein.

Evaluation

Often, the young athlete presents with a curve that was noted on a routine examination. The history and physical examination should focus on excluding significant causes and determine the risk of progression. This will assist in determining the need for more advanced imaging and testing. It is important to determine at which age it was first noticed for classification. The presence of pain or neurologic complaints is important. The family history of scoliosis should be determined. The highest risk of curve progression occurs during the adolescent growth spurt. This growth spurt precedes the onset of puberty in women, manifested with the onset of menses. Thus, the premenarchal (prior to the first menstrual cycle) woman is at a higher risk of progression. In the male athlete, the onset of puberty, with testicular enlargement and pubic hair development, precedes the growth spurt. Growth in the female athlete continues for up to 2 years after menarche.

The physical examination includes the height. This is important in following the adolescent to determine the cessation of growth. This occurs when there is less than 1 cm of growth in a 6-month time period. The physical examination is performed in the usually disrobed adolescent to look for skin abnormalities, such as café au lait spots, hairy patches, and dimpling, which may indicate underlying cord abnormalities such as neurofibromatosis and spina bifida. One should also examine for connective tissue disorders. The stigmata of Marfan syndrome should be assessed in the tall woman more than 5 feet (ft) 10 inches (1.75 meters [m]) and men more than 6 ft (1.8 m) in height. Tall athletes with two or more of the following major criteria of Marfan syndrome should be referred for genetic testing and echocardiography:

- *Ocular:* lens dislocation, myopia (nearsighted)
- *Cardiovascular:* mitral valve prolapse, aortic rupture
- *Musculoskeletal:* scoliosis, anterior chest wall deformities (pectus excavatum and carinatum), long thin fingers (arachnodactyly), arm span longer than the height, and a high-arched palate.
- Family history of *Marfan syndrome*

A neurologic examination should be complete, looking for abnormal reflexes such as Babinski reflexes (up-going toes with plantar foot stroking) and hyperreflexia. These may indicate a spinal cord abnormality.

The degree of scoliosis is initially evaluated with the evaluator standing behind the patient with the forward-bending test. With this maneuver, the curve becomes more obvious due to the rotational component, which makes the ribs more prominent on the convex side. This is more accurately assessed using the scoliometer. This is placed on the spine in the forward-flexed posture and quantitates the degree of rotation. When the scoliometer reads 7 or more, the patient should have an X-ray to determine the severity of the curve. If one uses a lower number such as 5, the specificity diminishes, and excessive numbers of radiographs are ordered. However, it is important to realize that not all scoliosis cases involve a rotational deformity. Thus, when the spine appears curved even without rotation, a radiograph should be considered.

When indicated, the initial imaging should be a full-length posteroanterior (PA) and lateral spine X-ray including the pelvis. Each curve is identified and quantified using the Cobb method (Figure 1). The top of the curve is determined at the level at which the vertebrae deviate the most from the central axis. The bottom of the curve is determined similarly. A line is drawn across the top of the uppermost vertebra, and one is drawn across the lowermost vertebra. Perpendicular lines to these are made to intersect. The intersection angle determines

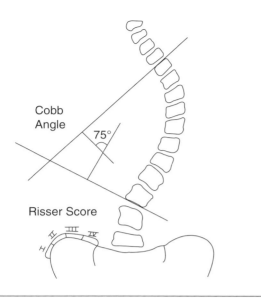

Figure I   Cobb Angle and Risser Score

Source: Pierre A. d'Hemecourt.

the extent of the curve. The curve must be greater than 10° to be classified as scoliosis. Lesser curves are referred to as spinal asymmetry.

The pelvic portion of the plain PA radiograph helps determine the remaining spinal growth potential by calculating the Risser score of the iliac crest growth cartilage (iliac apophysis). The iliac apophysis ossification appears from lateral to medial. Each 25% is divided into the first four scores. Risser I is the appearance of the first 25%. Risser II is the first 50% (Figure 1). Curves are more likely to progress in the early Risser scores of I or II.

The degree of the curve and the Risser score help determine the risk of progression. Curves less than 20° have a lower risk of progression unless the Risser score is less than I (22% risk of progression). A curve from 20% to 29% has a much higher risk of progression.

Further imaging with an MRI scan is considered when there are findings in the history and physical examination that indicate a neurologic concern as well as head, neck, or spinal pain. This should also be done on patients with juvenile onset and, according to some authorities, on patients with left-sided thoracic curves. The MRI scan should be a spinal screen that looks at the entire spine, including the junction with the occiput, to evaluate for a Chiari malformation (herniation of the cerebellar tonsils into the spinal canal).

Treatment

Observation

In mild curves, measuring less than 20°, observation is appropriate. The timing of this will depend somewhat on the age. Athletes less than 12 years of age or with a Risser score of I or less should be followed every 4 months. Older athletes can be followed every 6 to 8 months with a PA spine X-ray. Curves between 20° and 29° should be monitored more frequently, every 3 to 6 months. A progression of 5° may indicate a need for bracing.

Bracing

Curves that progress more than 5° should be considered for bracing. Curves more than 30° are also braced. Once initiated, the patient should have an initial PA radiograph of the spine in the brace to determine the degree of correction, as a value greater than 20% is a good prognostication for bracing efficacy. Bracing is continued until skeletal maturity, which is usually 1 to 2 years postmenarche.

Bracing may take several forms. The Boston overlapping brace is a commonly used thoracolumbarsacral orthosis (TLSO). It is worn ideally for 23 hours/day but has been used for 16 hours/day.

Rarely, a larger brace, the Milwaukee brace, is used to involve the cervical spine (cervicothoracolumbosacral orthosis [CTLSO]). This is used for high thoracic and double thoracic curves. Compliance is more difficult. There are two nighttime braces, the Charleston and Providence braces. Some studies indicate that they limit the progression of the curves. The data on the efficacy of all bracing are controversial and are being verified by ongoing clinical trials.

Surgical Intervention

Skeletally immature athletes who have a curve in excess of 50° are candidates for surgical stabilization, with consideration of the same for those with curves between 40° and 50°. Those adolescents who progress more than 5° while being managed in the brace are also considered for surgery. The surgical procedure usually involves segmental instrumentation and fusion. Curves that are very rigid may require an anterior thoracoscopic release.

Sports Participation

Sports participation is encouraged at all levels of scoliosis. Although physical therapy has not been shown to be helpful in managing the curve, the athlete should maintain cross-training and core stabilization for normal athletic conditioning. Full sports participation is encouraged. For some sports that emphasize repetitive asymmetrical spinal loading, such as rhythmic gymnastics, athletes are encouraged to cross-train to lessen these forces.

Many sports can be played while wearing a brace. In some sports such as gymnastics and swimming, the brace is removed during athletic competitions. However, if spinal instrumentation is performed, collision sports are contraindicated.

Pierre A. d'Hemecourt

See also Back Injuries, Surgery for; Cervical and Thoracic Disk Disease; Gymnastics, Injuries in; Lower Back Injuries and Low Back Pain; Musculoskeletal Tests, Spine; Slipped Disk; Young Athlete

Further Readings

Fiore N, Onimus M, Ferre B, Laurian JM. Treatment of lumbar and dorso-lumbar scoliosis using the Boston orthosis and the 3-valve orthosis. Comparative study of the results in the frontal and horizontal planes [in French]. *Rev Chir Orthop Reparatrice Appar Mot.*1988;74(6):569–575.

Gepstein R, Leitner Y, Zohar E, et al. Effectiveness of the Charleston bending brace in the treatment of a single curve idiopathic scoliosis. *J Pediatr Orthop.* 2002;22(1):84–87.

Haasbeek JF. Adolescent idiopathic scoliosis: recognizing patients who need treatment. *Postgrad Med.* 1997;101:207–209.

Huang SC. Cut-off point of the scoliometer in school scoliosis screening. *Spine.* 1997;22(17):1985–1989.

Lenssinck ML, Frijlink AC, Berger MY, Bierman-Zeinstra SM, Verkerk K, Verhagen AP. Effect of bracing and other conservative interventions in the treatment of idiopathic scoliosis in adolescents: a systematic review of clinical trials. *Phys Ther.* 2005;85(12):1329–1339.

Lonstein JE. Adolescent idiopathic scoliosis. *Lancet.* 1994;344(8934):1407–1412.

Lonstein JE, Winter RB. The Milwaukee brace for the treatment of adolescent idiopathic scoliosis. A review of one thousand and twenty patients. *J Bone Joint Surg Am.* 1994;76(8):1207–1221.

Newton PO, Wenger DR. Idiopathic scoliosis. In: Morrissy RT, Weinstein SL, eds. *Lovell and Winter's Pediatric Orthopaedics.* 6th ed. Philadelphia, PA: Lippincott Williams & Wilkins; 2006:693.

Noonan KJ, Weinstein SL, Jacobson WC, Dolan LA. Use of Milwaukee brace for progressive idiopathic scoliosis. *J Bone Joint Surg Am.* 1996;78(4):557–567.

Rowe DE, Bernstein SM, Riddick MF, Adler F, Emans JB, Gardner-Bonneau D. A meta-analysis of the efficacy of non-operative treatments for idiopathic scoliosis. *J Bone Joint Surg Am.* 1997;79(5):664–674.

Weinstein SL, Dolan LA, Spratt KF, Peterson KK, Spoonamore MJ, Ponseti IV. Health and function of patients with untreated idiopathic scoliosis: a 50-year natural history study. *JAMA.* 2003;289(5):559–567.

SCUBA Diving, Injuries in

Exploring the underwater world is a wonderful experience enjoyed by a wide variety of people. However, diving involves risks to health not encountered in other sporting activities and should not be attempted without certified instruction and assessment by a knowledgeable physician. This entry gives a brief overview of some common problems associated with diving and how to avoid them.

Diving can be done by swimming on the surface while breathing through a snorkel, holding your breath, or breathing compressed air from a tank or a hose (hookah). Problems can arise when the diver descends underwater because the pressure exerted by the water above the diver's body increases with depth. If this increased pressure unequally compresses the air and fluid spaces in the diver's body, an injury may result. In addition, breathing compressed gas at depths may cause another set of problems as gas is absorbed into the tissues, fluids, and spaces of the body. When the diver ascends to the surface, if the subsequent release and expansion of those gases occur in a rapid and uncontrolled manner, an injury known as decompression sickness may result.

Problems Caused by Water Pressure

Perhaps the most common problem in diving is the "ear squeeze," which results from the compression of the air behind the eardrum. Most of us experience this when diving to the bottom of a swimming pool. Special swallowing maneuvers can equalize the pressure in this middle part of the ear by opening the eustachian tube, which connects the throat with the middle ear. In a person with nasal congestion, the eustachian tube may be blocked, and equalization maneuvers may not work. Increasing the depth and pressure without equalization will eventually result in eardrum rupture and bleeding in the middle ear. While this may relieve the pressure difference and the pain, it can cause permanent damage or, worse, a sudden disequilibrium that could complicate a safe return to the surface. It is important not to dive when nasal congestion is present and middle ear equalization is not possible. Unless decongestants or allergy medications completely resolve nasal congestion and do not cause any side effects such as drowsiness, diving should be postponed. A similar, milder squeezing of the middle ear occurs when an airplane passenger descends to the higher air pressure at ground level.

The sinuses can similarly be "squeezed" and injured by increasing pressure as a diver descends, especially if nasal congestion blocks the sinus openings, preventing equalization. "Mask squeeze" occurs when the air in the mask is compressed and the mask presses on the face. It can cause headaches and bruising but is easily avoided with techniques learned in a diving course.

Problems Caused by Breathing Compressed Air

All gases, including the nitrogen and oxygen in ordinary air, can cause problems when they are breathed at increased pressures underwater. Compressed nitrogen can cause a mildly euphoric state with impaired judgment, which could be fatal for the diver or his buddy. This nitrogen narcosis is sometimes called the "rapture of the deep." Oxygen, which is lifesaving in many situations, can cause lung damage or even convulsions if breathed at high pressures. "Technical divers," who perform prolonged or very deep dives, often fill their tanks with special mixtures of oxygen, helium, nitrogen, or hydrogen to avoid these problems. But all gases have the potential to cause toxicity in certain situations.

Problems Caused by Ascent (Decompression Illnesses)

Self-contained underwater breathing apparatus (SCUBA) regulators, which were invented by Jacques Cousteau and Emile Gagnan, make SCUBA diving possible. As the diver descends to a higher-pressure environment, the regulator makes increasingly pressurized air available to fill the lungs. Surprisingly, it is the return to the lower pressure at the surface that is more dangerous than the descent. To understand this, let us review two laws of physics that you learned in high school and possibly forgot shortly thereafter.

Boyle's law states that at a constant temperature, the product of the pressure and volume of a gas is a constant. Thus, if the pressure increases, the volume decreases, and vice versa. The real-world application is that as a diver returns to the lower pressure at the surface, the volume of the gas in his or her lungs expands. For this reason, it is critically important that the return to the surface be slow, controlled, and with attention to exhaling this increased volume of gas. Otherwise, the alveoli, the tiny sacs in the lungs where blood and air meet, may burst, resulting in a pneumothorax. This is a leak that causes air to collect outside the lungs and compress it. In a similar fashion, air in the middle ear or sinuses may cause injury as the volume increases—a reverse squeeze.

Henry's law states that at a constant temperature, the amount of a gas dissolved in a liquid is directly proportional to the pressure of that gas above or around that liquid. As the pressure changes, the amount of gas dissolved in the liquid also changes. In diving, we are mostly concerned with the pressure of a gas in the alveoli and the amount of that gas dissolved in the blood capillaries surrounding each alveolus. Henry's law reminds us that as the pressure of nitrogen (the main gas in compressed air) increases in the lungs, the amount of nitrogen in the blood also increases. Conversely, when the diver ascends, and the pressure of nitrogen in the lungs decreases, the amount of nitrogen that can be kept dissolved in the blood and tissues also decreases. Some of this nitrogen, following Henry's law, must come out of solution, usually in the form of bubbles. While our bodies have other ways of quickly exchanging oxygen and carbon dioxide, the exchange of nitrogen is limited to simple diffusion.

Therefore, there are two mechanisms that change the gases in the body on ascent from a depth. Henry's law describes the increase in the amount of gas coming out of solution in body tissues such as fat, muscle, organs, and blood, and Boyle's law describes how the volume of that or any other gas increases. This may produce two main categories of decompression illnesses—decompression sickness and gas embolism.

The first, *decompression sickness*, results from the collection of gas where it does not usually exist—in and around joints, muscles, and nerves. It has been called "the bends" because of a doubled-over posture that may occur in the victims. A less serious condition occurs when gas collects in the skin.

The second, *gas embolism*, arises from bubbles in the blood causing the blockage of small arteries. Most people are familiar with embolic blockages of the blood vessels caused by blood clots in the heart or brain, which cause heart attacks or strokes. In a similar fashion, gas bubbles may cause embolic blockages in small arteries, with the same effects. While the heart and brain are the most common places for serious damage from gas emboli, other organs such as the kidneys and lungs can also be affected.

In addition to blocking the small arteries, the increasing size of the bubbles or gas collections may burst things. Even the small decrease in pressure that occurs when ascending in a pressurized aircraft might add to decompression from diving, and, therefore, air travel should not occur for several hours after diving.

Decompression sickness and gas embolism can usually be prevented through careful attention to diving techniques, especially ascending in an orderly, planned, and controlled fashion. If they do occur, initial treatment is breathing pure oxygen, which decreases the amount of nitrogen in the lungs, favoring the diffusion of nitrogen out of the tissues because of the resulting gradient.

A decompression illness that is not improving or results in serious symptoms should be treated in a hyperbaric (high-pressure) chamber, where the patient can be returned to high pressures in the hope of returning the gas to solution and then decompressing slowly, thereby allowing the gas to come out of solution gradually without causing damage. (One such hyperbaric center is The Duke Center for Hyperbaric Medicine and Environmental Physiology: 919–684–6726, Hospital 24 Hour 919–684–8111.)

Specific Injuries and Medical Concerns

Asthma may cause narrowing of the small airways, which could make equalization of pressures difficult and increase the chance of pneumothorax and gas emboli if alveoli burst in an area that cannot be equalized. Traditionally, persons with asthma were prohibited from diving. However, current recommendations are that well-controlled asthma is usually compatible with diving if the candidate is symptom-free with medication. What is critical is that the asthma be well controlled. All persons with asthma, but especially divers, must see a physician and take prescribed medications regularly to ensure optimal control. Conversely, on a related topic, anyone who has had a spontaneous pneumothorax should not dive. Chest X-rays are often done as part of a diving examination to look for this, but previous pneumothoraces are usually not detectable, and so a medical history is important in these cases.

Seizures, dizziness, migraine headaches with vision or balance changes, and panic attacks are other conditions that may not be too concerning in ordinary activities; however, if they occur under water, a safe return to the surface may be compromised, and their occurrence may be fatal. Similarly, symptoms of heart disease, which might be treated easily on the surface, may lead to drowning if they occur under water. Persons with these conditions are usually advised not to dive. In addition, a minimum level of physical fitness is required to dive safely because the diver may be confronted with unexpected challenges from weather, currents, temperature, and other physical conditions related to the diving environment. Also important is the possession and practice of good judgment to avoid situations that increase the risk of accidents.

Additional information can be requested from the Divers Alert Network, a nonprofit organization that maintains a comprehensive website and an emergency hotline for diving accidents (www.diversalertnetwork.org; 919–684–4DAN [4326]).

Ronald P. Olson and Jake Freiberger

See also Ear Infection, Outer (Otitis Externa); Surfing, Injuries in

Further Readings

Brubakk AO, Neuman TS, eds. *Bennett and Elliotts' Physiology and Medicine of Diving*. 5th ed. London, UK: Saunders; 2003.

Levett DZH, Millar IL. Bubble trouble: a review of diving physiology and disease. *Postgrad Med J.* 2008;84(997):571–578.

Websites

Divers Alert Network: http://www.diversalertnetwork.org
Duke Center for Hyperbaric Medicine and Environmental Physiology: http://hyperbaric.mc.duke.edu

SEASONAL RHYTHMS AND EXERCISE

Changes in seasons across the calendar year lead to variations in the weather and environmental conditions in most locations across the globe. Such variations exhibit a period of about 1 year ± 2 months and, thus, can be defined as "seasonal" rhythms. Seasonal rhythms are influential in determining patterns of behavior in a wide range of living organisms. These rhythms also have the potential to affect human behavior as we: (a) possess an internal body clock that is responsible for subtle rhythmic changes in a range of physiological functions across various time periods, and (b) are susceptible to the demands of external factors. The spatial distribution of humans across a wide range of climatic zones means that variability in environmental conditions across the calendar year is a common experience for most people. This makes understanding the potential impact of these seasonal changes on important social behaviors such as exercise, in both the recreational and the elite athlete, useful to the sport and exercise scientist. This knowledge may help inform the development of effective interventions to enhance health-related fitness, as well as highlight the best strategies for competitive athletes in optimizing performance.

The Basis for Seasonal Rhythms

Seasonal rhythms are linked to fluctuations in the prevailing climatic conditions observed at any given time of the year. These climatic conditions are, in their simplest terms, a direct consequence of the daily axis of rotation of the earth being inclined at 23.5° from the vertical and the elliptical orbit of the earth around the sun. This tilted orientation produces a seasonal variation in the duration of daylight from the equator to the poles. The angle at which the rays of the sun strike the surface of the earth also varies according to the season. This leads in turn to marked differences in the ambient temperature and other climatic and weather conditions that partly depend on the latitude and the prevailing topography. Such environmental changes, along with alterations in the amount of daylight, have the potential to be very influential on human social behavior. This is especially pertinent to activities, such as exercise, in which such environmental factors will affect important characteristics of the exercise stress (e.g., type, frequency, duration, and intensity). Changes in these variables will subsequently have consequences for both the acute physiological responses to exercise and the adaptations that follow chronic exposure to activity in both a health setting and a performance setting.

The potential theoretical importance of seasonal rhythms is not currently reflected in the amount of available research in the field. Methodological issues have undoubtedly had an effect as appropriate experimental designs and methodologies are very difficult to use in this field. More important though is our increasing ability to control both our climatic conditions and our exposure to light in our immediate surroundings. As a result, our habitual activities and behaviors are in theory no longer tightly bound to seasonal fluctuations in day length and climate and are more likely to depend on cultural, religious, and economic influences. These influences will clearly reduce the amount of the seasonal variability to be observed in human populations in Western industrialized societies and, thereby, potentially limit the ability of such rhythms to influence behavior. Nevertheless, seasonal variation can still affect many aspects of the work of the sport and exercise scientist, especially when the external environment strongly facilitates or acts as a barrier to exercise participation.

Seasonal Variation in the Physiological Responses to Exercise

The seasonal variation in ambient temperature and environmental conditions provides one basis for the existence of seasonal rhythms. Aspects such as metabolic rate and the physiological response to a given exercise stress are highly susceptible to such changes. This may either result in alterations in the social behavior of individuals or act to change the underlying physiology, a process known as acclimation. Characteristics of the human thermoregulatory system exhibit seasonal variation primarily as a consequence of acclimation. Sweating, a vital component of the body's heat loss response during exercise, is altered both with respect to its initiation and amount during summer because of the repeated exposure to elevated temperatures. Other thermoregulatory changes include variations in the core temperature response to an exercise stress and altered individual subjective thermal sensations to a given heat challenge. The time of the year can also affect other aspects of the exercise response, including causing changes in the hematocrit and alterations in the respiratory exchange ratio, with relatively more fatty acids being used as a fuel in the winter. Such changes may be partly mediated by the changes in body temperature associated with exercise because the core temperature is an important determinant of the metabolic response to exercise, elevating carbohydrate usage when levels are high.

Annual cycles in day length are also relevant to the existence of circannual rhythms as they have the potential to alter both the intrinsic elements of the body clock and exogenous behavioral factors. The relationship between seasonal changes in both day length (photoperiod) and night length (scotoperiod) and the behavioral, metabolic, and biochemical responses to exercise in humans remains uncertain. Seasonal changes of the natural photo- and scotoperiods at high latitudes have an effect on melatonin secretion in humans as discussed previously, though there is no consensus on whether humans generally display a seasonal rhythmicity in melatonin secretion. This limits the direct evidence that is available to support the theory that changes in the extent of melatonin control the effect of photoperiod, as occurs in animal models. Evidence that other circadian rhythms also display seasonal variation is also relatively weak in healthy humans. This may suggest that humans in industrialized countries live in environments in which the photoperiod may have lost its status of primary *zeitgeber* (a cue that synchronizes a person's "internal clock" to the earth's light/dark cycle).

Seasonal Variation in Physical Activity Patterns

Substantial evidence exists for significant seasonal variation in the physical activity of free-living adults in most industrialized countries. These changes display a sinusoidal pattern, with peak values occurring in summer for the majority of measures of physical activity. The most common habitual physical activities associated with leisure, such as walking for pleasure, gardening, lawn mowing, bicycling, hiking, and running, all display significant seasonal variation in industrialized populations. A variation in occupational activities seems to be able to explain less of the variability in activity patterns unless the local population is nonindustrialized and is, therefore, subject to specific periods of high levels of activity (e.g., during harvesting of crops). These reductions are also observed in humans who live at high latitudes during periods when one would assume that physical activity would be desirable to help protect against the climatic conditions. Changes in daylight hours seem to be important in these variations, though the more favorable environmental conditions in summer to carry out an active lifestyle will no doubt also play a role.

Seasonal Variation in Physical Fitness and Health

The maintenance of physical activity over the whole year is important for the health of individuals. Such changes in activity are also likely to have consequences for alterations in physical fitness. The best aerobic performances are frequently recorded in subjects at summertime—that is, unless individuals maintain high levels of physical activity in winter in specific recreational activities (e.g., winter sports such as skiing). These circumstances may limit the reductions observed in fitness and lead to more stable performance levels across relevant time periods. The impact of seasonality on health-related issues is, however, much more complicated as these relationships can be extremely variable and complex. It has been suggested that the month of birth may be related to the susceptibility to certain illnesses, though these associations should in no way be interpreted as being indicative of a direct relationship between different times of the year and disease risk. Changes in activity across the annual cycle may also compound problems with glycemic control in Type 2 diabetics. Epidemiological data do, however, highlight the idea that the incidence and mortality of cardiovascular disease, such as coronary heart disease, is increased in winter compared with the spring. This trend may be related to the seasonal variations in a number of risk factors (e.g., body weight, oxidant/ antioxidant processes, calorie intake) as a result of changes in temperature, lifestyle, and human physiology (e.g., blood pressure). These relationships would indicate that such variations in cardiovascular-related morbidity may be reduced by the careful modification of external environmental factors, such as better housing, improved heating, and changes to seasonally driven lifestyles.

Viral infections and influenzas are also more likely in the colder months, with the most commonly cited explanation being the increased "crowding" indoors of susceptible persons in the winter. Exercise-induced bronchospasm also shows seasonal variation, with a twofold increase in incidence in dry seasons compared with other times of the year. This would suggest that such conditions may be complicated by environmental factors such as dry air, the ambient temperature, and the presence of environmental allergens, such as pollen, in individuals. Mental health may also be more susceptible to challenges at certain times of the year. The long hours of darkness in winter, especially in the northern latitudes, can lead to a depression known as *seasonal affective disorder*. The seasonal effect on the diurnal rhythm in melatonin may partly explain these occurrences and open the possibility of the use of a combination of bright light and exercise as a therapeutic tool.

Seasonal Variation in Competitive Sports Performance

The types of sports in which athletes participate, as well as the training behavior of elite athletes, are clearly influenced by the seasonal changes in the weather. Skiing, ice skating, hurling, and ski jumping are naturally all "winter sports," while other sports, such as cricket and tennis, are primarily played in the warmer summer temperatures. The distinctness of the temporal location of such activities within the calendar year has recently become

blurred, with the development of indoor facilities that allow a variety of climatic conditions to be simulated. The accessibility of long-distance travel across hemispheres to reverse seasons has also enabled competitions to be scheduled at nontraditional times. As climatic conditions vary as a function of the time of year and geographical location, it is likely that athletic performances could be associated with additional physiological demands in some circumstances. For example, changes in environmental conditions, especially the ambient temperature, will alter the metabolic and physiological responses to a range of exercise stresses. The increased presence of seasonal allergens such as pollen may also compound any physiological changes. Travel across time zones will also not be without its own consequences if events are scheduled close to arrival times as the athlete groups involved may face additional difficulties in preparing for competition.

An understanding of the seasonal variation in sports performance is also complicated by exogenous factors that mask any inherent endogenous circannual rhythms. Elite athletes "periodize" or "cycle" their training throughout the year. Periodization involves the adoption of cyclic variations in the intensity and type of training stimuli and the amount of rest. The calendar year is traditionally divided into three distinct phases: the preparatory period, the competitive period, and the recovery phase, each of which has its own specific objectives and associated training load. It is therefore of little surprise that variations in performance in a range of physiological parameters (e.g., maximal oxygen consumption, anaerobic power, isometric and isokinetic strength, body composition) are associated with the different training phases that are adopted. This evidence would suggest that seasonal changes in performance are a consequence of external factors rather than any inherent internal seasonal rhythm.

More conclusive evidence for circannual rhythms in competitive sports performance may come from the observation of subtle differences within specific phases of the periodized year. Using this approach, a significant component of the exogenous changes in activity associated with the periodized year should be removed as the training stimulus should be much less variable. Team sports such as soccer show such subtle variations in the work rate completed by players during games at different stages of the competitive season. Such variations are not associated with alterations in the physical capabilities of players or their physiological characteristics as these do not tend to vary greatly within the competitive season. Large inter-individual differences in these data, as well as a failure to control other known determining factors of a player's work rate (e.g., opposition), do, however, preclude firm conclusions regarding the origin of these variations to be made on the basis of the data currently available.

Future elite performers may also be dictated partly by an observed seasonal birth bias. Age categories in youth sports are often managed by having a birth cutoff point to determine eligibility. Comprehensive evidence from a number of athletic groups (e.g., soccer, hockey, baseball) indicates that participants in underage teams tend to be born at the start of the competitive year. This provides these individuals with a chronological advantage over those born later in the year, which tends to be replicated in a maturational superiority. This early selection bias can carry through to those selected for elite adult competitions in later years. This phenomenon cannot be attributed to any endogenous circannual rhythm as the bias can be altered if the initial date for eligibility is changed. As such, coaches and selectors are advised to acknowledge the influence of such factors and compensate for them accordingly.

Another area directly relevant to competitive sports performance that displays a high degree of seasonal variation is the incidence of injury. There is clear seasonality in the frequency of injuries incurred by athletes participating in a wide range of sports, though this variation differs between sports. The highest injury rates seem to occur during the competitive season rather than the preparation periods. The multifactorial nature of the causes of sports injuries makes it very difficult to clearly attribute these differences in injury to any one specific factor. It is clear that a variety of exogenous factors, such as environmental conditions (both high and low temperatures can increase the risk of injury) and changes in the amount and intensity of activity, can predispose an individual to injury. Endogenous factors may also play a role. For example, vitamin D levels in the body can be increased in response to environmental light. This

fat-soluble vitamin promotes growth and mineralization of bones and increases the absorption of dietary calcium. This may mean that bone mineral density varies seasonally, with the lowest values observed in the winter months. This, when combined with the low levels of activity at this time of year, may lead to a weaker skeleton and increase injury disposition. Such changes may, however, be minimal in an athletic population that maintains high levels of activity across the calendar year.

Barry Drust

See also Circadian Rhythms and Exercise; Exercise and Disease Prevention; Performance Enhancement, Doping, Therapeutic Use Exemptions; Periodization; Shift Work and Exercise

Further Readings

Atkinson G, Drust B. Seasonal rhythms and exercise. *Clin Sports Med.* 2005;24(2):e25–e34.

Group TE. Cold exposure and winter mortality from ischaemic heart disease, cerebrovascular disease, respiratory disease and all causes in warm and cold regions of Europe. *Lancet.* 1997;349(9062): 1341–1346.

Peiser B, Reilly T, Atkinson G, Drust B, Waterhouse J. Seasonal changes and physiological responses: their impact on activity, health, exercise and athletic performance. *Int Sportmed J.* 2006;17:16–32.

Reilly T, Atkinson G, Waterhouse J. *Biological Rhythms and Exercise.* New York, NY: Oxford University Press; 1997.

Reilly T, Peiser B. Seasonal variations in health-related human physical activity. *Sports Med.* 2006;36(6): 463–485.

Simmons C, Paull GC. Season-of-birth in association football. *J Sports Sci.* 2001;19(9):677–686.

Uitenbroek DG. Seasonal variation in leisure time physical activity. *Med Sci Sports Exerc.* 1993;25(6):755–760.

SEIZURE DISORDER IN SPORTS

A seizure is a common, serious neurological event affecting approximately 10% of individuals during their lifetimes. Each year, an estimated 300,000 individuals in the United States, including 120,000 children and adolescents, will experience their first seizure. Team doctors and coaches should be familiar with caring for an athlete who has a seizure during an event. While athletic participation is generally encouraged for individuals who have had a single seizure or diagnosis of epilepsy, many factors are considered. This entry discusses recent guides for participation, safety and first-aid measures, and special considerations for athletes with a seizure disorder.

Definitions and Risk of Recurrence

The brain normally functions through a network of neurons that send and receive bioelectrical signals maintaining our homeostasis at rest and performing purposeful activities. In simple terms, a *seizure* is a neurological event during which normal brain messaging is interrupted by chaotic neuronal hyperactivity, resulting in loss of targeted function. *Epilepsy* is a condition in which an individual is susceptible to recurrent seizures.

Seizures originating in a discrete, localized region involving one side of the brain are called *focal* or *partial seizures*. Focal seizures are categorized into simple seizures, in which specific functions (e.g., unilateral muscle twitching) are affected, and complex seizures, in which the mental alertness and state of consciousness are affected. Typical clinical features include unresponsiveness, staring, or confusion, as well as gaze deviation, lip smacking, drooling, or semipurposeful hand movements. This abnormal bioelectrical activity can continue to spread to the opposite cerebral hemisphere, resulting in a secondarily generalized tonic-clonic seizure, historically described as a *grand mal* seizure or *convulsion*. Focal seizures may be caused by a variety of recognized pathology, including trauma, stroke, tumor, developmental structural abnormality, or infection irritating certain regions of the brain. Often, no clear cause or etiology can be determined.

A generalized seizure involves both cerebral hemispheres. The various subtypes of generalized seizures include absence, myoclonic, atonic (drop events), and generalized tonic-clonic. Absence seizures are brief, abrupt staring episodes or lapses in attention, most commonly seen in children. Myoclonic seizures are shocklike muscle twitches, most commonly presenting in adolescents. Primary generalized seizures often recur, typically have genetic etiologies, and commonly result in a diagnosis of epilepsy. Some conditions such as juvenile absence epilepsy and juvenile myoclonic epilepsy require lifelong therapy.

For the witness to a seizure, it is helpful to record the duration, recurrence, and clinical features of the seizure, such as the side of the body involved and the injuries sustained. A medical evaluation is required for anyone experiencing a first seizure. Through this evaluation, an electroencephalogram (EEG), neuroimaging, and consultation with a neurologist will determine the likelihood of recurrence and any necessary preventive therapy. A safety plan will also be devised in the case of a future seizure.

The overall risk of additional seizure in an individual having a single focal seizure is approximately 30% to 50%, while primary generalized seizures are very likely to recur without treatment. Some clinical factors may provoke a seizure, but it is important to make these determinations and any activity restrictions on an individual basis. Typical exacerbating factors include fever/infection, sleep deprivation, alcohol, some specific medications, and noncompliance with prescribed preventative anticonvulsant therapy. Many patients report stress and "overactivity" as factors, though these are hard to systematically evaluate and define. Rare cases of reflex epilepsy have been associated with aerobic exercise, reading, or other specific stimuli. Hyperventilation may provoke some generalized seizures though athletic participation and exertion typically do not. While traumatic brain injury can provoke a seizure, participation in contact sports, such as football or hockey, has not been shown to trigger seizures. Although precautions and an individualized plan are essential, aerobic exercise and athletic participation are recommended for individuals with a single seizure and for those with epilepsy.

Participation Guides

While athletic participation is encouraged and has clear health benefits, risks should be addressed in a thoughtful, practical manner in each individual setting. This risk-benefit analysis will consider the seizure type, likelihood of recurrence, present control, potential injury should a seizure occur, and reasonable safety precautions deployable. In 1997, the International League Against Epilepsy trimmed the list of restricted activities to self-contained underwater breathing apparatus (SCUBA) diving and sky diving. Obviously, some activities involve higher degrees of scrutiny and absolute seizure control, such as motor sports and precision shooting/archery and activities involving heights, such as rock climbing. Gymnastics, horseback riding, sailing, and swimming/diving are other sports requiring discretion, close supervision, and control of seizures prior to participation, due to risks of personal injury. Cycling, skating, and skiing also require seizure control and routine personal protection such as helmets. Contact sports such as football, hockey, and soccer do not have restrictions beyond close supervision and routine safety procedures. Aerobic activities and weight training should be undertaken with typical safety precautions. The speed, intensity, and setting of the activity will dictate the necessity of seizure control prior to participation as many individuals with active, uncontrolled epilepsy benefit from jogging, golf, and court sports such as tennis and basketball.

Safety and First Aid

In the event that an individual experiences a seizure, simple first-aid measures can be promptly implemented. Although a seizure can be initially alarming, a calm, reassuring manner is helpful. First, prevent any additional injury, protecting the patient from falls, collisions, or drowning. Time the duration of the event, and note clinical features if possible. Do not restrain the individual. Loosen tight clothing if possible. If safe, turn the individual on his or her side as some individuals have excess secretions and may vomit, although rarely. Also, do not place an object in the individual's mouth that could create the potential for choking or dental damage. The person having a seizure will not swallow his or her tongue, as is commonly misconceived. Stay with the individual and seek emergency medical care (911) if the seizure lasts longer than 3 minutes. Some individuals with epilepsy may have rescue medications available that are typically used after a 3-minute seizure duration. If the seizure is recurrent or provoked by head trauma or the individual fails to demonstrate recovery over a 10-minute duration following the event, the individual should also be evaluated on

an emergent basis. If it is the person's first seizure, a prompt evaluation is important. While emergency care is important for many, if the individual has recognized epilepsy and a self-resolving seizure lasting less than 3 minutes, emergency care may not be necessary. Many individuals feel tired, confused, and complain of headaches following a seizure; however, they should be able to be aroused and follow simple commands. It is important to stay with the individual until he or she has recovered. An individual who experiences a seizure should not return to immediate athletic participation. The Epilepsy Foundation of America has produced informative educational materials (www .epilepsyfoundation.org).

Prevention and Therapy Considerations

Therapeutic plans for individuals with epilepsy or for those who have experienced a single seizure often include a rescue medication in the event of a prolonged seizure lasting more than 3 minutes. These medications are typically a benzodiazepine such as diazepam or lorazepam, given by a rectal or buccal preparation. Nasal midazolam is beginning to be accepted as an alternative.

Preventative anticonvulsant medications, if necessary, should maximize the efficacy and tolerability. Clear cognitive function and alertness are critical to athletes. Lamotrigine and levetiracetam are medication options with infrequent sedation. Topiramate and zonisamide are effective medications for many types of epilepsy; however, for the athlete, special attention must be paid to hydration status and temperature control as these medications lead to a high incidence of kidney stones and reduced sweating, increasing the risk of hyperthermia and heat stroke.

Jason Doescher

See also Emergency Medicine and Sports; Fieldside Assessment and Triage; Physically and Mentally Challenged Athletes

Further Readings

Arida RM, Cavalheiro EA, da Silva AC, Scorza FA. Physical activity and epilepsy. *Sports Med.* 2008;38(7):607–615.

Fountain NB, May AC. Epilepsy and athletics. *Clin Sport Med.* 2003;22(1):605–616.

Websites

Epilepsy Foundation: http://www.epilepsyfoundation.org

SENIOR ATHLETES

Although some have suggested that the increased level of injuries diagnosed within the aging population is due to simply "outliving our warranties," a look into the subculture of senior—or masters—athletes reveals a number of individuals who are outperforming society's age-defined expectations. Athletes in the media spotlight, such as football player Brett Favre, cyclist Lance Armstrong, and swimmer Dara Torres, are redefining how we think about aging. However, these feats of enduring performance are not limited to elite-level athletes: Recreational athletes, including those who are abandoning the couch in pursuit of a more active lifestyle, have demonstrated some remarkable accomplishments of their own. Despite the fact that waiting rooms at doctors' offices across the country are filled with these "weekend warriors," sports medicine has largely ignored this group, preferring to focus on the child, collegiate, or professional athlete. The purpose of this entry is to illuminate the factors affecting performance and injury prevention in the aging athlete and to summarize the benefits of active aging, thereby dispelling the common notion that age is the sole factor contributing to an individual's activity level.

To maintain an active lifestyle as we age, it is important to understand the biology behind the aging process. At the cellular level, rapid cell division provides the human body with a remarkable regeneration capacity. It enables us to recover from injury rapidly throughout the childhood and early adult years. As we continue to age, our bodies become less efficient at these regeneration activities, resulting in stiffer tissues and a decline in overall performance. These changes occur not only at the macrolevel of muscles and joints but also at the microlevel of deoxyribonucleic acid (DNA). The way our genes are expressed also changes with age and activity level. The consensus among the general population is that this lapse in athletic prowess is an inevitable and irreversible part of the aging process. This consensus, however, is less grounded in science than in anecdote. Many studies are revealing the true capacity of our musculoskeletal system with aging and show that aging is not necessarily an irreversible decline from vitality to frailty.

We know from recent research efforts that "old" cells can be reprogrammed at the cellular level to behave like "young" cells by simply using exercise as medicine. In general, much more investigation into this decline and how much can be attributed to physical inactivity is needed. The high level of physical activity maintained by masters athletes throughout their lifespans make them model subjects for investigating healthy aging. By studying this population, we are able to eliminate the variable of physical inactivity or other health conditions when investigating the aging process.

The Longevity of the Masters Athlete

Masters athletes everywhere continue to debunk the common myth that turning 40 means slowing down. In a survey conducted by the Arthritis Foundation, 64% of masters athletes reported feeling an average of 11 years younger than their actual age, while 40% reported living a more healthy and physically fit lifestyle than in their 20s. Moreover, 33% of them boasted that they could beat their children in at least one sport. It is important to note that these people are not the exception but the standard. All individuals have the chance to maintain this high quality of life and functional capacity throughout their lifespans if they choose to avoid a sedentary lifestyle. Studies of performance decline in masters athletes indicate that the slowing phenomenon of the aging process does not have a significant impact until the seventh decade of life.

In a study of track athletes between the ages of 50 and 85 who participated in the 2001 National Summer Senior Games, running times across all distances declined with age. While this trend was expected, the surprising finding was the small degree of performance decline that occurred with age. Until the age of 75, the observed decline was slow and linear, with decreases of less than 2% per year. This decline was not found to be statistically significant. At age 75, however, the rate of decline jumped to approximately 8%. This trend of performance decline with age is shown in Senior Olympians competing at all distances, from the 100-meter (m) dash to the 10,000-m run. These results suggest that if disuse and disease are eliminated, individuals should be able to maintain high levels of functional independence until the age of 75. Therefore, the loss of independence before the age of 75 must be attributed to lifestyle habits, disease, or genetic predisposition.

Similar rates of maintained performance are also observed when investigating the scores of masters athletes on tests of aerobic capacity, such as the $\dot{V}o_2$max and the lactate threshold test. An analysis of the $\dot{V}o_2$max (peak oxygen uptake) scores of masters athletes over the age of 35 proposes that a 0.5% decline per year may be an intrinsic biomarker of the aging process. Women have displayed a slightly faster rate of decline than men in this area. These rates are much less than would be expected considering that a low $\dot{V}o_2$max is believed to be one of the fundamental reasons behind decreases in functional capacity in the aging population. Research investigating declines in endurance performance with aging attributed poor performance to a reduced $\dot{V}o_2$max and lactate threshold. In a study comparing healthy young adults, older sedentary individuals, and older endurance athletes, approximately 50% of the age-related differences witnessed in the $\dot{V}o_2$max score were found to be the result of a smaller stroke volume. The remaining differences were attributed to a lower maximal heart rate and reduced oxygen extraction. However, as shown within the masters athlete group, these trends can be greatly diminished through high levels of habitual exercise. This suggests that any exaggerated rates of decline are the results of lower energy levels, decreased training intensity, and less time spent training. Only modest portions of these declines in performance are age related.

These moderate rates of performance decline also depend on factors such as gender and type of physical activity. Investigation of track-and-field records to examine the rate of performance decline show that strength deteriorates before stamina does. This is best seen in sprinters, as their declines in running speed are paralleled with a decrease in stride length. This is believed to be the result of a decrease in muscle strength, which requires athletes to take a greater number of strides to cover

the same distance. However, when examining the times of Senior Olympian record holders, it was found that the rates of decline were most prominent among the endurance athletes. In swimmers, the sex differences were largest in the sprint events and smallest in the distance events. The data examining the rates of performance decline among types of swimming events also yield conflicting results, as some studies report a larger decline in sprint races while others find a larger decline in endurance races. Parallel to the runner's decrease in stride length, swimmers demonstrate a decreased stroke length, which results in an increase in stroke frequency. It is believed that the mechanisms of decline are different for each sport, depending on the demands of the activity; yet altogether, they remain gradual.

Injuries in Masters Athletes

The magnitude of evidence in favor of active aging raises an important question: If masters athletes are so healthy, why are they getting hurt? According to the U.S. Consumer Products Safety Commission, a 33% increase in injuries was witnessed within the masters athlete population from 1991 to 1998. Injuries are the number one reason for the stoppage of physical activity in this group and occur highest in sports such as cycling, basketball, baseball, and running. Investigation of the mechanism of these injuries reveals that 69% of masters athletes attempt to work through their pain to remain active. This is most likely why 60% of the injuries reported are the result of overuse and only 23% are the result of falls. Research has suggested a number of reasons for the increased incidence of injury witnessed within this group, the most notable of which is inappropriate training methods. Unpublished data from a study conducted by Wright and colleagues reveal that in a sample of masters athletes surveyed, 50% of the athletes devoted 5% or less of their total training time to stretching exercises. Of that group, 31.5% devoted only 0% to 2% of their time to stretching activities. This is without question an insubstantial amount of time. To avoid injury, masters athletes must train smarter than they did in their younger years. This includes proper nutrition, not overextending oneself when training, and adequate amounts of daily stretching, especially before intense bouts of exercise.

Muscle

Acute muscle strains account for a predominant portion of the injuries witnessed within the aging population. This is attributed to loss of flexibility as well as weak or fatigued muscles. The predisposition of masters athletes to these injuries is thought to be the result of their frequent participation in endurance sports. Investigation of the mechanism of these injuries reveals that the athletes often report changes in their training activities when recounting the onset of the injury. This supports the belief that older athletes do not transition from sport to sport as quickly as they did in their younger years and require a more extensive warm-up before commencing rigorous physical activity. Furthermore, all individuals have a responsibility to exercise, no matter at what age, to maintain stronger, resilient muscles that are more resistant to injury.

Tendon

Tendinosis in masters athletes commonly occurs as the result of overtraining. This subjects the tendon to repetitive microtrauma, which in turn causes it to stiffen. Other factors that can contribute to this age-related stiffening of connective tissues are decreases in water content, increases in elastin fibril thickness, and hormonal abnormalities, such as diabetes mellitus or an excess of corticosteroids. Three of the most prevalent types of tendinosis in masters athletes are rotator cuff tendinopathy, Achilles tendinitis, and tennis elbow. All this suggests that the gradual stiffening of tendons must be paralleled by changes in the masters athlete's training regimen if he or she is to avoid these injuries. Daily stretching exercises are paramount in avoiding tendon stiffening and the subsequent tendinosis.

Knee

In recent years, the consensus that exercise provides protective benefits to joints by reducing the incidence of degenerative diseases, such as osteoarthritis, has been a controversial issue. Traditionally, the prescribed therapy for knee pain has been modification of training activities, a technique not well received by many masters athletes. This makes the management of knee osteoarthritis one of the most challenging issues in sports medicine today since those affected by this disorder typically wish to maintain a high level of physical activity. Investigations of this disorder reveal that athletes symptomatic for knee osteoarthritis all demonstrated quadriceps weakness, reduced proprioception, and increased postural sway. Altered proprioception due to muscle fatigue may weaken the neuromuscular response and decrease the efficiency of protective muscular reflexes. This contradicts the paradigm that the aging athlete should not participate in activities that subject the knees to high levels of impact, such as running, as knee injuries can be avoided by maintaining quadriceps, core, and hip strength, as well as refraining from high-intensity workouts when fatigued.

Shoulder

Shoulder injuries, such as subacromial impingement and rotator cuff tears, are commonly associated with repetitive shoulder motion. Initially, the goal of shoulder surgery was to alleviate pain symptoms. Currently, the goal is to achieve a return to physical activities, which is becoming increasingly more common. Patients over 65 years demonstrate great success in recovering from subacromial decompression and rotator cuff repair, with a 94% satisfaction rate. The majority of these patients report a reduction in pain symptoms, independent living, and return to sports. Research investigating return to sports suggested that 80% of patients return to sports at their previous level of competition following surgery to their dominant shoulder. However, this becomes increasingly more difficult as patients pursue higher-intensity, higher-impact sports. Despite the success rates of these surgical procedures, these injuries are best treated through preventive efforts. Many athletes focus on building the "cosmetic" muscles, such as the biceps, triceps, and deltoids, while ignoring the exercises that work the smaller muscles, which are paramount for joint stability and avoiding injury.

Hip

Studies of women with lower extremity osteoarthritis revealed that fatigue was strongly associated with physical activity, while pain was more weakly associated with physical activity and was in the direction opposite to what was expected. This stresses the importance of fatigue management in helping masters athletes with osteoarthritis maintain high levels of physical activity. Hip arthroscopy is a method commonly used to treat labral tears and the early stages of osteoarthritis. It has yielded reproducible results in the diagnosis and treatment of intraarticular hip disorders in elite athletes. Hip arthroscopy could be a promising treatment for the aging population as many elite masters athletes refuse to modify their activities and do not have the degenerative changes to warrant joint replacement. Regardless of activity levels, the senior population will exhibit a redistribution of joint torques from plantarflexion to hip joint extension over time. However, the active elderly display a more pronounced increase of hip extension torque, which enables them to perpetuate the support torque at the level of young subjects. This age-related redistribution of joint torques is of pivotal importance since the active elderly use it as a means of compensating for diminishing muscle function. By maintaining flexibility, core, and gluteal strength, masters athletes may avoid hip injuries and continue to enjoy high levels of functional capacity.

Changes That Occur as We Age

Natural Aging: The Cardiovascular System

In the aging process, upkeep of cardiovascular function is imperative: Forty percent of deaths in people between the ages of 65 and 74 are the result of heart disease; for individuals over the age of 80, this proportion jumps to 60%. This is because many age-related physiological changes are witnessed in the cardiovascular system. For example, a 70-year-old heart has 30% fewer cells than the heart of a 20-year-old. The cardiac output of a 20-year-old is 3.5 to 4 times his or her resting capacity, while an 80-year-old can output only twice his or her resting capacity. During exertion, the maximum heart rate for a 20-year-old is between 180 and 200 beats per minute (bpm), while it is only 145 bpm for an 80-year-old. To some extent, these changes are part of the natural maturation of the heart. As part of the aging process, the maximum heart rate, the stoke volume, and the contractility of the heart will decrease. In

the arteries, a decreased elasticity occurs, which results in a narrower space for blood to flow from the heart. This produces a rise in blood pressure and forces the heart to pump harder, which eventually leads to a thicker left ventricle. All these changes disrupt the heart's delivery of oxygen to the tissues, which affects performance, metabolism, and energy levels. Although these physiological changes may appear alarming, chronic high-level exercise and a healthy diet have long been associated with healthy cardiovascular function and a slowing of these changes.

Masters Athletes: The Cardiovascular System

Through endurance conditioning, one is capable of modifying maximum oxygen consumption, diastolic filling and relaxation, and arterial stiffness. In a prospective study of masters athletes across 20 years, less than 14% evidenced risk factors for coronary heart disease at the 20-year evaluation point. In addition, a study of the effects of vigorous endurance training reflected a low prevalence of hypertension in masters athletes when compared with controls, with the masters athlete group being 27.8% less likely to have used medication for hypertension at any time. While a lower body mass and decreased body weight may explicate this effect, researchers believe that other mechanisms exist whereby exercise may induce a decreased rate of hypertension.

Natural Aging: The Muscular System

Sarcopenia, or the loss of lean muscle mass, is one of the major contributors to the loss of independence in the aging population. This is because large decrements in muscle mass will lead to an increased risk of injury. As with the heart, skeletal muscles will lose cells as they age, as well as exhibiting increased stiffness and a reduced size of the muscle fibers, beginning around the age of 50. These changes result in a decrease in muscle mass, which in turn produces an equal or greater decline in muscle strength and power. In the sedentary population, this loss of lean muscle mass is approximately 15% per decade between the ages of 50 and 70. After 70, this loss reaches approximately 30% per decade. The clinical impression is that these changes are the result of compositional changes of the muscle as research has shown an increased fat infiltration in the muscle of the aging sedentary population. However, recent studies of masters athletes have discovered that this is not the case.

Masters Athletes: The Muscular System

A study of masters weight lifters revealed a muscle deterioration rate of 1.0% to 1.5% per year. Additional studies determined that an 85-year-old weight lifter is as powerful as an inactive 65-year-old. This indicates that competitive performance throughout the later life stages is still feasible and that maintaining an increased level of physical activity in late life is imperative for healthy aging. Furthermore, analysis of anaerobic muscle performance indicated that age-related rates of decline in women exceed those of men but only in events requiring explosive power. It is in these events that we witness the largest rates of decline for both sexes. To contest the paradigm that muscle undergoes many age-related composition changes, Wright and colleagues are currently conducting a study that investigates the role of chronic high-level exercise in preventing the loss of lean muscle mass and strength. Preliminary findings support the observation that fat infiltration did not increase with age and that total muscle area and quadriceps strength did not decline with age. This offers further support that by maintaining muscle mass and strength, masters athletes are able to stave off falls, functional decline, osteoporosis, or other factors that lead to the loss of functional independence.

Natural Aging: The Skeletal System

The loss of bone mineral density (BMD) associated with aging is another major contributor to the loss of independence in the senior population. Decreases in BMD can lead to osteoporosis, subjecting the individual to an increased risk of fracture. Risk factors for osteoporosis include decreased calcium intake, low levels of active exercise, smoking, and low levels of testosterone in men. The loss of bone mass is a major problem for both men and women over the age of 40. Women lose bone mass twice as fast as men, at a rate of 1.5% to 2% per year. This rate reaches 3% per year postmenopause.

Masters Athletes: The Skeletal System

When comparing whole-body BMD values of masters athletes and sedentary adults, the athlete group exhibited significantly larger values of BMD. In a study of masters athletes participating in the 2005 National Senior Games, it was found that the majority of the women had more normal bone density than weak bone density, even those who were more than 80 years old. The incidence of osteoporosis among this group of woman masters athletes was less than in the general population at any age. In other studies, a 0.8% increase in hip BMD was associated with each hour-per-week difference of high-level exercise in women. These increases were most prominent among premenopausal women. A study of femoral neck, spine, and whole-body BMD in men over 65 years of age determined that bioavailable testosterone, physical activity level, and body mass index (BMI) all contributed to the variance of BMD values at the femoral neck. Independent analysis of these three variables revealed that bioavailable testosterone accounted for 20.7% of this variance, physical activity for 9.0%, and BMI for 6.5%. Bouts of high-intensity resistance training resulted in sharp increases in testosterone levels in middle-aged and older men, which may further alleviate decreases in BMD. All this demonstrates that BMD may be maintained in the aging population through high levels of chronic exercise.

Natural Aging: Cartilage and Tendon

Both cartilage and tendon can deteriorate through atrophy or overuse. Maintaining these tissues is of primary concern for the aging population. Tendinitis is a painful inflammation of the tendon that is quite common in athletes over 40. This condition develops as the tendon experiences repetitive microtears through excessive movements or inadequate stretching prior to physical activity. The lack of stretching causes the fibers of the tendon to gradually become shorter. Tendinitis is most commonly seen in the elbow, wrist, biceps, shoulder, leg, knee, and Achilles. Ultimately, it occurs in the areas of the body that the individual uses most. Healthy cartilage can deteriorate by softening or fissuring. High-impact activities have been shown to exacerbate this wear of deteriorated cartilage. Fortunately, this is not always the case.

Masters Athletes: Cartilage and Tendon

These conditions can be easily avoided with smart training methods, such as a proper warm-up and stretching prior to strenuous physical activity. The best way to protect cartilage and tendon is to adequately address issues such as pain and fatigue as they arise. Ignoring symptoms such as pain or weakness will only subject cartilage and tendon to further abuse. Rest and moderation of training activities are imperative to protect the health of the body's cartilage. If masters athletes adopt the right training methods, they will obtain the most favorable results. For example, a study of healthy middle-aged women athletes revealed that participation in exercise that produced an increased pulse rate for a minimum of 20 minutes was positively associated with the volume of medial tibial cartilage. None of the women in this study exhibited knee cartilage deficits as a result of this activity.

Additional Benefits of Active Aging

While chronic exercise is a known preventer and antidote to many of the problems that plague the sedentary aging population, there exist additional benefits that exercise brings to the aging population that are not often discussed in the literature.

Cancer

Recent research suggests that exercise can not only prevent cancer but also significantly reduce the risk of cancer-specific mortality in individuals who increase their levels of exercise postdiagnosis, specifically in breast and colorectal cancer. Adjusting for age at diagnosis, stage of the disease, state of residence, interval between diagnosis and physical activity assessment, BMI, menopausal status, hormone therapy, energy intake, education, family history, and treatment modality, researchers discovered that women who regularly participated in high levels of physical activity had a significantly greater chance of surviving breast cancer. Reduced mortality rates were also witnessed in women with Stages I to III colorectal cancer who participated in at least 18 metabolic-equivalent task hours of physical activity per week. Further research is necessary to evaluate this trend as related to other cancers as well as the precise amount of exercise necessary to obtain these benefits.

Cognitive Function

While many studies have investigated the benefits of active exercise for one's physical health, the benefits specific to cognitive function have received little recognition in comparison. This is staggering since declines in cognitive function have become one of the major contributors to the loss of independence in the aging population. Recent studies indicate that regular exercise can reduce reaction time and increase serum levels of testosterone and growth hormone in elderly men. These hormones are believed to exhibit a protective effect on the risk of dementia and Alzheimer disease. Associations between these diseases and low levels of physical activity were more distinct among carriers of particular genotypes. However, chronic exercise at midlife and beyond suggests an ability to delay the onset of dementia and Alzheimer disease despite genetic susceptibility. At present, Wright and colleagues are investigating the effects of chronic high-intensity exercise on specific areas of thought processing ability: working memory, sustained and selective attention time, response variability, nonverbal problem solving, and reaction time.

Depression

Depression is a common condition in the later life stages. Studies have shown that depression is most likely to emerge when an individual transitions from an active to a sedentary lifestyle. It is associated with the largest decrease in duration of physical activity. When mobility status was assessed, individuals who were able to maintain high levels of mobility throughout the aging process exhibited fewer depressive symptoms despite their decline in overall physical activity.

Diabetes

In recent years, Type 2 diabetes has emerged as one of the most rapidly growing public health concerns worldwide. It is well known that obesity, diet, and levels of physical activity combine with genetic factors to increase the risk of developing Type 2 diabetes. While all these factors contribute independently, obesity has been shown to be the largest contributor to the onset of the disease. Those with diabetes or at highest risk of developing the disease engage in rates of physical activity that are significantly below the national average, as determined by a nationally representative survey of the U.S. population conducted by the Medical Expenditure Panel Survey. Although genetics is an important contributing factor, it is important to note that it is only part of the problem and must usually be coupled with unhealthy lifestyle choices for the disorder to develop.

Stroke

Studies on the preventive benefits of physical activity for stroke revealed that increased activity levels are associated with a reduction in stroke mortality. Test subjects were assessed by self-reports of occupational and leisure activities. In addition, moderate levels of exercise exhibited benefits among individuals already diagnosed with heart conditions such as left ventricular hypertrophy.

It is of paramount importance for the senior population to maintain increased levels of physical activity if they wish to remain functionally independent throughout midlife and beyond. While there exist many age-related changes that we cannot avoid, exercise is a known preventer and antidote to the ravages of age-related disease. People everywhere are starting to realize these benefits as the number of individuals above 50 participating in high-level sports continues to increase. Records of the New York City Marathon from 1983 to 1999 reveal that the number of runners over the age of 50 is increasing more rapidly than is the number of any other age-group. In addition, the race times of the masters athlete group are demonstrating significantly greater improvement compared with the younger runners.

While injuries do occur within this masters athletes group, this is primarily because the athletes do not change their training regimens to accommodate the physiologic changes their bodies are experiencing. To avoid these changes and still participate in chronic high-level exercise, these athletes must FACE their future. FACE is an acronym for the four components of fitness after 40 that are essential to maximizing performance and training effectively:

F—Flexibility

A—Aerobic exercise

C—"Carry a load," or resistance training

E—Equilibrium and balance

Creating a balanced workout that touches on these cornerstones of physical fitness is a smart way to achieve one's fitness goals. FACE applies not only to competitive athletes but also to people of all ages and activity levels. Those who adopt an exercise regimen that embodies all these components will be able to reduce the slowing phenomenon that is so often thought to accompany life after 40.

Future efforts should focus on raising awareness about the benefits of active aging and preserving the longevity of masters athletes. This way, more individuals will be able to enjoy functional independence and the benefits of a healthy lifestyle into their later years. This is becoming increasingly more important each day as the baby boomer generation is now in their 60s and is starting to transition to the age of senior citizens. Therefore, time is running out for physicians to intervene and encourage the sedentary individuals within this group to start exercising before they reach the age of reduced functional capacity.

Andrew Wroblewski and Vonda Wright

See also Arthritis; Benefits of Exercise and Sports; Shoulder Arthritis

Further Readings

Ari Z, Kutlu N, Uyanik BS, Taneli F, Buyukuazi G, Tavli T. Serum testosterone, growth hormone, and insulin-like growth factor-1 levels, mental reaction time, and maximal aerobic exercise in sedentary and long-term physically trained elderly males. *Int J Neurosci.* 2004;114(5):623–637.

Bortz WM 4th, Bortz WM 2nd. How fast do we age? Exercise performance over time as a biomarker. *J Gerontol A Biol Sci Med Sci.* 1996;51(5): M223–M225.

Chen AL, Mears SC, Hawkins RJ. Orthopaedic care of the aging athlete. *J Am Acad Orthop Surg.* 2005;13(6):407–416.

Goodpaster BH, Park SW, Harris TB, et al. The loss of skeletal muscle strength, mass, and quality in older adults: the health, aging and body composition study. *J Gerontol A Biol Sci Med Sci.* 2006;61(10): 1059–1064.

Hanna F, Teichtahl AJ, Bell R, et al. The cross-sectional relationship between fortnightly exercise and knee cartilage properties in healthy adult women in midlife. *Menopause.* 2007;14(5):830–834.

Hassan BS, Mockett S, Doherty M. Static postural sway, proprioception, and maximal voluntary quadriceps contraction in patients with knee osteoarthritis and normal control subjects. *Ann Rheum Dis.* 2001;60(6):612–618.

Hernelahti M, Kujala UM, Kaprio J, Karjalainen J, Sarna S. Hypertension in master endurance athletes. *J Hypertens.* 1998;16(11):1573–1577.

Holick CN, Newcomb PA, Trentham-Dietz A, et al. Physical activity and survival after diagnosis of invasive breast cancer. *Cancer Epidemiol Biomarkers Prev.* 2008;17(2):379–386.

Lampinen P, Heikkinen E. Reduced mobility and physical activity as predictors of depressive symptoms among community-dwelling older adults: an eight-year follow-up study. *Aging Clin Exp Res.* 2003;15(3):205–211.

MacInnis RJ, Cassar C, Nowson CA, et al. Determinants of bone density in 30- to 65-year-old women: a co-twin study. *J Bone Miner Res.* 2003;18(9):1650–1656.

Mengelkoch LJ, Pollock ML, Limacher MC, et al. Effects of age, physical training, and physical fitness on coronary heart disease risk factors in older track athletes at twenty-year follow-up. *J Am Geriatr Soc.* 1997;45(12):1446–1453.

Meyerhardt JA, Giovannucci EL, Holmes MD, et al. Physical activity and survival after colorectal cancer diagnosis. *J Clin Oncol.* 2006;24(22):3527–3534.

Pitsavos C, Panagiotakos DB, Chrysohoou C, et al. Physical activity decreases the risk of stroke in middle-age men with left ventricular hypertrophy: 40-year follow-up (1961–2001) of the Seven Countries Study (the Corfu cohort). *J Hum Hypertens.* 2004;18(7):495–501.

Podewils LJ, Guallar E, Kuller LH, et al. Physical activity, APOE genotype, and dementia risk: findings from the Cardiovascular Health Cognition Study. *Am J Epidemiol.* 2005;161(7):639–651.

Pugh KG, Wei JY. Clinical implications of physiological changes in the aging heart. *Drugs Aging.* 2001;18(4): 263–276.

Rana JS, Li TY, Manson JE, Hu FB. Adiposity compared with physical inactivity and risk of type 2 diabetes in women. *Diabetes Care.* 2007;30(1):53–58.

Savelberg HH, Verdijk LB, Willems PJ, Meijer K. The robustness of age-related gait adaptations: can running counterbalance the consequences of ageing? *Gait Posture.* 2007;25(2):259–266.

van Gool CH, Kempen GI, Penninx BW, Deeg DJ, Beekman AT, van Eijk JT. Relationship between changes in depressive symptoms and unhealthy lifestyles in late middle aged and older persons: results from the Longitudinal Aging Study Amsterdam. *Age Ageing.* 2003;32(1):81–87.

Wright V, Winter R. *Fitness After 40: How to Stay Strong at Any Age.* New York, NY: AMACOM; 2009.

Wright VJ, Perricelli BC. Age-related rates of decline in performance among elite senior athletes. *Am J Sports Med.* 2008;36(3):443–450.

SESAMOIDITIS

The sesamoid bones of the foot were named because of their resemblance to sesame seeds. Unlike most bones, which are connected to each other through muscles and tendons, the two small sesamoid bones are found embedded in the muscle/tendon of the flexor hallucis longus muscle. Injury to these bones often occurs when great stresses are placed on the foot, such as in running and ballet dancing.

Anatomy

The flexor hallucis longus muscle is found on the undersurface (plantar surface) of the foot. It is responsible for flexing the great toe and is important in weight bearing and in transmitting forces through the foot, especially during push-off. The sesamoid bones act as a pulley for the muscle and, as such, allow much greater forces to be transmitted; a similar functional phenomenon elsewhere in the body is the kneecap (patella), which is also a sesamoid bone. The sesamoids also cushion and protect the joint where the big toe meets the foot (first metatarsalphalangeal joint).

Causes

Injury to the sesamoid bone/hallucis complex can occur as the result of a direct, acute injury or in a more chronic fashion, as in overuse or repetitive injuries. Either of the two sesamoid bones can be injured, but the medial sesamoid (closer to the inside of the foot or tibial side) is more commonly involved.

Fracture

Fracture of a sesamoid bone can occur as the result of a direct blow or forced hyperdorsiflexion (bending of the toe upward); alternatively, it can result from cumulative repetitive injury. A fracture results in immediate pain over the ball of the foot in the area underneath the great toe. There may or may not be swelling and bruising, and it may be difficult to bend or straighten the toe. Attempts at maintaining a normal gait will cause pain in this area of injury.

Stress Fracture and Sesamoiditis

Not uncommonly, however, pain develops gradually in the same area and may be the result of a stress fracture or sesamoiditis. A stress fracture results from repetitive injury, often during a period of more intense or frequent training. In a stress fracture, the repetitive, frequent microtrauma to the bone overwhelms the bone's ability to heal itself. It occurs more frequently in ballet dancers and long-distance runners, for whom frequent, forceful toe-offs are necessary. Additionally, football players are at risk, especially when playing on artificial surfaces.

In a similar manner, irritation and inflammation of the bone and surrounding soft tissue structures—the muscle, tendon, and bursa, collectively called the sesamoid complex—can occur. This condition is called *sesamoiditis* (Figure 1).

Diagnosis

History and Exam

Evaluation of this type of injury can be performed by a health care provider comfortable with disorders in the foot and ankle. The patient's main complaint is pain under the first metatarsalphalangeal joint (the "ball of the foot"), which worsens with weight-bearing activity and is somewhat relieved with getting off the injured foot. A thorough history is often the key to diagnosis, especially in chronic injuries. In addition to the location and character of the pain, important clues on history include any changes in training (frequency, intensity, duration) and in the footwear and surface used by the athlete.

Examination of course focuses on the area of the sesamoid bone but should include a complete

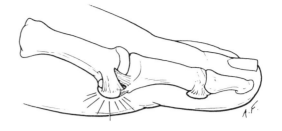

Figure 1   Sesamoiditis

Note: Sesamoiditis usually affects one or both of the sesamoid bones that lie within the tendon at the first metatarsalphalangeal joint.

exam of the foot, ankle, and gait (if pain allows) to search for predisposing factors. Pain is often elicited in bending and straightening the toe, particularly bending the great toe upward. Tenderness is prominent in the area of the sesamoid bones.

Imaging

With acute and chronic injuries, X-rays can be helpful in making the diagnosis. Interestingly, the medial sesamoid is composed of two parts (bipartite) in about 11% of the population, and this sometimes makes the diagnosis of an acute fracture difficult. X-rays of the other foot are sometimes then done for comparison, or additional imaging may be necessary.

Management

Nonsurgical

Initial management of injuries generally includes activity and weight-bearing modification, in addition to relative rest, ice, and nonsteroidal anti-inflammatory medications such as ibuprofen. Treatment of an acute fracture may require immobilization and non–weight bearing for 3 to 4 weeks or longer, followed by the use of orthotics for the shoe and a slow, gradual return to activity.

A stress fracture may also require casting for a short period of time, but chronic injuries, including sesamoiditis and some stress fractures, are best treated by eliminating the repetitive stress that caused the injury. This may involve a period of rest from the aggravating activity and modification of the shoe with orthotics and inserts. These are designed to remove the stress from the sesamoid complex and may be a gel insert or J-shaped pads. A stiffer-soled shoe may also be helpful. Activities often need to be modified for at least 6 to 8 weeks. If painfree by 6 to 8 weeks, the athlete may then begin a gradual return to activity. It may take 3 to 6 months for symptoms to completely resolve in some cases of acute or chronic injury. Patients should continue to wear appropriate orthotics during this time and resume activity as tolerated.

In sesamoiditis, a diagnostic and therapeutic corticosteroid injection of the sesamoid complex may be beneficial, in addition to the previously mentioned management.

Surgical

If there is no improvement after 6 months, surgery may be considered to improve comfort and function. Surgery may be discussed as an earlier option for a highly competitive athlete who desires a chance to return to competition sooner.

If an acute fracture has not healed properly (nonunion), then curettage and grafting of the bone may be attempted. Pinning with screws may also be an option. If these are not viable options, or are unsuccessful, it may be necessary to remove the bone.

Excision of a sesamoid bone may also be indicated in refractory cases of sesamoiditis or a stress fracture. It is important for the surgeon to identify which sesamoid bone (medial or lateral) is the troublesome one as removal of both bones has often been found to result in a significant deformity of the joint connecting the great toe to the foot.

Postoperatively, the patient can expect to be in a non–weight bearing cast for at least several weeks. After this, weight bearing may begin gradually, with a total casting time of approximately 6 weeks. Once the cast is removed, additional orthotics for a longer period of time may be necessary as the patient progresses back to activity.

Eugene S. Hong and Kathleen O'Brien

See also Foot and Ankle Injuries, Surgery for; Foot Injuries; Orthotics; Podiatric Sports Medicines

Further Readings

Cohen BE. Hallux sesamoid disorders. *Foot Ankle Clin.* 2009;14(1):91–104.

Goulart M, O'Malley MJ, Hodgkins CW, Charlton TP. Foot and ankle fractures in dancers. *Clin Sports Med.* 2008;27(2):295–304.

Prisk VR, O'Loughlin PF, Kennedy JG. Forefoot injuries in dancers. *Clin Sports Med.* 2008;27(2):305–320.

Vanore JV. Diagnosis and treatment of first metatarsalphalangeal disorders. *J Foot Ankle Surg.* 2003;42(3):143–147.

Young CC. Clinical examination of the foot and ankle. *Prim Care.* 2005;32(1):105–132.

SEVER DISEASE

Sever disease, also known as *calcaneal apophysitis*, was first described in the early 1900s. The calcaneal apophysis is a cartilaginous growth center located in the heel of the foot. Calcaneal apophysitis is a common cause of heel pain in growing, athletically active youth. Originally described as an inflammatory process, it has more recently been thought to result from overuse and weight-bearing injury to the growth center.

Anatomy

For descriptive purposes, the foot is divided into three areas: forefoot, midfoot, and hindfoot. The hindfoot contains two bones, the talus and the calcaneus. The calcaneus contains a vertically oriented C-shaped growth center located in the back of the heel. The growth center appears around age 5 to 9 and usually closes by age 13 to 16, when the calcaneus has achieved its mature adult shape. An additional cartilaginous growth center, the calcaneal ("traction") apophysis, is located where the Achilles tendon attaches to the bone.

Causes

Sever disease was originally described as an inflammatory process occurring within the calcaneal apophysis. Another proposed etiology was disruption of the blood supply to the growth center. Now, Sever disease is believed to be the result of repetitive mechanical stress applied to the apophysis by a tight heel cord (Achilles tendon) in an overactive young athlete.

This repetitive impact and shear stress on the growth center leads to microtrauma and injury at the junction of the bone and cartilage. This may occur during periods of rapid growth, such as a growth spurt, when the calf muscles and tendons cannot lengthen as quickly as long bones such as the tibia. An increased amount of athletic participation, including longer-duration, higher-intensity, and increased frequency of activities, contributes to the repetitive loading of the heel with weight-bearing activity. Sever disease does not occur after puberty, once the cartilage growth center fuses to become bone.

Symptoms

Sever disease is most common in active children 8 to 12 years old. It is slightly more predominant in boys. It presents with intermittent or daily heel pain and occurs on both feet in more than 50% of children. There is usually no history of an acute fall or direct injury to the heel. The child may describe the pain as located over the heel, and it may be severe enough to cause a limp, especially after participating in physical activity. While the pain may be present at rest or with daily activities such as walking, it is generally made worse with weight-bearing activities, such as running and jumping in sports activities. While all sports can make the symptoms of Sever disease worse, sports such as soccer, basketball, and running are common culprits. Heel pain may present at the beginning of a sports season or when the child is experiencing a growth spurt. The pain is usually absent in the morning, increases with activity during the day, and decreases with rest. Hard surfaces, such as a basketball court, or athletic shoes with little support and cushioning, such as soccer cleats, may worsen the symptoms.

Diagnosis

On physical examination, the most common finding is pain with compression of the inside and outside of the heel (the "squeeze test"). There should be no swelling, redness, or other skin or bone abnormalities. Usually, the gait is normal, but the child may walk with a limp. Many children also have a decreased flexibility or tightness of their calf muscles, resulting in limited dorsiflexion, the ability to pull or stretch a foot toward the head. The strength of the calf muscles is normal. Foot abnormalities such as pronation and flat feet may be present and worsen the condition. The child should otherwise be healthy, with no night pain or other signs or symptoms of systemic disease.

Plain radiographs are not routinely obtained because there are no findings that are diagnostic or specific for Sever disease. Findings such as irregularity of the growth center are often present on radiographs of asymptomatic feet. If the pain is unusual in character, other systemic symptoms are present, or the pain persists despite adequate rest and treatment, then plain radiographs may be considered to rule out other causes.

Treatment

The mainstay of treatment involves nonsurgical therapies. The most important treatment principle is to discontinue the repetitive activities that are causing the heel pain. This means completely avoiding or significantly limiting impact sports activities that involve running and jumping for some period of time.

The use of soft heel cups or heel lifts may help cushion and relieve the tension on the heel. Children should wear good-quality athletic shoes with an adequate shock-absorbent sole and avoid going barefoot at all times. Therapeutic exercises, such as stretching and strengthening of the calf muscles, may be prescribed under the supervision of a physical therapist.

As Sever disease is not an inflammatory process, anti-inflammatory medications are not indicated to decrease inflammation. Application of ice and the use of medications such as acetaminophen or ibuprofen may be helpful in reducing pain. Corticosteroid injections are not recommended. In rare cases, when the pain is severe and accompanied by a limp, crutches or immobilization may be used for a short period of time.

The majority of children are painfree and able to return to the desired physical activities within weeks to 2 months of proper treatment. A return to sports and physical activity is appropriate when the child can participate with minimal discomfort. Continued stretching, especially during growth spurts, may prevent initial or recurrent Sever disease. There are no known long-term sequelae of Sever disease.

M. Alison Brooks

See also Apophysitis; Foot Injuries; Osgood-Schlatter Disease; Sports Injuries, Overuse

Further Readings

Adirim TA, Cheng TL. Overview of injuries in the young athlete. Sports Med. 2003;33(1):75–81.

Ishikawa SN. Conditions of the calcaneus in skeletally immature patients. Foot Ankle Clin. 2005;10(3): 503–513.

Madden CC, Mellion MB. Sever's disease and other causes of heel pain in adolescents. Am Fam Physician. 1996;54(6):1995–2000.

Micheli LJ, Fehlandt AF Jr. Overuse injuries to tendons and apophyses in children and adolescents. Clin Sports Med. 1992;11(4):713–726.

Micheli LJ, Ireland ML. Prevention and management of calcaneal apophysitis in children: an overuse syndrome. J Pediatr Orthop. 1987;7(1):34–38.

Volpon JB, de Carvalho Filho G. Calcaneal apophysitis: a quantitative radiographic evaluation of the secondary ossification center. Arch Orthop Trauma Surg. 2002;122(6):338–341.

SHIFT WORK AND EXERCISE

Approximately 3.6 million people in the United Kingdom work mostly on shifts, representing 14% of the British workforce. This proportion is similar in most other developed countries. Shift workers predominate in heavy industries and emergency services, but they are also increasingly found in finance and service industries. Data from epidemiological studies suggest that shift work, and especially night work, is associated with insomnia, gastrointestinal problems, obesity, heart disease, and cancer. Disruption of circadian rhythms during shift work is thought to be important in explaining these increased health problems. Nevertheless, the differences between shift workers and day workers in lifestyle factors, including participation in physical activities, have been generally underresearched.

On a behavioral level, shift work can restrict the opportunities to be physically active, although this can depend on individual choice of leisure pursuit (group or individual based). On a biological level, the disruptions to circadian rhythms and sleep that are associated with shift work can alter the normal physiological responses to a bout of physical activity as well as how well a particular exercise bout is tolerated. The latter issue might have implications for long-term adherence to physical activity regimens during shift work. Unfortunately, studies in which physical activity interventions are administered to shift workers are rare.

Physical Activity Behaviors During Shift Work

Workers and their families can alter their habits to cope with the disruption to domestic life that is associated with shift work, although women shift workers seem to have particular problems in balancing their work and domestic lives. Unlike the malleable domestic environment, organized leisure activities and training sessions for sports clubs are generally scheduled in the early evening and weekends to accommodate the day-working majority. This scheduling conflict makes it very difficult for the shift worker to participate in organized activities and has been found to contribute to the decision of some people to leave shift work altogether. Those shift workers who enjoy solitary or individual activities are probably not so disadvantaged. Individual shift workers who join fitness and health clubs can enjoy the benefits of "off-peak" membership costs and can use the facilities at less crowded times. Activities such as cycling, swimming, and jogging can also be carried out on an individual basis in the shift worker's own spare time. Nevertheless, organized competitions in these sports are still normally scheduled in the weekend, when it is more likely that a shift worker is at work. Moreover, the transient negative experiences of exercising while partially deprived of sleep and at times that are out of kilter with the "body clock" (e.g., in the early morning) might be perceived to be significant enough for the shift worker to stop these individual activities. Such attrition at an early stage in an exercise program would be unfortunate since there are, as discussed below, likely benefits of exercise to the shift worker.

Benefits of Physical Activity to the Shift Worker

Physical activity, when timed appropriately, may consolidate human circadian rhythms. Although purely correlational in nature, there is evidence that good tolerance to rapidly rotating shift work is associated with large amplitudes (mean-to-peak differences) of circadian rhythms, which tend to be observed more in physically active and fitter individuals than in sedentary people. Nevertheless, it may well be that those people who are naturally more tolerant of shift work are able to be more physically active, rather than vice versa. This "chicken or the egg" conundrum is common in many descriptive studies on shift work. There is no direct evidence to suggest that any unique circadian characteristics of physically fit shift workers mediate fewer short-term tolerance problems and better health compared with less fit workers.

It is known that habitual bouts of physical activity increase both the duration and the quality of nocturnal sleep in diurnally active people. The amount of slow-wave sleep (SWS), which is thought to be important for brain restoration and recovery during nocturnal sleep, is also increased by physical activity. It is possible that physical activity is beneficial via a reduction of anxiety, a sleep-inducing thermogenic effect, or long-term antidepressant effects or by mediating a circadian phase that is more amenable for sleep. Increases in sleep quality following exercise may be mediated by temperature elevation, which, in turn, increases SWS. Chronic physical activity promotes the sleep-onset process by inducing more proficient temperature downregulation. In a recent study on the effects of exercise on daytime sleep during partial sleep deprivation, it was found that sleep latency (the time it takes to enter sleep after retiring to bed) and wrist activity were reduced by exercise taken 4 hours prior to the sleep period, offering support that the favorable effects of physical activity on sleep quality translate to a shift work context. Nevertheless, shift workers who are motivated enough to exercise might attempt to exercise closer than 4 hours to a given sleep period or even at night. The exact consequences of these unusual timings of exercise bouts relative to the unusual timings of sleep periods are not known. Recently, it was found that there are no negative effects of exercise when taken close (within 2 hours) to the start of a sleep period, although this sleep period was taken at night by people living diurnally.

The temporal placement of physical activity may also affect the adjustment to shift or night work via advancing or delaying an individual's circadian rhythms. If circadian rhythms can be adjusted to times more amenable to the particular shift that is being worked, it is possible that feelings of fatigue, tiredness, sleepiness, and other short-term effects of working unusual hours can be attenuated. These improvements in shorter-term tolerance might, in turn, make exercise more tolerable to the shift worker and so aid the maintenance of participation in physical activity regimens. Nocturnal exercise can induce phase delays in the onset of melatonin secretion, but exercise-induced phase advances have not been confirmed in humans. At best, the phase-shifting effects of exercise on the body temperature rhythm are very small, and the substantial levels of activity (possibly 3 hours of exercise at 50% to 60% of maximal oxygen uptake) needed to obtain these small phase shifts are impracticable and may even be unattainable by the majority of shift workers.

Physical Activity Interventions During Shift Work

It has been speculated that improved workplace-based recreational facilities, to promote physical activity, might be useful for general tolerance to shift work. Nevertheless, there is little empirical support for such views. To date, there has been only one study in which a physical training intervention was administered specifically to shift workers. Mikko Härmä, and his colleagues in Finland, designed a training program for 119 women shift workers. Exercise sessions were administered between two and six times per week, between 60% and 70% of maximal heart rate, and for a 4-month period. It was found that this moderate physical training mostly benefited aspects of sleep. General fatigue decreased significantly in the training group during the whole cycle of rotating shift work, and scores on some tests of performance improved. The authors suggested that moderate exercise should be performed several hours before the main sleep period when on a morning or day shift schedule. Physical activity was advised before an evening nap, during a period of night work, although the researchers did not investigate the specific issues about the timing of the exercise.

Although there are predicted benefits of physical activity for the shift worker, there is evidence that the majority of shift workers do not follow the general guidelines to take more exercise. Whether this is due to the disruptive nature of shift work, feelings that an unhealthy lifestyle is acceptable providing that shift work continues to pay well, or the general reluctance to adopt a healthy lifestyle is, at present, unclear.

Greg Atkinson

Author's Note: The author's research work on shift work and health is currently funded by the National Prevention Research Initiative: http://www.npri.org.uk.

See also Seasonal Rhythms and Exercise; Sleep and Exercise; Sleep Loss, Effects on Athletic Performance

Further Readings

Atkinson G, Edwards B, Reilly T, Waterhouse J. Exercise as a synchroniser of human circadian rhythms: an update and discussion of the methodological problems. *Eur J Appl Physiol.* 2007;99(4):331–341.

Atkinson G, Fullick S, Grindey C, Maclaren D. Exercise, energy balance and the shift worker. *Sports Med.* 2008;38(8):671–685.

Costa G. Shift work and occupational medicine: an overview. *Occup Med (Lond).* 2003;53(2):83–88.

Härmä M. Ageing, physical fitness and shift work tolerance. *Appl Ergon.* 1996;27:25–29.

Harrington JM. Health effects of shift work and extended hours of work. *Occup Environ Med.* 2001;58:68–72.

Shoulder Arthritis

Glenohumeral arthritis, or shoulder arthritis, is a rare but potentially debilitating condition in the young athlete. A number of treatment options are available, depending on the etiology of the condition, the extent of joint damage, and the functional deficit present.

Etiology

Degenerative arthritis can be classified as either primary, implying an unknown causative agent, or secondary, in which the underlying pathological mechanism has been established. Primary osteoarthritis is primarily an age-related disorder associated with repetitive stress on a normal joint. Athletes most at risk include those engaged in repetitive overhead activities, such as in cricket, baseball, weight lifting, and racquet sports. In contrast, secondary arthritis, which is more common in the younger athlete, usually has an underlying cause, such as a previous shoulder surgery, trauma, infection, ischemia, or inflammation. Capsulorrhaphy arthropathy can occur if the anterior shoulder capsule has been excessively tightened during stabilization surgery, thereby limiting movement, principally external rotation. Posterior translation during external rotation results in posterior glenoid erosion and capsular damage. Osteonecrosis (avascular necrosis) may be traumatic or atraumatic in origin. In traumatic cases, there is usually disruption of the vascular supply to the humeral head following a proximal humeral fracture. Atraumatic osteonecrosis may be idiopathic or secondary, resulting from smoking, steroid and alcohol use, or hematological disorders (sickle cell anemia and thalassemia). The patients are normally younger and may present with few diagnostic indicators besides pain. Inflammatory arthritides such as gout, systemic lupus erythematosus (SLE), psoriatic arthritis, and ankylosing spondylitis, though less common in athletes, form the second largest category of glenohumeral arthritis. In these conditions, multiple joints may be involved. Clinical findings of cervical spine pathology, the presence of a cuff tear, or bilateral glenohumeral involvement should prompt further hematological investigation. Glenohumeral septic arthritis is uncommon except in immunocompromised individuals. Localized erythema and warmth are highly suggestive of infection, and if confirmed by aspiration, urgent arthroscopic irrigation and debridement is required.

Assessment of the Arthritic Shoulder

A patient with glenohumeral arthritis usually presents with a history of progressive pain and stiffness. The pain commonly intensifies with use and interferes with sleep, especially when lying on one side. There may be crepitus on glenohumeral movement and an inability to perform tasks requiring shoulder rotation. Specific consideration must be given to symptoms and signs suggesting the possible underlying etiology. Initial examination of the shoulder should include inspection of the upper torso for signs of muscle atrophy and asymmetry. Careful assessment of the cervical spine is mandatory to identify sources of referred pain. The active and passive ranges of shoulder motion must be recorded. Examination usually reveals pain with a restricted range of movement, often accompanied by crepitus. Limited external rotation is a common finding in osteoarthritis and may require adjunctive therapy. The integrity and strength of the rotator cuff muscles should be assessed as this may influence the choice of treatment offered. This may, however, be difficult due to pain. Unlike in rheumatoid arthritis, most patients with osteoarthritis have preserved or only slightly diminished strength, indicating only mild, if any, rotator cuff dysfunction. It is also important during the assessment process to ascertain the nature of the sport played by the athlete, hand dominance, level of performance, and intention to return to competition.

Imaging the Arthritic Shoulder

The three preferred radiographic projections of the glenohumeral joint are a true anteroposterior view, a scapular outlet view, and an axillary view. The radiographic features of glenohumeral osteoarthritis typically include joint space narrowing, osteophyte formation, subchondral sclerosis, and cyst formation. Further imaging modalities are not always necessary, but computed tomography (CT) may be a useful aid in preoperative planning to assess the patient's bone stock and glenoid version. Magnetic resonance imaging (MRI) may be indicated when there is clinical suspicion of a rotator cuff tear, which may influence future management: For example, a major tear may rule out total shoulder replacement.

Conservative Treatment

There is wide variability in the presentation of degenerative glenohumeral disease. Significant destructive radiographic changes may be present, but an individual may continue to function well if his or her demands are low. On the other hand, individuals with limited radiographic findings may find themselves substantially incapacitated by pain. Given this inconsistency, the success of nonoperative therapy cannot be based on radiological findings but rather must be based on the patient's own views of his or her functional capabilities. Recognizing that the most common arthritides are progressive in nature, conservative management should be based on maintenance of function as well as improvement. The principles of conservative management in glenohumeral osteoarthritis include: (a) activity modification, (b) medication for pain relief, and (c) a self-conducted physiotherapy program. Activity modification requires a commonsense approach, whereby the patient limits symptom-provoking activity. Activities such as racquet sports should be discouraged unless they are tolerable to the patient. This may seem a simple request; however, with such a large emphasis on continued participation in sports, many athletes are unwilling to forego playing despite the pain. The success of drug therapy in treating osteoarthritis is variable. Nonsteroidal anti-inflammatory drugs (NSAIDs) are often given to relieve symptomatic pain, but there is no evidence of its having any affect on disease progression. It is widely suggested that opiates should be avoided due to their potential for dependence. Omega 3 and glucosamine supplementation may be beneficial, although data regarding their efficacy are scarce despite widespread over-the-counter use. Intraarticular corticosteroid injections may provide temporary symptomatic relief in recalcitrant cases. Repeated injections are discouraged due to their catabolic effect on articular tissue and, therefore, should not be used as a mainstay of treatment. Intraarticular hyaluronan injections, although more costly, have been shown to have longer beneficial effects compared with corticosteroids, with fewer side effects. Physiotherapy typically involves gentle range-of-movement exercises to preserve and, if possible, improve joint motion, strengthen the rotator cuff muscles, and maintain glenohumeral stability.

Arthroscopic Treatment

Arthroscopic debridement may be employed to treat early glenohumeral osteoarthritis that has failed to respond to conservative management. Arthroscopy allows careful examination of the degree of cartilage damage and the integrity of the soft tissue envelope. Unstable chondral fragments and osteophytes can be removed and microfracture performed to stimulate cartilage regeneration. Associated pathology can be addressed by additional procedures such as the repair of labral/rotator cuff tears, subacromial decompression, or acromioclavicular joint resection. Arthroscopic debridement is principally a temporary treatment measure for shoulder arthritis, and its results depend greatly on the severity of the disease. It is however, a valid option for younger athletic patients, in whom more definitive procedures such as arthroplasty may be contraindicated due to the risk of component deterioration and subsequent failure.

Shoulder Arthroplasty

The principle indication for glenohumeral arthroplasty (joint replacement) is pain refractory to conservative and arthroscopic treatment. The procedure offers reliable pain relief and may result in secondary recovery of strength and function. Arthroplasty should be considered with caution in mild to moderate arthritis, in younger patients with high functional demands, and where there is a lack of glenoid bone stock or rotator cuff deficiency. It is important when counseling a patient with regard to prosthetic reconstruction that realistic expectations be set. The type of arthroplasty chosen must take into account patient factors such as age and activity levels, as well as the nature of the underlying pathological process, the pattern of joint destruction, and the integrity of the soft tissue envelope. Choices include humeral head resurfacing (total or partial), stemmed hemiarthroplasty, and total shoulder replacement (including reverse polarity). Where good bone quality remains, humeral head resurfacing using a pegged metal cap is a relatively simple technique providing a valid alternative to stemmed hemiarthroplasty, particularly in younger patients. This form of surgery is less invasive than traditional shoulder replacement and, therefore, recovery is typically much faster. Resurfacing can help prolong or avoid altogether the need for future joint replacement. It is therefore an attractive option for young athletes in whom undergoing arthroplasty at an early age carries a greater risk of future revision surgery. More normal anatomical relationships are maintained; potential errors in determining the humeral head

height, glenoid version, and implant alignment are minimized; and stem-related complications are avoided.

Glenohumeral Arthrodesis

This is a fairly crude technique involving fusion of the humeral head to the glenoid and acromion, thereby relying solely on scapulothoracic rotation to move the upper limb. It is now rarely employed as cases unsuitable for modern replacement techniques are limited. Indications include severe septic arthritis and previous failed joint reconstruction with severe bone loss. Patients undergoing this type of procedure generally have significant functional limitation.

Conclusion

In the active individual, most cases of glenohumeral arthritis should be managed using the conservative methods detailed above. Once these are exhausted, surgical treatment must be selected on a case-by-case basis, considering the individuals functional demands, type and severity of arthritis, and residual bone stock. Patients with only minor arthritic changes may benefit from arthroscopic treatment initially, whereas those with extensive damage may require total arthroplasty. In these cases, where possible, less invasive techniques such as cementless resurfacing of the glenoid should be employed. Further long-term randomized studies are required to compare cementless humeral head arthroplasty with stemmed hemiarthroplasty and total shoulder arthroplasty if a conclusion about the optimal treatment of young arthritic athletes is to be reached.

Angus Robertson and Richard O. N. Evans

See also Arthritis; Shoulder Injuries

Further Readings

Reineck JR, Krishnan SG, Burkhead WZ. Early glenohumeral arthritis in the competing athlete. *Clin Sports Med.* 2008;27(4):803–819.

Williams MD, Edwards TB. Glenohumeral arthritis in the athlete: evaluation and algorithm for management. *Oper Tech Sports Med.* 2008;16(1):2–8.

SHOULDER BURSITIS

Bursae are flattish, fluid-filled sacs lined with synovial membrane that typically lie between bone and tendons or adjacent tendons; bursa sacs provide a smooth gliding surface for tendons to move along and may lessen the irritating friction that could otherwise occur between the tendon and other structures. At baseline, the fluid in the bursa is minimal. When the bursa becomes inflamed (as indicated by the suffix "itis"), it enlarges and the fluid contents increase. There are eight bursae in the shoulder. The primary or largest bursa, the subacromial bursa, is located just under the acromion, the rounded-off bony prominence located most laterally on the shoulder. While understanding the concept of *shoulder bursitis* is useful, it may not completely describe the root cause of the problem. The inflamed bursitis condition commonly occurs due to or in response to rotator cuff tendon inflammation from poor mechanics and/or overuse. The rotator cuff muscles are anatomically directly underneath the subacromial bursa; when one structure is inflamed, the adjacent structure becomes inflamed as well (Figure 1).

Causes

When the bursa becomes inflamed, it swells up and occupies more space. In doing so, the swollen bursa can further limit the size of the space (the subacromial space) in which the rotator cuff tendon moves. In certain extremes of motion, this can cause a painful impingement phenomenon. This mechanism can lead to further irritation and pain. Rotator cuff tendinopathy may often be the underlying mechanism causing shoulder bursitis. The rotator cuff muscles, which become tendons when attached to bones, are the dynamic structures that allow for the tremendous range of motions in multi-directions that the shoulder is capable of producing. There are four muscles that make up the rotator cuff: supraspinatus, infraspinatus, teres minor, and subscapularis. The shoulder is referred to as a ball-and-socket joint—the rounded ball of the humerus fits into the shallow, saucer-like socket of the glenoid. A golf ball resting on a tee is an appropriate analogy. This great mobility of the shoulder joint does come at a price, with the

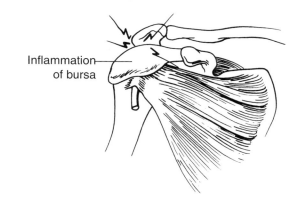

Figure 1 Inflammation of the Bursa Occurs Between the Rotator Cuff Tendons and the Shoulder Blade

shoulder joint having increased susceptibility to injury and overuse.

Clinical Evaluation

Rotator cuff problems generally occur in older populations, ages 40 to 50, who may or may not be athletically inclined. It can present either insidiously, which may or may not involve an increase in certain shoulder movement activities, or in a more acute setting after a specific injury. Any change in the intensity, frequency, or duration of an activity, be it at work or at home, as well as any new activity could contribute to developing an overuse injury. Age-related changes to tendons result in their less pliable or elastic (rubber band–like) quality; this can lead to fraying, swelling in the tendon, calcified deposits, and frank tears. Thus, as we get older, we may be more prone to overuse injuries such as rotator cuff tendinopathy and shoulder bursitis, and unfortunately, we may recover less well from them.

In the athletic population, rotator cuff tendinopathy can develop in any overhead throwing or motion sport such as baseball and softball, racquet sports such as badminton and tennis, swimming, and water polo.

Examples of activities that patients describe are a weekend playing softball or playing fetch with a dog and carrying more than the usual bags of groceries or heavy suitcases on a trip. Occasionally, they may recall a specific incident, such as a fall on an outstretched hand or a sudden jerking or traction from catching a heavy falling object. Most of the time, however, a patient cannot say how the pain started.

Most commonly, the pain affects a fairly large area, directly over the shoulder, in the posterior neck/upper back, and, not uncommonly, down the arm over the deltoid region. Rarely does shoulder bursitis pain radiate past the elbow. The pain or soreness is not only exacerbated by heavy lifting or very strenuous activities, but it can also result from simple maneuvers performed in activities of daily living. This would include reaching up into a cabinet, lifting an arm up to the head to brush or shampoo one's hair, reaching behind to slip a hand into a jacket sleeve, pulling up a pair of pants, and turning a steering wheel, to name some of the most common exacerbating actions.

One common symptom of rotator cuff tendinopathy is nighttime pain that occurs with lying on the affected arm/shoulder. It can wake a person up if he or she should unintentionally roll over to that side. Usually, the "weakness" patients may have is the result of guarding against the pain, which would reflexively limit how much load they place on the shoulder. This is in contrast to any inherent or primary loss of muscle strength, intrinsic to the muscles or nerves itself.

Management

Rehabilitation

The mainstay of treatment for rotator cuff tendinopathy/shoulder bursitis is effective physical therapy/rehabilitation. Initial exercises would involve stretching, correcting muscle imbalance and improving coordination, and eventually strengthening of the rotator cuff muscles. For athletes, an evaluation of biomechanics and the entire kinetic chain function, as well as pinpointing of training errors, should be incorporated to prevent recurrence of problems.

Medication

For pain relief, nonsteroidal anti-inflammatory drugs (NSAIDs) such as ibuprofen or naproxen are often prescribed. There is some evidence to suggest that NSAIDs may slow or harm the healing process in tendons; additionally, care must be taken to prevent gastritis/stomach ulcers. Liberal application of

ice for 15 to 20 minutes three times a day is recommended for pain control without the risk of any significant adverse effects. An option for pain control, especially pain causing significant disruption in sleep or work, is a cortisone injection. An advantage of corticosteroid injection is that pain reduction may allow the patient to participate in physical therapy more effectively. Cortisone is a powerful anti-inflammatory and can be injected directly into the affected joint or area—for example, directly into the inflamed subacromial bursa.

Imaging

For diagnostic purposes, imaging can be obtained. Although plain films or X-rays will not show bursitis or rotator cuff tendons, they are helpful to look for bony abnormalities that are indirect signs of rotator cuff problems, such as calcifications in the tendon, down-sloping or hooked acromion, and other bony processes that can cause similar symptoms such as arthritis. If more advanced imaging is desired, either because a frank and complete tear is suspected and/or the patient is not improving or the diagnostic picture is more complicated, magnetic resonance imaging (MRI) can be considered. MRI is the imaging modality of choice to directly visualize and evaluate the rotator cuff tendons. The presence of a complete tear is not an automatic indication for surgery, as many patients do quite well with a course of aggressive rehabilitation and there are people with rotator cuff tears who have good range of motion, have good strength, and are functionally asymptomatic.

Operative

Operative treatments can be considered if there is no progress, unrelenting pain, or inadequate function. Most rotator cuff tendon surgeries can be done with arthroscopy, whereby small incisions and thin pencil-like instruments are used, and most often on an outpatient basis.

Calcific Bursitis

On occasion, calcium crystals may accrue in the bursa. This "calcific bursitis" can be very painful and subject to flare-up of severe pain. Surgery is sometimes required to remove the calcified bursa.

Eugene S. Hong and Laura Anderson

Further Readings

Andrews JR. Diagnosis and treatment of chronic painful shoulder. *Arthroscopy.* 2005;21(3):333–347.

Kibler BW. Rehabilitation of the athlete's shoulder. *Clin Sports Med.* 2008;27(4):821–831.

McFarland EG. Examination of the shoulder in the overhead and throwing athlete. *Clin Sports Med.* 2008;27(4):553–578.

Meister K. Injuries to the shoulder in the throwing athlete. *Am J Sports Med.* 2000;28(4):587–601.

Woodward TW. The painful shoulder. *Am Fam Physician.* 2000;61(11):3291–3300.

SHOULDER DISLOCATION

The shoulder is the most frequently dislocated joint, and the injury is common in contact sports and activities with a potential for falling accidents, such as skiing or biking. It occurs commonly in young adults and can lead to significant disability for an athlete. Most dislocations result from trauma, and the majority (>90%) occur anteriorly.

Anatomy

The shoulder is a ball-and-socket joint. The humeral head (ball) sits in the glenoid (socket) and allows the large range of motion that humans have at the shoulder. This range of motion allows extremes of motion, such as those that an elite pitcher uses to throw the ball.

There are a number of structures that help stabilize the glenohumeral joint. First, to help the humeral head fit more snugly in the glenoid, the glenoid is surrounded by a ring of cartilage called the labrum. Second, the glenohumeral ligaments add further stability to the joint. These ligaments are thickened areas of the shoulder capsule, which encompasses the entire joint. Both the labrum and the glenohumeral ligaments can be injured when the humeral head dislocates out of the glenoid.

In addition, important arteries and nerves travel in this area and can be injured from a shoulder dislocation.

Causes

As mentioned, more than 90% of traumatic shoulder dislocations are anterior, with the head of the humerus dislocating out of the front of the glenoid. This usually occurs as the result of a fall with the arm in the abducted (held away from the body) and externally rotated position or when the arm is hit from the front when held in this same position, as can happen in a football tackle.

Less frequently (2–4%), the dislocation is posterior, with the humeral head dislocating out of the back of the joint. This usually occurs when the arm is forward elevated and internally rotated. These dislocations are less likely to occur from sports (although they can occur with the pass block in football) and are more likely the result of a motor vehicle accident, seizure, or electric shock (Figure 1).

Symptoms

The patient with an acutely dislocated shoulder is usually in a good deal of distress. He or she holds the arm slightly away from the body and in internal rotation. The patient avoids moving the joint due to the pain, and on examination, it will be found that there is little ability to rotate the shoulder.

If the patient has had previous shoulder dislocations, he or she may present without an acute dislocation but with complaints of the shoulder "popping in and out," especially when his or her arm is in the throwing position.

Diagnosis

In the acute setting, the history of the mechanism of the injury, as well as the physical exam, is usually enough to make the diagnosis. The examiner should always perform a good neurovascular exam (checking the pulses and nerve supply to the arm both in the central and peripheral distribution) as damage may have been done to important structures. The axillary nerve, which supplies the large deltoid muscle of the shoulder, is not uncommonly damaged from a shoulder dislocation. Axillary nerve integrity can be assessed by testing the sensation of the skin over the deltoid muscle on the outside of the arm.

It is also necessary to obtain X-rays to confirm the dislocation and the direction of the dislocation and to evaluate for other bony abnormalities such as fractures. Two specific fractures are commonly associated with a shoulder dislocation. A Hill-Sachs lesion is an impaction fracture of the back of the humeral head, and a bony Bankart lesion occurs when the labrum at the front of the glenoid is disrupted and pulls off a piece of bone. At least two views, and preferably three different views, of the shoulder should be obtained and are usually sufficient to make the diagnosis.

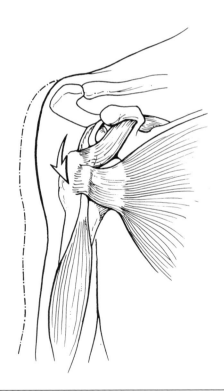

Figure 1   Shoulder Dislocation

Notes: Shoulder dislocations are relatively common because of the structure of the shoulder joint, which gives it great mobility. Unlike other joints in the body, the socket has almost no bony support, making it susceptible to injury in sports.

Management

Reduction

There are many different methods of reducing the dislocated shoulder (putting it back in place). The reduction is much easier to do if performed within a few minutes of the injury. After 15 to 30 minutes or so, muscle spasms and swelling make the reduction more difficult and painful and may necessitate patient sedation. Because of this, some providers may choose to forego X-rays (after ensuring a normal neurovascular exam) and attempt the reduction on the sidelines. This is especially true if the dislocation is a recurrence for the athlete.

Various reduction techniques can be done with the patient sitting or lying on his or her back and stomach. All methods use a countertraction force along the arm to help get the humeral head back over the glenoid rim. A simple method involves the patient lying on a table face down with the affected arm dangling off the side. A weight is tied to the arm to apply the force needed over time. Other methods involve the physician pulling gently downward on the arm while an assistant pulls upward on a sheet or towel wrapped around the patient's chest and under the armpit. As the shoulder relocates, a clunk may be felt.

Postreduction Care

After reduction, it is imperative to reassess the blood and nerve supply to the arm. X-rays should be taken to document that the reduction was successful and to assess for any bony abnormality in the setting of a first-time acute shoulder dislocation. A sling can be provided for the patient's comfort as well as to let the capsule and ligaments heal, especially if this is the first dislocation. For recurrent dislocations, the sling can be used as long as symptoms persist. The patient should be instructed in and begin early range-of-motion exercises, such as pendulum swings, to prevent shoulder stiffness and to allow a quicker return to function.

Rehabilitation after shoulder dislocation involves achieving range of motion and strengthening the muscles of the shoulder, in particular the rotator cuff and scapular stabilizers. These muscles help stabilize and support the shoulder joint.

Bracing may be used in athletes to protect them from the "at-risk" position of abduction and external rotation. There are a variety of braces on the market available to the athlete, all of which attempt to keep the arm from finding that at-risk position.

Surgery

Controversy exists regarding surgical correction of first-time dislocations. The statistics show that in young patients under the age 20, the rate of recurrence is 65% to 95%. In 20- to 40-year-olds, the rate is 60%, and above 40, only 10% will recur. This has led some to encourage young, active patients to consider surgical correction after the initial dislocation. The complications of recurrent dislocation include neurovascular injury, fracture, and degenerative arthritis of the shoulder joint.

Various surgical procedures for shoulder stabilization exist and can be performed open or arthroscopically. Open procedures use a large incision through which the surgery is performed, while arthroscopic surgery involves several small incisions made around the shoulder, with an arthroscope, or camera, used to visualize the shoulder joint.

Procedures to correct the unstable shoulder involve reattaching the torn ligaments and labrum and often eliminating any capsular redundancy. Unfortunately, sometimes a loss of external rotation of the shoulder results from the surgery. This can be detrimental to certain athletes, such as pitchers, who rely on excessive external rotation for their sport. The success rates for the two procedures are about equal now, with recurrence rates after surgery of 5% to 15%. The arthroscopic method affords less morbidity and the ability to see more of the joint itself.

Postoperative care involves a period of immobilization with a rapid introduction of range-of-motion exercises to prevent stiffness. As with nonoperative management, once painfree range of motion is achieved, gradual strengthening exercises are added.

Eugene S. Hong and Katherine Beck

See also Shoulder Injuries; Shoulder Injuries, Surgery for; Shoulder Instability; Shoulder Subluxation

Further Readings

Chahal J, Kassiri K, Dion A, MacDonald P, Leiter J. Diagnostic and treatment differences among experienced shoulder surgeons for the instability conditions of the shoulder. *Clin J Sport Med.* 2007;17(1):5–9.

Deitch J, Mehlman CT, Foad SL, Obbehat A, Mallory M. Traumatic anterior shoulder dislocation in adolescents. *Am J Sports Med.* 2003;31(5):758–763.

Quillen DM. Acute shoulder injuries. *Am Fam Physician.* 2004;70(10):1947–1954.

Wang RY, Arciero RA. Treating the athlete with anterior shoulder instability. *Clin Sports Med.* 2008;27(4): 631–648.

SHOULDER IMPINGEMENT SYNDROME

Shoulder impingement syndrome is a common source of shoulder pain in the general population as well as in the athletic community. Like other syndromes, shoulder impingement syndrome refers to a group of symptoms and diagnostic signs. As the name implies, this syndrome is caused by the compression of structures within the shoulder joint.

Athletic participation that requires overhead arm motion puts an athlete at risk for developing shoulder impingement syndrome. These sports include swimming, tennis, baseball, golf, volleyball, and gymnastics. In addition to overhead activity, a "loose" shoulder joint, the anatomy of the acromion, and disease within the acromioclavicular joint place an athlete at risk of developing this syndrome.

Anatomy

The shoulder joint is a very complex joint, with many structures. A good knowledge of the anatomy of this joint is essential for understanding shoulder impingement syndrome (Figure 1). There are two joints to be aware of, the *glenohumeral joint* and the *acromioclavicular joint*. The glenohumeral joint is composed of the glenoid fossa (socket) of the scapula (wing bone) and the head of the humerus bone (upper arm bone). The

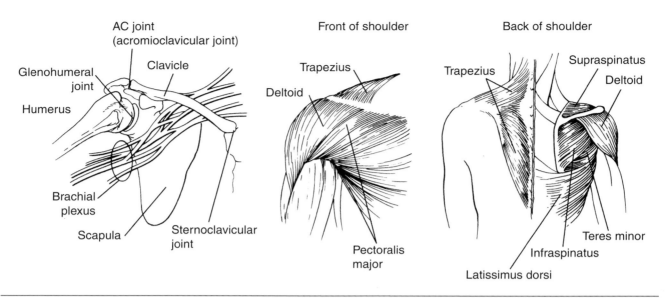

Figure 1   Anatomical Structures of the Shoulder

acromioclavicular joint is formed by the attachment of the outer part of the clavicle and the acromion process, a forward projection of the scapula.

Surrounding these bones are multiple tendons, ligaments, and muscles. More specifically, though, the following are anatomical structures important to a discussion of shoulder impingement syndrome: the rotator cuff complex (made up of four muscle-tendon units, the supraspinatus, infraspinatus, teres minor, and subscapularis), the subacromial bursa (a sac of fluid that lies underneath the acromion process), the labrum (a ring of cartilage in the glenohumeral joint), and the biceps tendon. All these structures may be internally compressed, causing shoulder impingement syndrome.

As mentioned, the anatomy of the acromion process has a role in causing shoulder impingement syndrome. This relationship was first noted by Dr. Charles Neer in 1972 in the *Journal of Bone and Joint Surgery*. He described three acromion types: Type I, flat; Type II, curved; and Type III, hooked (Figure 2).

Causes

Shoulder impingement syndrome is caused by the compression of structures surrounding the glenohumeral joint. Any source of weakness or dysfunction of the joint will result in instability and excessive motion of the humeral head. Surrounding

the humeral head is the rotator cuff complex, together with the subacromial bursa. These structures are typically the ones impinged on. Compression commonly occurs between the humeral head and the acromion. A Type III, hooked acromion is mostly associated with shoulder impingement, but it may occur with any type of acromion morphology. Other structures in the shoulder may be the source of compression besides the acromion, however, and include the acromioclavicular joint as well as structures surrounding the coracoid process, another forward projection of the scapula.

Throwing athletes (baseball pitchers, javelin throwers, football quarterbacks) are at increased risk for shoulder impingement syndrome due to the extreme range of motion that is required of the shoulder to participate in their positions. The range of motion that places these athletes at risk is referred to as the "cocked position." The cocked position is the point at which the athlete's arm is maximally rotated overhead and extended behind the body. With the arm in this position, the stability of the shoulder is maximally stressed, causing excessive motion at the glenohumeral joint and subsequent compression of internal structures. Participation in these sports requires repetitive throwing motions, which may cause fatigue, weakness, and additional dysfunction of the glenohumeral joint, resulting in worsened compression and more severe impingement.

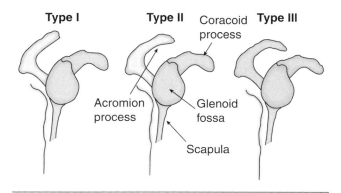

Figure 2   Anatomical Variants of the Acromion Process

Source: Adapted from Fongemie AE, Buss DD, Rolnick SJ. Management of shoulder impingement syndrome and rotator cuff tears [Figure 2m]. *Am Fam Physician.* 1998;57(4):667–674.

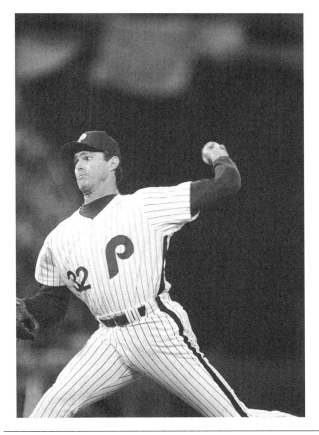

Cocked position for throwing. Philadelphia Phillies pitcher Steve Carlton delivers a pitch in the early innings of a World Series game against the Baltimore Orioles, Friday, Oct. 14, 1983, Philadelphia, Pennsylvania.

Source: AP.

Symptoms

Pain with overhead activity is the most common complaint. As the impingement worsens, pain is present outside activity and is typically located along the outside or back of the shoulder and occurs at night, especially when the patient lies on the affected shoulder. In addition to sports activities, the athlete may complain of pain when putting on a shirt or brushing his or her hair.

Initially, throwing athletes complain of increased stiffness in the shoulder and have difficulty with their warm-up activities. The pain is worse during the cocked position of throwing, as described above.

Diagnosis

As with all sports injuries, a diagnosis of shoulder impingement syndrome requires a thorough review of the history of the athlete's pain and an extensive physical exam. The physical exam starts with a thorough neck exam to make sure that a neck abnormality is not the cause of the shoulder pain. At the start of the shoulder exam, the athlete is asked to move the shoulder through all ranges of motion, looking for abnormalities or pain. If shoulder impingement syndrome is present, the athlete will have pain with movement and in particular when bringing his or her arm over the head, a motion commonly referred to as the "painful arc." Sometimes, with shoulder pain, strength can be diminished compared with the uninjured shoulder. However, in athletes, strength is typically preserved. Other special tests can be used to diagnose the presence of impingement on exam: These include a positive Neer test, Hawkins-Kennedy test, or Yocum test. The Neer, Hawkins-Kennedy, and Yocum tests attempt to cause external compression of internal shoulder structures, re-creating the athlete's pain. In a throwing athlete, pain can also be re-induced by moving the athlete's arm into an extended and rotated position, re-creating the cocked position of throwing. Reproduction of the troublesome pain is consistent with a diagnosis of a type of impingement called *posterior impingement.*

Plain radiographs (X-rays) may be obtained to look for bony abnormalities causing internal compression of shoulder structures. Radiographs will demonstrate the shape of the acromion as well as abnormalities in the acromioclavicular joint and coracoid process. All these, as mentioned above, can be a source of impingement, and their presence on X-rays makes a diagnosis of impingement for an athlete with shoulder pain more likely.

In addition to X-rays, additional imaging techniques may be used to diagnose shoulder impingement syndrome. Magnetic resonance imaging (MRI) is commonly used. In an athlete with shoulder impingement syndrome, MRI is used mostly to evaluate for the presence of specific causes or abnormalities in the shoulder that may be the source of pain, such as a rotator cuff tear or tear of cartilage in the glenohumeral joint. In the absence of specific abnormalities, the MRI scan of a shoulder with impingement syndrome will show some generalized inflammation or collections of fluid in the area of compression. Ultrasound, like MRI, can also be used to exclude other specific abnormalities as the source of pain.

Treatment

The treatment of most athletic injuries, including shoulder impingement syndrome, can be divided into *acute* and *subacute* therapy. In the absence of long-standing pain and dysfunction or the presence of other specific shoulder abnormalities (e.g., rotator cuff tear), the treatment of shoulder impingement syndrome does not include surgery. Some potential surgical interventions are discussed below.

Acute Therapy

At the time of initial evaluation, there may be significant pain and/or dysfunction. For this, acute therapy may consist of rest, cryotherapy (ice), and nonsteroidal anti-inflammatory medications (NSAIDs) such as ibuprofen. For appropriate rest, the athlete must avoid any aggravating activity, including all overhead motion or any sport-specific activity that re-creates his or her pain. Cryotherapy can be initially used to aid in pain relief and help reduce inflammation. In addition to cryotherapy, NSAIDs are also used to reduce pain and inflammation. These medications are typically used for 10 to 14 days and only as needed thereafter.

Additional acute therapies may be used for the reduction of pain and inflammation. These may be performed by a certified physical therapist (PT or DPT) or certified athletic trainer (ATC) and may include electrical stimulation (E-stim), phonophoresis, iontophoresis, or therapeutic ultrasound. Phonophoresis and iontophoresis use sound waves and an electrical current, respectively, to push anti-inflammatory medication through the skin to the site of injury.

Subacute Therapy

Physical Therapy

After the initial pain and inflammation are addressed, physical therapy should be focused on the achievement of full and nonpainful range of motion of the affected shoulder. Once this range of motion is achieved, physical therapy is then used to restore the strength and function of the shoulder musculature. The rehabilitation program is used to restore the function of all the muscles surrounding the shoulder, including those that control the movement of the scapula.

For a nonathlete patient, the rehabilitation program is complete once the patient returns to normal activities of daily living without pain. An athlete, however, must then be guided back to sport-specific activities after full range of motion and strength are regained. Certain sport activities place a much higher demand on the shoulder joint than normal daily activities. During a return-to-sports program, the athlete is taken through exercises that simulate the demands of the athlete's sport. For example, a football quarterback is asked to re-create his throwing motion, initially with light resistance and then using lightweight dumbbells.

Other Treatments

Completion of the above treatment programs will commonly result in full recovery for most athletes. However, if a full return to his or her sport activity is not accomplished in 2 to 3 months, the following treatment options may be considered.

Steroid Injection. Sports medicine physicians often use an injection of a steroid solution into the shoulder joint or subacromial space (an area between the acromion and the head of the humerus) if chronic inflammation is thought to be the cause of shoulder impingement syndrome. The goal of the injection is to reduce the inflammation and pain to help facilitate recovery and the ability to perform the rehabilitation program. Glucocorticoid solutions are used for injection in combination with a local anesthetic, lidocaine or marcaine.

Surgery. As stated before, in the absence of long-standing problems or specific abnormalities, surgery is rarely indicated for shoulder impingement syndrome. Long-standing shoulder impingement syndrome is defined as any dysfunction that has not improved with the above therapies or has lasted longer than 3 months. If there is no improvement in the athlete's shoulder pain after 3 months of the above treatments, surgical exploration with minimally invasive arthroscopic surgery may be considered. During this procedure, the surgeon will attempt to localize the source of the athlete's pain and repair damaged tissue. Also, if a Type III acromion is noted on plain radiographs, an acromioplasty procedure may be performed. During this procedure, the surgeon removes part of the undersurface of the acromion bone to help "decompress" the area of impingement—in other words, to make more room for internal structures to avoid future compression and impingement. Following surgery for shoulder impingement syndrome, in the absence of an extensive repair for a specific abnormality, the athlete can be expected to complete a course of physical therapy in 2 to 4 weeks and begin a return to sport-specific activities in 4 to 6 weeks.

David W. Kruse

See also Musculoskeletal Tests, Shoulder; Principles of Rehabilitation and Physical Therapy; Rotator Cuff Tendinopathy; Shoulder Bursitis; Shoulder Injuries; Shoulder Injuries, Surgery for

Further Readings

Jobe FW, Pink M. Classification and treatment of shoulder dysfunction in the overhead athlete. *J Orthop Sports Phys Ther.* 1993;18(2):427–432.

McFarland EG. Examination of the shoulder. In: Kim TK, Park HB, Rassi GE, Gill H, Keyurapan E, eds. *The Complete Guide.* New York, NY: Thieme; 2006:142.

Meister K. Internal impingement in the shoulder of the overhand athlete: pathophysiology, diagnosis, and treatment. *Am J Orthop.* 2000;29(6):433–438.

Michener LA, Walsworth MK, Burnet EN. Effectiveness of rehabilitation for patients with subacromial impingement syndrome: a systematic review. *J Hand Ther.* 2004;17(2):152–164.

Neer CS. Anterior acromioplasty for the chronic impingement syndrome in the shoulder: a preliminary report. *J Bone Joint Surg Am.* 1972;54(1):41–50.

van der Windt DA, Koes BW, de Jong BA, Bouter LM. Shoulder disorders in general practice: incidence, patient characteristics, and management. *Ann Rheum Dis.* 1995;54(12):959–964.

SHOULDER INJURIES

Shoulder injuries occur as a result of both acute trauma and chronic overuse and affect both bony and soft tissue structures. Acute injuries as a result of falling or collision are seen mainly in collision, contact, and extreme sports, such as hockey, football, snowboarding, and skateboarding. Overuse injuries are becoming more frequent as a result of year-round competition and sport-specific training. Overuse injuries are seen commonly in sports such as swimming, baseball, volleyball, softball, and tennis. Shoulder pain occurs in 40% to 80% of swimmers and 50% to 95% of baseball players.

Overuse injuries result from microtrauma from repetitive movements of large rotational forces. They are often associated with joint looseness, mobility impairment, or muscle imbalances. Several risk factors contribute to such injuries. These risk factors include poor mobility, muscle weakness, muscle imbalance, and shoulder blade asymmetry. Additional risk factors in children and adolescent athletes include open physeal (growth) plates, joint laxity, and underdeveloped musculature.

Injury patterns to the athlete's shoulder are sport specific. In football, the shoulder is the second most commonly injured body part, next to the knee. Shoulder injuries are most often shoulder dislocations, shoulder separations, and collarbone fractures. Bicycling results in many shoulder injuries, usually collarbone fractures and shoulder separations from falling on the shoulder. Shoulder injuries are the most common injury to the upper extremity in wrestling, with shoulder separations being the most common. Repetitive microtrauma frequently results in multidirectional instability in swimmers and gymnasts.

Anatomy

There are four bony articulations in the shoulder: (1) the glenohumeral joint, (2) the acromioclavicular (AC) joint, (3) the sternoclavicular (SC) joint, and (4) the scapulothoracic articulation. The glenohumeral joint is a ball-and-socket joint. The glenoid cavity is relatively shallow and, therefore, inherently unstable. Additional stability is provided by the glenohumeral ligaments, glenoid labrum, and capsule, as well as the rotator cuff and scapular-stabilizing muscles.

The labrum is a ring of fibrous tissue that attaches directly to the glenoid fossa. It expands the size and depth of the glenoid cavity. The superior portion of the labrum inserts directly onto the biceps tendon, and the biceps tendon inserts on the supraglenoid tubercle. The shoulder capsule has three primary bands, called the superior, middle, and inferior glenohumeral ligaments. The anterior and posterior bands of the inferior glenohumeral ligament prevent anterior and posterior translation of the humeral head. The superior margin of the anterior band of the inferior glenohumeral ligament attaches to the glenoid fossa at the two o'clock position. When the shoulder is abducted and externally rotated, this broad ligament rotates anteriorly to prevent subluxation (partial dislocation) of the humeral head.

The rotator cuff muscles are the dynamic stabilizers of the shoulder and include the supraspinatus, infraspinatus, teres minor, and subscapularis. These muscles stabilize the position of the humeral head in the glenoid fossa, rotate the humerus, and help elevate the upper extremity. They also act to depress the humeral head as a counterforce to the deltoid, which acts to elevate the arm and force the humeral head superiorly. The rotator cuff muscles rely on optimal functioning of the deltoid and scapular-stabilizing muscles. The scapular-stabilizing muscles include the trapezius, serratus anterior, rhomboids, levator scapulae, and pectoralis minor.

Normal shoulder movement requires that the scapulothoracic joint, the AC joint, and the SC joint all move together smoothly. Smooth, integrated movement of these joints is necessary to achieve full upper limb elevation. Scapular movement removes the acromion from the path of the humeral head so that it does not become impinged.

There are unique differences in structure in the pediatric shoulder compared with adult shoulders. In the skeletally immature athlete, there is a growth plate at the proximal end of the humerus where new bone is formed. Approximately 80% of the growth of the upper extremity occurs at this physeal plate. The epiphyseal plates are relatively weaker than the surrounding ligaments, predisposing children and adolescents to growth plate fractures and avulsion fractures not seen in adults. Proximal humeral closure occurs by age 14 to 16 years in girls and age 16 to 21 years in boys.

Another difference in the immature shoulder is the higher proportion of Type III collagen. As growth and development progress, Type III collagen is steadily replaced by the more stable Type I collagen seen in adults. The presence of Type III collagen in younger athletes results in more shoulder laxity, which can contribute to shoulder instability, particularly in throwing and overhead athletes.

Evaluation of Injuries

Details of Injury

Details that can diagnose shoulder injuries include the date of onset of symptoms, whether there was a specific traumatic event, the mechanism of injury, the location of pain, the presence of mechanical symptoms or instability, and management of the injury to date. Previous shoulder injuries may predispose an athlete to future injuries, particularly if the injury was not fully healed. In overhead athletes, additional information, including what sport is played, the level of competition, the number of repetitions, and where in the overhead motion pain occurs, can help determine the exact injury.

Physical Findings

Injuries to the shoulder can result in muscle atrophy, asymmetry, discoloration, or deformity, as well as winging of the shoulder blade. There may be tenderness to palpation of the bony and soft tissue structures, including the SC joint, AC joint, clavicle, acromion, scapula, greater tuberosity of the humerus, deltoid, and proximal biceps tendon.

The range of motion of the injured shoulder may be decreased or painful in forward flexion (elevation), abduction, and external and internal rotation. The range of motion of the injured shoulder may be decreased in comparison with the uninjured side. The movement of the shoulder blade may also be abnormal with a shoulder injury (dyskinesia).

Muscle strength may be decreased with a shoulder injury. Specific muscles can be tested to determine any weakness or pain. The supraspinatus strength (thumb-down abduction at 30° horizontal flexion or "empty-can" test), infraspinatus strength (external rotation with the arm adducted), external rotation with the arm in a neutral position, subscapularis strength (lift-off test performed with the hand at the lower back and pushing away from the spine against resistance), and deltoid strength (abduction with the arm at the side) against resistance may all be affected by an injury.

Biceps tendinopathy can be assessed with the Speed test and the Yergason test. The Speed test is performed with the patient standing and the shoulder forward flexed against resistance with the elbow extended and the forearm supinated. Pain or tenderness in the bicipital groove indicates a positive test. The Yergason test is performed with the elbow flexed to 90° and the forearm pronated (hand turned upward). The patient actively tries to supinate (palm of the hand turned downward) the wrist against resistance. A positive test elicits pain in the bicipital groove.

Special tests for the shoulder include the anterior apprehension relocation test, the load and shift test, the O'Brien test, the anterior slide test, the sulcus test, and impingement tests. The anterior apprehension relocation test assesses anterior instability. With the patient supine and the arm hanging off the bed, the patient's shoulder is passively moved into external rotation until guarding is appreciated (positive test) or capsular-end feel is reached. After a positive apprehension test, a posteriorly directed force is applied to relocate the humeral head in the glenoid fossa (relocation test). Apprehension disappears, and there is an increase in passive external rotation.

The load and shift test assesses for anterior as well as posterior instability. With the patient sitting, the humeral head of the affected shoulder is grasped in the examiner's hand and anterior, and

posterior force is applied to determine the amount of translation within the glenoid fossa. The following grading system is helpful: Grade 0 = *no translation*, Grade 1 = *translation up to the glenoid rim*, Grade 2 = *translation onto the rim (subluxation)*, and Grade 3 = *translation over the rim or dislocation*. A comparison should be made with the uninjured shoulder.

The O'Brien test can be used to assess superior labral anterior-posterior (SLAP) injuries. With the patient standing, the injured arm is flexed forward to 90° with the thumb pointed down. The examiner applies a downward force to the arm while the patient resists. Pain in the shoulder joint is considered a positive test. The thumb is then turned upward, and the maneuver is repeated. This should not be painful. Unfortunately, pain can result from this maneuver in the presence of an AC injury, biceps tendinitis, or posterior instability, resulting in a false positive. SLAP lesions can also be evaluated by the anterior slide test. The athlete stands with hands on the hips. The examiner places one hand over the athlete's shoulder, and the other hand is placed behind the elbow. The examiner then applies a force anteriorly and superiorly while the athlete pushes back against the force. A positive test results in pain localized to the anterosuperior aspect of the shoulder, a pop or click in the same area, or reproduction of the athlete's symptoms.

The sulcus sign assesses for the presence of inferior instability. The patient should be seated and completely relaxed. With the shoulder in the neutral position, the examiner exerts a downward force on the humerus, looking for the presence of a depression or sulcus at the glenohumeral joint (positive test). A positive sulcus sign may indicate generalized ligamentous laxity or multidirectional instability. If generalized ligamentous laxity is suspected, patients should be assessed for hyperextension of the elbows and metacarpal-phalangeal joints and hyperflexion of the first carpometacarpal/wrist joint.

Sometimes pain in the shoulder can result from the humeral head butting up against the acromion (impingement). Impingement tests include the Neer and Hawkins signs. They evaluate the rotator cuff and subacromial bursae. The Neer test is performed with the athlete in the seated position. The examiner places one hand on the shoulder and passively flexes the shoulder forward until pain is experienced by the athlete. The Hawkins test is also performed with the athlete seated. The examiner stabilizes the shoulder with one hand while passively internally rotating the arm with the arm forward flexed and the elbow flexed to 90°. Pain in the shoulder indicates impingement of the humeral head by the acromion. An additional impingement sign is the crossover test, which confirms AC pathology. With the patient seated, the arm of the affected shoulder is adducted across the chest. A positive test elicits pain in the AC joint.

Investigations

Investigations that may be necessary to help determine the diagnosis in shoulder injuries include X-rays, a computed tomography (CT) scan, an ultrasound scan, a bone scan, and a magnetic resonance imaging (MRI) scan. In acute injuries, X-rays including anteroposterior views with internal and external rotation as well as axillary views should be performed to look for fractures. Calcific tendinopathy, arthritis, subluxation, or dislocation, as well as impingement, may be seen on X-rays. A CT scan can provide greater bony definition.

An ultrasound scan can be used to help confirm the suspicion of a muscle or tendon tear.

Examination can be performed as a static or dynamic investigation. The size of the tear and the thickness of the intact tissue can be measured. A dynamic examination may confirm impingement.

MRI scans have become increasingly helpful with the diagnosis of rotator cuff and labral tears, although arthroscopy remains the gold standard. MRI arthrography (injection of dye into the shoulder joint) is currently the recommended diagnostic study of choice for labral tears.

Types of Injury

Various types of shoulder injuries are listed in Table 1.

Prevention of Injury

Proper technique is important to avoid injury, particularly in overhead athletes. It should be taught early and reinforced throughout an athlete's career. Year-round conditioning should be encouraged,

Table 1 Shoulder Injuries

Common	Uncommon	Must Not Be Missed
Rotator cuff strain/tendinopathy	Rotator cuff tear	Tumor
Glenohumeral dislocation	Biceps tendinitis	Referred pain from thoracic/ abdominal structures
Glenohumeral instability	Fracture (scapula, humeral neck, proximal humerus in children)	Thorax outlet syndrome
Labral tears (superior labral anterior-posterior [SLAP])	Arthritis	
Clavicle fracture	Neurapraxia (burner)	
Acromioclavicular (AC) joint separation/dislocation	Sternoclavicular (SC) separation/ dislocation	
Little League shoulder	"Frozen shoulder"	
Shoulder subluxation	Bursitis	
Impingement syndrome		

Source: Author.

with emphasis on core strengthening and lower extremity strengthening.

In overhead sports such as football, baseball, softball, and tennis, proper technique should be reinforced to ensure that athletes are using their lower extremity strength to help impart force to the ball and limit the stress to the shoulder. Avoid "overthrowing."

To avoid overuse injuries, appropriate rest and recovery should be ensured. Athletes should take advantage of the off-season to allow muscle recovery. Athletes should not play the same sport all year round or participate on more than one team. In children and adolescents, restrictions in the number of repetitions, such as the number of pitches and types of pitches (no sliders or curve balls), can help reduce shoulder injuries.

Return to Sports

Before an athlete with a shoulder injury returns to sports, he or she should have attained full range of motion of the shoulder and full strength of the rotator cuff and scapulothoracic muscles, as well as core and lower extremity strength. Pain should be resolved. The athlete should have progressed through a functional exercise program consisting of sport-specific activities and drills that mimic the stresses that the athlete will encounter in practice and competition. The athlete must also demonstrate the appropriate mechanics for his or her particular sport to minimize the risk of reinjury and to achieve maximal performance.

Laura Purcell

See also Acromioclavicular (AC) Joint, Separation of; Clavicle (Collarbone) Fracture; Frozen Shoulder; Glenoid Labrum Tear; Little League Shoulder; Shoulder Bursitis; Shoulder Impingement Syndrome; Shoulder Instability; Shoulder Subluxation; Superior Labrum From Anterior to Posterior (SLAP) Lesions

Further Readings

Guido JA Jr, Brown T. Adolescent shoulder injuries. In: Micheli LJ, Purcell LK, eds. *The Adolescent Athlete.* New York, NY: Springer; 2007:165–193.

Hackney RG. Advances in the understanding of throwing injuries of the shoulder. *Br J Sports Med.* 1996;30(4):282–288.

Kibler WB, Murrell GAC. Shoulder pain. In: Brukner P, Khan K, eds. *Clinical Sports Medicine.* 3rd ed. Sydney, Australia: McGraw-Hill; 2007:243–288.

Kocher MS, Waters PM, Micheli LJ. Upper extremity injuries in the pediatric athlete. *Sports Med.* 2000;30(2):117–135.

Mazoue CG, Andrews JR. Injuries to the shoulder in athletes. *South Med J.* 2004;97(8):748–754.

Meister K. Injuries to the shoulder in the throwing athlete. Part one: biomechanics/pathophysiology/classification of injury. *Am J Sports Med.* 2000:28(2):265–275.

Meister K. Injuries to the shoulder in the throwing athlete. Part two: evaluation/treatment. *Am J Sports Med.* 2000;28(4):587–601.

Roger B, Skaf A, Hooper AW, Lektrakul N, Yeh L, Resnick D. Imaging findings in the dominant shoulder of throwing athletes: comparison of radiography, arthrography, CT arthrography, and MR arthrography with arthroscopic correlation. *AJR Am J Roentgenol.* 1999;172(5):1371–1380.

Wang HK, Cochrane T. Mobility impairment, muscle imbalance, muscle weakness, scapular asymmetry and shoulder injury in elite volleyball athletes. *J Sports Med Phys Fitness.* 2001;41(3):403–410.

Wilk KE, Meister K, Andrews JR. Current concepts in the rehabilitation of the overhead throwing athlete. *Am J Sports Med.* 2002;30(1):136–151.

SHOULDER INJURIES, SURGERY FOR

The shoulder plays a major role in athletic competition. "Overhead sports" athletes are those whose primary sport involves much activity with the arm overhead. These sports include, but are not limited to, football, basketball, baseball, tennis, swimming, lacrosse, and gymnastics. These sports place particularly significant stresses and strains on the athlete's shoulder. Baseball pitchers, due to the high energy of the pitch, are a unique group of athletes who place particularly high demands on their dominant shoulder. Swimmers also rely heavily on repetitive exaggerated shoulder motions to swim fast. Shoulder injuries are more common in overhead sports athletes and occur most frequently in baseball pitchers and swimmers.

This entry reviews the anatomy of the shoulder and the types of injury that commonly occur in athletes and explains the surgeries used to repair the affected structures.

Anatomy

The shoulder is a ball-and-socket joint in which the ball is the head of the humerus and the socket is called the *glenoid*. The glenoid socket is directly attached to the scapula, or shoulder blade. Both the ball of the humerus and glenoid socket are covered in smooth cartilage that resembles the shiny white end of a chicken bone. The smooth cartilage allows the ball-and-socket bones to move against each other with minimal friction. The glenoid socket resembles a dish and is surrounded on its edges by a circular rim of rubbery cartilage called the labrum. The labrum can be thought of as an O-ring that attaches to the outer edges of the glenoid socket. The labrum serves to make the glenoid socket deeper and helps keep the ball of the humerus from moving outside the socket. The *shoulder capsule* is made up of strong elastic tissue that surrounds the head of the humerus and glenoid socket. The shoulder capsule prevents the ball of the humerus from moving outside the glenoid socket. The shoulder capsule is reinforced by *ligaments,* or areas of condensed fibrous bands, that run between the head of the humerus and glenoid socket to provide strength to the shoulder capsule.

The rotator cuff is a group of four muscles that lie on top of the shoulder capsule, surrounding the ball of the humerus and the glenoid socket. These muscles sit on top of the shoulder like the cuff of a shirt. Two rotator cuff muscles lie on top of the shoulder and are called the *supraspinatus* and the *infraspinatus*. One rotator cuff muscle sits in front of the shoulder and is called the *subscapularis*. The *teres minor* is the fourth rotator cuff muscle, and it lies in the back of the shoulder. The rotator cuff muscles all form muscle tendons that attach to the head of the humerus. The rotator cuff functions to move the shoulder in all directions. The top muscles (supraspinatus and infraspinatus) work to bring the arm above the head and are most important in overhead sports.

Surrounding the rotator cuff muscles is the *deltoid* muscle. The deltoid muscle begins at the collarbone and shoulder blade and attaches to the humerus. The deltoid muscle helps the rotator cuff move the shoulder. The *biceps* muscle lies in the front of the arm and helps bend the elbow. The biceps muscle in the arm becomes a cordlike *biceps tendon* near the shoulder. In the shoulder, the biceps tendon attaches to the glenoid socket at the top of the labrum. There are also multiple *bursa* around the shoulder. A bursa is a small fluid-filled sac that occurs around tendons and allows the tendons to move without generating friction with nearby bones. The most prominent bursa in the shoulder lies below the deltoid muscle and above the rotator cuff tendons.

Shoulder Joint Function

The ball-and-socket nature of the shoulder allows the shoulder to move more than any other joint in the body. The labrum, capsule, and ligaments of the shoulder must strike a delicate balance between allowing the shoulder to move in all directions and preventing the ball of the humerus from moving out of the glenoid socket. The strength and power of the shoulder come from the rotator cuff muscles and the deltoid muscle. Athletes must develop their shoulders' strength and mobility to accommodate the demands of their sports. Baseball pitchers normally have significantly more strength and different motion ranges in their throwing shoulder as compared with their other shoulder. The best swimmers tend to have loose shoulder joints on both sides, which allows for great shoulder motion. Shoulder injuries can occur when the stress and strain of the sport or activity prevail over the ability of the shoulder to perform its function.

Shoulder Joint Injuries

Most athletic shoulder injuries are muscle strains, tendinitis, or bursitis. Muscle strains represent microscopic muscle tears that occur when the muscle is stretched more than it can withstand. Muscle strains can occur in the rotator cuff, biceps, and deltoid muscles. These injuries are treated with rest and heal on their own over time. Tendinitis occurs when the muscle tendon (the part of the muscle that attaches to the bone) becomes irritated or inflamed. Tendinitis occurs most commonly in the rotator cuff muscle tendons near where they attach to the head of the humerus. Rotator cuff tendinitis is often seen in repetitive overhead sports such as tennis, swimming, and baseball. Many times, a small injury to the rotator cuff tendon is ignored by the athlete, who continues to stress and strain the tendon through playing the sport. Over time, the body responds by sending blood cells to the rotator cuff tendon in an attempt to repair the injury. An inflammatory response is generated by the blood cells, which causes pain and swelling in the area of the rotator cuff tendon. Rotator cuff tendinitis is treated with rest, ice, anti-inflammatory medications (e.g., ibuprofen), and physical therapy focusing on shoulder muscle strengthening. Bursitis is a similar inflammation of a shoulder bursa. This can occur when the nearby tendon is inflamed, as is often the case in rotator cuff tendinitis. Shoulder bursitis is treated like rotator cuff tendinitis. In addition, the physician may elect to inject a corticosteroid (an injectable anti-inflammatory medication) into the shoulder bursa to help decrease inflammation in that area.

The most common shoulder injuries in sports that may require surgery are rotator cuff tendon tears, labrum tears, and shoulder dislocations. Rotator cuff tendon tears occur when the rotator cuff tendon pulls away from its attachment to the humerus. This can occur when a sudden force is placed on the arm, pulling the arm away from the body. Rotator cuff tendon tears can also occur in the setting of rotator cuff tendinitis if the athlete continues to stress the inflamed tendon. Rotator cuff tendon tears most commonly occur in overhead throwing athletes in the supraspinatus tendon at the top of the shoulder. Rotator cuff tears can be diagnosed by a physical exam as the athlete will have weakness with overhead shoulder motion. When a physician suspects a rotator cuff tear, an MRI scan of the shoulder is usually obtained and can be used to diagnose a rotator cuff tear. Rotator cuff tendon tears can be of partial thickness (where only a part of the thickness of the tendon has pulled off its attachment on the humerus) or full thickness (where the entire thickness of a portion of the tendon has pulled off the humerus). Many partial-thickness rotator cuff tendon tears will heal on their own and can be treated without surgery. Full-thickness tendon tears often require surgical repair.

Labral tears are most common in overhead throwing athletes such as baseball pitchers. These injuries usually cause deep pain and popping of the shoulder joint with overhead activities. Labral tears occur in many different forms and sizes. When the

labrum tears at the top of the glenoid socket, it is called a SLAP tear (which in medical terms stands for superior labrum anterior-posterior). These labral tears are important because the biceps tendon attaches to the labrum in this region. When the physician suspects a labral tear, an MRI scan is often obtained to evaluate the shoulder labrum. Sometimes dye is injected into the shoulder prior to the MRI scan to help the radiologist identify the labrum and determine if there is a tear. Many labral tears do not require surgery. Surgery is usually reserved for overhead throwing athletes who have deep shoulder pain and popping that does not improve after a period of rest and rehabilitation.

Shoulder dislocations occur when the ball of the humerus slips outside the glenoid socket. Because of its inherent mobility, the shoulder is the joint that is most likely to dislocate in the body. Shoulder dislocations most commonly occur when the ball of the humerus moves outside the glenoid socket and toward the front of the shoulder (an anterior shoulder dislocation). This occurs when the arm is extended and a force pushes the arm backward while levering the head of the humerus forward. When the shoulder dislocates, the head of the humerus must be "reduced" or put back in the glenoid socket. This can sometimes be done on the playing field by the athletic trainer. At other times, shoulder muscle spasms prevent the shoulder from being reduced easily. In these cases, the athlete is usually taken to the emergency room, where medication is used to relax the muscles while a physician manipulates the shoulder back into place.

When the humeral head dislocates out of the glenoid socket toward the front, the shoulder capsule and ligaments, and occasionally the front of the labrum, are usually torn. An MRI scan may be obtained to determine exactly what structures have been injured by the dislocation. Many shoulder dislocations are treated without surgery. The athlete is usually placed in a sling for a period of time before undergoing a course of physical therapy to restrengthen the shoulder. When a shoulder dislocation occurs in a young athlete who participates in overhead contact sports, the chance of the shoulder dislocating again is very high. Also, in patients who have had shoulder dislocations in the past, the chance of having another dislocation is very high. In these and other cases of shoulder instability, surgery may be recommended to repair the torn labrum and to retighten the front of the shoulder capsule and ligaments to prevent future shoulder dislocations.

Surgery: Rotator Cuff Repair

Surgery for a full-thickness rotator cuff tear involves repairing the torn rotator cuff tendon back to where it attached on the humeral head. This surgery can be done through a large incision (open technique) or through multiple tiny incisions with the aid of an arthroscope (arthroscopic technique). The choice of technique depends on the pattern of the tear and the preference of the surgeon. Open techniques require that part of the deltoid muscle be detached and then repaired to allow access to the torn rotator cuff tendon. Recently, arthroscopic equipment and skills have improved considerably, allowing many tears to be repaired using this technique. Arthroscopic rotator cuff repair often results in less pain immediately after surgery, although the overall recovery time and time to tendon healing are not changed.

During rotator cuff repair, in most cases, one or more tiny metal or absorbable anchors are inserted into the bone of the humeral head where the torn rotator cuff is supposed to attach. The anchors are connected to strong suture material that is used to tie the torn rotator cuff back to where it attached on the humeral head. The number of anchors used depends on the size of the tear. After surgery, patients are placed into a sling that is typically worn for approximately the first 3 weeks after surgery. For the first 6 weeks after surgery, no active lifting of the arm over the head is allowed. Full recovery from rotator cuff repair back to sporting activities often takes 4 months or much longer for overhead throwing athletes.

Surgery: Labral Repair

When surgery is necessary for labral tears in the shoulder, an arthroscopic technique is most commonly employed. In these cases, multiple small incisions (termed arthroscopic *portals*) are made around the shoulder. The arthroscope (a small, thin camera) is placed through one of these portals and into the shoulder joint (between the humeral head and glenoid socket). With the arthroscope in the shoulder, the surgeon is able to look at a monitor

and identify the labrum (the rubbery O-ring around the glenoid socket) to determine if there is a tear. The surgeon decides how to proceed based on the size, shape, and location of the labral tear.

For smaller tears or tears that are frayed and degenerated, the surgeon may elect to remove only the torn portion of the labrum and leave the rest of the labrum alone. This is done with the aid of a miniature motorized shaver that is placed through an arthroscopic portal. For larger tears or tears that involve the labrum on the top of the shoulder (where the biceps tendon attaches), the surgeon may elect to repair the torn portion of the labrum back to where it belongs on the glenoid socket. This is done by placing tiny metal or absorbable anchors through an arthroscopic portal and into the glenoid socket at the location of the tear. Strong suture material is attached to the anchor, and this suture is then passed around the torn labrum and used to tie the torn labrum back down to the glenoid socket. After labral repair surgery, most patients are kept in a sling for approximately 3 weeks before starting a course of physical therapy. Return to sports takes approximately 3 to 4 months as the repair site has to heal. For baseball pitchers and overhead throwing athletes, return to full throwing can take as long as 9 to 12 months.

Surgery: Shoulder Instability

Surgery for shoulder instability involves repairing the structures that were injured when the head of the humerus dislocated out of the glenoid socket. These injured structures usually include a combination of the shoulder capsule, ligaments, and front part of the labrum. Repair of these structures can be done through one large incision on the front of the shoulder (open technique) or through multiple small incisions around the shoulder (arthroscopic technique). In the past, the open technique has produced the best results, but recent advancements in arthroscopic equipment and skill have made arthroscopic surgery an equal or better alternative in many cases.

The goal of surgery for shoulder instability is to repair the torn structures caused by the dislocation and to tighten the shoulder capsule just enough to prevent the humerus from dislocating again. If the shoulder capsule is overtightened by surgery, some shoulder motion will be lost, and the athlete will have trouble returning to high-level sports. If the shoulder capsule is not tightened enough, the humeral head may dislocate again. Regardless of whether an open or an arthroscopic technique is used, the front part of the labrum is first examined. A tear in the front part of the labrum is often seen and is termed a *Bankart tear* (named after the physician who discovered it). This part of the labrum has the shoulder capsule ligaments attached to it and must be repaired back to the glenoid socket. Repair is usually done by placing tiny metal or bioabsorbable anchors in the front part of the glenoid socket. Strong suture material attached to the anchors is then used to tie the front part of the labrum back to the front part of the glenoid socket (a *Bankart repair*). This helps restore the bumper effect of the front part of the labrum on the glenoid socket, which helps keep the humeral head from coming out of the front of the shoulder. In addition, Bankart labral repair tightens the front shoulder capsule ligaments that are attached to this part of the labrum. If further tightening of the shoulder is necessary, sutures are then placed in the front part of the shoulder capsule to retighten it.

After surgery for shoulder instability, most patients are placed in a sling for 3 to 4 weeks. The arm is kept near the body, and active motion of the arm away from the body is not allowed for the first 6 weeks after surgery. Approximately 3 months of physical therapy is necessary after surgery to restore shoulder motion and strength. Return to sports generally occurs at about 4 to 6 months after surgery.

Dennis E. Kramer

See also Acromioclavicular (AC) Joint, Separation of; Clavicle (Collarbone) Fracture; Frozen Shoulder; Glenoid Labrum Tear; Shoulder Injuries; Shoulder Instability; Superior Labrum From Anterior to Posterior (SLAP) Lesions

Further Readings

Chen FS, Diaz VA, Loebenberg M, Rosen JE. Shoulder and elbow injuries in the skeletally immature athlete. *J Am Acad Orthop Surg.* 2005;13(3):172–185.

DeBerardino TM, Arciero RA, Taylor DC, Uhorchak JM. Prospective evaluation of arthroscopic stabilization of acute, initial anterior shoulder dislocations in young athletes. Two- to five-year follow-up. *Am J Sports Med.* 2001;29(5):586–592.

Jones KJ, Wiesel B, Ganley TJ, Wells L. Functional outcomes of early arthroscopic Bankart repair in adolescents aged 11 to 18 years. *J Pediatr Orthop.* 2007;27(2):209–213.

McConville OR, Iannotti JP. Partial-thickness tears of the rotator cuff: evaluation and management. *J Am Acad Orthop Surg.* 1999;7(1):32–43.

Meister K. Injuries to the shoulder in the throwing athlete. Part two: evaluation/treatment. *Am J Sports Med.* 2000;28(4):587–601.

Mileski RA, Snyder SJ. Superior labral lesions in the shoulder: pathoanatomy and surgical management. *J Am Acad Orthop Surg.* 1998;6(2):121–131.

Nam EK, Snyder SJ. The diagnosis and treatment of superior labrum, anterior and posterior (SLAP) lesions. *Am J Sports Med.* 2003;31(5):798–810.

Walton J, Paxinos A, Tzannes A, Callanan M, Hayes K, Murrell GA. The unstable shoulder in the adolescent athlete. *Am J Sports Med.* 2002;30(5):758–767.

Yamaguchi K. Mini-open rotator cuff repair: an updated perspective. *Instr Course Lect.* 2001;50:53–61.

SHOULDER INSTABILITY

Glenohumeral instability is a common shoulder disorder, particularly among young athletes. Traditionally, shoulder instability has been divided into two types: those that were initially caused by a traumatic event and those associated with generalized ligamentous laxity.

Peak incidences of traumatic shoulder dislocation occur in a bimodal distribution. Men are at the highest risk of dislocation between 20 and 30 years of age, whereas women more frequently experience dislocation of the shoulder between 61 and 80 years of age. Risk factors for shoulder dislocation include falling on an outstretched arm; a direct blow to the shoulder, as in an automobile accident; force applied to an outstretched arm, as in a football tackle; and forceful throwing, lifting, or hitting. Sports that place an athlete at a higher risk of shoulder dislocation include football, wrestling, and hockey.

Generalized ligamentous laxity can also place an athlete at a higher risk of dislocation. Although ligamentous laxity can be congenital, activities such as swimming, gymnastics, and weight lifting, which frequently subject the shoulder to extremes of glenohumeral motion, can stretch out the capsule and place the shoulder at a higher risk of dislocation.

Anatomy

The glenohumeral joint is made up of a ball-like humeral head rotating on a shallow, dishlike surface, the glenoid. The bony anatomy of the glenohumeral joint allows the shoulder the widest range of motion of any joint in the body. Because of this wide range of motion, the shoulder is very dependent on soft tissue restraints to prevent dislocation.

The soft tissue restraints of the shoulder include the glenoid labrum, the surrounding capsule and ligamentous structures, and the rotator cuff musculature.

The glenoid labrum is a border of soft tissue that surrounds the bone of the glenoid and effectively deepens the glenohumeral articulation. The glenoid labrum may provide stability against humeral head translation.

The capsule extends from the periphery of the glenoid around the humeral head to the periphery of the articular cartilage. The capsule is thickened in three distinct areas. These thickenings make up the glenohumeral ligaments. The ligaments function to stabilize the shoulder by becoming taut in different positions of shoulder motion.

The superior glenohumeral ligament and middle glenohumeral ligament stabilize the shoulder against inferior subluxation or dislocation when the arm is at the patient's side. They also assist in resisting posterior translation. The primary function of the middle glenohumeral ligament is to limit external rotation with the arm at 45° of abduction. The inferior glenohumeral ligament forms a sling with an intervening axillary pouch that tightens anteriorly as the shoulder extends, preventing anterior dislocation, and tightens posteriorly as the shoulder flexes, preventing posterior dislocation.

The surrounding rotator cuff musculature provides dynamic shoulder stabilization. Weakening of the rotator cuff musculature can contribute to shoulder instability.

In 1923, Bankart described a lesion that occurs during a shoulder dislocation and ultimately leads to shoulder instability. The lesion is a detachment of the anterior-inferior portion of the labrum from the rim of the glenoid. The lesion occurs as the labrum is sheared from the glenoid rim during a shoulder dislocation.

In multidirectional instability, the capsule is often enlarged and may be weakened from multiple episodes of subluxation or dislocation.

Causes

It is important to understand the difference between laxity and instability. Laxity refers to the extent to which the humeral head can be translated on the glenoid. Instability is an abnormal increase in glenohumeral motion that causes symptoms such as pain, subluxation, and dislocation and functional symptoms such as catching or locking.

Individuals who have congenitally lax joints are at an increased risk for shoulder instability. Laxity can also be acquired through activities that involve extremes of glenohumeral motion that may stretch out the shoulder capsule, such as swimming, gymnastics, and weight lifting.

The most common direction of traumatic dislocation is anterior. Traumatic anterior dislocation commonly occurs with the arm in a position of abduction/external rotation. Activities that place the shoulder at risk for dislocation and subsequent instability include contact sports, falls on an outstretched arm, direct blows to the shoulder, and forceful throwing, lifting, or hitting. Traumatic dislocations that occur in patients less than 20 years old are at a significant risk for redislocation. A youth or adolescent with a first-time dislocation is at a 70% to 100% risk of dislocating again.

Posterior dislocation occurs when an axial load is placed on a flexed, adducted, internally rotated shoulder. Posterior instability can occur as a result of repetitive episodes of loading the posterior capsule, as is common with an offensive lineman. Other causes of posterior instability include seizures and motor vehicle accidents.

Inferior instability is most commonly associated with multidirectional instability.

Symptoms

An athlete who presents after a traumatic dislocation will often complain of pain that is usually worse with activity or with the arm in certain positions.

The pain is often associated with the direction of the dislocation (i.e., posterior shoulder pain with posterior dislocations). Symptoms may be aggravated by overhead activities, carrying objects at the side, or overuse. Other complaints may include weakness, a sensation of the shoulder slipping out of place, or numbness and tingling of the affected extremity. Nocturnal pain is variable.

As instability worsens, symptoms begin to occur in midranges of glenohumeral motion common to activities of daily living.

Diagnosis

Physical Examination

The physical examination of shoulder instability should begin with an inspection of the shoulder and its surrounding musculature. Findings that may be common with glenohumeral instability include atrophy of the biceps, supraspinatus, or infraspinatus.

The range of motion of the involved shoulder should then be compared with the opposite shoulder. Restrictions to motion as well as hypermobility should be noted.

Special tests for the shoulder include the sulcus sign, the drawer test, the anterior and posterior apprehension test, the relocation and release tests, the load and shift test, and the jerk test.

The drawer test is useful for evaluating increased anterior and posterior shoulder laxity. The examiner performs this test by stabilizing the scapula and clavicle with one hand while gently pushing the humeral head as far forward and then as far back as possible with the other hand. Normal humeral head translation is approximately 50% of its anterior-to-posterior dimension.

Inferior laxity is demonstrated by the sulcus sign. This test is performed with the examiner standing at the patient's side. The patient is encouraged to relax as the examiner grasps the patient's arm just above the elbow and gently pulls distally while observing the lateral acromion. As the humeral head translates inferiorly, a sulcus is formed between the acromion and the humeral head. The size of the sulcus should be compared with the opposite shoulder.

The anterior apprehension test is the classic provocative test for anterior instability. It is performed by placing the arm in 90° abduction,

extension, and external rotation with the elbow flexed to 90°. The examiner then progressively externally rotates the shoulder. A patient with anterior instability will complain of pain in the anterior shoulder or apprehension of impending dislocation.

The relocation test increases the specificity of the anterior apprehension test for cases of subtle instability. It is performed by placing the shoulder in a position of apprehension and then applying a posteriorly directed force over the humeral head. A patient with instability will feel decreased pain and reduced apprehension. When the examiner removes the posterior force, the pain and apprehension return (release test).

Anterior and posterior instability can also be tested with the load and shift test. This test is performed with the patient lying on the examination table. The table serves to stabilize the scapula. The patient's arm is slightly abducted from his or her side. The examiner then stabilizes the scapula with one hand and grasps the proximal humeral shaft with the other hand. While slightly compressing the humeral head against the glenoid, the examiner attempts to slide the proximal humerus off the anterior and then the posterior glenoid rim. In the stable shoulder, anterior or posterior translation of approximately half the distance of the humeral head will occur.

The jerk test is an additional test for posterior shoulder instability. It is performed by placing the patient's arm in 90° flexion, adduction, and internal rotation with the elbow flexed to 90°. The examiner applies a posteriorly directed force at the elbow, attempting to push the humeral head posteriorly off the glenoid. A jerk or clunk is felt as the humerus slips over the edge of the posterior glenoid rim.

Imaging

Imaging of the unstable shoulder should include the three standard views: anterior-posterior (AP), scapular Y, and axillary. Although the dislocated shoulder frequently only involves soft tissue injury, as many as 55% of traumatic dislocations have an associated bony injury.

Additional views that may be helpful in visualizing bony injury include the West Point view and the Stryker notch view. The West Point view is taken with the patient prone, with the arm abducted to 90° and hanging over the side of the table. The radiograph is taken with the X-ray beam aimed anteriorly and 25° medially. It is most helpful in detecting anterior-inferior glenoid rim fractures (bony Bankart lesions).

The Stryker notch view brings Hill-Sachs lesions (humeral head impaction lesions) into view. The radiograph is taken in an anterior-to-posterior direction, aiming the beam 10° cephalad with the patient supine with his or her hand on top of his or her head with the elbow flexed.

Because instability most commonly involves a soft tissue component, magnetic resonance imaging (MRI) is usually performed for diagnosis and surgical planning. To improve visualization of soft tissue avulsions (labral tears), a dye can be injected into the glenohumeral joint prior to the MRI scan (an MR arthrogram). Recent literature states that the sensitivity of an MRI scan alone in diagnosing a labral tear is 91% to 93%. The addition of dye in the glenohumeral joint (MR arthrogram) improves the sensitivity to 96%.

Treatment

Nonsurgical

Treatment of instability is primarily nonsurgical. Rehabilitation usually begins with a period of activity modification and rest. A short period of immobilization may be required for pain control in a patient with multidirectional instability. After a traumatic dislocation, younger patients (less than 30 years old) should be immobilized in a sling for 3 weeks to allow the tissues to heal prior to exercises to restore strength and motion. Older patients are at greater risk for shoulder stiffness but with a reduced risk of developing recurrent instability. Some physicians therefore have patients begin exercises to restore range of motion after only 1 week of immobilization.

Modalities to help reduce pain such as ice, anti-inflammatory medications, and electrical stimulation can also be of great use. Overhead activities are initially avoided. Once the patient's pain is well controlled, an exercise program is instituted to help restore normal, painfree range of motion. Exercises should include strengthening of the deltoid, periscapular, and surrounding rotator cuff musculature.

Surgical

Arthroscopy

Arthroscopy can be used as an effective tool for both diagnosing and treating shoulder instability. Some of the benefits of shoulder arthroscopy include avoiding the morbidity associated with a large incision and releasing the subscapularis muscle from its attachment site on the proximal humerus required in an open surgical approach.

Arthroscopy is additionally beneficial because it allows the physician to visualize the relationship of the humeral head to the glenoid and the integrity of the ligaments and capsule as the shoulder is taken through a range of motion. The labrum can be inspected and probed for any areas of detachment. The shoulder capsule, which is often enlarged and weakened from multiple dislocations, can also be evaluated.

Shoulder instability is treated by tightening the loose shoulder capsule. This is done by placing plicating stitches in the capsule and typing them through special arthroscopic cannulas. The labrum, if torn from its attachment on the glenoid, can be repaired by placing small anchors along the edge of the glenoid. The anchors have a suture attached to them that allows the surgeon to secure the torn labrum back to the bone while it heals.

Open Treatment of Shoulder Instability

Several methods have been developed to treat shoulder instability through an open (nonarthroscopic) procedure. Some of these involve repairing the capsule in a shortened fashion, while others are meant to limit the patient's external rotation to prevent her or him from getting into a position of potential dislocation.

An open procedure is performed by making a longitudinal incision in the axillary crease. Dissection is carried down through the subcutaneous tissues to an interval between the pectoralis major and the deltoid muscles. The subscapularis muscle is then identified and released from its attachment on the proximal humerus. The capsule is then split. Labral tears, if present, are identified and repaired. The capsule can then be tightened on closure.

After Surgery

As a general rule, the shoulder is protected in a sling for 4 to 6 weeks after surgical repair. The sling should be removed several times each day for elbow and wrist range-of-motion exercises.

During the first 2 weeks after surgery, the patient is allowed to perform pendulum-type exercises with the arm hanging at his or her side while he or she gently swings the arm in small circles.

Formal physical therapy begins after the 2-week postoperative visit. Initially, the patient is allowed to forward-flex his or her shoulder to 90°. External rotation is limited to neutral for the first 6 weeks. At 6 weeks, the patient is allowed to increase the external rotation to 30°. Full external rotation range of motion is allowed at 4 months postoperatively. Progressive strengthening exercises are begun at 6 weeks postoperatively. Return to sports is allowed at 4 months postoperatively once 90% of the strength and a functional range of motion have been regained.

Jeffrey Vaughn

See also Acromioclavicular (AC) Joint, Separation of; Clavicle (Collarbone) Fracture; Frozen Shoulder; Glenoid Labrum Tear; Shoulder Injuries; Shoulder Instability; Superior Labrum from Anterior to Posterior (SLAP) Lesions

Further Readings

Bahk M, Keyurapan E, Tasaki A, Sauers EL, McFarland EG. Laxity testing of the shoulder: a review. *Am J Sports Med.* 2007;35(1):131–144.

Gill T, Zarins B. Open repairs for the treatment of anterior shoulder instability. *Am J Sports Med.* 2003;31(1):142–153.

Tennent TD, Beach WR, Meyers JF. A review of the special tests associated with shoulder examination. Part I: the rotator cuff tests. *Am J Sports Med.* 2003;31(1):154–160.

Tennent TD, Beach WR, Meyers JF. A review of the special tests associated with shoulder examination. Part II: laxity, instability, and superior labral anterior and posterior (SLAP) lesions. *Am J Sports Med.* 2003;31(1):154–160.

SHOULDER SUBLUXATION

The shoulder joint is more complex than other joints because it has a full 360° of motion. This is made possible by the structures making up the joint itself. The joint is made up of the placement of the ball of the humerus on the glenoid portion of the scapula. This can be likened to a "bowling ball sitting on a golf tee," where the top portion of the humerus, or head, is the bowling ball and the smaller glenoid is the tee. Just as the ball is held in place by the rim of the tee, the humerus is held in place by sitting on the glenoid and is supported by a rim of cartilage called the labrum, just as a golf tee has a rim. Because this does not allow much stability, there are numerous soft tissue structures to hold this joint together. Ligaments, with the most important being the inferior glenohumeral ligament, hold the humeral head on the glenoid. A soft tissue capsule holds the structure together. Muscles called the supraspinatus (needed for forward flexion), infraspinatus and teres minor (needed for external rotation), and subscapularis (needed for internal rotation) move the humerus and, thus, allow the humerus to move on the glenoid. In most patients, this is a stable arrangement; however, in some, there can be instability or too much perceived movement. Such instability can be intrinsic to an individual. When the instability produces symptoms, then it becomes pathologic and problematic to the patient. When this instability allows the shoulder to ride up on the labrum, producing feelings in the patient as if the shoulder is going to "pop out" or dislocate, which it does not do, the action of the shoulder is referred to as having undergone a subluxation.

Symptoms

Shoulder subluxation is perceived by the patient as a shoulder that is "moving too much," "moving in ways it should not," or "making noise" during activity. Patients often report that the shoulder *feels* as though it were "popping out" but is not actively dislocating. This is especially evident in shoulder-dependent sports such as swimming or throwing sports. In addition to these "unstable" feelings, patients can also feel pain deep in the glenohumeral joint or sometimes numbness going down the same-sided arm. This can be due to the movement of the humerus on the glenoid and by associated contact of nerves close to the joint by the moving humerus. Often, the subluxation will worsen with each successive motion that places the shoulder in the dependent position. This position has the affected arm in 90° flexion and 90° abduction and external rotation. The shoulder does not necessarily have to be in this position for subluxation to be perceived, but it is the more common position in which to feel the shoulder begin to subluxate. Increasing symptomatology, associated numbness, and a feeling as though the shoulder is going to dislocate often bring patients to the physician's office.

Types of Perceived Instability

It is the physician's job to recognize in which way the patient perceives subluxation and what the underlying cause of the movement is. The most common way that patients feel the shoulder moving is with increasing motion forward, or anterior subluxation. Backward, or posterior, motion is relatively rare. Some patients can feel movement more out of the bottom of the shoulder joint, or inferior. Still others can have multidirectional movement, in which they feel the shoulder move in a combination of all these motions. The reasons for a subluxating shoulder can include a genetic predisposition to abnormally loose cartilage that makes up the supporting soft tissue structures, injury to the joint or its surrounding structures, or a combination of both. Sports with a high demand on the shoulder, such as throwing sports, often make subluxating shoulders worse.

History and Physical Examination

The history is often the most important factor in the diagnosis of shoulder subluxation. This aids the physician in determining in which direction the shoulder is moving to produce the feelings of subluxation. Physical examination is also extremely important. Range of motion and strength are assessed to determine if there is a neuromuscular reason for the subluxation. Certain structures, such as a tear in the rim of the glenoid labrum, are tested physically to see if injury to these structures is the cause of the instability. Finally, the physician manipulates the shoulder in various planes in an effort to reproduce the feeling of subluxation within the patient or actively move the shoulder in a position that can make the patient feel as if the shoulder is about to "come out of joint." Often the physician checks one position at a time for movement or complaints of subluxation.

Diagnostic Testing

Diagnostic testing for shoulder subluxation is often directed at the shoulder structures to determine if they are the cause of the abnormal movement. X-rays can determine if there is damage to the bony structures of the shoulder, leading to subluxation. Computed tomography (CT) is also a good test to examine bone. Magnetic resonance imaging (MRI) with the addition of contrast material, called an *MR arthrogram*, can allow the physician to visualize any damage to soft tissue structures as a possible reason for subluxation.

Treatment

Nonsurgical

Treatment for shoulder subluxation is directed toward stabilizing the shoulder and preventing excess movement. The first and least invasive course of treatment is to perform physical therapy to attempt to have the muscles of the shoulder stabilize the humerus and glenoid tighter within the joint. Assistive braces or harnesses can be used for stabilization of the shoulder by preventing movements that would lend the shoulder to dislocation. These can only be used in sports or positions in certain sports that would not require the arm to be in full forward flexion, full abduction, or full external rotation. Return to play can follow physical therapy, provided that the patient has diminished symptoms, full active range of motion of the shoulder, and full strength within the shoulder.

Surgical

If stability cannot be maintained with physical therapy, surgery is often considered. With surgery, if there is a damaged structure, the physician will attempt to repair the damaged structure. With cases of nontraumatic origin, such as genetically "loose" soft tissue, surgery will be attempted to make the shoulder joint soft tissue tighter to hold the humerus on the glenoid to prevent subluxation. Surgery is usually successful. Return to play after surgery for recurrent subluxation is often possible 4 to 6 months after the procedure and associated physical therapy. There is often the risk of recurrent symptoms within the shoulder if the patient returns to sports, especially one that is very shoulder dependent. This is often seen in swimmers. Athletes who were stable postsurgery often again become unstable because of the high demands placed on the shoulder joint by their sport.

R. Robert Franks

See also Acromioclavicular (AC) Joint, Separation of; Shoulder Dislocation; Shoulder Instability

Further Readings

Hunt SA, Kwon YW, Zuckerman JD. The rotator interval: anatomy, pathology, and strategies for treatment. *J Am Acad Orthop Surg.* 2007;15(4):218–227.

Mahaffey BL, Smith PA. Shoulder instability in young athletes. *Am Fam Physician.* 1999;59(10):2773–2782.

McCarty EC, Ritchie P, Gill HS, McFarland EG. Shoulder instability: return to play. *Clin Sports Med.* 2004;23(3):335–351.

McKeag DB, Moeller JL, eds. (2007). *ACSM's Primary Care Sports Medicine.* Philadelphia, PA: Lippincott Williams & Wilkins; 2007.

Sherbondy PS, McFarland EG. Shoulder instability in the athlete. *Phys Med Rehabil Clin N Am.* 2000;11(4):729–743.

Walton J, Paxinos A, Tzannes A, Callanan M, Hayes K, Murrell GA. The unstable shoulder in the adolescent athlete. *Am J Sports Med.* 2002;30(5):758–767.

SICKLE CELL DISEASE

Sickle cell disease (SCD) is caused by a mutation in hemoglobin, the oxygen-carrying component of red blood cells (RBCs). This change in hemoglobin causes RBCs to become abnormal. Normally flexible and oval-shaped, RBCs in SCD lose their flexibility and assume a rigid, "sickle" shape. This change in shape hinders the ability of RBCs to travel through vessels. Since the role of RBCs is to carry oxygen throughout the body, sickling prevents oxygen from getting to vital areas, leading to a number of major complications.

Those who receive two sickle cell genes from their parents present with SCD, while those who receive one sickle cell gene and one normal hemoglobin gene are referred to as sickle cell trait (SCT) carriers. Although carriers possess one sickle gene, they often do not present with the major complications seen in those with two genes due to the one normal hemoglobin gene. Both SCD and SCT protect individuals from malaria, making the sickle cell gene predominant in people (or their descendants) in places where malaria is widespread, such as sub-Saharan Africa. An estimated 8% of African Americans are SCT carriers, and other populations with the sickle gene include the Mediterranean, Middle Eastern, Caribbean, Indian, and South and Central American populations.

Impact on Athletes

The majority of people with SCD do not participate in strenuous physical activity due to the increased risk of sickling caused by lower oxygen levels and anemia resulting from RBC destructions. Although most people with the SCT do not experience any symptoms, intense physical activity can produce exertional sickling. The causes of this exertional sickling are low levels of oxygen, metabolic acidosis, overheated muscles, and RBC dehydration. It is most likely to begin after 2 to 3 minutes of any all-out exertion, and as with SCT, the sickling leads to blockage of the blood vessels and eventual muscle breakdown due to the lack of blood supply. This muscle breakdown can threaten the lives of athletes.

Exertional sickling is extremely dangerous to athletes and ranks as the number four cause of nontraumatic sports deaths in high school and college athletes. In the past 40 years alone, exertional sickling has killed at least 15 football players and accounted for 5% of sudden, nontraumatic sports deaths in high school and college athletes in the past decade. When comparing SCT with normal controls, the relative risk of exercise-related death was 30 times greater with SCT. The data show that the more strenuous the activity is, the greater the sickling.

Signs and Symptoms

Sickling collapse due to exertional sickling is often confused with cardiac or heat collapse. However, there are subtle differences. Athletes with sickling collapse do not lose consciousness, and they often experience cramping, not seen with cardiac collapse. Unlike heat collapse, the core temperature in those with exertional sickling is not greatly elevated.

Other signs and symptoms include the following:

- Cramping with no prior muscle twinges
- Pain
- Inability to catch one's breath
- Fatigue
- Generalized muscle weakness

If treated appropriately, sickling players recover quickly.

Safety

Sickling collapse due to exertional sickling is a medical emergency. The athletes should immediately have their vital signs checked and should be administered oxygen. The administration of oxygen often can prevent further worsening of symptoms as the sickling cells will return to their normal shape. If the athlete's condition does not improve, he or she should immediately be brought to the hospital.

Although SCT athletes are at increased risk of sudden death, this should not prevent them from participating in sports. If simple precautions are taken, the risk of exertional sickling greatly decreases. The following are some of these precautions:

- Gradual progressions in training with longer periods of rest
- Stopping participation in the activity if any of the above symptoms present themselves
- Emphasizing hydration
- Avoiding heat stress
- Having supplemental oxygen available
- Educating athletes on the signs and symptoms

Screening

All newborns in the United States are screened for the sickle cell gene. Athletes who are carriers of the trait should inform their coaches as well as trainers of their condition to ensure a safe environment. Screening is inexpensive and reliable. In the absence of screening or if an athlete is unsure of his or her status, screening should be completed prior to any strenuous exercise regimen.

Jeffrey R. Bytomski and Harvey E. Montijo

See also Epstein-Barr Virus, Infectious Mononucleosis, and Splenomegaly; Infectious Diseases in Sports Medicine; Presports Physical Examination

Further Readings

Eichner ER. Sickle cell trait. *J Sport Rehabil.* 2007;16(3):197–203.

Holmes PS, Kerle KK, Seto CK. Sickle cell trait and sudden death in athletes. *Am Fam Physician.* 1998;58(8):1760–1761.

Kerle KK, Runkle GP. Sickle cell trait and sudden death in athletes. *JAMA.* 1996;276(18):1472.

Monchanin G, Connes P, Wouassi D, et al. Hemorheology, sickle cell trait, and alpha-thalassemia in athletes: effects of exercise. *Med Sci Sports Exerc.* 2005;37(7):1086–1092.

Side Stitch

Side stitches are associated with vigorous physical activities such as walking fast, running, swimming, cycling, and aerobic exercise. The longer medical term—*exercise-related transient abdominal pain*—is both a definition and a description of the symptoms: a painful but temporary condition associated with exercise that affects the lower (right) side of the abdominal wall.

A study conducted by Morton and colleagues (2005) in Australia, and published in the *Journal of Science and Medicine in Sport*, showed that among 848 distance runners, 27% experienced side stitches and 46% felt pain on the right side. Side stitches seem to affect exercisers below the age of 20 more than they do older adults, women more often than men, and those who are not in good physical condition more than well-conditioned individuals. Relatively few major studies have investigated the topic, and while information coming from those studies is relevant, it cannot be considered conclusive.

Causes

Side stitches among runners may be the result of the pumping action of legs putting pressure on the diaphragm from below, with the rapid breathing associated with strenuous physical activity expanding the lungs and placing pressure on the diaphragm from above at the same time. The combined effect is one of pinching the diaphragm, reducing the flow of blood and oxygen, and causing noticeable pain in the side. While this scenario seems plausible, it is a theory that has not been proven by scientific research and one that does not seem to account for side stitches in exercisers who do not walk or run.

When a fitness walker or distance runner pounds his or her legs against the ground while taking rapid breaths, the connective tissue that extends from the diaphragm to the liver can be stretched. That stretched, stressed tissue could also be responsible for causing pain in the side.

The amount and type of food consumed before an exercise session may place an additional stress on the diaphragm, again potentially causing side stitches. Whether the food-exercise association is real, there are ways to minimize the negative effects of foods and beverages on exercise without compromising athletic performance. These strategies are discussed below, in the Prevention section.

Although not warming up adequately before exercise has been mentioned as a possible cause of side stitches, there is no evidence to support that claim. In fact, the Australian study found that the incidence of side pain occurred equally during the first, middle, and latter segments of the 14-kilometer race. If the side stitches had occurred only during the initial part of the race, an inadequate warm-up might have been the cause. That was not the case.

In spite of some logical explanations and a few well-designed studies, the exact cause of side stitches remains an exercise science mystery. Nevertheless, scientists, sports medicine physicians, elite athletes, and weekend exercisers agree that the pain is as real as it is temporary and that the discomfort can be minimized, if not eliminated.

Symptoms

Side stitches have two distinguishing symptoms. The first is a stabbing pain on the lower right side of the abdomen, and the second is pain that subsides almost immediately after the cessation of exercise. Side pain that persists regardless of exercise patterns is not exercise-related transient abdominal pain, and people who have that symptom should seek medical attention.

Treatment

The immediate treatment for side stitches is simply to stop doing whatever causes the pain, wait a couple of minutes, and resume the activity. Some people try to temporarily decrease the pain by stopping, bending forward, and tightening the abdominal muscles. There is no long-term treatment, but there are ways to lessen the probability that the condition will develop in the first place.

Prevention

The measures a person takes to avoid side stitches may be effective for that individual but not necessarily for all exercisers. Ten suggestions for preventing side stitches follow:

1. To focus on breathing patterns that might be associated with side stitches, exhale through pursed lips.

2. Before exercising, stretch by extending the left arm upward and leaning toward the right. Hold for 20 to 30 seconds, and repeat the stretch with the right arm up while leaning to the left.

3. Practice breathing deeply during exercise to stretch the diaphragm.

4. Change patterns of breathing while running or walking. For example, inhale, hold for one second, exhale. Then inhale, hold for 2 seconds, exhale. Next, inhale, hold for 3 seconds, exhale.

5. Change the pace of walking or running during an exercise session.

6. To address potential nutrition-exercise interaction, eat moderately sized, low-fat meals 2 to 3 hours before a training session or event.

7. Experiment with various sources of calories to discover the ones your body can tolerate without developing side stitches. Examples include energy gels, sports drinks, fruits, and grains.

8. Do not test a new or different kind of food or beverage the day of an important event.

9. Eat a familiar, easily digested, low-fat or no-fat snack an hour before a workout. Half a sandwich, a sports drink, fig bars, and granola bars are possible choices.

10. Drink 10 to 16 ounces (oz; 1 oz = 29.57 milliliters) (two cups) of cold fluid approximately 15 to 30 minutes before practice sessions or athletic events, and drink 4 to 8 oz of cold fluid every 10 to 15 minutes during exercise.

Jim Brown

See also Abdominal Injuries; Dietitian/Sports Nutritionist; Nutrition and Hydration

Further Readings

Morton DP, Callister R. Factors influencing exercise-related transient abdominal pain. *Med Sci Sports Exerc.* 2002;34(5):745–749.

Morton DP, Richards D, Callister R. Epidemiology of exercise-related transient abdominal pain at the Sydney City to Surf community run. *J Sci Med Sport.* 2005;8(2):152–162.

SINUSITIS IN ATHLETES

Sinusitis (or rhinosinusitis) is the inflammation of the sinus airspaces and epithelial lining within the bones of the face. The symptoms associated with it are responsible for a significant percentage of athletes' visits to training rooms and physicians throughout the year. It can be difficult to differentiate between sinus infections and other upper respiratory infections because the symptoms overlap. Understanding the difference, however, can help an athlete return to play and perform at a normal level more quickly.

Anatomy

The sinuses are air pockets within the skull that include the maxillary sinuses, located within the cheek bones; the ethmoid sinuses, located behind the bridge of the nose; the frontal sinuses, located above the eyes in the center of the eyebrows; and the sphenoid sinus, located behind the ethmoid sinuses and behind the eyes. When the mucus-clearing cilia of the epithelial tissue that lines the sinuses cannot function due to swelling and inflammation, mucus is trapped, and an excellent growth medium for bacteria is provided, resulting in symptoms usually correlating with the location of each sinus. Because the epithelial lining of the sinuses and nasal passage is the same as that seen in much of the respiratory system, sinusitis can also cause problems anywhere in the respiratory tract.

Diagnosis

Although bacteria and viruses account for a majority of cases, allergens, smoke, pollution, and cold air can also cause rhinosinusitis. A careful history can usually elicit the likelihood of the latter diagnoses. Sinusitis is a self-limiting condition 80% to 90% of the time. To avoid unnecessary antibiotic use and expensive testing, clinical prediction rules have been developed on the basis of meta-analyses of numerous studies. According to the Cochrane Database and the Agency for Health Care Research and Quality (AHRQ), the most significant clinical predictors for the diagnosis of sinusitis, regardless of symptom duration, and therefore for the consideration for antibiotics, are unilateral purulence, predominantly unilateral facial pain, bilateral purulence, and the presence of pus in the nasal cavity. When other minor symptoms such as fever, headache, anosmia, facial congestion, fatigue, cough, and dental or ear pain have been present for more than 7 days, antibiotics should also be considered. The use of sinus radiographs and limited computed tomography (CT) scans of the sinuses for the diagnosis of sinusitis should be reserved for recalcitrant cases lasting more than 30 days and/or two antibiotic treatment failures.

Asthma and allergy sufferers can have an allergic rhinosinusitis with symptoms mimicking those of acute sinusitis. If any of the acute sinusitis clinical predictors become evident, then antibiotics should be prescribed. Migraines can often be mistakenly attributed to sinusitis when the main complaint is either sinus pain or headache in the absence of other symptoms. A careful history and physical exam should screen out the athletes with sinusitis.

Treatment

The *Sanford Guide to Antimicrobial Therapy* and most primary care and otolaryngology organizations recommend mucolytics, analgesics, decongestants, and sinus irrigation in the early stages of infection. With athletes who may undergo drug testing, providers should be aware of current banned substances such as pseudoephedrine. A list of these can be found on the U.S. Olympic Committee (USOC) and sports governing board websites. In most cases of uncomplicated acute sinusitis, amoxicillin for 7 to 10 days provides adequate coverage. There is no evidence that non–penicillin-based antibiotics offer any additional benefit over penicillins. In penicillin-allergic patients, sulfa drugs, macrolides such as azithromycin and clarithromycin, cephalosporins, and quinolones are good substitutes, but providers should be aware of the potential tendinopathic side effect of quinolones. In more serious cases or treatment failures, amoxicillin-clavulanic acid for 14 to 21 days is recommended. In athletes diagnosed with sinus infections who have comorbid asthma and allergic rhinitis, nasal steroids may enhance mucociliary clearance and reduce nasal congestion. Aggressive long-term treatment in these athletes with nasal steroids, nonsedating antihistamines, nasal irrigation with saline, and/or leukotriene inhibitors can reduce the frequency of sinus infections and improve lung volumes, fatigue, and overall athletic performance.

Return to Sports

Most athletes with a diagnosis of sinusitis can return to practice immediately. Unless they have a fever, severe fatigue, or a significant symptomatic drop in peak flows, there is no specific reason to hold them out from competition or training. Swimmers and divers with sinusitis, significant eustachian tube dysfunction, serous otitis media, or bilateral facial congestion have increased risk for tympanic membrane rupture and should be watched closely. These athletes also appear to be more susceptible to sinus infections, possibly due to the effect of chlorine as an irritant. A tympanogram to monitor tympanic membrane mobility may be useful in providing clearance to divers with persistent symptoms. Ear plugs are not recommended for water athletes, but nose plugs can be used in athletes susceptible to sinusitis.

James Dunlap

See also Allergies; Infectious Diseases in Sports Medicine; Physiological Effects of Exercise on Cardiopulmonary System

Further Readings

Agency for Health Care Policy and Research. *Diagnosis and Treatment of Acute Bacterial Rhinosinusitis. Summary, Evidence Report/Technology Assessment.* Rockville, MD: Agency for Health Care Policy and Research; 1999 (AHCPR Publication No. 99-E015).

Leipzig JR, Slavin RG. Sinusitis in athletes. In: Weiler JM, ed. *Allergic and Respiratory Disease in Sports Medicine.* New York, NY: Informa Health Care; 1997:207–222.

Williams JW Jr, Aguilar C, Makela M, et al. Antibiotic use for acute maxillary sinusitis. *Cochrane Database Syst Rev.* 2000;(2):CD000243.

SKIING, INJURIES IN

Skiing, an alpine sport and popular winter pastime, is enjoyed in many countries by millions of people at more than 300 facilities in the world's mountainous regions. The skier slides down a naturally or artificially snow-covered hill on skis attached to the foot through boots and bindings. *Telemark skiing* refers to a skiing style and a specific nomenclature in which the only connection to the ski is through a binding attachment of the ski boot at the toes with the heel being free, as is the case with all cross-country skis. The emergence of new technologies and ski designs as well as skiing techniques and interests have led to the further development of alpine or downhill skiing and its numerous sport disciplines, together with cross-country skiing and, most recently, snowboarding, an alternative form in which both the athlete's feet are placed on a single board. The rapid evolution of these sports has been spurred by the innovation and creativity of sport enthusiasts as well as advances in equipment design and manufacture. New disciplines are continually being introduced as the sport continues to develop over time.

Ski Disciplines

The International Ski Federation (FIS) administers the following sport disciplines:

Alpine Skiing. This includes Downhill (DH), Super-G (SG), Giant Slalom (GS), and Slalom (SL). Downhill is considered to be the showcase sports event, with the longest distance and the greatest speed. Downhill and Super-G are considered the speed events, while Giant Slalom and Slalom are considered the technical events. Slalom is the shortest of the tech events, with a zigzag race across the ski hill carving a path around gates. There is also an event termed the Combined (CO; in Europe, K), composed of the combined efforts of two separate races—the Downhill and Slalom—which are run on courses that are shorter than normal. More recently, an event called the Super Combined (SC) was introduced with a shorter downhill and a single slalom, both run on the same day.

Cross-Country Skiing. This is the original and most popular Nordic ski sport. Initially cross-country skiing meant only one technique, in which a "diagonal stride" was performed in prepared ski tracks. In the 1980s, the "skating" technique was popularized and was considered to be more of a free technique than a "classical" stride, in which skiers today use a trackless course except during tricky turns or transitional sections. Cross-country skiing is a rugged mix of endurance and speed, with a variety of race distances ranging from 800-meter (m) sprints to 50-kilometer (km) events.

Nordic Combined Skiing. This is a combination of the two main elements of Nordic skiing, cross-country skiing and jumping. The traditional competition entailed a 90-m jumping competition followed by 15 km of skiing. Ski jumping is one of the most spectacular winter sports because athletes fly through the air traveling distances greater than a football field down a snowy slope.

Freestyle Skiing. This in its earliest form was named for the creative elements and "free" components of skiing performance, which included ballet, moguls, and an aerial maneuver. In 2000, ballet was dropped, and the disciplines of moguls and aerials flourished. In aerials, skiers are launched 50 feet (17 m) or more into the air off a "kicker" to land on a steep slope while performing intricate twists and flips. Moguls is the pulsating sport event where skiers maneuver through a treacherous course of bumps, with two obligatory air jumps that are scored by the judges along with the speed of the run to determine the winner.

Skiing for the Physically Disabled. This gained momentum in the 1960s and was originally called "handicapped skiing." Disabled skiing began as a rehab and recreational activity for people with mobility impairments. Eventually, it also became a competitive environment with disciplines in alpine races and cross-country events. Disabled skiers are classified according to their disability, which includes 12 basic classes along with 3 blind classifications. The FIS uses a 3-class system: sit-skiers, stand-ups, and blind.

Promoting Safety

The United States Ski and Snowboard Association (USSA) is the national governing body of the United States for Olympic Skiing and Snowboarding and is the parent organization of U.S. Ski Team and U.S. Snowboarding.

The promotion of safety and the enhancement of the overall experience for skiing enthusiasts is undertaken by an association called the National Ski Patrol (NSP), which follows a creed of "service and safety." The NSP was originally organized as a committee of the USSA (formerly known as the National Ski Association) back in 1938. In 1980, this nonprofit organization was recognized with a federal charter by the U.S. Congress to promote safety and health in skiing and other outdoor winter recreational activities. Today, its membership exceeds 26,000, with more than 600 ski patrols throughout the United States. NSP has evolved from its infancy as a service organization to a professional education association responsible for the development of, and education in, safety and emergency care training methods.

Although skiing and snowboarding are commonly depicted as highly dangerous, deaths associated with the sport are rare. During the period from 1991 to 2003, a total of 469 traumatic deaths occurred at ski resorts in the United States. Collisions of all sorts, but chiefly with trees, account for 90% of the fatalities.

The issue of helmet use in skiing and snowboarding continues to be debated. Helmet use is currently accepted by approximately 38% of skiing enthusiasts but has been steadily on the rise at a rate of nearly 4% annually. Although helmet use has been shown to reduce the number of head injuries by 30% to 50%, this is limited to less serious injuries. Non–helmet users' risk of death from head injuries is two times greater than the risk for those involved in accidents while wearing helmets. In very high-speed collisions, helmet use has not resulted in a reduction of fatalities because helmets are not designed to encounter the extreme forces involved at high speeds.

Orthopedic Ski Injuries

The most common injury in skiing is attributed to the knee joint. Injuries to this particular joint are typically identified as soft tissue and ligamentous type injuries, with the anterior cruciate ligament (ACL), the ligament inside the knee joint that prevents anterior displacement, being the most commonly injured tissue. An injury to this ligament is typically the result of a fall that causes a distribution of forces and an increase in the torque absorbed by the knee. The ski itself acts as a lever arm that significantly increases these forces transmitted through the knee during a fall. This is why proper equipment and maintenance of ski bindings are essential. It is important that the binding-release mechanisms activate during a fall to prevent significant injury to the knee.

The medial collateral ligament (MCL), which is the supporting ligamentous structure on the inside aspect of the knee, and the meniscus, the cartilage tissue inside the knee joint, are the next commonly damaged tissues in the lower leg. The ACL and the meniscus are typically repaired with surgical intervention to prevent long-term consequences to the knee joint. MCL injuries are not typically treated surgically but require a rehabilitation intervention strategy for full recovery. The relative frequency of lower leg fractures continues to decline, which can be attributed to better equipment, better binding

technology, and shorter skis, particularly the shorter tail on carving skies, which has revolutionized the recreation industry.

Injuries to the head and face are typically the next most common in skiing. Concussions and contusions acquired when a skier falls and comes into contact with the snow surface at significant forces result in a higher frequency of reported trauma. Fractures of the skull and closed-head injuries are the most frequent traumas that result in head-related traumatic deaths. Attention to concussions and any mild traumatic brain injuries is essential to recovery so that the athlete does not return to the sport before proper recovery has been confirmed. Many head injuries are complicated by the fact that they recur over the course of a day or an entire ski trip, leading to complications and long-term consequences. Another frequent injury to the facial region is due to t-bars and poles and accidents that occur while getting on and off lifts. This includes facial cuts, knocked-out teeth, bloody noses, eye injuries, and ear cuts or abrasions following contact with the snow.

Upper extremity injuries in the skiing population occur much less frequently than in the snowboarding population. Most commonly, typical injuries reported in the literature include fractures of the wrist and forearm as a result of falling on an outstretched limb. Shoulder dislocations predominate for the same reason but more typically to an outstretched arm reaching backward. The shoulder essentially becomes unstable and pops out of joint completely. A dislocation is quite different from a shoulder separation because it involves the shoulder joint (known as the *glenohumeral joint,* the articulation of the head of the humerus with the glenoid fossa of the scapula) and requires a much greater traumatic force for injury to occur. A dislocation is different from a subluxation because the joint actually displaces completely—it doesn't just slide to the edge of the rim and return to its normal position. A separation usually involves the *acromioclavicular (AC) joint,* a supporting structure at the end of the clavicle.

The so-called *skier's thumb* is caused by injury that results when a ski pole and, more conspicuously, the wrist strap force the thumb away from the axis of the hand, resulting in a ligamentous injury. There are two common strap grips, the traditional and the saber, resulting in injury because the thumb cannot get out of the way during the fall, causing trauma to the ulnar collateral ligament of the thumb. This ligament connects the bones on the inside aspect of the thumb (more specifically the metacarpal and the proximal phalanx) and is typically the most commonly injured extremity next to the knees, which are sprained. Because it plays a major role in our grasping, pinching, and stabilizing objects in our hand, the injury is often very debilitating. Typical treatment following proper evaluation and diagnosis is immobilization for up to 6 weeks in less traumatic situations. In severe cases, however, surgery is recommended to repair the injured ligament. The best prevention strategy would be to use strapless poles so that one falls on the palm of the hand rather than a thumb-restricted hand with a pole in between. Fractures of the lower arm are also common, including fractures to the radius, the ulna, and the scaphoid bone in the hand.

Spinal injuries are not very common, but they still account for almost 5% of the fatalities that occur on the slopes. Injuries to the cervical spine are the most traumatic. Cervical vertebrae may be fractured as the result of a fall, whether it be due to compression, rotation, or hyperextension. Such injury potentially results in damage to the spinal cord, which is life threatening.

Nonorthopedic Ski Injuries

Other common skiing injuries that are less serious but still debilitating include frostbite, dehydration, and sunburn. Sunburn results from solar ultraviolet (UV) radiation, not from the heat. Sun exposure on cold, snowy days without any protection often results in sunburn, particularly in young children. It is essential that prevention be emphasized while skiing anytime. Hypothermia results when the core body temperature drops below 95 °F. Exposure to cold environments, particularly in the presence of wet, windy conditions, can lead to the loss of body heat very quickly. Recognizing the signs and symptoms, such as confusion, slurred speech, fatigue, exhaustion, shivering, and loss of motor control, necessitates immediate action. The key is to eliminate the exposure and warm the individual. Hypothermia may lead to cardiac arrest; therefore, close observation is extremely important. Frostbite is literally frozen body tissue. Children are at a much greater risk than adults because they lose body heat more rapidly and are reluctant to protect against exposure. Treatment typically includes removing the wet clothing and warming the exposed body parts in warm—not hot—water and prevention from additional exposure. Following an appropriate immediate treatment strategy, medical care is advised.

Preventing Ski Injuries

There are several ways to prevent serious injuries as a skier. This includes maintaining your equipment every season by having a certified ski technician service your skis and bindings every year. Proper binding release and new advances in binding technology are the main reason for ski injuries declining. The skier should always make sure that his or her boots fit properly. Use of protective eyewear and a helmet is recommended. One of the best ways to prepare for the upcoming ski season and to prevent injury on the slopes is to maintain a strength-and-endurance exercise program. Skiing requires aerobic power and strength, even at the beginning of the season; trying to "ski oneself into shape" is not recommended. Some strength exercises that will prove useful are leg presses, squats, hamstring curls, lateral leg raises, and core exercises such as crunches, sit-ups, and side bends. For enhancing aerobic capacity, cycling with the seat adjusted high at >80 revolutions/minute (rpm), running, swimming, and using a jump rope, ski machines, stepping machines, and elliptical trainers are recommended.

Richard Quincy and Grant Armour

See also Conditioning; Frostbite and Frost Nip; Snowboarding, Injuries in

Further Readings

Alpine ski injuries. http://www.ski-injury.com/specific-sports/alpine. Accessed June 24, 2010.

American Academy of Orthopedic Surgeons. Position statement: Helmet use in skiing and snow boarding. http://www.aaos.org/about/papers/position/1152.asp. Accessed June 21, 2010.

Burtscher M, Gatterer H, Flatz M, et al. Effects of modern ski equipment on the overall injury rate and the pattern of injury location in Alpine skiing. *Clin J Sport Med.* 2008;18(4):355–357.

Chaze B, McDonald P. Head injuries in winter sports: downhill skiing, snowboarding, sledding, snowmobiling, ice skating and ice hockey. *Phys Med Rehabil Clin N Am.* 2009;20(1):287–293.

Ekeland A, Rodven A. Injury trends in Norwegian ski resorts in the 10 year period 1996–2006. *J ASTM Int.* 2008;5(6). http://www.astm.org/digital_library/journals/jai/pages/jai101620.htm. Accessed June 21, 2010.

Goulet C, Hagel BE, Hamel D, Légaré G. Self-reported skill level and injury severity in skiers and snowboarders. *J Sci Med Sport.* 2010;13(1):39–41.

Johnson R, Ettlinger C, Shealy J. Update on injury trends in Alpine skiing. *J ASTM Int.* 2008;5(10). http://www.astm.org/digital_library/journals/jai/pages/jai102046.htm. Accessed June 21, 2010.

McBeth PB, Ball CG, Mulloy RH, Kirkpatrick AW. Alpine ski and snowboarding traumatic injuries: incidence, injury patterns, and risk factors for 10 years. *Am J Surg.* 2009;197(5):560–564.

Stay safe in snow. http://www.ski-injury.com/latest_news. Accessed June 24, 2010.

Skill Acquisition in Sports

Humans acquire skills, sometimes deliberately, sometimes incidentally, and often by necessity. Skill can be defined as the achievement of an intended outcome repeatedly, with economy of both time and effort (which is logical, given that conservation of energy has been the primary driver in the evolution of most organisms). In sports, acquisition of skill can refer to movement (learning specific ways in which to move in order to achieve a movement goal) or the cognitions associated with movement (e.g., learning when and where to move). In both instances, the "skill" shows improvement as a function of appropriate practice, accompanied by increasingly consistent performance associated with greater persistence and, eventually, adaptable performance in a wide range of situations or contexts.

Our understanding of skill acquisition has its beginnings in work that examined the way in which people acquire telegraphy skills—the ability to transmit and translate the complex dots, dashes, and pauses of Morse code—which was the Internet of the 1800s. The work established that it takes many years of training to become truly skilled, variability of performance decreases over time, and events that disrupt the performance of beginners are less likely to disrupt the performance of experts. The work also suggested that skill acquisition is not necessarily continuous but that plateaus can occur, during which practice does not appear to take effect. Shortly afterward, a universal law of learning was realized. This was the power law of practice, which characterizes skill acquisition as having the greatest rate of change early in practice, with gradual reductions in rate of change occurring as a function of increasing amounts of practice. The role of practice in skill acquisition has received much consideration, not surprisingly given the remarkable feats of skill so often seen in sport. While it is unlikely that there will ever be a definitive clarification of whether those of us who display such high levels of skill are a freak of nature or the function of nurture, there is no doubt that the level of skill that most of us achieve is closely associated with the degree to which we devote time and effort to practice the skill.

Two approaches dominate the study of skill acquisition in sport: information processing approaches and ecological-dynamical approaches.

Information Processing Accounts of Skill Acquisition

The information processing approach to skill acquisition evolved from cognitive psychological characterizations of the human brain as a computer that processes data from the stream of information elicited by the sensory organs and produces an output specific to the "software" that has been loaded. The approach supposes that the flow of information from our senses is of no value until it is converted to symbolic representations that guide movement with commands that are programmed either in advance as some sort of movement plan or schema (open-loop models) or modified on the basis of comparing available afferent information with central representations of the sensory feedback generated by previous successful movements (closed-loop systems).

The approach implies that repetition allows the internal representations to be updated, adapted, and refined (e.g., with knowledge of the results) to produce increasingly efficient movement that progresses from a consciously controlled, cognitive stage of information processing that is rule based, slow, and erratic to an unconsciously controlled, automatic stage that is procedural, fast, and effortless. This fundamental, stages-of-learning distinction is common across the numerous psychological theories of skill acquisition. Recently, it has been argued that the cognitive stage may be superfluous to motor learning and that the learner does not therefore need to progress through such a stage before reaching later autonomous stages that reflect expert performance. It has even been suggested that advantages accrue from avoiding the cognitive stage. By using *implicit* motor learning techniques that prevent the accumulation of explicit or declarative knowledge during the cognitive stages of skill acquisition, researchers have trained people in skills that are more stable under conditions of psychological stress, multitasking, and even fatigue.

Ecological-Dynamical Approaches to Skill Acquisition

An ecological approach to skill acquisition grew out of dissatisfaction with the view that there is a need to process information from the senses before movement can be produced efficiently. In *The Ecological Approach to Visual Perception*, J. J. Gibson (1979) argued that the direct interaction between an organism and its environment specifies *affordances* (the personal possibilities for an action or behavior); information obtained by perception, therefore, does not require elaboration in the manner suggested by information processing accounts, implying that movements can be initiated directly by perception and that perception and action are mutually dependent.

Coupled with the ecological approach, a dynamical systems view of motor behavior has emerged that views biological organisms as capable of dynamically self-organizing in response to constantly interfacing with their environment, much in the way that the study of thermodynamics deals with open systems that self-organize into spatial and temporal patterns that can be defined by one or two specific order parameters.

This view progressed from the work of N. A. Bernstein, who in his book *The Coordination and Regulation of Movement* (1967) suggested that the human body (the motor apparatus) has evolved with an almost limitless array of coordination possibilities to respond with dexterity to the host of motor problems that constantly emerge in the environment. Bernstein viewed skill acquisition as a degrees-of-freedom problem in which the learner must find a way to coordinate the many degrees of freedom available within the motor system. He suggested that this is done by constraining the muscles to act as synergies (i.e., coordinative structures) that can be controlled without cognition. Initially, this requires execution of the movement/skill to be simplified by freezing some of the degrees of freedom (i.e., by locking up various joints) and releasing the degrees of freedom as movement competence proceeds and later by exploiting the energetic forces that exist within the actor-environment interface (e.g., inertia, momentum). This focus on movement constraints within an ecological framework that models the human movement apparatus as a dynamic system attracted to a stable coordination pattern offers an alternative to the traditional information processing approach to skill acquisition in sports.

Rich S. W. Masters and Bruce Abernethy

See also Attention Focus in Sports; Sport and Exercise Psychology

Further Readings

Bernstein NA. *The Coordination and Regulation of Movement.* London, UK: Pergamon Press; 1967.

Ericsson KA, Krampe R, Tesch-Römer C. The role of deliberate practice in the acquisition of expert performance. *Psychol Rev.* 1993;100:363–406.

Fitts PM, Posner MI. *Human Performance.* Belmont, CA: Brooks/Cole; 1967.

Gibson JJ. *The Ecological Approach to Visual Perception.* Boston, MA: Houghton Mifflin; 1979.

Handford C, Davids K, Bennett S, Button C. Skill acquisition in sport: some applications of an evolving practice ecology. *J Sports Sci.* 1997;15(6):621–640.

Kelso JA. Phase transitions and critical behavior in human bimanual coordination. *Am J Physiol.* 1984;246(6, pt 2):R1000–R1004.

Kugler PN, Kelso JAS, Turvey MT. On the concept of coordinative structures as dissipative structures: I. Theoretical lines of convergence. In: Stelmach GE, Requin J, eds. *Tutorials in Motor Behavior.* New York, NY: North-Holland; 1980:3–47.

Masters RSW, Maxwell JP. Implicit motor learning, reinvestment and movement disruption: what you don't know won't hurt you. In: Williams AM, Hodges NJ, eds. *Skill Acquisition in Sport: Research, Theory and Practice.* London, UK: Routledge; 2004:207–228.

Schmidt RA. A schema theory of discrete motor skill learning. *Psychol Rev.* 1975;82:225–260.

SKIN CONDITIONS IN WRESTLERS

No other sport is probably more closely associated with skin lesions and infections than the sport of wrestling. Because wrestling involves direct contact, the chances of transmission to an athlete are higher than in most sports. Transmission can occur most obviously by skin-to-skin contact, but can also be spread by contact with objects such as a mat or headgear. While skin infections were once considered a nuisance, they can now be deadly or debilitating, and their proper identification and treatment have never been more important. As discussion of every skin condition seen in wrestling is beyond the scope of this article, the most common conditions seen in the sport are addressed here.

Bacterial Infections

Impetigo

The most common bacterial infection seen in wrestling is impetigo. The bacteria usually responsible are *Staphylococcus* or *Streptococcus*. The bacteria are spread from person to person or by shared equipment or surfaces. The most common place to see impetigo is in areas where the skin is exposed. Honey-crusted lesions that are often seeping fluid characterize the disease. The area around them may be red, and the patient may have itching. The infection is highly contagious. When the condition is discovered, the athlete should be removed immediately from competition. A culture can definitively identify the organism, but diagnosis is often based on the uniqueness of the lesion. Treatment consists of topical antibiotics for small lesions and oral antibiotics for larger patches of lesions. Return to sports is generally after 5 days of antibiotic treatment, and when all the lesions have dried and crusted over. They should also be covered with a gas-permeable bandage.

Folliculitis

Folliculitis is a common term referring to infection of the hair follicles by bacteria. It often occurs after a wrestler suffers an abrasion from the mat or from clothing. Small, pus-filled follicles characterize the infection. Treatment is imperative to prevent secondary infection. Topical antibiotics are often prescribed to treat this infection. A gas-permeable dressing should cover the affected area while the athlete is actively infected. In most instances, athletes do not need to be removed from competition when suffering from folliculitis.

Furunculosis

Furunculosis is a form of folliculitis in which a "boil" develops. The bacteria usually responsible for this infection are *Staphylococcus* or *Streptococcus*. Again, it commonly occurs from an abrasion from the mat or from clothing. It is characterized by a large, red, often pus-filled raised lesion on exposed areas of the skin. Topical and, if warranted, oral antibiotics are used to treat this infection. If pus is present, often physicians will open the lesion and allow it to drain while the patient is being treated with antibiotics. If the lesion can be adequately covered, there is no pus drainage, and the athlete does not have any ill effects from the lesion, then he or she can participate in sports during treatment.

Methicillin-Resistant Staphylococcus Aureus

The emergence of methicillin-resistant *Staphylococcus aureus* (MRSA) has become a great concern in wrestling. These bacteria are resistant to some of the most common antibiotics prescribed for skin infections. MRSA is often believed to start as a lesion that looks like a "spider bite" or boil. It is often a raised, red lesion that may or may not have pus at its center. If not identified and treated quickly, the infection can advance through a limb or disseminate through the body. If this happens, patients may have some of the typical signs of systemic infections, including a fever and chills. Identification of the bacteria can be done via a culture. Treatment includes opening and drainage of the wound followed by antibiotic therapy. More general antibiotics are given first and tailored to drugs that the MRSA is susceptible to once the bacteria are identified and susceptibility to antibiotics is determined via culture. Treatment is begun with a high suspicion of MRSA infection before the cultures are returned. Again, return to sports is allowed when all the lesions have dried and crusted and any systemic symptoms have resolved after antibiotic treatment. Some patients, however, are chronic carriers of MRSA. Doing swabs of the nasal passages, groin, or axillae, where MRSA is known to colonize, often leads to their discovery. These patients are often placed on antibiotics, either topically or orally, to try to definitively eradicate the infection.

Acne Vulgaris

Athletes are not immune to acne vulgaris, one of the most common bacterial infections found in the general population. Acne vulgaris is caused by bacterial growth in the pores of the skin secondary to androgen stimulation that results in unorganized keratinization and irritation of the skin. Stress, both mechanical and emotional, as well as certain drugs, cosmetics, and foods, can make the acne worse. Acne is typified by the blackheads and whiteheads on a red base seen most commonly on the face but also found on any surface of the body. The acne lesions are often characteristic, and no further laboratory work-up is needed to identify the condition. Acne is treated using topical bactericidals, topical and oral antibiotics, topical and oral retinoids, hormonal treatments, phototherapy, or laser therapy. These treatments may be carried out alone or in combination to try to control the outbreaks. It is critical to try to control these outbreaks to prevent secondary bacterial infection in wrestlers with more severe cases of acne. Acne alone is not reason enough to stop a wrestler from competing. Acne can be lessened by wearing clean, dry, loose, cotton clothing in a cool, well-ventilated environment. Wet clothing should be changed as soon as possible. Proper-fitting equipment is also necessary as acne can be made worse by ill-fitting equipment. Scarring from continued irritation of areas of acne is often a complication of this common athletic skin condition.

Viral Infections

Herpes Simplex

The most common viral infection seen in the sport is herpes simplex. In wrestling, this infection is often referred to as herpes gladiatorum. The virus that is often responsible for this disease is herpes simplex I. This virus is spread in the same manner as bacteria, but the infection is not treatable with antibiotics. The lesion from herpes simplex is described as a "blister on a red base." It is often seem in the area of the lips but can appear anywhere on the body. There are often systemic symptoms that occur approximately 1 week before the eruption of the lesions, which include flulike symptoms, malaise, fatigue, and itching or tingling at the site of the infection. The virus can be identified by a culture, but this is usually not performed as the lesions are so specific to this virus. Treatment is often supportive and addresses individual symptoms. If identified early, antiviral medicines can be given that can decrease the symptoms and duration of the outbreak. These drugs work best if given within 72 hours of identification of the virus. Wrestlers with chronic infections are often placed on oral antiviral medications. Return to sports occurs when all the lesions have dried and crusted over. This can take anywhere between 4 and 7 days. The lesions should then be covered with a gas-permeable bandage for competition.

Molluscum Contagiosum

Molluscum contagiosum is another common viral infection seen in wrestlers. It is spread in the same manner as the other viral infections. Wrestlers who are infected should immediately be removed from competition. Raised lesions with a hollow center characterize the disease. They are often seen in clusters and have a waxy appearance. They are often found on exposed areas of the skin. Treatment is by removal of the lesions via modalities such as freezing with liquid nitrogen or scraping off using a specific tool. There are also medications that can treat the disease. Once the lesions are removed and the athlete is free of new lesions, the wrestler can return to activity.

Warts

Warts are caused by the human papillomavirus and can be found on any part of the athlete. They are characterized by raised, scaly lesions and are often characteristic in their appearance. They are spread by direct contact. There is usually no laboratory testing attempted as the lesions themselves are diagnostic. Treatment is via removal of the lesions by substances such as salicylic acid or liquid nitrogen or by direct excision. As long as the lesions are covered, wrestlers need not be removed from competition.

Fungal Infections

Tinea

The most common fungal infection is due to the tinea fungus. Tinea can be found in any location on the body and thrives in a warm, moist environment. Infection in the scalp is referred to as *tinea capitis*. Infection at the foot is referred to as *tinea pedis*, or athlete's foot. Infection in the groin is referred to as *tinea cruris*, or jock itch. Infection on the trunk or extremities is termed *tinea corporis*, or ringworm. The most commonly isolated organism causing infection is *Trichophyton tonsurans*. These infections are spread by skin-to-skin contact and by sharing of equipment, uniforms, or towels.

A ringworm infection is most often recognized on the body by its characteristic ring formation. The fungus generally appears in a red patch that is scaly and has a distinct border with a clear center. This patch generally does not have little "satellite" lesions around it but can appear on other areas of the body. A scraping of the fungal infection can allow its identification when it is observed under a microscope; however, this is rarely done as the lesion often has a characteristic appearance. Athletes discovered with these lesions should be immediately withdrawn from competition as the infection is highly contagious. Tinea lesions are also likely to get secondarily infected with bacteria if left untreated. Treatment is generally by topical antifungal medications. If topical antifungal medications cannot control and treat the infection, then systemic antifungal medications are used. Caution needs to be used when these are prescribed as they may be toxic to the liver. Some athletes who are highly susceptible to tinea and develop chronic infections are often placed on chronic antifungal medications. Return to sports should not be attempted until after approximately 5 days of treatment with antifungal medication and drying of the lesions. These should be covered with a gas-permeable bandage when returning to competition.

Infestations

Scabies

Scabies is caused by an infestation of the body by a small living organism. The living organism burrows itself in the skin, leaving droppings along the burrows, causing persistent itching. The hallmark symptom of infestation is a persistent itch followed by redness of the affected skin. This is often first seen in the skin between the fingers but can also be seen in other areas of the body. The rash is identified by the characteristic burrows. This skin condition is easily spread from person to person. Usually, the athlete is not the only person affected as he or she brings the infection home, causing the infection of other family members. Treatment is washing with a solution that is left on overnight to kill the organism. Treatments are carried out every 3 days until the infection is cleared. Individuals without symptoms are treated twice, with 1 week between treatments. Athletes should be removed from competition at the first signs of infestation and can return to sports the next day after the overnight treatment.

Noninfectious Skin Conditions

Contact Dermatitis

This skin condition is not due to an organism but is due to an allergic reaction to an object such as a headgear. The skin lesion generally begins as a red patch with a border that approximates the size of the item exposed to the skin to which the athlete is allergic. This redness may evolve to scaling and weeping of the area with continued exposure. Small fluid-filled blisters may also appear. There are no lab tests to perform as the skin signs usually alert physicians to the diagnosis. Treatment is by using topical corticosteroids on the affected areas. If the outbreak is significant, oral steroids may be necessary. There is often no reason to withdraw the athlete from competition. The key to treatment is to eliminate that item to which the athlete is allergic, substitute the affected item with an item the athlete is not allergic to, or put a barrier between the irritating item and the athlete's skin.

Prevention

Good hygiene is the key to prevention of common dermatological conditions associated with wrestling. The following rules should be followed:

1. Removal from competition at the first sign of an infectious lesion.

2. Showering after all practice and competition sessions.

3. Thorough drying of all body areas.

4. No sharing of equipment or uniforms.

5. Use of breathable athletic clothing.

6. Consistent laundering of athletic clothing.

7. Consistent cleaning of athletic surfaces.

8. Being aware that body shaving exposes the skin to infection.

R. Robert Franks

See also Fungal Skin Infections and Parasitic Infestations; Skin Disorders Affecting Sports Participation; Skin Infections, Bacterial; Skin Infections, Viral; Wrestling, Injuries in

Further Readings

Adams BB. New strategies for the diagnosis, treatment, and prevention of herpes simplex in contact sports. *Curr Sports Med Rep.* 2004;3(5):277–283.

Derma A, Ilgen E, Metin E. Characteristics of sports-related dermatoses for different types of sports: a cross-sectional study. *J Dermatol.* 2005;32(8): 620–625.

Dworkin MS, Shoemaker PC, Spitters C, et al. Endemic spread of herpes simplex virus type 1 among adolescent wrestlers and their coaches. *Pediatr Infect Dis J.* 1999;18(12):1108–1109.

Johnson R. Herpes gladiatorum and other skin diseases. *Clin Sports Med.* 2004;23(3):473–484.

Mast EE, Goodman RA. Prevention of infectious disease transmission in sports. *Sports Med.* 1997;24(1):1–7.

Mellion MB, ed. *Team Physician's Handbook.* 3rd ed. Philadelphia, PA: Hanley & Belfus; 2002.

SKIN DISORDERS, METABOLIC

Metabolic skin disorders include several conditions that may cause discomfort and impaired performance. Conditions such as eczema, psoriasis, and urticaria can affect a significant proportion of the athletic community. The pathophysiology of all these disorders can be traced back to the participant's immune system working abnormally. Although treatment of these skin problems is not difficult, they must be first correctly identified and diagnosed to enable the timely return of the athlete to active participation.

Eczema

Eczema is an extremely common skin condition and has the potential to affect athletic participation. Although *eczema* is often used synonymously with the term *atopic dermatitis*, true eczematous reactions can occur in people with or without other findings of atopy, such as allergic conjunctivitis, bronchial hyperreactivity, or allergic rhinitis. Nonallergic sources account for 10% to 25% of eczematous reactions, and most are associated with atopy. In recent years, the term *atopic eczema/dermatitis syndrome* was coined to encompass several varieties of atopic dermatitis that are clinically related.

The effect that eczema has on athletes is a function of its prevalence in the population. Up to 10% of school-age children in the United States have eczema; furthermore, many school-age children participate in organized athletics. As a result, there is a significant likelihood that school-age children who play sports will also have eczema.

Diagnosis

Diagnosing eczema is a challenging task because of the many noneczematous disorders that mimic its skin lesions and symptoms. In addition, the skin manifestations of eczema itself are varied, appearing erythematous, papular, macular, or pruritic depending on its severity. Milder lesions are characterized by erythematous, maculopapular microvesicles. More severe outbreaks display crusted-over lesions that may or may not weep. Over time, the lesions become increasingly dry and result in lichenification. Regardless of the lesion's severity or chronicity, the hallmark of eczema is the intense pruritus (itching) that accompanies the rash and often results in excoriation due to repetitive scratching.

Eczema is usually localized to the flexor creases of the arms and legs, with occasional distribution to the genitalia and face. However, as the condition becomes more severe, it may spread to any body surface.

Treatment

Most cases of mild eczema will respond to more benign treatments such as topical steroid creams or over-the-counter moisturizing lotions. Caution should be advised with chronic topical steroid use,

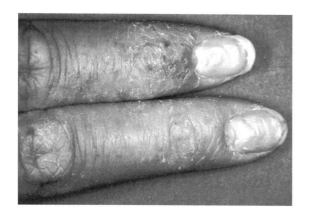

Eczema

Source: From DermNet NZ. Reproduced with permission.

since there is risk of pigmentation changes, striae formation, and atrophy of the skin. Because of these complications, treatment with steroid creams around the eyes and face should be avoided. Pruritus that is associated with eczema is usually well controlled with antihistamines.

Newer therapies aimed at suppressing the immune response, such as cyclosporine, have also been used. In recent years, the medication pimecrolimus has been marketed as a first-line agent against mild to moderate eczema. Although this nonsteroidal medication is effective in inhibiting the inflammatory cytokines of eczema, physicians should attempt to use more conventional treatments first, because pimecrolimus suppresses T-cell function and may make individuals more susceptible to viral infections.

Return to Sports

Eczematous eruptions can be a significant impairment for athletes. The discomfort of not only the pruritus but also the physical contact of athletic gear against the affected skin can negatively affect athletic performance. Furthermore, the team physician must recognize the risk of secondary bacterial infection of eczematous skin, usually caused by *Staphylococcus aureus* or Group A beta-hemolytic *Streptococci*. It is this secondary bacterial infection in eczema that may require withholding the athlete from participation, especially in sports that require skin-to-skin contact between competitors.

Return-to-play decisions must be individualized based on a number of considerations. The location of eczematous outbreaks on the body and the feasibility of covering the lesions, clinical improvement with treatment, and the likelihood of physical contact between athletes should all be factors in determining an athlete's return. Because misdiagnosis and/or ineffective treatment of eczema are a common occurrence, habitual return to play after immediate initiation of antibiotics should be discouraged.

Psoriasis

Psoriasis is an autoimmune condition that affects approximately 2% of the U.S. population. It is characterized by erythematous, scaly patches that are sometimes silvery in color. The patches usually have very well-defined edges and often appear symmetrically on the body. As with eczema, the performance of athletes afflicted with this disorder is often impaired because of the discomfort of the rash, the chronic arthritis associated with the condition, or secondary bacterial skin infections, which may preclude participation in sports.

Diagnosis

The key to diagnosing psoriasis is being able to identify its pathognomonic rash from other dermatologic conditions. Psoriatic lesions are usually covered with a silvery white scale as a result of the increased turnover of the skin cells. Although this appearance is unique to psoriasis, it may not always manifest in this way and can easily be misdiagnosed as eczema, dermatophytic infection, or lichen planus.

Athletes with psoriasis may display the Koebner phenomenon, in which psoriatic plaques appear on previously unaffected areas as a result of trauma. This may be especially disabling for athletes if the affected site is the plantar surface of the foot. Although this phenomenon waxes and wanes with athletic activity, it may become uncomfortable enough to discourage an athlete from participating in sports.

Another complication of psoriasis that may affect athletes is psoriatic arthritis. This chronic manifestation affects about 5% of patients with psoriasis. Classically, the axial skeleton and the metacarpophalangeal (MCP) and proximal interphalangeal

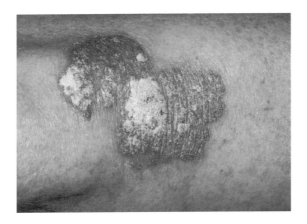

Psoriasis

Source: From DermNet NZ. Reproduced with permission.

Notes: The most common ages for psoriasis to first appear are the late teens, but it is possible for children to be affected as well. It affects men and women equally, although among children, girls are more commonly affected than boys. There does appear to be a genetic predisposition to psoriasis, but it is also known to be influenced by many environmental factors. Usual sites of involvement include the scalp, eyebrows, knees, elbows, ears, genitalia, and nails. Psoriatic fingernails can become yellowish in color and display pitting, which can often aid physicians in diagnosis.

(PIP) joints of the hands are involved. On X-ray, erosion of the articular surfaces of the involved joints is observed.

Treatment

There is a wide spectrum of agents used to treat psoriasis. The more traditional methods such as selenium formulations, topical corticosteroids, or coal tar preparations are effective against mild cases of psoriasis.

As the psoriatic outbreak becomes more severe, the use of systemic or newer biologic agents may be indicated. Although quite effective, these newer medications and treatment modalities carry a certain degree of risk. Methotrexate is hepatotoxic and has been shown to interact with nonsteroidal anti-inflammatory drugs (NSAIDs). Cyclosporine combined with psoralen-ultraviolet light treatment (PUVA) increases the risk of squamous cell carcinoma. Oral retinoids have been shown to be highly teratogenic. Thus, the team physician may decide to take the help of other specialists in prescribing these agents and managing more severe cases of psoriasis in athletes.

Return to Sports

Return-to-sports decisions regarding outbreaks of psoriasis are quite similar to those regarding outbreaks of eczema. The risk of secondary bacterial infection is present in psoriasis, and decisions regarding return to play should take into account the same precluding factors as those concerning eczema. Therefore, the team physician should determine the appropriate time for return to competition on a case-by-case basis.

Exercise-Induced Urticaria

Exercise-induced urticaria, also known as *cholinergic urticaria*, is a physically mediated allergic condition that has been increasingly reported in recent years. This type of reaction occurs much less commonly than those arising from allergen exposure; however, for active individuals and athletes, this disorder may be extremely debilitating.

Diagnosis

The physiologic mechanism underlying exercise-induced urticaria is unknown, although the clinical manifestations appear to arise due to an exaggerated cholinergic response to rapid increases in core body temperature. Acetylcholine release followed by mast cell degranulation and histamine release precede the urticarial response. People with this condition may experience the urticaria not only after exercise but also after hot showers, during times of emotional stress, or when afflicted with a fever.

The classic response is characterized by the development of generalized flushing, coupled with discrete, punctuate, extremely pruritic 2- to 4-mm wheals surrounded by a red flare. Fortunately, vascular collapse is not commonly associated with this condition. Other clinical signs of parasympathetic activation such as lacrimation, salivation, or diarrhea may also aid in diagnosis.

Urticaria usually begins approximately 6 minutes after the onset of exercise and reaches a peak in 12 to 25 minutes. However, recovery may take from 2 to 4 hours. This condition primarily affects young active individuals between the ages of 10

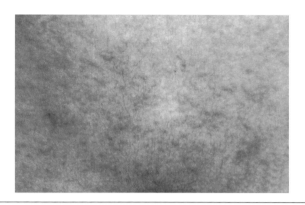

Exercise-induced urticaria

Source: From DermNet NZ. Reproduced with permission.

and 30, although it may recur for many years after initial onset. Although diagnosis is usually made clinically, methacholine skin challenge tests have been used to help confirm the presumed diagnosis.

Treatment

Treatment of cholinergic urticaria consists of withdrawing the precipitating factor and using antihistamine medications/creams to relieve the urticaria. Use of a mast cell–stabilizing medication such as cromolyn sodium or beta blockers such as propranolol has also been reported, but antihistamines such as hydroxyzine are more universally recommended.

Return to Sports

The degree of discomfort and willingness to return to participation dictate the decision to allow an athlete to continue playing. However, if exercise is the essential trigger of the condition, it may be prudent to withhold the player from participation until prophylactic antihistamine medications can be given to help blunt the urticarial response.

Lucien Parrillo

See also Dermatology in Sports; Skin Conditions in Wrestlers; Skin Disorders Affecting Sports Participation; Urticaria and Pruritus

Further Readings

Adams BB. Dermatologic disorders of the athlete. *Sports Med.* 2002;32(5):309–321.

Blumenthal MN. Managing allergies in active people. *Phys Sportsmed.* 1997;25(8):129–134.

Del Giacco SR, Manconi PE, Del·Giacco GS. Allergy and sports. *Allergy.* 2001;56(3):215–223.

Hosey RG, Carek PJ, Goo A. Exercise-induced anaphylaxis and urticaria. *Am Fam Physician.* 2001;64(8):1367–1374.

Pedersen BK, Hoffman-Goetz L. Exercise and the immune system: regulation, integration, and adaptation. *Physiol Rev.* 2000;80(3):1055–1081.

Veale DJ, Fitzgerald O. Psoriatic arthritis—pathogenesis and epidemiology. *Clin Exp Rheumatol.* 2002;20 (6, suppl 28):S27–S33.

SKIN DISORDERS AFFECTING SPORTS PARTICIPATION

Sports-related skin disease is quite common with a wide variety of causes. Broadly categorized as infections, dermatitis, or trauma, several skin disorders directly affect sports participation. Early recognition and treatment are crucial in determining the athlete's ability to return to play and preventing the occurrence of outbreaks among team members.

Infections

Skin infections cause the most disruption to individual and team activities. Many of the skin infections that affect athletes are transmitted by close contact. A variety of other factors contribute, including macerated skin from sweating, abrasions, and occlusion from equipment. These risk factors are present in many sports. The National Federation of State High School Associations Sports Medicine Advisory Committee and the National Collegiate Athletic Association have set specific guidelines for return to sports after a skin infection is diagnosed in wrestlers; these guidelines can help guide treatment and return-to-play decisions for other sports as well. Athletic skin infections can be fungal, bacterial, or viral.

Fungal Infections

Fungal infections of the skin are caused by dermatophytes that invade and reproduce in the outermost layer of the skin, as well as the hair and nails. They cause superficial infections commonly referred to as "ringworm" or *tinea*. Tinea affects the scalp, body, groin, and feet. Fungal infections are easily spread between athletes. Therefore, an athlete should have the affected areas covered and oral or topical antifungal treatment initiated. Wrestlers specifically need to be treated for a minimum of 72 hours for the skin and 2 weeks for the scalp prior to return to play.

Bacterial Infections

Bacterial disease can range from impetigo to cellulitis. Impetigo appears as a honey-colored scab and is caused by *Staphylococcus* or *Streptococcus* bacteria. Treatment should be initiated after soaking the area to remove the lesion's crust. Topical antibacterial agents are then applied for localized disease. Oral antibiotics are considered if the disease is extensive or if methicillin-resistant *Staphylococcus aureus* (MRSA), a serious condition, is suspected.

Boils (abscess) typically begin near the hair follicles. Infection is introduced by skin injury and is typically caused by *Staphylococcus* or *Streptococcus*. Abscesses, typically described as painful, red, soft tissue masses, most commonly occur in moist areas where hair follicles are present, such as the groin, posterior thighs, and face. Athletes at risk include those who are diabetic, are obese, use steroids, or have poor hygiene. Treatment consists of draining the lesion. Oral antibiotics are not typically needed unless there is concern for overlying skin infection (cellulitis) or MRSA. Cellulitis presents as diffuse red, warm, tender, and swollen areas of skin. Cellulitis is particularly dangerous as it may spread rapidly. Athletes with the condition can become quite ill. Antibiotic treatment and close monitoring are crucial until resolution.

Bacterial infections need to be considered "noncontagious" prior to return to play. This requires that no new lesions develop for 2 days. All current lesions should be scabbed over, with no oozing or drainage. An athlete needs to have been on an oral antibiotic for a minimum of 3 days. If new lesions develop or there is continued drainage, a diagnosis of MRSA should be considered, which requires prolonged treatment, defined as a minimum of 10 days, with all lesions scabbed over.

Viral Infections

Viral disease can take many forms, but most frequently, athletes are plagued by the herpes simplex virus (HSV). HSV appears as a cluster of skin blisters with a reddened base. Athletes may have associated symptoms such as a fever, chills, and muscle aches. Patients often notice a tingling or burning sensation before the onset of HSV lesions. Athletes with abrasions or lacerations of the skin are at high risk for transmission. HSV is self-limiting and will spontaneously improve but can recur and is easily spread. Outbreaks can be prevented by keeping athletes out of competition while treatment is initiated. A low index of suspicion and early detection are crucial for preventing spread. Careful inspection of each athlete before practices and competitions is vital to prevention. Prior to returning to play, the athlete should have no new lesions for 2 days, and all current lesions should be scabbed over, with no oozing or drainage. An athlete's first episode of herpes needs to be managed with antiviral treatment for a minimum of 10 days. This should be extended to 14 days if associated symptoms such as a fever, chills, and muscle aches are present at diagnosis. Recurrent episodes require a minimum of 5 days' antiviral treatment prior to return to play. In athletes with a recurrent infection, suppressive treatment should be considered.

Molluscum contagiosum is caused by the poxvirus and is spread by skin-to-skin contact. This infection is typically seen in swimmers, gymnasts, and wrestlers. Molluscum appears as a skin-colored papule with a central dimple, commonly seen on the face, neck, and trunk. These lesions are usually asymptomatic and resolve spontaneously. However, spontaneous resolution can take many months, and most athletes desire to expedite resolution in order to return to play. Molluscum can be removed by scraping, cryotherapy, or local application of medicated creams.

Parasitic Infections

Scabies is caused by *Sarcoptes scabiei*. A scabies infection occurs when a female mite burrows under the skin, leaving eggs in the tract she creates. Scabies infections are characterized by severe nighttime itching that usually occurs between 1 and 4 weeks after infection. Burrows appear as tracts in the skin and are commonly found between the web spaces of the fingers or over the wrists, breasts, axillae, scrotum, penis, or knees. Transmission occurs through close contact for a substantial period of time. Treatment typically involves a topical lotion. The lotion is spread over the entire body, kept on for 8 to 12 hours, and then washed off. A repeat application in 1 week is usually adequate for eradication. The clothing and bedding of the infected individual should be washed and dried at high temperatures. Household contacts of those infected with scabies should also wash their clothing and bedding and be treated as noted above.

Infection Prevention

In athletes, skin infection prevention is crucial. This requires athletes to pay close attention to personal hygiene, such as not sharing personal items or equipment, washing clothes and personal gear regularly, showering immediately after practice and competition, and regular use of shower shoes. Education and skin surveillance are essential for early recognition and treatment and to expedite return to play.

Dermatitis

Allergic or irritant dermatitis can cause significant redness, swelling, and itching of an affected body part. Diagnosis is often readily apparent in individuals on the basis of the distribution of the rash and a history of repeated skin eruptions after exposure. Recognition of environmental irritants and allergens is critical for appropriate treatment.

Trauma

Abrasions need to be cleansed with antibacterial soap, and protective dressings need to be applied. Return to play for lacerations should occur once active bleeding is stopped and the wound is properly dressed. Calluses and blisters occur secondary to shearing forces and perspiration. Frequently due to ill-fitting footwear, treatment of these conditions involves frequent sock changes, antiperspirants, and new, properly fitted shoes. Similarly, jogger's toe is caused by painful bleeding beneath the toenails in an athlete wearing improper shoes.

Properly fitted shoes again are the mainstay of treatment.

Matthew Leroy Silvis and Amy Sucheski

See also Allergic Contact Dermatitis; Cholinergic Urticaria; Fungal Skin Infections and Parasitic Infestations; Jogger's Nipples; Prickly Heat; Skin Disorders, Metabolic; Skin Infections, Bacterial; Skin Infections, Viral; Skin Infestations, Parasitic; Sunburn and Skin Cancers; Toenail Fungus

Further Readings

Adams B. Strategies for the diagnosis, treatment, and prevention of herpes simplex in contact sports. *Curr Sport Med Rep.* 2004;3(5):277–283.

Benjamin H, Nikore V, Takagishi J. Practical management: community-associated methicillin-resistant *Staphylococcus aureus* (Ca-MRSA): the latest sports epidemic. *Clin J Sport Med.* 2007;17(5):393–397.

Cordoro K, Ganz J. Training room management of medical conditions: sports dermatology. *Clin Sports Med.* 2005;24(3):565–598.

Johnson R. Herpes gladiatorum and other skin diseases. *Clin Sports Med.* 2004;23(3):473–484.

Kockentiet B, Adams BB. Contact dermatitis in athletes. *J Am Acad Dermatol.* 2007;56(6):1048–1055.

Mathiew ME, Braunstein WB. *"Scabies" Principles and Practice of Infectious Diseases.* 6th ed. Philadelphia, PA: Elsevier; 2001.

Pleacher MD, Dexter WW. Cutaneous fungal and viral infections in athletes. *Clin Sports Med.* 2007;26(3):402–409.

Sedgwick PE, Dexter WW. Bacterial dermatoses in sports. *Clin Sports Med.* 2007;26(3):383–396.

SKIN INFECTIONS, BACTERIAL

Bacterial skin infections are a common occurrence among athletes and range from simple "sweaty-sock syndrome" to potentially life-threatening methicillin-resistant *Staphylococcus aureus* (MRSA) infections. Conditions that favor infection, such as skin abrasions, moist environments, and skin contact with other players, are all present in the athletic environment. This entry discusses some common and some unusual causes of bacterial skin infections among athletes.

MRSA Infections

There is a growing prevalence of this infection in the athletic community, and although deaths are extremely uncommon, they have been reported. The hallmark of these infections is that they do not respond to the antibiotics traditionally used for skin infections and may progress more rapidly than do "normal" skin infections to severe illness requiring hospitalization. It is important to distinguish between hospital-acquired methicillin-resistant *Staphylococcus aureus* (HA-MRSA) and community-acquired methicillin-resistant *Staphylococcus aureus* (CA-MRSA). HA-MRSA has been an issue for many years and affects primarily those in hospitals and nursing homes, those with immune disorders, and those with recent antibiotic usage. CA-MRSA has been of concern only for two decades or so and does not need any of these requirements to infect individuals and thus even causes infections in otherwise healthy athletes.

MRSA can be the pathogen involved in many of the skin conditions described below. Treatment depends on the prevalence of MRSA in the community, the severity of infection, and the type of infection (MRSA is more likely to cause abscesses, although this is not a reliable identification measure). Oral antibiotics such as trimethoprim/sulfamethoxazole, clindamycin, doxycycline, or linezolid may be used to treat these infections, although more severe cases may need hospitalization with intravenous vancomycin. A full discussion of MRSA is found in the encyclopedia entry dedicated to that topic.

Folliculitis

Folliculitis is a superficial infection or irritation of the base of the hair follicles anywhere on the body. Athletes usually complain of mild to moderate tenderness or itchiness and have small pustules located at the base of the hair shafts, usually with a small amount of redness at the base of each pustule. Folliculitis in athletes can be broken down into three types: *Staphylococcus* L (either MRSA or methicillin-sensitive *Staphylococcus aureus* [MSSA]), *Pseudomonas folliculitis*, or *Pseudofolliculitis barbae*.

Staphylococcus folliculitis is the most common type of folliculitis and is usually found on areas of the skin under equipment pads, although it can occur anywhere on the body. Most of these infections are from MSSA strains of organisms, but MRSA can be an issue even in these small lesions. Treatment of these infections should include oral antibiotics and the use of antibacterial soaps to help prevent recurrence. The type of antibiotics given depends on the severity of the infection and the level of concern for MRSA. Treatment is usually for 7 to 10 days.

Pseudomonas folliculitis, also called "hot tub folliculitis," occurs most commonly as clustered lesions under swimming gear. As the name implies, poorly cleaned hot tubs or whirlpools are usually the cause of the infection. This is a self-limiting condition that typically lasts 5 to 7 days and usually does not respond to either topical or oral antibiotics. Appropriate cleaning of whirlpool facilities is essential to prevent infection and transmission.

Pseudofolliculitis barbae is not truly an infection but rather a reaction of the skin to ingrown hairs at sites of shaving. It has a presentation similar to that of true folliculitis but often does not have pustules that are as inflamed as in that condition. Treatment involves using fresh razors, manually releasing ingrown hairs with a sterile needle, or stopping shaving for several days to allow the hairs to grow out. Occasionally, there will be bacterial superinfection, in which case the condition should be treated as a true folliculitis.

Pitted Keratolysis

Also called "sweaty-sock syndrome," this is a condition presenting as sliminess and intense malodor of the feet, with a characteristic pitting of the skin of the foot almost exclusively at the pressure-bearing areas. It is commonly initially misdiagnosed as a fungal infection. Treatment of pitted keratolysis is to ensure a dry environment through the use of synthetic socks and an aluminum chloride antiperspirant (Drysol) and frequent changing of socks and footwear. Persistent lesions should be treated with topical antibiotics such as clindamycin or erythromycin. This is not usually considered a contagious condition, and players do not need to be held back from practice or play.

Erysipelas/Cellulitis

Cellulitis is differentiated from erysipelas by the fact that it involves the subcutaneous tissue, whereas erysipelas is essentially a superficial infection. Both involve redness, swelling, and pain of the involved tissue, and there may be red streaking found extending from the infection (called lymphangitis). In severe cases, there may be a fever, chills, and malaise.

These infections are usually caused by *Streptococcus* and *Staphylococcus* species in athletes, although many different types of bacteria may be responsible. Oral antibiotics are the treatment of choice, and strong consideration should be given to treating for MRSA in regions with a high prevalence or infections involving risky areas such as the groin, hands, and face.

Abscesses

Abscesses are closed pockets of infection within the skin and often underlying tissue. Friction is a high risk factor for developing these lesions, as are warm, moist environments. Unlike cellulitis and erysipelas, there is rarely any fever or chills unless the abscess is extensive or there is significant surrounding cellulitis. Abscesses are almost always caused by *Staphylococcus* species, and MRSA is of particular concern with these types of infections. Incision and drainage of the abscess under sterile conditions is highly recommended in most cases when feasible. Cultures should be obtained from the abscess contents. If the lesion is small, if the patient is otherwise healthy, and if he or she has a close follow-up with a medical provider, this alone may be sufficient treatment. Often, however, oral antibiotics are needed in addition to incision and drainage—particularly if surrounding cellulitis is present.

Erythrasma

Patients with this skin infection complain of discolored, reddish plaques between their toes or in their groin or armpits or between their buttocks. There is little to no pain, and often only mild itching or irritation. People with depressed immune systems, obesity, or excess sweating are more at risk of developing this infection. The diagnosis can be confirmed by shining a special fluorescent (Wood's) lamp on the patches, with a coral-red appearance indicating erythrasma.

The causative bacteria for these infections are *Corynebacterium* species, although there is a high association with concomitant fungal infections. Treatment consists of topical antibiotics, a combination of topical antibiotics and antifungals, or

even oral antibiotics. This is a contagious condition, and so players should avoid contact, group showers, or shared footwear if any lesions are present.

Impetigo

One of the most contagious of bacterial skin infections affecting athletes, it is unfortunately also one of the most common. Impetigo can affect any area of skin but is most often found on the face. There are two types: bullous (bubble-forming) and nonbullous. Both types have a classic "honey-crusted" appearance to the lesions, although the lesions can also mimic cold sores, poison ivy, or even simple acne.

For simple cases, treatment can be simply the use of topical mupirocin (Bactroban), an antibiotic cleanser. This cannot penetrate any crust that is present, however, so any crust must be soaked off prior to application. Occasionally, oral antibiotics are needed to treat more severe infections. It is of utmost importance to quarantine any infected individual for at least 2 to 3 days after starting treatment to prevent spread among a team or region.

Mycobacterium Marinum Infections

Caused by bacteria related to those that cause tuberculosis, *Mycobacterium marinum* is a very rare skin condition that aquatic athletes can contract from infected freshwater or saltwater swimming areas. After several days to weeks after exposure, patients may present with nonhealing ulcerated lesions. Treatment is oral antibiotics for up to a year's duration.

Necrotizing fasciitis

Despite being extremely rare, this condition of "flesh-eating bacteria," as it is sometimes referred to in the popular press, is fairly well known. Athletes may present with a mild cellulitis, which can progress rapidly over hours to days to severe infection and death. Any such rapid progression or severe pain out of proportion to the appearance of an infection warrants immediate hospitalization for intravenous antibiotics and surgical debridement of the wound. Even with such precautions, as many as 1 in 4 patients die.

Peter E. Sedgwick

See also Methicillin-Resistant *Staphylococcus Aureus* Infections; Skin Conditions in Wrestlers; Skin Disorders Affecting Sports Participation

Further Readings

Adams BB. Dermatologic disorders of the athlete. *Sports Med.* 2002;32(5):309–321.

Benjamin HJ, Nikore V, Takagishi J. Practical management: community-associated methicillin-resistant *Staphylococcus aureus* (CA-MRSA): the latest sports epidemic. *Clin J Sport Med.* 2007;17(5): 393–397.

Cohen PR. Community-acquired methicillin-resistant *Staphylococcus aureus* skin infections: implications for patients and practitioners. *Am J Clin Dermatol.* 2007;8(5):259–270.

Sedgwick PE, Dexter WW, Smith CT. Bacterial dermatoses in sports. *Clin Sports Med.* 2007;26(3):383–396.

SKIN INFECTIONS, VIRAL

Viral infections of the skin are commonly seen in athletes. Excessive sweating, tight clothing, and close skin-to-skin contact may contribute to the occurrence of infection. Because many of these diseases are potentially contagious to other athletes, a rapid diagnosis and initiation of treatment is important to prevent spread to teammates or opponents. Although most of the lesions resolve with no treatment, athletes often do require treatment in view of the high rate of transmission to other athletes if the condition is left untreated. Additionally, to reduce the spread of infection, the major sports organizations have set guidelines that require treatment of the lesion(s) and confirmation of resolution before allowing participation.

Verruca Vulgaris (Warts)

Warts most commonly affect the hands and feet and are caused by a strain of the human papilloma virus. The virus can enter through breaks in the skin, as in the case of an abrasion. The wart infects a superficial layer of the skin (the basal layer) and does not travel into the deep layers. The warts tend to grow slowly over 4 to 6 months. They can be

spread either by direct contact with the virus or contact with an object that has come in contact with the virus (i.e., the mat in wrestling). If left alone, a majority of warts tend to resolve after about 2 years.

Treatment of warts focuses on direct destruction or surgical removal. The virus actively replicates at the base of the lesion, and so it may be necessary to remove the superficial layers before treatment is initiated to allow improved success of resolution.

Warts do not require that athletes be restricted from play. However, it will be necessary to have the lesions covered during competition. The National Collegiate Athletic Association (NCAA) rules that lesions should be "adequately covered."

Herpes Simplex Virus

The herpes simplex virus (HSV) is classified into two strains: Type 1 and Type 2. In general, HSV-1 is associated with lesions around the mouth. The lesions are very common in childhood. Occasionally, the lesions are asymptomatic, though they can be very painful and cause significant difficulty with eating. The initial infection often shows up from 1 to 3 weeks after contact with the virus. At the time of the first infection, the person may have a fever, headaches, and muscle aches and feel ill. After the initial infection, the virus lies dormant in the nerves of the face and has the potential to reactivate at a later point in life. Reactivation is often associated with physical or emotional stress, ultraviolet light, or fever (immune system stress). Usually, the person does not feel ill with a recurrent infection.

The infection appears as tiny blisters (called *vesicles*) with clear fluid and redness of the skin. Often, before the skin findings, an infected person may recall a feeling of tingling or burning in the location where the infection has settled. After the vesicle stage, the lesion may form a painful ulcer. Eventually, the lesions scab and dry up and self-resolve after 3 to 5 days. It is generally accepted that high doses of antiviral medications such as acyclovir or valacyclovir may help resolve the lesions. In some cases, a persistent use of the same medication in a lower dose can potentially help prevent recurrence of the infection.

The infection is so common in wrestlers that a particular name has been given to an HSV infection in that subset of athletes: *herpes gladiatorum.* In rugby players, HSV infection is known as scrum pox. It has been reported that 7.6% of college wrestlers and 2.6% of high school wrestlers are infected annually with the disease.

The NCAA has set guidelines for treatment and rules regarding return to play for athletes. Wrestlers who have HSV must be free of signs of infection (fever, muscle aches, feeling ill) for 72 hours and must not have any new lesions for 72 hours; all lesions must be dry, and the athletes should have been treated for at least 120 hours with oral antiviral medications before they can be released to practice or competition. For this reason, many athletes with the condition prefer to continue preventive therapy with antiviral agents throughout their season.

Varicella

Varicella is more commonly known as chicken pox and is part of the Herpesviridae family of viruses. As it is genetically similar to HSV-1 and HSV-2, it tends to produce lesions that are similar in appearance. The virus can grow rapidly and cause many lesions to show up in a short period of time. The entire body can be affected. Prior to the institution of immunization against varicella, it was a very common childhood infection. The lesions show up about 2 weeks after exposure to the virus. The skin rash proceeds in a predictable way—first as red flat spots, then raised spots, then small blisters, and finally a scab. Since the virus reproduces itself so rapidly, it is possible to see all stages of the lesions in an individual person at the same time. The condition is highly contagious and is probably spread most efficiently starting 2 days before the rash starts up until 7 days after the rash has started. Most children infected with varicella improve within a short period of time and have no permanent effects. Varicella is particularly dangerous to pregnant women in their first 5 months because of fetal damage. Adults tend to have a more serious illness at times, resulting in pneumonia or a brain infection.

Herpes Zoster (Shingles)

Once a person has had chicken pox, he or she tends to be protected from a second infection.

However, the virus can lie dormant in the nerves of the body and may resurface in times of stress or in the elderly. This resurgence is known as herpes zoster or, more commonly, *shingles.* Shingles returns in a single nerve root and follows the course of the nerve. In many instances, this produces a red rash with small blisters in a line. Often this is seen across the neck, chest, or abdomen. A more serious recurrence can occur in the nerves of the face. With facial involvement, there can be paralysis of the muscles of the face that is usually temporary but can result in permanent deformity. Recently, an immunization against shingles has become available, and it could decrease this risk of recurrence.

Molluscum Contagiosum

Molluscum contagiosum is caused by a virus in the Poxviridae family. It appears as a painless bumpy rash with multiple small lesions. After contact with the virus, it may take from 1 to 6 months for the lesions to develop. The bumps are often of a pearly color and have a center that appears pressed in on itself. Most of the time, there are no symptoms associated with the rash. The infection is particularly common in children and tends to occur on their trunk, thighs, or upper arms. Children tend to pass the virus by direct contact with lesions. Adults can manifest the disease in their genital area, and the condition is often considered sexually transmitted. Most often the lesions regress in about 6 to 9 months. If the lesions are single, they can resolve in as short a period as 2 months. If treatments are recommended, they are focused on directly destroying the lesions by freezing them, chemically destroying them, or cutting them off. There are topical creams that can help resolve the lesions as well, but they tend to take about 1 month to clear the lesions.

The NCAA requires that lesions be removed in some manner before clearance for competition. Localized or solitary lesions can be covered with a dressing and taped. After removal, it is recommended that the athlete be removed from competition for 24 hours.

Allyson S. Howe

See also Skin Conditions in Wrestlers; Skin Disorders
    Affecting Sports Participation

Further Readings

Pleacher MD, Dexter WW. Cutaneous fungal and viral infections in athletes. *Clin Sports Med.* 2007;26(3):397–411.

Ruocco E, Donnarumma G, Baroni A, Tufano MA. Bacterial and viral skin diseases. *Dermatol Clin.* 2007;25(4):663–676.

Habif TP. Warts, herpes simplex, and other viral infections. In: Habif TP, ed. *Clinical Dermatology: A Color Guide to Diagnosis and Therapy.* 4th ed. Philadelphia, PA: Mosby; 2003:Chapter 12.

SKIN INFESTATIONS, PARASITIC

Parasitic skin infestations are infections of the skin caused by small organisms that require human hosts for a portion of their life cycle. These skin infections, including lice and scabies, rarely affect athletes when compared with viral or bacterial infections. Though these infestations are rare, any of them may affect an athlete's ability to participate in practice or competition. Symptoms include intense itching and the development of a rash or bite marks. Diagnosis is based on a clinical exam. The most common treatment for these conditions is topical medications. Scabies and lice are transmitted from person to person, meaning that actively infected athletes cannot be allowed to participate until treatment is complete.

Anatomy

The skin is the largest organ of the body. It covers an area of approximately 2 square yards (yd^2; 1 yd^2 = 0.84 square meters [m^2]). The skin ranges in thickness from 0.5 millimeters (mm) on the eyelid to more than 4 mm on the palms of the hands and soles of the feet. Up to 15% of a person's body weight is made up by the skin.

The skin has several major functions. It plays a major role in regulating the body temperature with a vast network of small blood vessels below the skin surface. The skin helps protect the body from damage, dehydration, and systemic infections. This protection is obtained by having a relatively impervious external layer of skin called the epidermis. Supporting the epidermis is an internal layer called the dermis. The dermis forms the support structure for the external layer.

Organisms that cause parasitic skin infestations have adaptations including special claws and suckers that can aid attachment to the epidermis. Lice exert their clinical effects on the skin surface, whereas scabies organisms burrow into the epidermis itself.

Lice

Causes

Lice are parasitic insects about 2 mm in length that survive by feeding on human blood. Lice infestations are caused by one of three different organisms, named for the human anatomic site that is affected. Pediculosis capitis refers to head lice, pediculosis corporis refers to body lice, and pediculosis pubis refers to genital lice. Transmission of the infection requires close skin-to-skin contact with another infected person. Rarely, the infection can be transmitted from clothing or equipment that was recently used by an infected person. Close skin contact can occur during athletic participation. Lice infestations are classically reported in sports such as wrestling, where there are prolonged periods of skin-to-skin contact. However, lice remain a rare cause of skin problems in the athlete. One-tenth percent of skin infections in college wrestlers are due to lice.

Symptoms

The bites of the lice lead to complaints of itching up to 10 days after exposure. The itching can be severe and is due to a local allergic reaction to the bite. Other symptoms can include a tickling sensation or a sensation of movement on the affected area. Sores can develop from repeated scratching.

Diagnosis

Diagnosis is made by observing the area of concern. The body part affected is examined for live lice or lice eggs, called "nits." Nits are small, white nodules attached at the base of a hair shaft. Nits can be mistaken for dandruff, hair spray droplets, or dirt particles. Use of a fine-toothed comb can facilitate visualization of an affected area. If live lice are seen, then the diagnosis of lice infestation is confirmed.

Treatment

Treatment of an affected athlete involves the use of topical medications to eradicate the infestation or make the skin inhospitable for the lice. Commonly used topical medications include permethrin 5% cream, pyrethrin cream, and lindane shampoo. There are multiple forms of the topical treatments, and each form has individual instructions for application. Some treatments require a doctor's prescription, while others are available over the counter in the pharmacy. Topical medications can typically be repeated 1 week after the initial treatment.

All clothing, hats, sporting equipment, and bedclothes used for 5 days prior to use of the topical medication require special handling. All items should be cleaned in a washing machine set to the hot cycle and dried at a high temperature. Any item that cannot be cleaned in this fashion should be placed in an airtight container for 3 to 5 days. These measures are designed to diminish the risk for reinfestation by an athlete's personal items.

Prevention

Preventing the spread of lice from one athlete to another can be promoted by employing several simple measures. Any athlete who has an active lice infestation should not practice or compete in any sport that requires skin-to-skin contact with other participants. Athletes need to have infestations fully treated before returning to play. The National Collegiate Athletic Association (NCAA) has special rules for wrestlers with skin infections. Collegiate wrestlers with lice are required to be fully treated before they are allowed to compete. At the time of a precompetition skin check, a physician or certified athletic trainer may disqualify a wrestler if there is evidence of active lice infestation.

Scabies

Causes

Scabies is a parasitic infestation caused by small parasitic organisms called *Sarcoptes scabiei* mites. The mite burrows into the epidermal layer of the skin. As the mite burrows into the skin, it deposits its eggs and fecal matter. The fecal matter of the mite is also called *scybala*. Transmission of the infestation is most often through close skin-to-skin contact with another infected person. Rarely, the infection can be transmitted from clothing or equipment that was recently used by an infected person. Scabies infestations are classically reported in wrestling, where there are prolonged periods of skin-to-skin contact during matches or practice. However, scabies remain a rare cause of skin problems in the athlete when compared with bacterial, viral, and fungal infections. Only 0.5% of skin infections in college wrestlers are due to scabies.

Symptoms

Athletes present with complaints of severe itching, especially at night. The affected athlete develops characteristic skin lesions within several weeks of exposure. These skin lesions can occur in the webbing of the fingers or on the hands, arms, legs, trunk, or groin. The lesions are classically thin, linear, red, slightly raised plaques but can also be diffusely spread red bumps or papules. In athletes who have had prior episodes of scabies, the symptoms can appear within a few days of reexposure. This can happen due to the host's immune system being reactivated quickly to the infestation.

Diagnosis

Diagnosis is made by carefully examining the lesions for characteristics of scabies as described earlier. A black speck that can just be seen by the naked eye at the end of a linear lesion represents the burrowing mite.

To confirm the diagnosis, a scabies preparation is performed. This preparation is done by scraping the linear plaques three or four times each with a scalpel blade in the direction of the visible black speck. The scrapings are then placed in a drop of mineral oil on a microscope slide. The slide is then examined with a microscope on a low-magnification setting. The presence of mites, eggs, or scybala is considered a positive result.

Treatment

Treatment of an affected athlete involves the use of topical or oral medications to eradicate the scabies infestation. A commonly used topical medication is permethrin 5% cream, applied to every surface of the body. The cream is left in place overnight and washed off in the morning. The topical medication therapy is typically repeated 1 week after the initial treatment. An alternative treatment is an oral medication called ivermectin. A single dose is given and then repeated 7 to 14 days later. The severe itching typically resolves within 1 or 2 days following the first treatment. However, a topical corticosteroid cream can be applied for cases of persistent severe itching.

All clothing, hats, sporting equipment, and bedclothes used for 5 days prior to the use of the topical medication require special handling. All items should be cleaned in a washing machine set to the hot cycle and dried at a hot temperature. Any item that cannot be cleaned in this fashion should be placed in an airtight container for 3 to 5 days. These measures are designed to diminish the risk for reinfestation by an athlete's personal items.

Prevention

Preventing the spread of scabies from one athlete to another athlete can be promoted by employing several simple measures. Any athlete who has an active scabies infestation should not practice or compete in any sport that requires skin-to-skin contact with other participants. Athletes need to have infestations fully treated before returning to play. The NCAA has special rules for wrestlers with skin infections. Collegiate wrestlers with scabies are required to be fully treated and have a negative scabies preparation before they are allowed to compete. At the time of a precompetition skin check, a physician or certified athletic trainer may disqualify a wrestler if there is evidence of active scabies infestation.

John P. Colianni

See also Fungal Skin Infections and Parasitic Infestations; Skin Conditions in Wrestlers; Skin Disorders Affecting Sports Participation; Skin Infections, Bacterial; Skin Infections, Viral

Further Readings

Adams BB. Dermatologic disorders of the athlete. *Sports Med.* 2002;32(5):309–321.

Adams BB. *Sports Dermatology.* New York, NY: Springer; 2006.

Centers for Disease Control. Parasitic disease information. http://www.cdc.gov/ncidod/dpd/parasites/scabies/default. Published 2003. Accessed August 15, 2008.

Centers for Disease Control. Lice. http://www.cdc.gov/lice. Published May 16, 2008. Accessed August 15, 2008.

SKULL FRACTURE

Sports and recreation–related head injuries, such as concussions, are relatively common. Fortunately, skull fractures occur very infrequently from athletic participation. With improvements in head gear and protective equipment, it has become rare that enough force is imparted to the skull to result in a fracture during athletic events. When a skull fracture does occur, however, it is important that it be promptly recognized and treated. Skull fractures typically result in injury to the brain, which may require emergent treatment.

Anatomy

The skull consists of a total of 27 bones that constitute two main regions. The first region is the bony covering around the brain (cranium), and the second region is formed by the bones constituting the face (Figure 1). The facial bones consist of the upper portion, which houses and protects the eyes and nose, and the lower portion, which helps form the jaws. This entry focuses on fractures to the first region of the skull, the cranium, which covers the brain.

During growth, the bones of the skull are connected by growth plates, which are also known as "sutures," that eventually fuse together. The bones are named based on their location. As shown in Figure 1, the bones covering the brain include the frontal bones, at the front of the skull; the sphenoid and temporal bones, at the side; the parietal bones, on the top; and the occipital bones, at the back of the skull. The major bones of the face include the nasal bone, forming the nose; the maxilla and the zygomatic bone, forming the upper jaw; and the mandible, forming the lower jaw. The mandible is technically not considered a part of the skull but rather a separate bone that connects to the skull via the temporomandibular joint or TMJ.

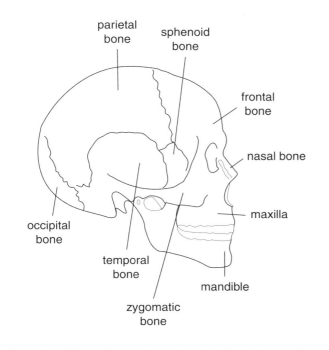

parietal bone

sphenoid bone

frontal bone

nasal bone

maxilla

occipital bone

temporal bone

zygomatic bone

mandible

Figure I   Some of the Major Bones Constituting the Face and Skull

Causes

A skull fracture is simply a break in a skull bone. The majority of skull fractures are not related to sports but result from motor vehicle accidents, falls, or violence. Skull fractures are grouped into four main types: linear, depressed, diastatic, and basilar. Linear skull fractures are the most common, accounting for about 70% of all skull fractures and virtually all fractures resulting from sports activities. With a linear fracture, there is a break in the bone, but the break does not result in any movement of the bone. With a depressed skull fracture, the area of the skull that is broken is pushed inward or appears sunken. This type of fracture has a higher risk of injury to the underlying brain. Diastatic skull fractures are fractures that occur along the growth plates or sutures of the skull. These fractures tend to occur in newborns and infants and are not typically seen after sporting activities. Basilar skull fractures are fractures that occur at the base of the skull or the portion underneath the brain. This type of fracture can occur even with helmet use in high-energy automobile racing accidents.

In sporting activities, fractures to the facial bones occur much more commonly than do fractures to the cranial bones. Improvements in head-and-face protection in sports such as football and hockey have led to a substantial decline in the number of cranial and facial fractures. Even in sports where very high impacts may be imparted to the head, resulting in injury to the brain, such as automobile racing, modern helmets have made the incidence of skull fractures quite low. Sports in which no protection is worn, such as soccer or rugby, actually account for a significant number of facial fractures and occasionally fractures to the cranium. A fracture can be caused by direct contact against another athlete, such as in a head-to-head contact in soccer. Fractures can also result from contact between the head and a piece of athletic equipment, such as the goalpost in soccer, or less commonly from contact against the ground. Fractures at the base of the skull (basilar fracture) can result from high-energy automobile racing accidents due to sudden compression forces imparted to that portion of the skull.

Symptoms

The symptoms resulting from a skull fracture depend on the type of fracture sustained. Athletes who have suffered a depressed skull fracture may be rendered unconscious due to underlying brain injury. With a linear skull fracture, the athlete may not lose consciousness but often will display symptoms consistent with a concussion, such as headache, confusion, and lethargy. Postconcussion symptoms can last for days to weeks and are listed below. Athletes who have suffered a linear skull fracture have pain and tenderness overlying the area of the fracture.

Diagnosis

The diagnosis of a skull fracture begins with a history and physical exam. The history usually reveals a high-energy mechanism, especially if the athlete wears protective headgear, as in auto racing. In some cases the headgear may not have been fit or functioned properly, as with a baseball player hit on the head by a pitch. In rare cases, the athlete may not have worn headgear at all, such as a soccer goalie who contacts the goal post with his

Postconcussion Signs/Symptoms	
"Bell rung"	Nausea
Depression	Nervousness
"Dinged"	Numbness/tingling
Dizziness	Poor balance/coordination
Excessive sleeping	
Fatigue	Poor concentration, easily distracted
Feeling "in a fog"	Ringing in the ears
Feeling "slowed down"	Sadness
Headache	"Seeing stars"
Inappropriate emotions or personality changes	Sensitivity to light
	Sensitivity to noise
Loss of consciousness	Sleep disturbance
Loss of orientation	Vacant stare/glassy eyed
Memory problems	Vomiting

head, resulting in a fracture. Most athletes who have sustained a skull fracture are rendered unconscious from the initial impact to the skull and underlying brain. Although the neurologic injury and other associated injuries take precedence over the skull fracture in initial treatment, diagnosis of the skull fracture is important to minimize potential late complications. Depressed and open skull fractures should be apparent in a physical exam; however, linear skull fractures may not be obvious.

A diagnosis of linear skull fractures and fractures at the base of the skull is typically made on radiographic imaging. Plain radiographs have essentially been supplanted by the computed tomography (CT) scan in the imaging of the skull and brain. The CT scan is much more sensitive in detecting subtle fractures of the skull, especially those at the base of the skull. Unlike plain radiographs, a CT scan also images the brain and will detect bleeding in or around the brain. A magnetic resonance imaging (MRI) scan will also show skull fractures but is best for evaluating the brain for bleeding, contusion, or a shearing-type injury.

Treatment

Nonsurgical Treatment

The initial treatment for an athlete with a skull fracture focuses on the ABCs (airway, breathing, and circulation) of advanced trauma life support. The athlete's cervical spine should be immobilized with a rigid collar until spine injury can be ruled out. The athlete should be transported to a medical center that provides neurosurgical services. In the rare event of an open skull fracture, the wound should be covered with sterile gauze and intravenous antibiotics administered.

Linear skull fractures are typically treated nonoperatively. Ice can be applied to the area of contact to minimize swelling. A computed axial tomography (CAT) scan should be obtained to evaluate the underlying brain tissue for injury or bleeding. The CAT scan also accurately shows the extent of the fracture. Patients should be monitored for at least 24 hours to assess for deterioration in neurologic functioning. Narcotic pain medication should be avoided or given in limited quantities to minimize difficulty in diagnosing changes in neurologic status.

Surgery

Depressed skull fractures require surgery to eliminate pressure on the underlying brain tissue. Open skull fractures also require surgery to wash out the wound, elevate the depressed portion of the skull, and close the wound. These injuries represent surgical emergencies to minimize further brain injury and decrease the risk of infection. Since depressed and open skull fractures tend to result from very high-energy injuries, surgery may also require evacuation of underlying hematoma.

Rehabilitation

Nonsurgical Rehabilitation

Linear skull fractures heal without any surgical intervention. The fractures typically unite by 6 to 8 weeks after the injury. The type and extent of rehabilitation depend mostly on the degree of associated brain injury. Athletes who have sustained a concussion can return to athletic activity once the fracture has healed and all postconcussive symptoms have resolved both at rest and during activity.

After Surgery

Return to athletic competition after a skull fracture that requires surgery is controversial. Whether an athlete attempts to return depends on multiple factors, including the extent of brain injury and the nature of the sport that resulted in the injury. It is not the fracture, which typically heals without incident, but the extent of damage to the brain that is the most important factor in the athlete's long-term prognosis. To even consider returning to athletic competition, the athlete must have a complete neurologic recovery and not be at increased risk for repeat brain injury. Given that this is such a rare occurrence, there are no studies to help guide physicians in managing a patient.

Robert Victor Cantu and Robert C. Cantu

See also Concussion; Emergency Medicine and Sports; Fieldside Assessment and Triage; Head Injuries

Further Readings

Antoun JS, Lee KH. Sports-related maxillofacial fractures over an 11-year period. *J Oral Maxillofac Surg.* 2008;66(3):504–508.

Bak MJ, Doerr TD. Craniomaxillofacial fractures during recreational baseball and softball. *J Oral Maxillofac Surg.* 2004;62(10):1209–1212.

Boden BP, Tacchetti R, Mueller FO. Catastrophic injuries in high school and college baseball players. *Am J Sports Med.* 2004;32(5):1189–1196.

Delaney JS. Head injuries presenting to emergency departments in the United States from 1990 to 1999 for ice hockey, soccer, and football. *Clin J Sport Med.* 2004;14(2):80–87.

Exadaktylos AK, Eggensperger NM, Eggli S, Smolka KM, Zimmermann H, Iizuka T. Sports related maxillofacial injuries: the first maxillofacial trauma database in Switzerland. *Br J Sports Med.* 2004;38(6):750–753.

Roccia F, Diaspro A, Nasi A, Berrone S. Management of sport-related maxillofacial injuries. *J Craniofac Surg.* 2008;19(2):377–382.

Tozoglu S, Tozoglu U. A one-year review of craniofacial injuries in amateur soccer players. *J Craniofac Surg.* 2006;17(5):825–827.

SLEEP AND EXERCISE

Exercise has been proposed as offering a safe and healthy means of alleviating insomnia and other sleep disorders. This entry discusses the impact of sleep disorders, reviews the surveys and epidemiologic evidence supporting the benefits of exercise, and discusses the potential mechanisms by which exercise can promote healthy sleep patterns.

In industrialized countries, the annual global incidence of insomnia is approximately 30%. The prevalence of sleep problems increases with age, such that more than 50% of adults over age 60 have some sleep-related complaint.

Insomnia has been associated with physical and mental illness, impaired quality of life, and increased risk of automobile accidents. Moreover, in the United States, the costs associated with the resulting worker absenteeism, declines in work productivity, and increases in health care utilization have been estimated at approximately $14 billion.

Individuals' reactions to disturbed sleep and self-help strategies can often exacerbate and perpetuate insomnia. For example, excessive worry about insomnia and attempts to compensate by spending extra time in bed can lead to a vicious cycle dynamic of further sleep problems.

Many physicians who are untrained in dealing with sleep problems are most inclined to treat patients with sleeping pills. However, sleeping pill use has been associated with daytime sedation, "sleep driving," and impaired cognition; and chronic nightly use has been associated with a mortality risk comparable with that associated with smoking a pack of cigarettes per day.

Hence, there has been an increased interest in cognitive/behavioral treatments for insomnia. There is compelling scientific evidence that these treatments are superior to sleeping pills for chronic treatment of insomnia. However, the treatments are costly and time-consuming, and there are not enough clinicians who are trained to administer these treatments. Thus, other self-administered treatments would be helpful.

Exercise is almost invariably included in both expert and lay recommendations for improving sleep. The expectancy that exercise promotes sleep is centuries old; moreover, the notion that exercise promotes sleep has been consistent with historical theories about the function of sleep. For example, theories that sleep serves an energy conservation or body restitution function naturally led to hypotheses that energy utilization and body tissue breakdown associated with exercise could elicit unique needs for sleep. These theories influenced much of the earlier research on exercise and sleep. However, they have been largely discredited on the basis of evidence, for example, supporting the idea that sleep is associated with only a minimal reduction in oxygen consumption and no particular increase in protein synthesis or replenishment of adenosine triphosphate (ATP) stores.

Undoubtedly, some of the interest in this topic stems from anticipation that exercise could be a very attractive alternative or adjuvant treatment for insomnia. Exercise has profound health benefits and would be a comparatively safe, inexpensive, and simple means of improving sleep. Besides affecting insomnia and sleep quality, there are also theoretical and empirical rationales for expecting that exercise could be a useful alternative or adjuvant treatment for several other sleep disorders, such as sleep apnea, restless legs syndrome, and circadian rhythm sleep disorders.

Insomnia/Sleep Quality

Survey Results

Surveys have consistently shown that exercise promotes sleep. For example, in a National Sleep Foundation poll, people who reported exercising regularly also reported fewer complaints of difficulty falling asleep, difficulty staying asleep, waking up unrefreshed, or daytime sleepiness compared with people who reported exercising less frequently than once per week, and these associations showed a dose-response pattern.

In other population surveys, people have consistently reported that exercise helps them sleep better. For example, Urponen and colleagues studied a random sample ($n = 1,090$) of people in Tampere, Finland, who were prompted thus: "Please state, in order of importance, three practices, habits, or actions which you have observed to best promote your falling asleep or your quality of sleep." The respondents (men, 33%; women, 30%) reported that exercise was the most important behavior, more important than reading or listening to music

(men, 15%; women, 23%), taking a sauna/shower (men, 9%; women, 9%), and psychological factors (men, 8%; women, 9%).

Although these survey results are provocative, it is plausible that they might overestimate the benefits of exercise for sleep. Physically active people tend to have better physical and mental health, which are conducive to sleep, and they tend to engage in other healthy behaviors that are conducive to sleep, such as avoidance of smoking and excessive alcohol consumption.

Moreover, people are not always accurate in their assumptions about sleep. For example, although the "nightcap" is commonly used to promote sleep, it is well established that alcohol actually impairs sleep. Likewise, people might assume that exercise promotes their sleep on the basis of a common, but incorrect, assumption that physical fatigue is synonymous with sleepiness.

Interestingly, survey data have unanimously failed to support the common assumption that late-evening exercise will disrupt sleep. For example, assessing a random sample that includes people who reported exercising after 8 p.m. ($n = 320$), Vuori and colleagues in Finland found that the majority of these people reported that after exercise, they fell asleep more quickly (65%), had deeper sleep (62%), and woke up feeling better (60%).

Epidemiologic Results

Epidemiologic studies could theoretically provide stronger evidence that exercise promotes sleep because they can statistically control for some of the potential confounds listed above. Epidemiologic studies have consistently found that self-reported exercise is significantly independently associated with less insomnia and other sleep complaints. These associations have been observed across all age-groups and various ethnicities around the world. The association of exercise with better sleep has generally been modest compared with other predictors (e.g., depression and stress/anxiety), but the association has been more consistently established than for perhaps any other behavior. Moreover, if exercise indirectly promotes sleep via its antidepressant/anxiolytic effects, then these studies might underestimate the effect of exercise.

Nonetheless, there are a number of limitations of the epidemiologic studies linking exercise with better sleep. First, with few exceptions, these studies have relied on self-reported measures of exercise and sleep. These measures have often had unknown reliability and validity. Second, as discussed above, causality cannot be definitively inferred from epidemiologic associations. The epidemiologic associations could be explained by external factors, such as incidental outdoor light exposure, which has been associated with better sleep. Moreover, fatigue is a barrier to exercise, so people who sleep better might be more inclined to exercise. Third, the studies often have not adequately measured or controlled for health status and other behaviors that can affect sleep.

Experimental Studies

Acute Exercise

Approximately 50 experimental studies have examined the effects of acute exercise on sleep in comparison with sedentary control treatments. These studies have focused predominantly on laboratory polysomnographic measures. Our meta-analysis of this literature summarized the effect and explored potential moderating factors. The meta-analysis found that acute exercise elicited virtually no effect on how long it took subjects to fall asleep or how much they were awake during the night and that exercise elicited a statistically significant but modest increase in total sleep duration (median 10 minutes), a significant but small increase in slow-wave sleep (SWS) (1.6 minutes), a significant increase in rapid-eye-movement (REM) latency (11.6 minutes), and a significant decrease in total REM duration (6 minutes).

The effect of acute exercise on sleep duration was significantly moderate by exercise duration, with negligible effects for exercise durations of less than 1 hour (2 minutes) and progressively greater effects following exercise of 1 to 2 hours (11 minutes) and more than 2 hours (15 minutes). This finding raises some questions about the practical utility of exercise for promoting sleep since many people are unwilling to exercise for 1 hour. On the other hand, no moderating effects of fitness or exercise intensity were found, which is consistent with survey and experimental evidence that exercise promotes sleep across the population.

Also consistent with surveys, experimental evidence indicates that late-evening exercise does not impair sleep for most individuals. This lack of impairment has been found in sedentary individuals as well as physically active individuals and has been seen even following vigorous exercise of 1 to 3 hours' duration, ending only 30 minutes before bedtime.

In summary, experimental studies have found significant, but quite modest, beneficial effects of acute exercise on sleep. However, there have been a number of limitations of these studies that might explain the modest effects. First, the studies have often had small sample sizes. Second, the studies have typically been limited to one or two nights. Because sleep is sensitive to many factors, more assessment nights might be needed to delineate the effects of exercise. The most important limitation is that the studies have focused almost exclusively on good sleepers, who have little room for improvement. Indeed, it has been shown that acute exercise and sleeping pills have quite comparable effects in good sleepers. Whether exercise will also have an effect similar to sleeping pills in insomniacs is a question worthy of future research.

Chronic Exercise

Chronic exercise studies have also generally revealed only modest beneficial effects of exercise on sleep. However, most of these studies have also been limited to normal sleepers. Several recent studies have examined whether exercise training could improve sleep in older adults, who tend to have worse sleep compared with young adults. In general, the results do not suggest more beneficial effects of chronic exercise in older versus young adults. There is some limited evidence of greater benefits of chronic exercise in older adults with insomnia, as might be expected. However, this evidence is limited mostly to self-reported sleep, which could be confounded by expectancy effects and demand characteristics. Further research involving insomniacs and objective sleep measures is needed.

Obstructive Sleep Apnea

Obstructive sleep apnea (OSA) affects about 10% of the adult population and has been associated with cardiovascular disease, diabetes, and mortality. The primary treatment for OSA, continuous positive airway pressure (CPAP), has limited efficacy and is associated with dismal compliance. There is recent interest in the notion that exercise could help reduce OSA severity or at least offset some of its hazardous consequences.

Epidemiologic studies have consistently shown an association of exercise with reduced symptoms and diagnoses of OSA. For example, Peppard and Young of the University of Wisconsin-Madison found that the relative risk of polysomnographically determined sleep apnea (>5 events per hour) was 0.62, 0.39, and 0.31 in respondents (n = 1,104) who reported exercising 1 to 2 hours, 3 to 6 hours, and 7 hours or more, compared with 0 hours per week. Although weight loss is an obvious potential mechanism by which exercise could indirectly reduce apnea, the association of exercise with reduced apnea has persisted following control for body mass index and skin fold thickness.

Uncontrolled experimental studies have revealed that exercise training can reduce OSA severity, and these effects were not correlated with weight loss. A recent randomized controlled study found that exercise training significantly reduced central sleep apnea (a rarer type of apnea) in patients with chronic heart failure.

Restless Legs Syndrome

Restless legs syndrome (RLS) is associated with excruciating "creepy-crawly" sensations in the legs, which cause an irresistible urge to move the legs, primarily at night when one is trying to sleep. The presence and severity of RLS has been strongly linked to genetic factors, as well as iron and dopamine deficiencies. Anecdotally, people who suffer from RLS report that moderate daytime exercise can help prevent or reduce the severity of RLS symptoms at night. Moreover, exercise involving the legs is the best remedy for acute RLS symptoms. Epidemiologic research by Phillips and colleagues of the University of Kentucky has also indicated that exercise is associated with reduced RLS. Finally, randomized controlled research has shown that both acute and chronic exercise can reduce the symptoms of RLS. In one study by de Mello and colleagues in Sao Paulo, Brazil, the effects of exercise were comparable with those of L-dopa, one of the primary pharmacologic treatments for RLS.

Mechanisms by Which Exercise Could Promote Sleep

Anxiolytic Effect

Exercise could promote sleep via anxiety reduction. Clearly, anxiety disturbs sleep, and there are dozens of studies that indicate that acute exercise can reduce state anxiety and chronic exercise can reduce trait anxiety. The anxiolytic effect of acute exercise provides some rationale for expecting that the evening might be the best time to exercise since the anxiolytic effects are best established during the first few hours after exercise.

Antidepressant Effect

Since depression is also clearly linked with poor sleep, exercise could also promote sleep, indirectly, via its well-established antidepressant effects. Singh and colleagues at Harvard University conducted a 16-week exercise training study of depressed individuals and found that sleep-promoting effects were significantly correlated with antidepressant effects. Some evidence suggests that the efficacy of antidepressant drugs might be mediated partly by decreases in REM sleep and increases in REM latency, and so it is plausible that the antidepressant effects of chronic exercise might also be partly mediated by the REM changes that have been observed after acute exercise.

Thermogenic Hypothesis

One of the most widely accepted hypotheses in this area is that exercise could promote sleep via body-heating effects. This hypothesis is supported by evidence that the anterior hypothalamus/pre-optic area of the brain is associated with both sleep regulation and body cooling and that passive heating (e.g., in hot tubs) can promote sleep. Most compellingly, Horne and colleagues at Loughborough University in the United Kingdom have shown that experimental blunting of temperature elevation during exercise (via body cooling) can attenuate some of the beneficial effects of exercise on sleep. Chronic exercise could also potentially promote more rapid temperature down-regulation at night, which has been linked with sleep onset.

Circadian Phase-Shifting Effect

Exercise could also have a positive effect on sleep via its influence on the circadian system. One of the hallmark features of primary insomnia is an erratic sleep-wake schedule. There is evidence that exercise can help stabilize the circadian system, which could, in turn, stabilize and improve sleep.

Moreover, there is compelling evidence that exercise can shift the circadian system, which could help correct circadian rhythm sleep disorders. Exercise and bright light have also been shown to have additive phase-shifting effects, both in animals and humans. Delayed sleep phase syndrome, which often prevents one from going to sleep before 2 a.m. or arising before 10 a.m., is particularly prevalent in adolescents and young adults. This condition can result in profound sleep deprivation, absenteeism and tardiness, and impaired academic and work performance. The circadian phase–advancing effects of morning exercise could help correct this problem. Conversely, the phase-delaying effects of evening exercise could help treat advanced sleep phase syndrome, which tends to cause one to go to bed before 9 p.m. and wake up before 4 a.m.

About 20% of the U.S. workforce are shift workers. Shift work is associated with chronic sleep problems as well as many other morbidities, including heart disease, cancer, mood disturbance, and gastrointestinal distress. In a randomized, controlled experiment involving a simulated "graveyard shift," we found that nighttime exercise facilitated circadian adjustment to the shift and resulted in a significant reduction in symptoms.

Conclusion

It is commonly assumed that exercise is one of the most important behaviors promoting sleep. Surveys and epidemiologic studies have supported this assumption. Experimental studies have shown more modest effects of acute and chronic exercise on sleep. However, these studies have been limited to good sleepers. More promising results have been found in studies of exercise in people with sleep problems. Further randomized controlled research of this type is needed. Moreover, there should be verification of the exciting evidence that exercise might be an effective treatment for sleep apnea, RLS, and circadian rhythm sleep disorders.

Shawn D. Youngstedt

Note: Preparation of this entry was supported by HL71560 and a VA (VISN-7) Career Development Award.

See also Circadian Rhythms and Exercise

Further Readings

Peppard PE, Young T. Exercise and sleep-disordered breathing: an association independent of body habitus. *Sleep*. 2004;27(3):480–484.

Urponen H, Vuori I, Hasan J, Partinen M. Self-evaluations of factors promoting and disturbing sleep: an epidemiological survey. *Soc Sci Med*. 1988;26(4):443–450.

Youngstedt SD. Effects of exercise on sleep. *Clin Sports Med*. 2005;25(2):355–365.

Sleep Loss, Effects on Athletic Performance

Sleep has always been thought of as a critical factor for optimal performance in athletics. Research has established that sleep is an active physiological state and not a passive process and is as complex as wakefulness. Critical cognitive, immunological, and metabolic processes occur during sleep, but its direct relationship to athletic performance is still unproven.

Both sleep and athletic performance are extremely individual activities and are influenced by many factors and variables, making research on this subject difficult to perform. However, scientific evidence is emerging that confirms a connection between sleep and athletic performance.

This entry describes the basic circadian rhythms and stages of sleep; the causes of sleep deprivation; sleep requirements; the effects of sleep deprivation through cognitive, immunological, and metabolic impairment; sleep quality; and recovery.

Circadian Rhythms

Circadian rhythms, or biological rhythms, are physiological parameters that fluctuate in specific ways over a 24-hour cycle. Sleep and wakefulness are among those rhythms. Circadian rhythms are genetically and environmentally determined in humans. Each athlete has a preferred sleep schedule that best suits his or her circadian phase. If a circadian preference and sleep schedule are not harmonized, or get out of phase, it will affect the amount and quality of sleep of the athlete.

Overview of Stages of Sleep

The American Academy of Sleep Medicine (AASM) uses a standardized method for describing sleep. This was revised in 2007. The modified stages of sleep and general outline include the following:

- Sleep is analyzed in 20- to 30-second epochs, with each epoch being assigned a single sleep stage.
- Sleep is subdivided into two general states: rapid eye movement (REM) sleep and non–rapid eye movement (NREM) sleep. NREM sleep is further subdivided into four stages.

  o *REM:* Electroencephalogram (EEG) findings show rapid, low voltage, similar to an active, awake EEG pattern. High-frequency beta waves occur with frequent bursts of REM. Most vivid dreaming occurs during this stage.

  o *NREM:* This accounts for up to 80% of total sleep time in human adults.

    - *Stage 1:* In this stage, the brain transitions from wakefulness to sleep or from alpha waves to theta waves. The muscle tone is lost, and the person loses awareness of the external environment. This stage lasts for only minutes, before the person moves on to the next stage.

    - *Stage 2:* EEG findings are characterized by higher "sleep or theta spindles" and "k-complexes," which are thought to be associated with arousal. This stage accounts for up to 55% of total sleep and lasts only a few minutes.

    - *Stages 3 and 4:* (the new AASM guidelines combine Stages 3 and 4). These are characterized by "deep sleep" or "slow-wave sleep." Delta waves are more pronounced. This is the last and deepest of the sleep stages before REM sleep. If a

person is deprived of this stage of sleep, it rebounds once sleep is allowed again, suggesting that this stage is essential to the sleep process.

The true function of REM sleep is uncertain, although some data suggest an important role in memory consolidation. Some data indicate that NREM sleep has an association with the restorative functions of sleep, that is, restoration of alertness and energy. The data indicate that deep sleep is increased in athletes after significant physical effort.

Causes of Sleep Deprivation

Many circumstances can contribute to sleep disturbance and disruption of normal sleep cycles in an athlete. Some of these are work, academic and practice schedules; difference in time zones while traveling; pre-event anxiety or excitement causing early sleep arousal; early start of an event; diet; lifestyle choices; or jet lag.

Though many studies have produced mixed results or show methodological flaws in establishing whether optimal performance is influenced by transmeridian flights, one study showed that an appropriate choice of itinerary and lifestyle did indeed reduce the negative effects of jet lag in athletes.

Sleep Requirements

There is great interest in the ideal sleep requirement for an athlete to "rest and recuperate." Individuals respond differently to workout routines, and sleep deprivation and their sleep need vary.

In a 1994 National Institute of Mental Health study, participants with a "stabilized" sleep pattern averaged 8 hours and 15 minutes—a figure that is often interpreted as the amount of sleep that most adults require. Recent studies show that teenagers need as much, if not more, sleep as younger children (an average of 9.25 hours per night).

Though significant differences exist among individual athletes in their degree of vulnerability and responses to sleep deprivation, eventual negative effects have been shown to be cumulative. Sleep restriction practiced on a chronic basis induces performance deficits of the same order and magnitude as those observed during a large single event of total sleep deprivation. For example, if a person with a usual nightly sleep quota of 8 hours sleeps only 7 hours, there is a 1-hour sleep deficit that is carried over to the next day. A 7-hour sleep debt accrues after 7 days of losing 1 hour of sleep a night, nearly equal to a full night without sleep.

Effects of Sleep Deprivation

Though the direct effects of sleep deprivation on an athlete's performance are unproven, their relationship to the human body's metabolic processes, immunological function, and cognitive processing is more established and is related to a variety of adverse consequences.

Cognitive Impairment

Studies demonstrate a causal relationship among sleep, memory, and performance. Though not related to sports, major catastrophes such as In a 2008 study published in *Neurologic Clinics,* Three Mile Island accident, Chernobyl nuclear plant disaster, Exxon Valdez oil spill, and Space Shuttle Challenger disaster have been attributed to the poor judgment of sleep-deprived workers.

Dr. Charles Samuels cites previous research that has shown that sleep restriction (sleep deprivation) is linked to cognitive impairment with distinct interindividual variability. Cognitive performance (psychomotor vigilance) is directly affected by sleep deprivation. The impact of sleep disturbance on learning and neural plasticity (changes that occur in the brain as a result of experience) has also been established.

Sleep-deprived patients have reported decreased energy levels. They have difficulty with short-term memory, attention, alertness, speed, hand-eye coordination, and decision making—all of which are relevant to optimal athletic performance. These symptoms often disappear when normal sleep is restored.

Immunological Impairment

Chronic reduction in sleep can lead to immunosuppression. The integrity of normal immunological functions is negatively affected by sleep restriction. Studies have shown that partial or total sleep deprivation resulted in increased plasma levels of immune system "messengers" (tumor necrosis factor alpha [TNF-α] and interleukin 6 [IL-6]), which are involved in immune regulation. These "messengers" serve to connect the nervous, endocrine, and immune systems.

According to Samuels, there is a critical relationship between physiological recovery during sleep and an athlete's ability to train at maximum capacity with optimal results. The phenomenon of overtraining syndrome or chronic training fatigue is believed to result chiefly from immunological, neuroendocrinological, and musculoskeletal factors. The athlete's total sleep need and ongoing sleep debt are key factors in postexercise recovery, performance, and susceptibility to overtraining syndrome.

Metabolic Impairment

In a 1999 article published in *Lancet,* K. Spiegel and colleagues showed that sleep-deprived participants metabolized glucose less efficiently, leading to a reduced ability to manage glucose (similar to what is found in the elderly), decreased activity of human growth hormone, and elevated serum cortisol. Theoretically, elevated cortisol levels may interfere with tissue repair and growth and may lead to overtraining and injury.

Other detrimental changes in normal body metabolism due to sleep deprivation have been published, including delay in the healing of wounds, which has been shown in a study of rats with burn wounds. One night of sleep deprivation shows abnormal findings in electrocardiogram (EKG) testing (significant increase in QT max, QTd, cQTd, and P waves) in healthy young adults. These EKG changes can contribute to the development of arrhythmias. The effects of sleep deprivation on P waves may contribute to atrial fibrillation.

Sleep Quality

It is not enough to have an adequate quantity of sleep. An athlete may sleep for 8 hours or more and still be sleepy, secondary to disturbances in sleep quality. Sleep quality is another factor affecting performance in athletes. The full "restorative" benefit of sleep may not be received if sleep is fragmented by recurrent arousal without full awakening or light sleep with recurrent awakening.

Athletes experiencing "nonrestorative sleep" may become more tired from training, which affects performance and recovery. Optimal sleep quality may facilitate optimal athletic performance.

Recovery

When overcoming the effects of sleep deficit, any possible sleep "disturbance" should be minimized to allow normal and full sleep cycles to produce a full restorative benefit.

A positive or mitigating effect of "recovery sleep," that is, strategic napping, has been established as well in sleep deprivation studies, and it helps improve alertness and aspects of physical performance.

A Stanford University study showed that "extra" or extended sleep may boost athletic performance. Subjective reports of improved sprint times, increased free throw percentage, higher energy, and improved mood were obtained in six members of the men's basketball team who were instructed to "get as much sleep as possible" over a 2-week period. Studies with a larger sample may provide more meaningful results.

Conclusion

Determining an athlete's sleep patterns and ideal sleep needs and optimizing opportunities to allow optimal sleep quality so that the full restorative benefit of sleep can be achieved should be the current goal of coaches and athletes.

Coaches and athletes can make reasonable decisions to reduce the negative impact of sleep loss and encourage sleep quality as well as quantity. Traveling athletes can minimize the negative effects of readaptation when traveling over time zones by strategically planning their itinerary and lifestyle choices. Above all, further research must be conducted on the effect of sleep on athletic performance.

Mitchell Pratte

See also Circadian Rhythms and Exercise; Sleep and Exercise

Further Readings

American Academy of Sleep Medicine. Extra sleep improves athletes' performance. *ScienceDaily.*

Abstract presented at: SLEEP 2007, 21st Annual Meeting of the Associated Professional Sleep Society (APSS); June 13, 2007; Baltimore, MD.

Dinges DF, Kribbs NB. Performing while sleepy: effects of experimentally induced sleepiness. In: Monk TH, ed. *Sleep, Sleepiness and Performance.* New York, NY: John Wiley; 1991:97.

Iber C, Ancoli-Israel S, Chesson A, Quan SF. *The AASM Manual for the Scoring of Sleep and Associated Events: Rules, Terminology, and Technical Specification.* 1st ed. Westchester, IL: American Academy of Sleep Medicine; 2007.

Lamberg L. Sleep may be athletes' best performance booster. *Psychiatr News.* 2005;40(16):21.

Mitler MM, Carsskadon MA, Czeisler CA, Dement WC, Dinges DF, Graeber RC. Catastrophes, sleep, and public policy: consensus report. *Sleep.* 1988;11(1):100–109.

Pressman MR. Stages and architecture of normal sleep. http://www.uptodate.com/patients/content/topic.do?topicKey=~psuFiJzHRll/Js. Accessed June 15, 2010.

Samuels C. Sleep, recovery, and performance: the new frontier in high-performance athletics. *Neurol Clin.* 2008;26(1):169–180.

Shearer WT, Reuben JM, Mullington JM, et al. Soluble TNF-alpha receptor 1 and IL-6 plasma levels in humans subjected to the sleep deprivation model of spaceflight. *J Allergy Clin Immunol.* 2001;107(1):165–170.

Speigel K, Leprodult R, Van Cauter E. Impact of sleep debt on metabolic and endocrine function. *Lancet.* 1999;354(9188):1435–1439.

Van Dongen HP, Baynard MD, Maislin G, Dinges DF. Systematic interindividual differences in neurobehavioral impairment from sleep loss: evidence of trait-like differential vulnerability. *Sleep.* 2004;27(3):423–443.

Van Dongen HP, Maislin G, Mullington JM, Dinges DF. The cumulative cost of additional wakefulness: dose-related response effect on neurobehavioral functions and sleep physiology from chronic sleep restriction and total sleep deprivation. *Sleep.* 2003;26(2):117–126.

Vgontzas AN, Zoumakis E, Bixler EO, et al. Adverse effects of modest sleep restriction of sleepiness, performance, and inflammatory cytokines. *J Clin Endocrinol Metab.* 2004;89(5):2119–2126.

Walker MP, Stickgold R. It's practice, with sleep, that makes perfect: implications of sleep-dependent learning and plasticity for skill performance. Clin Sports Med. 2005;24(2):301–317.

Waterhouse J, Atkinson G, Edwards B, Reilly T. The role of a short post-lunch nap in improving cognitive, motor, and sprint performance in participants with partial sleep deprivation. *J Sports Sci.* 2007;25(14):1554–1566.

Waterhouse J, Edwards B, Nevill A, et al. Identifying some determinants of "jet lag" and its symptoms: a study of athletes and other travelers. *Br J Sports Med.* 2002;36(1):54–60.

Youngstedt SD, O'Connor PJ. The influence of air travel on athletic performance. *Sports Med.* 1999;28(3):197–207.

SLIPPED CAPITAL FEMORAL EPIPHYSIS

Slipped capital femoral epiphysis (SCFE) is an orthopedic emergency. It must always be considered in an adolescent with hip pain. Any young patient presenting with knee pain should always have his or her hips examined for SCFE. Treatment suggested is primarily surgery to prevent further damage and destruction to the femur (thighbone).

Anatomy

SCFE occurs at the femur in the hip joint. Specifically, the femoral head is the area that is part of the hip joint; the pelvic portion is called the acetabulum. The femoral head has a growth plate or epiphyseal plate, which is wider and weaker than normal bone. The slip is actually a Salter-Harris fracture (the classification for fractures involving the growth plate) that occurs in that growing and weakened area of bone.

Causes

SCFE happens in about 1 to 10 per 100,000 people. It is nearly 2.5 times more common in males than in females. It usually occurs in boys between 10 and 16 years of age and girls between 12 and 14 years. African Americans have a higher incidence of SCFE. About 25% of SCFEs are bilateral or affect both hips.

Obesity is a risk factor, because it increases the shear forces on the growth plate in the femoral head. Genetics may play a role as well. Of the patients with SCFE, 5% to 7% have another family member with the injury.

Metabolic and endocrine disorders also increase the risk of SCFE. Any patient with SCFE who is less than 10 years of age should have a metabolic and endocrine evaluation. These disorders include hypothyroidism, hypopituitary disorders, growth hormone deficiency, hypogonadal syndromes, and renal osteodystrophy. Bilateral SCFE is more common in young patients.

Clinical Evaluation

SCFE should be diagnosed and treated as quickly as possible to decrease the risk of long-term complications.

History

Most patients will complain of hip pain with decreased range of motion and difficulty weight bearing. Some will complain of knee pain (the pain radiates down the obturator nerve, which can confuse the examiner). The duration of symptoms should be obtained. If it is longer than 3 weeks, it is deemed chronic, whereas if it is less than 3 weeks, it is considered acute SCFE. Occasionally, patients will present with hip pain that has lasted longer than 3 weeks along with an acute worsening of pain or limp. This is termed *acute on chronic SCFE.*

It is important to inquire about family history and about symptoms consistent with the metabolic and endocrine disorders mentioned above.

Physical Exam

Some, but not all, patients may be obese. They classically hold the affected leg in external rotation or the foot pointed away from the body. This outward rotation may worsen with forward bending (flexion) of the hip. Testing of hip range of motion will be painful. It should be determined whether they can weight bear. It is always important to examine the opposite hip. Finally, the physical exam should also look for clues to endocrine and metabolic disorders.

Diagnostic Imaging

X-rays should be obtained. It is necessary to obtain X-rays of the opposite hip not only to rule out bilateral disease but also to use it for a comparison with the injured hip. Radiographs should include two views, usually a front-to-back film (AP or anteroposterior) and a "frog leg" view. However, if the patient is known to have SCFE, the frog leg view may potentially worsen the slippage, so a cross-table lateral view should be obtained.

The X-rays should be assessed to classify the amount of slippage and to see if there is other damage to the femoral head.

Blood testing for endocrine and metabolic disorders is necessary only in patients younger than 10 years or patients with other signs or symptoms of the disorders. Magnetic resonance imaging (MRI) and computed tomography (CT) are not helpful with diagnosis.

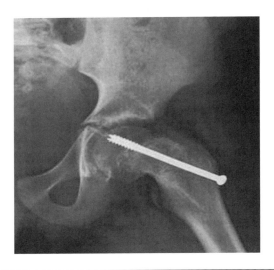

Postsurgical radiograph of a patient with an SCFE

Source: Kevin D. Walter, M.D., Children's Hospital of Wisconsin.

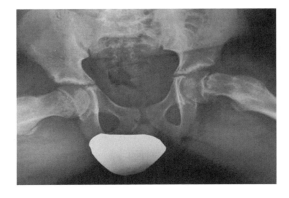

Patient's right side shows the normal femoral head; the left side shows SCFE.

Source: Kevin D. Walter, M.D., Children's Hospital of Wisconsin.

Classification

There are three ways to classify SCFE. The most important is stable or unstable. A stable SCFE means that the patient is able to weight bear. An unstable patient cannot put any weight on the affected leg because of the pain. An unstable SCFE means that the patient is likely to get progressively worse.

The next classification is based on the duration of symptoms. This includes chronic, which is greater than 3 weeks, and acute, which is less than 3 weeks of symptoms. The term *acute on chronic* refers to greater than 3 weeks' duration of symptoms but with a recent worsening of symptoms.

Finally, the amount of slippage can be determined by looking at the X-rays. Type I is less than 33% displacement. Type II is 33% to 50% displacement. Type III is more than 50% displacement. The larger the degree of displacement, the more likely the patient will have complications.

Treatment

SCFE is an orthopedic emergency. The patient should be non–weight bearing at all times. An orthopedic surgeon should be immediately contacted to evaluate the patient.

The most common treatment is surgery or internal fixation. The surgeon will use screws to fix the femoral head to the femur. This screw goes through the growth plate. The screw will provide stabilization, which can reduce the risk of further slipping. The screw also can cause the growth plate to close earlier than usual, which increases stability.

This procedure is done shortly after diagnosis to reduce the risk of avascular necrosis (AVN) or bone death of the femoral head. The femoral head is supplied by a single blood vessel that runs through the hip joint. As SCFE worsens, there is a chance that the blood flow will be disrupted, which causes AVN. The cartilage on the joint surface of the femur (articular cartilage) can be damaged as well. This is called chondrolysis. These two complications can lead to disability, pain, and early arthritis.

Since the blood vessel that supplies the femoral head is very sensitive, the slipped portion is rarely repositioned in the anatomically correct position. It is usually just fixated in its slipped position, due to fears that repositioning may damage the blood vessel.

Prophylactic bilateral fixation is controversial. Some surgeons feel that the risk of the opposite hip becoming affected is an indication for surgery on both hips. Other surgeons feel that it is not necessary to operate both sides unless the patient is younger or has an endocrine disorder, because both these issues have a higher risk of bilateral involvement.

Casting and other surgical procedures have been done in the past, but they have a high rate of complication, and thus have fallen out of favor.

After Surgery

The surgeon will discuss after-surgery care. Usually, patients are non–weight bearing or partial weight bearing on crutches for about 6 to 8 weeks after the surgery. Rehabilitation exercises after surgery can minimize weakness and improve strength.

X-ray follow-up until the growth plates close is recommended. During this time, leg lengths should be observed as well. Since the goal of surgery is to prematurely close the growth plate in the proximal femur (near the hip), the affected leg may be shorter than the unaffected leg.

There is some controversy about return to sports and contact sports. Some surgeons allow return after the growth plate has closed, some do not allow a return to contact sports, while others may allow return before growth plate closure. This is best discussed on a case-by-case basis with the surgeon.

Of course, if there are concerns for endocrine or metabolic disease, it may be worthwhile to follow up with a primary care provider or an endocrinologist for further evaluation.

Most patients who have a smaller percentage of slippage do quite well with early diagnosis and treatment. However, patients who are diagnosed late, as well as patients with severe slippage, may have more complications. The complications of AVN and chondrolysis may lead to chronic pain and early onset arthritis, both of which can lead to significant disabilities.

Kevin D. Walter

See also Hip, Pelvis, and Groin Injuries; Hip, Pelvis, and Groin Injuries, Surgery for; Hip Fracture; Musculoskeletal Tests, Hip; Orthopedist in Sports Medicine, Role of; Referred Pain

Further Readings

Frick SL. Evaluation of the child who has hip pain. *Orthop Clin North Am.* 2006;37(2):133–140.

Katz DA. Slipped capital femoral epiphysis: the importance of early diagnosis. *Pediatr Ann.* 2006;35(2):102–111.

Lehmann CL, Arons RR, Loder RT, Vitale MG. The epidemiology of slipped capital femoral epiphysis: an update. *J Pediatr Orthop.* 2006;26(3):286–290.

Uglow MG, Clarke NMP. The management of slipped capital femoral epiphysis. *J Bone Joint Surg Br.* 2004;86(5):631–635.

Slipped Disk

Spinal pain is a common reason for preventing athletes from participation in sports. The spine is composed of the cervical (neck), thoracic (upper back), and lumbar (low back) vertebrae. Approximately 20% of athletes will experience back pain during a 1-year period. Neck pain will occur in about 10% of athletes overall during this time period. Of course, this will vary from sport to sport. The cyclist will have a much higher prevalence of neck pain, while the gymnast will complain more of low back pain.

The sources of spinal pain are multiple and include the surrounding muscles, the ligaments, the facet joints, and the intervertebral disk. The disk accounts for up to 25% of spinal pain. However, there are a number of pathologic processes that are associated with the disk. It may degenerate with loss of fluid and height. Or the disk may rupture, which is called a *herniated disk* or, in lay terms, a "slipped disk." To prevent and to properly rehabilitate an athlete with this injury, one must understand the biomechanics of both the sport and the individual athlete.

Anatomy

The spinal column descends from the skull to the pelvis with 7 cervical vertebrae, 12 thoracic vertebrae, and 5 lumbar vertebrae. The articulation of the adjacent-level vertebrae occurs via the intervertebral disk in the front and the facet joints in the back (Figure 1). The lumbar vertebrae end on the sacrum, which is a fused V-shaped vertebra that

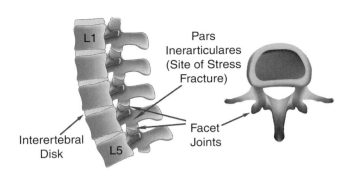

Figure 1   Lumbar Vertebrae (*lateral view*) and Single Vertebra (*top view*)

Source: Illustration by Michael d'Hemecourt.

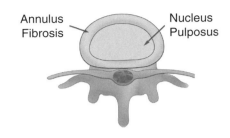

Figure 2   Cutaway View of Intervertebral Disk, Showing the Nucleus Pulposus at the Center, Surrounded by Annular Ligaments

Source: Illustration by Michael d'Hemecourt.

articulates with the pelvis to transfer forces from the trunk to the legs.

The disks become progressively larger from the cervical spine down through the lumbar spine. The disks provide shock absorption to the spine as well as motion. These disks are composed of three basic components: the annular ligaments on the outside (annulus), the colloidal gel (nucleus pulposus) on the inside, and the end plates of the vertebrae above and below. The *annulus* is composed of well-organized ligamentous sheaths (10–20 layers; Figure 2). The *nucleus pulposus* is a hydrous gel with few cells and some inflammatory enzymes. The *end plates* are at the top and bottom of the vertebrae, where the disk attaches. Since there is no blood supply to the disk, the end plate provides the nutrition to the disk by way of hydrostatic pressure during motion. In the child and adolescent athletes, these end plates are composed of soft growth cartilage and are susceptible to injury.

The disks are round and crescent shaped, with the posterior curved away from the posterior spinal column. The one exception is the lowest disk at the lumbar-sacral juncture (L5-S1), which is round. In the adult, the disk has the weakest ligamentous constraints on the posterolateral side, where the nerve roots exit. As such, a rupture here will affect the nerve. Conversely, the child and young adolescent may rupture into the soft end plate growth cartilage.

Etiology

A slipped disk represents a herniation of the nucleus through a tear in the outer annular ligaments.

When a small isolated tear occurs, the nucleus stays in place except for mild bulging. This annular tear will appear as an intense white line on some magnetic resonance imaging (MRI) scans. This is called a high-intensity zone (HIZ) and has been correlated with pain.

When the annular tear is more complete, a herniated disk will occur with expression of the nucleus material through the tear in the annulus. The slipped disk may be subdivided into a protrusion, an extrusion, and a sequestration. A protrusion occurs with a partial focal tear of the ligaments, and there is a broad-based disk protrusion of the nuclear gel. An extrusion represents a complete focal annular ligament tear with a more narrow-based gel extrusion, but it remains in contact with the central gel (Figure 3). A sequestration occurs when this extrusion separates from the disk.

Risk Factors

Risk factors include smoking, obesity, genetic factors, lack of core conditioning, hard labor, and sedentary lifestyles. A genetic component is felt to be one of the most important considerations. Certain motions in sports are highly associated with disk involvement due to the biomechanics of the sport. When the spine is loaded in flexion, the disk on the front of the lumbar spine is placed under the greatest pressure. Examples of this loaded flexion include wrestling, power lifting, and crew (catch phase). Cycling can also load the spine in flexion when the fatigued cyclist loses the normal lordosis or sways back and slumps forward.

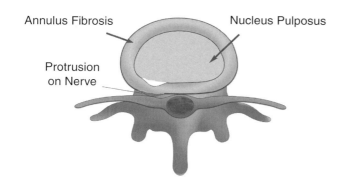

Annulus Fibrosis   Nucleus Pulposus

Protrusion
on Nerve

Figure 3   Herniated Disk, Showing Extruded Part of
the Nucleus Pulposus Impinging on the
Pathway of the Nerve Root

Source: Illustration by Michael d'Hemecourt.

The cervical disk may rupture in the wrestling take-down position. Collision sports such as American football and rugby also have some association to disk rupture due to direct impact and torsional loads. Long-distance cyclists place the spine in extension with a strong shear force, which can also cause disk rupture. Up to 40% of cyclists will complain of neck pain after a week of riding.

Clinical Presentation and Evaluation

The athlete with the disk herniation will present with pain either centrally or peripherally into the extremities. A herniated disk may occur next to the nerve roots. When it affects the nerve roots, pain and weakness of muscle groups in the distribution of the nerve supply may occur. In the neck, this will often produce symptoms along the shoulder, scapular, arms, or hand. In thoracic disk herniation, the symptoms will often distribute to the anterior chest or abdomen. In the lumbar spine, the distribution involves the buttocks, thighs, lower leg, and/or feet. These radiating symptoms are called *radicular symptoms.* They may be secondary to nerve compression from the mechanical bulk of the herniation or simply nerve irritation from leakage of inflammatory enzymes from inside the disk. Conversely, when the disk does not affect the nerve roots, there will be central pain in the neck, upper back, or lower back, depending on the level involved. This is called *axial pain syndrome.*

Disk herniations in the cervical spine mostly occur at the lowest cervical levels: C5-C6 and C6-C7. These levels produce symptoms into the arms and hands. Similarly, the lower lumbar spine is also affected, L5-S1 and L4-L5, which can affect the lower legs and feet. Thoracic disks are very uncommon but usually occur in the lower thoracic spine.

The peripheral pain often far exceeds the central neck or back pain. Certain motions are often provocative of the symptoms, while other motions will relieve the symptoms. Neck pain is often aggravated by activities that place the neck in hyperflexion or hyperextension. Classically, the cyclist or computer worker with the neck extended and chin forward will suffer aggravation of symptoms. Chin retraction may alleviate the symptoms. Lumbar or thoracic pain is often aggravated in the sitting or bending forward posture. In some cases, lumbar extension will relieve the pain.

It is essential to inquire about any worrisome red flags in the athlete that may prompt an immediate imaging evaluation. These would include loss of ability to hold the urine or stool, fever, chills, weight loss, weakness of an extremity, or constant night pain. In the absence of these, full imaging would be warranted if the symptoms last for longer than 6 weeks in the adult or 3 weeks in the young athlete. An MRI scan is usually the most appropriate imaging method to detect disk disease, but a CT scan is useful if the MRI scan is not possible.

Treatment

Treatment is based on the acuity of onset and the level of neurologic involvement. If there are signs of nerve root involvement, the progression is slower but usually follows a specific sequence. During the first few days, there is relative rest with utilization of analgesics. Rest should not exceed more than a few days. As the initial inflammation quiets, the subacute phase of isometric strength is used, where the core muscles or upper trunk muscles, if the neck is involved, are activated without motion. This often involves the use of calisthenic exercises, such as bridges for the lower back. Gradually, more dynamic low-resistance exercises are used, with progression of resistance as tolerated. Finally, as the athlete regains full strength, the sport-specific phase is started, with conditioning aimed at simulating sport-specific motions with attention to proper form. It is important to realize that cervical spine disk involvement typically requires more gradual progression initially as motion is poorly tolerated.

Because the herniated nucleus of the disk includes inflammatory components, an anti-inflammatory medication is very useful along with analgesics. In refractory cases, epidural injections of corticosteroids are very useful in accelerating the recovery phase. The adolescent athlete will often benefit from bracing to allow better rehabilitation.

Finally, surgery may be considered in three situations: (1) progressive muscle weakness, (2) loss of bowel or bladder control (emergent), and (3) refractory symptoms. The latter situation is somewhat subjective. In cases of severe pain, this may be as early as 6 to 8 weeks. In moderate cases, it may be months before surgery is considered. If surgery is needed, the athlete with a simple disk excision may possibly be ready for sports participation in 6 to 8 weeks.

Pierre A. d'Hemecourt

See also Back Injuries, Surgery for; Cervical Disk Degeneration; Intervertebral Disk Disease; Lower Back Injuries and Low Back Pain; Musculoskeletal Tests, Spine; Neck and Upper Back Injuries

Further Readings

Bogduk N. The inter-body joints and intervertebral discs. In: *Clinical Anatomy of the Lumbar Spine.* 3rd ed. London, UK: Churchill Livingston; 1991:13–31.

d'Hemecourt P, Gerbino P, Micheli L. Back injuries in the young athlete. *Clin Sports Med.* 2000;19(4): 663–675.

Frontera WR, Micheli LJ, Herring SA, Silver JK, eds. *Clinical Sports Medicine: Medical Management and Rehabilitation.* Philadelphia, PA: Saunders Elsevier; 2007.

SNAPPING HIP SYNDROME

Coxa saltans, or *snapping hip,* is a condition in which one feels a snapping sensation with movement of the hip. This may be accompanied by an audible pop and sometimes pain. There are three types of coxa saltans: external, internal, and intraarticular. Coxa saltans is common between the ages of 15 and 40 and is more often found in women. It is particularly common in athletes and dancers who undergo repetitive twisting motions about the hip.

Anatomy

The hip joint is the junction between the pelvis and the thighbone. The bony anatomy involves a ball-and-socket joint, with the head of the femur (thighbone) comprising the ball and the socket being formed by a groove in the pelvis called the acetabulum. This groove is deepened by a rubbery structure around the rim, called the *labrum.* The cartilage between these two surfaces serves as a cushion to absorb the stress transmitted between the surfaces.

There are many muscles around the hip that attach on the femur and pelvis. The muscles attach to the bones via ropelike fibrous tissue called *tendons.* Some of these tendons cross over bony prominences, which are normal protrusions in the bone. The natural consistency of healthy tendon fibers allows them to glide over these prominences with joint movement. Between the tendons and the bony prominences, there are sacs of fluid, called *bursae,* which minimize the friction between the bones and the tendons that pass over them.

The *iliotibial (IT) band* is a fibrous structure that extends from the pelvis to the knee. It functions to flex and rotate the thigh. The *gluteus maximus* is a large muscle that extends across the buttock and rotates the hip. Both the IT band and the gluteus maximus muscle cross over a bony prominence on the femur called the *greater trochanter.* This bony prominence can be easily felt in most people by pushing on the bone over the outer aspect of the thigh. With normal walking motions about the hip, the muscles and tendons glide over the greater trochanter without difficulty.

The hip flexor complex is a set of muscles formed by the iliacus and psoas muscles, which fuse to form the iliopsoas tendon. This connects the spine with the femur and functions to flex the hip. The iliopsoas tendon crosses over the hip joint, near the groin. In doing so, it passes in a groove next to the femoral head (the ball of the hip joint) and over the pelvis at a point called the *iliopectineal eminence.* With hip movement, the tendon slides from one side of the femoral head to the other (see Figure 1).

Causes

Coxa saltans can be divided into three different types. The external and internal types are generally caused by overuse and irritation of the muscle groups, which can lead to snapping of the tendons over the bony prominences. The two types are distinguished by their locations and the groups of muscles and tendons involved. The third type is intraarticular, in which the snapping can originate from within the hip joint itself. This is much less common but tends to be a more serious problem.

The external snapping hip is the most common type. Here, the IT band or the muscle of the gluteus maximus can catch and cause a snapping sound while crossing over the greater trochanter during normal motions of the hip. This may be due to tightening of these structures, caused by lack of flexibility. This can also happen if the greater trochanter protrudes more than normal. If the underlying bursa becomes irritated, one may have pain associated with the snapping as well.

In the internal snapping hip, the snapping occurs in the groin. The iliopsoas tendon becomes irritated due to overuse and can catch or snap while moving over the iliopectineal eminence or the femoral head. Inflammation from overuse of the iliopsoas tendon, called tendinitis, is often found in athletes or dancers who repetitively flex and externally rotate the thigh.

The intraarticular type of snapping hip stems from problems within the hip joint itself. This type is more commonly related to an injury rather than to chronic overuse. One of the more common injuries in this category includes labral tears, which are injuries to the cartilage rim around the joint. Other injuries may cause pieces of the cartilage, termed *loose bodies*, to be entrapped within the hip, causing a clicking noise with movement.

Symptoms

Typically, snapping hip develops over the course of months or years. Patients will describe an audible snap that is often reproducible at the time of the exam. An associated bursitis may cause tenderness or pain accompanying the snapping sensation.

In contrast, patients with intraarticular snapping may note a sudden onset of symptoms, usually

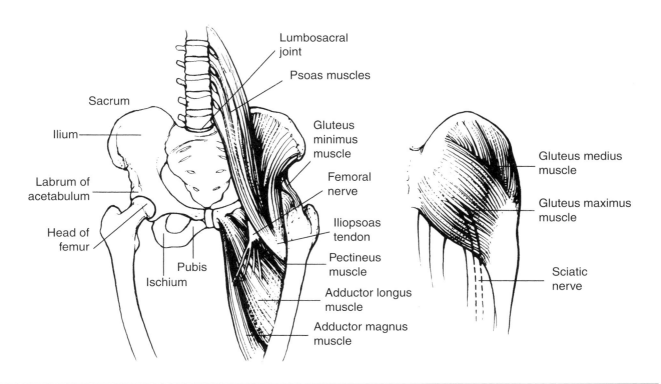

Figure I   Anatomy of the Hip, Pelvis, and Groin

related to a specific injury. Patients may describe their symptoms as a clicking rather than an audible snapping sound. This type is more likely to be associated with pain and may also include locking or catching sensations while moving the hip.

Diagnosis

The diagnosis of internal and external coxa saltans is typically made by observing the snapping and identifying the area involved. The external type can be diagnosed by feeling the snapping of the IT band over the greater trochanter as the patient flexes and extends the hip. Tightness of the IT band on examination may also point to this diagnosis. Those with internal snapping hip will have similar symptoms near the iliopsoas tendon in the groin.

X-rays are generally not helpful in the diagnosis of snapping hip, as the soft tissues involved cannot be assessed on radiographs. Magnetic resonance imaging (MRI) may be used to rule out injuries to the intraarticular cartilage but are not routinely obtained.

Rarely, internal and external coxa saltans may require diagnostic procedures. An ultrasound test is a noninvasive method of using sound waves to image the hip. Iliopsoas bursography (injecting dye into the bursa) can also be used to diagnose internal coxa saltans. Both techniques can detect abnormal motion of the tendon over the bony prominences, as well as identify any inflamed bursal tissue or tendons.

Treatment

Nonsurgical Treatment

The typical treatment for most cases of internal and external snapping hip is nonoperative, as the snapping motion of the hip is considered normal. If symptoms persist and become painful, then the physician may give a cortisone injection directly into the area that is inflamed. Rest, anti-inflammatory medications, and physical therapy will also help stretch and heal the muscles and tendons that are irritated. Most patients respond well to conservative therapy and are able to resume normal activities within 6 to 12 weeks.

Surgery

Surgical treatment of the internal and external types of snapping hip is rarely indicated, but it may be performed in cases of severe and persistent symptoms. Surgical treatment of external coxa saltans involves removal of the inflamed bursa and lengthening of the IT band. This removes tension from the tendon and allows it to glide over the bony prominences without snapping.

For the internal type, a similar procedure involving lengthening of the iliopsoas tendon is available. This can be done through a small incision in the groin or through a procedure called arthroscopy, which is a minimally invasive method using small incisions and a camera. Both procedures are typically done as outpatient surgeries.

Unlike the internal and external types, intraarticular causes of snapping hip generally require surgery. Many types of disorders contribute to intraarticular snapping, and these require therapies that are specific to the disorder. In cases of injury to the cartilage, surgery may be indicated to either remove or repair the problem. Most procedures of the hip are done with a standard open surgery. However, the advent of arthroscopic surgery has provided a minimally invasive way to address many of these problems.

After Surgery

Physical therapy after surgery depends on the type of surgery that is performed. Tendon-lengthening procedures will cause some hip weakness for several weeks until the muscle begins to heal. The first few weeks of physical therapy should focus on protecting the hip and reducing pain with range-of-motion exercises, as well as exercises to increase control of the leg. At the rate determined by the physician, therapy should later progress to strengthening and gait training, with eventual return to normal activities.

Miho J. Tanaka and Dennis E. Kramer

See also Hip Flexor Tendinitis; Iliotibial Band Syndrome; Trochanteric Bursitis

Further Readings

Allen WC, Cope R. Coxa saltans: the snapping hip revisited. *J Am Acad Orthop Surg.* 1995;3(5):303–308.

Gruen GS, Scioscia TN, Lowenstein JE. The surgical
treatment of internal snapping hip. *Am J Sports Med.*
2002;30(4):607–613.

Kelly BT, Williams RJ 3rd, Philippon MJ. Hip
arthroscopy: current indications, treatment options,
and management issues. *Am J Sports Med.*
2003;31(6):1020–1037.

Provencher MT, Hofmeister EP, Muldoon MP. The
surgical treatment of external coxa saltans (the
snapping hip) by Z-plasty of the IT band. *Am J Sports
Med.* 2004;32(2):470–476.

Snowboarding, Injuries in

The origin of snowboarding is somewhat debatable, yet most historians of the sport agree that the first snowboard was made out of a plywood plank in 1929 by M. J. "Jack" Burchett, who strapped the wood to his feet using a clothesline and horse reins. Some historians attribute snowboarding's origins to Sherman Poppen back in 1965, when he tinkered with the invention of a toy called a "snurfer" for his daughter, which consisted of two skis bound together and then tied a rope to the front for steering downhill to mimic the combined components of surf and snow. The early entrepreneurs Jake Burton Carpenter and Demetrije Milovich designed and produced the modern-day version of snowboards. The sport's modest beginning can be traced back to the production of snowboards and bindings back in 1977, although the sport did not really flourish until the 1990s. It made its Winter Olympic Games debut in 1998 in Nagano, Japan, and is today the fastest-growing winter sport with more than 3.4 million participants. There is some speculation that snowboard will take over skiing in popularity by as early as 2015.

The Sport and Its Equipment

The appearance of the snowboard on the scene was initially met with much resistance, for its enthusiasts were characterized as rebellious teenagers in baggy clothing, looking for an outlet that was devoid of respect and etiquette and disrupted the natural flow of skiing. Snowboarding in its infancy appealed to surfers, skateboarders,

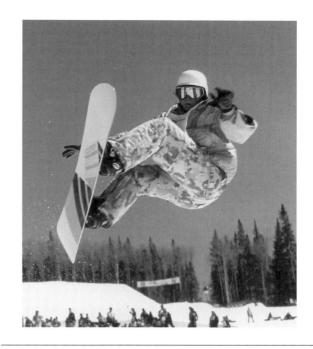

Snowboarding is the fastest-growing winter sport, with more than 3.4 million participants.

Source: Eric Limón/iStockphoto.

and backcountry idealists, who were often characterized as overly aggressive youths with a foolhardy attitude that negatively affected safety, although such characterizations might be attributed to age bias.

Snowboarding is typically identified in three major categories according to the particular style of riding or the type of board: (1) freestyle board, (2) freeride (all-mountain) board, and (3) Alpine (carving) board. Each board is uniquely characterized by the specific construction technique, the material of the board, and the unique shape, pattern, and flex for each specialty.

A freestyle snowboard is typically the one a beginner uses because it is more stable, wider, and more forgiving and thus easier to ride. Due to the softer flex and the shape, as well as the uniform symmetry, forward motion can occur in both directions, as is typically seen in the twin tip boards. These boards are meant for performing tricks such as airs, spins, grabs, and fakies (motion in a reverse direction) in terrain parks and half pipes. The contrasting directional freestyle snowboard has a stiffer tail than the nose of the board and is more beneficial when primarily going in one direction with a particular footed dominance.

Freeride (all-mountain) snowboards are typically the most popular type of snowboard, as illustrated by the sheer number of sales of these types of boards. These specialty boards are designed to be used for powder snow conditions and are identified as all-terrain mountain boards because they can be used not only on the hill but also in a terrain park and in a half-pipe. Freeride snowboards have a more directional shape, with a tail that is narrower, shorter, and flatter than the tip of the board. The stance position of these boards also differs in that they are typically offset toward the tail of the board. These boards are soft enough for beginners to maneuver in the snow and stiff enough to carve some turns.

Alpine (carving) snowboards, in contrast, look like larger versions of skis with a shoveled front tip and asymmetric appearance. They are characterized as carving snowboards because of their ability to make sharp, clean turns and their great edging abilities on hard snow for stability and speed. Alpine snowboards are designed for high-speed performance, such as in racing, and for moving in a more uniform direction; therefore, they are much more difficult for beginners to manage and learn due to the advanced body mechanics required to maneuver on harder snow surfaces.

Competition snowboarding includes numerous sporting events that are sanctioned by the International Ski Federation, abbreviated in all languages as FIS. FIS was founded on the eve of the first Olympic Games in 1924 in France with 14 member nations. Today, 107 National Ski Associations constitute the membership of FIS, which oversees the World Cup competitions and the World Championships. The federation organizes a number of disciplines in alpine, parallel giant slalom (PGS), and freestyle, which include subcategories such as half-pipe, snowboard cross, big air, and, more recently, slope style.

Following the collapse of the National Association of Professional Snowboarders in 1990, five nations and 120 athletes established the International Snowboarding Federation (ISF) with the goal of keeping the officiating by riders and for riders. The ISF set the standard for snowboarding competition, which contributed to snowboarding becoming an Olympic sport in 1998. Controversially, the International Olympic Committee did not recognize the ISF as the governing body for snowboarding but recognized FIS as the sport's official governing body. Many snowboarders boycotted the Olympics as a result, concluding that the FIS rules were inappropriate for snowboarding. The FIS has maintained its control over the Olympics, giving credence to the position that snowboarding is a discipline of skiing and not its own, individual sport.

Injuries in Snowboarding

The pattern of injuries in snowboarding differs from that in skiing primarily because of significant differences in sport mechanics. Skiing typically demonstrates a significant number of injuries, from torque-type injuries such as tears of the anterior cruciate ligament (ACL) of the knee to other lower extremity pathologies induced by the free rotation and often uncontrollable trauma of the lower extremities during falls. Snowboarding, in which two feet are planted firmly on the same board, does not demonstrate the same frequency of rotational torque-type injuries. Instead, falls on an outstretched arm typically lead to more injuries of the upper extremity. The wrist is the most commonly injured body part, with wrist fractures accounting for almost half of upper extremity injuries. Wrist sprains and elbow fractures, along with clavicle fractures and shoulder dislocation, contribute to the upper extremity percentages being predictably higher for snowboarders than for skiers.

The use of helmets has reduced the frequency of head injuries to between 30% and 50%. Injuries to the head typically occur as a result of a direct blow to the head when making contact with the hard-packed snow surface. As a result, the injuries that occur are less serious in nature and are limited to head lacerations, contusions to the head, and milder versions of concussions. There continues to be a reduction in the number of fatalities due to increased helmet use, which has been shown to drastically reduce the severity of concussions and minimize the number of skull fractures as well as lessen the likelihood of severe closed-head injuries. The overall rate of injury has increased for snowboarding more recently due to the greater number of beginners who have taken up the sport. The research literature has clearly demonstrated that the highest frequency of injury is typically found in young novice snowboarders. More than 50% of novice skiers have the greatest likelihood of being injured in their first season of snowboarding. Additional contributing factors include failure to wear appropriate protective gear or receive appropriate instruction. Injury prevention is of extreme importance in snowboarding and entails the selection of specific gears such as wrist guards, elbow guards, back protectors, and tailbone butt protection along with helmets and proper boot fitting and equipment maintenance.

Boots and bindings are also of particular interest in snowboarding due to the different types of styles. There are three styles of boots: (1) soft, (2) hard, and (3) hybrid. Most of the boots today are softer in form and function, making it easier to maneuver specific snowboard moves due to the increased flexibility of the boot material. Hard boots are typically used only for racing and are the most common cause of boot type injuries and fractures. Most bindings on snowboards are nonreleasable and are made of plastic molding, with buckles to strap the boots onto the boards. The number of ankle injuries has been reduced due to the advanced technology of boots and bindings, but fractures remain the predominant ankle injury. The most common fracture is the so-called snowboarders' ankle, which is a fracture of the lateral process of the talus and is often undiagnosed on a typical X-ray. Treatment of a nondisplaced fracture typically consists of casting for 6 to 8 weeks. Displaced fractures are usually characterized by a displacement of 2 millimeters and are typically treated by open reduction internal fixation repair of the bone tissue.

Other common injuries in skiing that are less serious but still debilitating include frostbite, dehydration, and sunburn. Sunburn results from ultraviolet radiation and not from heat. Sun exposure on cold snowy days without any protection often results in sunburn, particularly in young children. Sunburn prevention should be practiced when skiing at any time. Hypothermia results when the core body temperature drops below 95 °F. Exposure to cold environments, particularly wet, windy conditions, can lead to rapid loss of body heat. Recognizing the signs and symptoms of hypothermia, such as confusion, slurred speech, fatigue, exhaustion, shivering, and loss of motor control, necessitates immediate action. The key is to eliminate the exposure and warm the individual. Hypothermia can often lead to cardiac arrest, so observation is also of great importance. Frostbite is literally frozen body tissue. Children are at a much greater risk than adults because they lose heat more rapidly and are often reluctant to protect against exposure. Treatment typically includes removing wet clothing, warming the exposed body parts in warm water, and preventing additional exposure. Following an appropriate treatment strategy and medical care are advised.

Richard Quincy and Grant Armour

Further Readings

Bladin C, McCrory P. Snowboarding injuries. An overview. *Sports Med.* 1995;19(5):358–364.

Hagel B. Skiing and snowboarding injuries. *Med Sport Sci.* 2005;48:74–119.

Johnson RJ, Shealy JE, Yamagishi T, eds. *Skiing Trauma and Safety.* Vol. 16. Philadelphia, PA: American Society for Testing and Materials; 2006. (ASTM STP 1474).

Young CC, Niedfeldt MW. Snowboarding injuries. *Am Fam Physician.* 1999;59(1):131–136.

Websites

International Society for Skiing Safety: http://www.isssweb.com

Snowboarding Injuries: http://www.ski-injury.com

Stay Safe in Snow: http://www.ski-injury.com/specific-sports/snowboard-injuries

SOCCER, INJURIES IN

The physical demands of soccer can result in a wide variety of injuries to athletes. Youth and adult soccer players of all skill levels are at risk for both traumatic and overuse injuries. The types of injuries that may occur during soccer participation include sprains, strains, contusions, abrasions, fractures, and head injuries.

Mechanisms of Injury

Both contact and noncontact injuries occur during soccer participation. Contact injuries may result from contact with another player or equipment (i.e., ball, goal post). Noncontact injuries occur due to the high frequency of pivoting, running, and jumping activities performed by soccer players. Contact injuries more commonly occur during games, whereas noncontact injuries are more common during practice. For injuries that result in missed playing time, injury rates for both men and women are higher during games than during practice.

Acute Lower Extremity Injuries

The majority of soccer injuries occur in the lower extremities, with ankle sprains and knee ligament injuries occurring most frequently. Muscle strains of the hip adductors, hamstrings, and quadriceps are also very common. The contact nature of the sport also increases the frequency of contusions and abrasions to the lower extremities.

Ankle

A common ankle injury in soccer is a lateral ankle sprain. The ligament most commonly injured in an ankle sprain is the anterior talofibular ligament; this is caused by forced ankle plantarflexion and inversion. The calcaneofibular ligament is the second most commonly injured ligament in a lateral ankle sprain, followed by the posterotalofibular ligament. When the foot is forced into dorsiflexion and eversion, the deltoid ligament on the medial aspect of the ankle can be injured.

A high ankle sprain is a more severe type of ankle sprain. In this injury, the ligaments above the ankle (the syndesmosis) are torn. A high ankle sprain includes injury to the anterior inferior tibiofibular ligament, posterior talofibular ligament, and interosseous ligament. Pain at the ankle with compression of the tibia and fibula above the ankle (squeeze test) or a Maisonneuve fracture (proximal fibula) are positive findings of a high ankle sprain. High ankle sprains that are determined to be unstable are treated with stabilization of the fibula to the tibia with one or two screws while the injury heals.

When evaluating an athlete with an ankle sprain, the possibility of a Jones fracture (at the base of the fifth metatarsal) must also be considered.

Knee

Knee ligament and meniscal injuries result from pivoting, rapid direction changes, rapid deceleration motions, or contact with another player. Knee ligament injuries can occur with or without meniscal damage. Soccer players, especially women, are at a high risk for noncontact anterior cruciate ligament (ACL) injuries. The ACL is injured when the lower extremity is in a position of femoral internal rotation, genu valgum, and tibial external rotation. A valgus stress to the knee will injure the medial collateral ligament (MCL). Less commonly injured is the lateral collateral ligament (LCL). LCL injuries result from a varus stress to the knee. Multiple ligament knee injuries can occur with higher forces (see Figure 1).

Chronic Lower Extremity Injuries

Excessive amount of running during soccer can lead to chronic, overuse injuries. Achilles and patellar

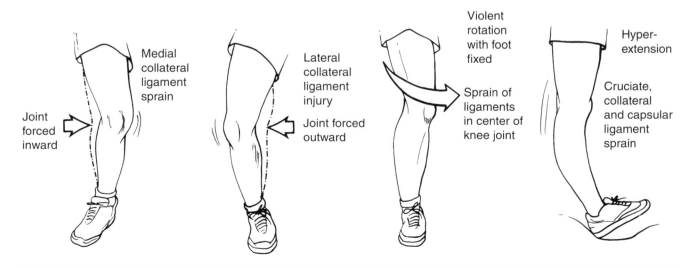

Figure I   Knee Ligament Injuries

Notes: Which of the knee ligaments are injured depends on how the injury occurs. The most common mechanisms of knee injuries and the specific ligaments that most often get damaged are shown in the figure in each case.

tendinitis are common in adult soccer players. Although rare, stress fractures can develop from factors such as a hard playing surface, poor shoe wear, improper mechanics, and training errors.

Upper Extremity Injuries

Although not as common as lower extremity injuries, upper extremity injuries do occur during soccer. Direct contact with another player or a fall on an outstretched hand can result in upper extremity injuries, including acromioclavicular joint sprains, clavicle fractures, glenohumeral joint dislocations, elbow sprains and dislocations, and wrist sprains.

Injuries to Skeletally Immature Athletes

Year-round training combined with a high number of training hours increase the risk for injury in any sport. In a skeletally immature athlete, the apophysis, an ossification center where a tendon attaches to the bone, can be injured by traction forces or from a sudden muscular contraction. The forceful running and kicking motions during soccer play can cause avulsion fractures of the pelvic apophyses, including the anterior superior iliac spine (ASIS), the anterior inferior iliac spine (AIIS), the ischial tuberosity, and, less commonly, the pubic symphysis and the iliac crest. An avulsion of the ASIS is due to a forceful stretch or contraction of the sartorius muscle, whereas an avulsion of the AIIS is related to the rectus femoris muscle.

In addition to an acute avulsion fracture, overuse-type injuries to the apophysis can also occur from excessive running and jumping in young soccer players. Repetitive traction forces cause inflammation at the apophysis, known as *apophysitis*. Common sites of apophysitis in soccer players include the tibial tuberosity (Osgood-Schlatter disease), calcaneus (Sever disease), inferior pole of the patella (Sinding-Larsen-Johannson), and iliac crest.

Head Injuries

Concussions during soccer play most often result from player-to-player contact but may also occur from contact with the playing surface or goal post. Although there has been some concern that the repetitive low-impact stress of heading the ball may possibly have injurious effects to the brain, there is no conclusive evidence for this. Heading the ball is considered a safe skill when done properly.

Return to Sports After an Injury

Once an athlete has sustained an injury, a qualified health care professional should assess the athlete to determine if he or she is ready to return to play. The athlete should be painfree, have no swelling, have full range of motion, and have normal strength testing done before considering return to sports. Isokinetic strength testing can be used to objectively identify and evaluate smaller strength deficits that are not detectable by manual muscle testing. Sport-specific functional testing also needs to be performed to determine if the athlete is ready to return to sports. Lower extremity functional testing should progress from bilateral to unilateral and from straight-plane activities to multiplanar activities. Examples of functional tests include balance/proprioceptive tests, broad jump, unilateral hop test, triple hop test, crossover hop test, and sport-specific drills (running, lateral movements, pivoting, and cutting maneuvers).

Injury Prevention

Although the risk of contact and noncontact injuries with soccer participation cannot be eliminated, it is possible to decrease the risk of injury. General guidelines to minimize the risk of injury during soccer participation include the following:

- Always perform a proper warm-up (general cardiovascular warm-up, dynamic stretches, sport-specific drills).
- Perform lower extremity stretches to improve muscle flexibility.
- Wear proper shoes.
- Use protective equipment.
- Maintain good field conditions.
- Maintain an adequate fitness level (muscle strength and cardiovascular endurance).
- Have proper hydration and nutrition.
- Enforce game rules.
- Properly supervise young athletes.

Since most soccer injuries occur to the lower extremities, training programs specifically for minimizing the risk of ankle and knee injuries can be beneficial. Training programs may include all or any combination of the following components: warm-up, lower extremity stretching, lower extremity and core strengthening, proprioceptive and neuromuscular training, plyometrics, and sport-specific agility drills.

Anna Thatcher and Jeffrey Vaughn

Further Readings

Agel J, Evans TA, Dick R, Putukian M, Marshal SW. Descriptive epidemiology of collegiate men's soccer injuries: National Collegiate Athletic Association Injury Surveillance System, 1988–1989 through 2002–2003. *J Athl Train.* 2007;42(2):270–277.

Dick R, Putukian M, Agel J, Evans TA, Marshall SW. Descriptive epidemiology of collegiate women's soccer injuries: National Collegiate Athletic Association Injury Surveillance System, 1988–1989 through 2002–2003. *J Athl Train.* 2007;42(2):278–285.

Gilchrist J, Mandelbaum BR, Melancon H, et al. A randomized controlled trial to prevent noncontact anterior cruciate ligament injury in female collegiate soccer players. *Am J Sports Med.* 2008;36(8): 1476–1483.

Hewett TE, Ford KR, Myer GD. Anterior cruciate ligament injuries in female athletes: part 2. A meta-analysis of neuromuscular interventions aimed at injury prevention. *Am J Sports Med.* 2006;34(3):490–498.

Leininger RE, Knox CL, Comstock RD. Epidemiology of 1.6 million pediatric soccer-related injuries presenting to US emergency departments from 1990 to 2003. *Am J Sports Med.* 2007;35(2):288–293.

Yard EE, Schroder MJ, Fields SK, Collins CL, Comstock RD. The epidemiology of United States high school soccer injuries, 2005–2007. *Am J Sports Med.* 2008;36(10):1930–1937.

SPEED, AGILITY, AND SPEED ENDURANCE DEVELOPMENT

The goal of all team and individual sports athletes is to have great speed, agility, and speed endurance to outperform their opponents. To develop these conditioning adaptations to their full potential, the athletes have to be ready for rigorous training and must be disciplined when not training to allow the body to recover properly; otherwise the risk of injury from overtraining is imminent. This entry will provide insight on the necessary training variables to become not only faster but also faster for longer periods and more agile on the court, field, or floor.

Defining Speed, Agility, and Speed Endurance

To develop speed, agility, and speed endurance, it is necessary to assess the needs of the athlete in the sport or position that he or she plays. First, it is important to fully understand each of these terms.

Speed

Speed is the ability of an athlete to create a lot of velocity through recruiting muscles rapidly. Speed must come from all joints and segments of the body working sequentially (see the entry Resistance Training). Pure speed is often seen in sports as straight-line speed, such as the 100-meter (m) sprints or a fastball in baseball. Just as important for the ability to develop speed through the segments of the body is developing the muscles, joints, tendons, and ligaments for the rapid deceleration of the joints once the speed-producing movement is complete. If the body is not able to decelerate itself, then serious injury will occur. For example, if the muscles did not decelerate when throwing a fastball, then the arm would likely dislocate.

Agility

Agility, also known as sports speed, is an athlete's ability to rapidly accelerate, stop, and change directions and accelerate again. Agility training is a priority for sports played on a field in team settings such as soccer, rugby, and American football. The focus of agility training should be on the ability to slow down the body rapidly and accelerate the body as fast as possible in as little time possible. Developing speed for sports requires an immense amount of power coupled with eccentric and concentric strength of the antagonist and agonist musculature.

Speed Endurance

Speed endurance means that the athlete is able to sustain high velocity and able to reproduce the acceleration and deceleration multiple times without a significant drop-off in power output multiple times for more than 6 to 7 seconds. This would mean that the athlete has a high threshold for pyruvate-lactate accumulation. The dominating energy system supporting high-intensity work for durations greater than 10 seconds is the anaerobic glycolysis system.

The rate of force development (RFD) implies how quickly a movement can be produced. This is the measure that will indicate how successful off-season conditioning is for the athletes on the field. To increase the RFD in a movement pattern that ultimately increases speed, agility, and speed endurance, the ratio of fast-twitch glycolytic (Type IIa) muscle fibers and fast-twitch oxidative (Type IIab) muscle fibers to slow-twitch oxidative (Type I) muscle fibers need to increase more on the side of Type IIa.

This will result in an increase in the impulse production, according to Steven Plisk (in *Essentials of Strength Training and Conditioning*, 2000), by generating a greater force in a given time or by improving the RFD.

Speed Technique Development

For an athlete to reach his or her true potential in top-end speed, form, or technique must be developed along with the athlete's muscular strength and power. A needs analysis for the athlete's power profile is necessary before prescribing the correct ratio of volume to intensity of conditioning for the athlete's respective sport or position. The ratio of pure speed drills to strength-speed drills for an offensive lineman in football would be drastically different from that of a wide receiver. Coaches must conduct video analysis of the amount, if any, of contact the athlete has with opposition, how many quick changes in direction the athlete executes in competition, how long it takes for the athlete to decelerate, and the number of times that an athlete performs sprints at maximal effort. To develop the optimal speed endurance program, the strength coaches need to know what the work-to-rest ratio throughout the sporting event typically is. Once the aforementioned data have been collected, the team strength coach and team head coach are able to combine the information on movement and performance with the information on skill of the athlete(s). Having this information all together allows the coaches to develop the best sequence of movement, performance, and skill drills and the best work-to-rest ratio between these types of drill before, during, and after a given competitive season to optimize on-field performance and to decrease the risk of injury.

Sprinting technique drills will teach the athlete the correct form to use when accelerating away from an opponent or when trying to catch or pass an opponent. If the athlete's form is impaired, more energy than is necessary is being expended to produce a movement, ultimately causing fatigue. In the case of sprinting, two variables dictate the forward projection of the athlete's body: stride length and stride frequency. Stride length is the distance between the feet each time a foot makes contact with the ground. If the athlete's stride length is too long or too short, it will take more effort than is necessary. The length of the stride will vary depending on the athlete's height and limb length. Stride frequency is the number of times that the legs can turn over in a maximal sprint. Steven Plisk points out that both stride frequency and length are equally important when an athlete is accelerating; however, the stride rate has the most influence at maximal speed. When the athlete's speed picks up, impulse production becomes more dependent on the ability to create force rapidly.

There are a multitude of techniques that coaches use to develop straight-line speed. Form drills such as "high-knee drills" and "butt-kickers" train the hips and knees in the rapid turnover. Different styles of skipping and bounding help with stride length frequency development. Hill training is another very useful training modality. When athletes run up gradual hills, their leg drive technique is developed; focusing on high knee strikes will develop impulse. Running down gradual hills will assist the athlete in increasing stride frequency and stride rate. It is important to note that the incline/decline of a hill should not be too steep so that the athlete's form is not compromised.

Agility Technique Training

Having great straight-line speed does not necessarily translate into great sports speed. The most important components in developing sports speed are acceleration and deceleration development. Stability and efficiency are essential when training the right body mechanics so that the transitions between stopping, quick change of direction, and acceleration are more balanced. Agility training can be taught through form drills, using set parameters such as cones, lines, or poles. Agility training can also be taught openly through reaction drills such as mirror drills, tag, or reacting to cues from the coaches, such as a whistle or signal indicating a change of direction. Agility must be trained in all plains of motion—sagittal, frontal, and transverse—to provide the athlete with the necessary conditioning for movements that may occur during competition.

Speed and Agility Training Methods

There are several ways to develop an athlete's speed and agility. Hill training is one example. Others include the following:

- Footwork and form drills
- Assisted and resisted sprinting drills
- Resistance training
- Flexibility training

Footwork and Form Drills

Footwork drills and form drills are necessary to conduct at the beginning of training sessions. Examples are ladder drills, crossovers, turns, and cuts using traffic cones. The body is sensitive to neuromuscular feedback and is able to adapt to the detailed drills so that the body keeps the correct form even when it is fatigued.

Assisted and Resisted Sprinting Drills

Hill training is a form of assisted running because the athlete is running with the downward pull of gravity. Another way to train an athlete to run faster is to use stretched rubber tubing with a harness around the athlete's waist or torso to pull him or her forward. Rubber tubing may also be used for resisted running. When the tubing stretches, it creates greater resistance. Parachutes, running uphill, and weighted sleds that are pushed or pulled by the athlete are other tools to provide resistance while running forward, backward, and laterally.

Resistance Training

General total body strength and power training must complement the aforementioned drills. Resistance training must be used to maintain overall kinetic chain symmetry and to prevent overtraining injuries that may occur. (For more information on the proper methods of training and sequencing, see the entries Periodization and Resistance Training.)

Flexibility Training

Strength and conditioning coaches must know the work-to-rest ratio in the sport of the athletes they are training to optimize the adaptations of speed endurance. Sports such as rugby and soccer have different work-to-rest ratios in comparison with American football or ice hockey. Rugby and soccer athletes do not have as much opportunity to rest between high-intensity plays unless play has been stopped due to penalty, injury, or halftime. It is important to note that the energy system that must be trained, and is affected the most by speed-endurance training, is the anaerobic glycolysis system. When repetitive bouts of high-intensity sprints or tackling occur in rapid succession, lactate-pyruvate concentrations increase in the body's cells because the mitochondria (the organelle responsible for cellular respiration) are unable to clear out the by-products produced. Implementing the aforementioned speed and agility drills with little or no rest at submaximal (80–90% of maximal intensity) efforts when the athletes are slightly fatigued will produce a positive adaptation for speed endurance. Having the athletes perform obstacle courses that integrate footwork drills with sprints and low-intensity jogging are popular ways to train athletes for improved speed endurance. (For more information on speed-endurance training, refer to the entry Interval Training/Fartlek.)

Samuel L. Berry

See also Cardiovascular and Respiratory Anatomy and Physiology: Responses to Exercise; Exercise Physiologist; Exercise Physiology; Interval Training/ Fartlek; Periodization; Resistance Training

Further Readings

Brown LE, Ferrigno V. *Training for Speed, Agility, and Quickness.* 2nd ed. Champaign, IL: Human Kinetics; 2005.

Faccioni A. Assisted and resisted methods for speed development (part I). *Mod Athl Coach.* 1994; 32(2):3–6.

Faccioni A. Assisted and resisted methods for speed development (part II). *Mod Athl Coach.* 1994; 32(3):8–11.

Plisk SS. Speed, agility, and speed-endurance development. In: Baechle TR, Earle RW, eds. *Essentials of Strength Training and Conditioning.* 2nd ed. Champaign, IL: Human Kinetics; 2000: 471–490.

Sandler D. *Sports Power.* Champaign, IL: Human Kinetics; 2004.

SPEED SKATING, INJURIES IN

Speed skating is a sport that held its first competition over 300 years ago in the Netherlands. There are two disciplines in speed skating—long track and short track. Short-track skaters race in a pack around a smaller oval, while long-track skaters race in their own lane. All speed skating athletes are at risk of sustaining injuries during training and competition, although the short-track skaters are at higher risk.

History

Ice skating originated thousands of years ago, when Scandinavian men attached animal bones to their footwear to help glide across frozen waterways. The metal blade was invented in the late 1500s. That helped spur the popularity of speed skating. The first world championship was held in the Netherlands, with four events: 500, 1,500, 5,000, and 10,000 meters (m). Short-track speed skating began in the early 1900s.

Olympic long-track speed skating debuted in 1924, at the first Winter Games in Chamonix, France. Short-track speed skating was introduced at the 1988 Winter Games in Calgary, Canada. Both disciplines are governed by the International Skating Union.

Long-Track Speed Skating

Equipment

The body of the ice skate is called the boot. Many elite athletes have custom boots created using the molds of their feet. The boot is constructed with leather and carbon graphite. A long-track boot is cut lower on the ankle than a short-track boot.

The blades are made from carbon steel. They are very flat and thin, allowing long-track skaters to glide in long, straight lines. Most elite skaters use a clap skate. This blade detaches at the heel and has a spring-loaded hinge at the ball of the foot. As the skater lifts his or her foot, the hinged blade remains on the ice longer. This improves speed and traction.

Most skaters wear eye protection to prevent tearing and drying secondary to wind. Many also wear skin-tight clothing with hoods designed to make them more aerodynamic. Long-track speed skaters do not wear helmets.

Events

Long-track speed skaters race counterclockwise on a two-lane, 400-m oval. The winner is the person with the fastest time. The athletes will cross over, or change lanes, every lap on the back stretch. Thus, long-track skaters do not race in the same lane.

The traditional events are the 500, 1,000, 1,500, 3,000, 5,000, and 10,000 m. A 100-m sprint event has been recently added. Team pursuit is also a newer event. In team pursuit, each team begins at opposite points on the track. A team of three or four skaters race in a single-file line, allowing the skater in the back to conserve energy by not having to break the wind. They rotate positions in the single-file line to try to get the fastest time for six to eight laps.

Short-Track Speed Skating

Equipment

The short-track boot rises higher on the ankle than a long-track boot to give more stability with turning.

The blades are made from carbon steel. They are shorter and thicker than long-track skates to withstand the stress of turning. The blades are offset and bent to allow skaters to lean into turns without allowing the boot to contact the ice.

All skaters must wear protective gear. This includes a helmet, a neck protector, cut-resistant gloves, knee pads, and shin guards. Most skaters wear protective eyewear, which also helps prevent tearing. The skaters wear tight-fitting skin suits like the long-track skaters. However, many short-track suits are made of Kevlar, making them cut resistant and safer.

Events

There are normally four to six skaters racing counterclockwise around a 111-m oval. The outcome of the race is not based on time, but the first person to cross the finish line is the winner. The racers all share the same space, so there is great potential for contact between skaters, falls, and subsequent collision into the wall of the rink.

The main events are the 500-, 1,000-, 1,500-, 3,000-, and 5,000-m relay. In relay events, there are usually four teams of four skaters. The skaters must take at least one lap on the track, but there is no set number of laps that each racer must complete.

Injuries

Very few data are available on injury rates in speed skaters. While injuries can occur during training and competition, it is thought that short-track skaters are at higher risk of injury due to the higher risk of collision. There is a higher risk of asthma symptoms due to exposure to cold, dry air. As with all athletes who compete in international events, there is a risk for infectious disorders common to the region hosting the event, as well as common viral syndromes.

Skaters are at risk for overuse injuries, particularly of the lower extremities. This is secondary to the repetitive motions required for the sport. Back pain can be secondary to mechanical and muscular issues, as well as lumbar disk disease. Hip pain is commonly related to iliotibial band tendinopathy and groin strains. Knee pain is frequently secondary to patellofemoral pain syndrome and patellar tendinopathy.

Foot and ankle disorders frequently occur due to irritation from the skate boot. A tightly laced boot can apply pressure to the muscles around the ankle, causing Achilles tendinopathy, as well as "lace bite," which is a common name for tendinitis of the anterior tibialis and toe extensor muscles. Due to the amount of time spent in the skates, athletes may develop athlete's foot or tinea pedis. Interestingly, peroneal tendinopathy is seen much more frequently in short-track speed skaters due to the force required to complete sharp, high-speed crossover turns.

All speed skaters are at risk for arm and wrist injuries such as contusions, fractures, and sprains secondary to falls. Short-track skating carries a higher risk for upper extremity injuries due to the high-speed, pack-style skating format. This leads to a great deal of contact and can precipitate falls. Therefore, injuries such as shoulder dislocations, concussions, and lacerations (from contact with the skate blades) are seen much more frequently in short-track speed skaters.

Injuries can potentially be reduced by ensuring that athletes use proper equipment and maximize their off-ice conditioning. Athletes should also warm up well and remain warm throughout their practice and competition. It is important that they have well-maintained skates that fit properly. The blades should be sharpened frequently to improve traction. Of course, loose clothing that can get caught on the blades should not be worn.

Kevin D. Walter

See also Ankle Injuries; Concussion; Conditioning; Contusions (Bruises); Knee Injuries; Lower Leg Injuries; Tendinopathy

Further Readings

2007 Canada Winter Games. Media information package long track speed skating. http://www.canadagames.ca/Images/Games/2007%20Media%20Packages/FINAL%20LONG%20TRACK%20ENGLISH.pdf. Accessed August 24, 2008.

2007 Canada Winter Games. Media information package short track speed skating. http://www.canadagames.ca/Images/Games/2007%20Media%20Packages/FINAL%20SHORT%20TRACK%20ENGLISH.pdf. Accessed August 24, 2008.

Quinn A, Lun V, McCall J, Overend T. Injuries in short track speed skating. *Am J Sports Med.* 2003;31(4):507–510.

SPINAL CORD INJURY

Spinal cord injury (SCI) is a rare but potentially devastating occurrence in sports. In the general population, motor vehicle crashes are the most common cause at around 40%. Sports and recreation injuries are responsible for about 12% of

SCI, diving accidents being the most common cause in this category. However, any sport involving speed, contact, or collision presents an environment where SCI can occur. This includes, but is not limited to, ice hockey, football, motor sports, and cycling.

Anatomy

The spinal cord extends from an opening in the base of the skull (the *foramen magnum*) to the second lumbar vertebra in the lower back. Beyond this level, it continues as a bundle of nerve roots called the *cauda equina*, or "horse's tail" because of its appearance. The spinal cord resides in a canal formed within the bony vertebral column of the back, which provides protection for the delicate tissue.

The spinal cord is divided into 31 segments or levels: 8 cervical (neck), 12 thoracic (upper and midback), 5 lumbar (lower back), 5 sacral, and 1 coccygeal. The latter two are so named because the nerve roots for these segments exit the spinal canal via the sacrum and coccyx, which are part of the pelvis. Viewed in cross section, each segment gives rise to motor nerve roots that exit the spinal cord from the front and sensory nerve roots that exit dorsally (from the back). The motor and sensory roots from each segment combine to form a spinal nerve corresponding to that segment, one to the left and one to the right. These spinal nerves carry motor and sensory information from the spinal cord to the periphery and back.

The spinal cord's job is to transmit information from the brain to the body (e.g., coordinating the motions of one's arm and hand to pick up a cup) as well as to transmit feedback from the body to the brain (once one's hand grasps the cup, this sensory information is sent to the brain to let it know that it can proceed with the instructions to lift it from the table).

Etiology

Most injuries to the spinal cord are traumatic in origin. Traumatic SCI frequently occurs in association with dislocation or fracture of the surrounding vertebrae in the neck or back. However, a special consideration in the pediatric population is SCI without radiographic abnormality (SCIWORA), where the increased flexibility of the developing spinal column allows for trauma to be inflicted on the spinal cord in extreme neck flexion or extension without any apparent fracture or dislocation occurring. In such an injury, the spinal cord is contused (bruised) by the impinging vertebrae. Depending on the severity of the impingement and the resulting inflammatory reaction, this injury can be temporary or permanent. The clinical exam will reveal diminished motor or sensory function consistent with the segmental level of injury. However, X-ray and computed tomography (CT) will reveal no bony or ligamentous injury. Magnetic resonance imaging (MRI) may show the cord contusion itself, but diagnosis and management are best guided by the clinical exam.

SCI may also be the result of compression of the cord, without actually cutting or bruising it. This is possible in the case of dislocation of vertebrae, progressive narrowing (stenosis) of the bony spinal canal, bulging of one or more intervertebral disks (the cushions between vertebrae), or several other, more progressive conditions. Spinal cord function is affected by the direct compression and/or by reduced blood flow and nourishment of the cells. Clinically, a patient will have reduced sensory and motor functions consistent with the level affected, which may be progressive over time, starting with an occasional "numbness and tingling" and progressing to complete loss of motor function.

Injury Patterns and Symptoms

SCI is a broad term referring to any injury that either temporarily or permanently prevents the spinal cord from performing its job of transmitting motor and sensory information between the brain and the rest of the body. More specific terms are generally defined by anatomic location of the injury (paraplegia vs. tetraplegia) and its severity (complete vs. incomplete). Paraplegia is an injury to the spinal cord in the thoracic, lumbar, or sacral segments. The most obvious deficit is loss of function of both lower limbs; however, sensation will be affected below the level of the injury (e.g., an injury at T2 would affect sensation from the chest all the way to the feet). Tetraplegia is an injury to the cord in the cervical region, which results in loss of function of all four extremities. In addition, an injury in the cervical region can have profound effects on one's ability to breathe, as motor control of the diaphragm originates from the C3-C5 segments. Both paraplegia and tetraplegia cause varying degrees of loss of bowel and bladder function.

Complete SCI is usually associated with a severe vertebral fracture and/or dislocation, with bony fragments transecting, or cutting, the spinal cord. While paraplegia and tetraplegia are considered complete injuries (as evidenced by loss of both motor and sensory function), it is also possible to have an incomplete injury where only motor or sensory function is lost or where only one side of the body is affected. For example, *anterior cord syndrome* is characterized by loss of motor function but preservation of many sensory functions, which travel primarily in the back of the spinal cord. *Brown-Sequard syndrome* is a unique condition in which the left or right half of the spinal cord is transected. Given the manner in which motor and sensory information cross from right to left at different levels, a person with this injury characteristically presents with loss of position sense and motor function on the same side of the body as the injured side of the cord and loss of pain and temperature sensation on the opposite side.

Treatment

Although research is ongoing, there is little to be done to repair a damaged spinal cord. Therefore, management is directed toward pain control, prevention of worsening of symptoms, and recovery of function where possible. This is done through medication, physical therapy and rehabilitation, and, in some cases, surgery.

Medication is an area of intense debate and research. There is little disagreement regarding pain control. Analgesics ranging from acetaminophen and nonsteroidal anti-inflammatory drugs such as ibuprofen to narcotics such as morphine and hydrocodone are all useful in managing pain. However, care must be taken to prevent development of dependence on these drugs and to avoid side effects associated with overuse.

Steroids have played a role of varying prominence with regard to treatment of SCI. More recent evidence shows that steroids may be helpful in reducing the secondary effects of acute SCI, that is, the inflammatory reaction that occurs after injury and is thought to be responsible for some of the longer-lasting damage. Significant improvements in neurologic outcome have been demonstrated with initiation of steroid administration very soon after injury (within 8 hours). However, more research needs to be done in this area to determine efficacy. Also, steroid administration has side effects that may outweigh the neurologic benefits, such as immune suppression, which makes a patient susceptible to severe infection.

Physical therapy can be very effective in both mild and severe injury. In more mild cases, a therapy regimen that improves flexibility may reduce compressive symptoms, including helping a herniated disk "slide" back into place. Also, strengthening of the core muscles (e.g., abdominal muscles and the muscles that stabilize the spine) may be helpful in reducing symptoms by providing an "assist" to the vertebrae and intervertebral disks. In more severe cases where a lasting motor deficit is present, intensive therapy and rehabilitation can help a patient learn to use different muscle groups to compensate or even help a previously affected muscle group and nerve pathway to "relearn" its function.

Another therapy receiving much attention is the intravenous (IV) infusion of very cold saline solution. Saline with a normality of 0.9% has a similar salt concentration to the water present in the body and is used routinely for IV hydration. With regard to SCI, as well as to prehospital management of trauma patients in general, the infusion of ice-cold saline drops the body's temperature by several degrees, which is thought to reduce the body's oxygen and energy demands and is a way to preserve the delicate and damaged tissue, particularly until more definitive management can be initiated. Cooling is another way to reduce the postinjury inflammatory reaction. However, more research must be done to determine the precise effects that produce benefit as well as the appropriate algorithm for implementation. For example, there is a fine line between enough cooling to preserve tissue and too much cooling that triggers failure of, and damage to, other organs. Also, following injury there is likely to be a time after which the benefit of cooling is lost and the effect is perhaps detrimental.

Surgical repair of the spinal cord itself is not currently possible. However, there are several procedures to treat persistent insults to the spinal cord. Laminectomy is a procedure in which the lamina, part of the vertebra that forms a protective ring around the spinal cord, is removed. This allows swelling of the cord or surrounding the soft tissues to bulge outward and away from the spinal cord rather than compress the cord. The more bone that is removed, the more unstable the spine becomes, increasing the risk for future injury to the spinal cord. As a result, spinal fusion may be required. Supplemental bone tissue (from either the patient or another donor) is used to stimulate the body's own bone building to fuse the adjacent vertebrae and limit their mobility. The goals are decreased pain and risk of further injury but at the expense of overall mobility of the back.

Because of the risks associated with surgery in general and because of the likelihood of reduced function after surgery, decompressive procedures are reserved for cases of severe neurologic compromise (particularly in cases of direct pressure on the spinal cord) or in cases where more conservative therapy provides little or no improvement.

Prognosis

SCI is a potentially devastating injury. Incomplete injuries generally have a better prognosis than complete injuries. Patients with complete injuries have a 5% or less chance of recovery, which drops to nearly 0% at 72 hours postinjury. Preservation of some sensory function indicates a 50% chance of recovering the ability to walk. In terms of long-term survival, the mortality rate has steadily improved over the years, mostly as a result of gains in infection control with early diagnosis and better treatment of conditions such as pneumonia and urinary tract infection.

In general, the sooner the SCI individual receives acute intervention (i.e., decompression, steroids, IV cooling) and is stabilized, the better the prognosis. Acute interventions aimed at curbing the inflammatory response are believed to prevent secondary tissue damage and, therefore, further loss of function.

Regarding return to play following a sports-related SCI, the first consideration is whether the patient is dealing with a permanent deficit and that deficit's implications in sports selection and participation. Second, the patient's injury and functional exam must be stable in the case of a permanent deficit or completely resolved in the case of a temporary deficit.

Gregory Steencken and Amanda C. Conta

Further Readings

Bagley LJ. Imaging of spinal trauma. *Radiol Clin North Am.* 2006;44(1):1–12.

Branco F, Cardenas DD, Svircev JN. Spinal cord injury: a comprehensive review. *Phys Med Rehabil Clin N Am.* 2007;18(4):651–679.

Eddy D, Congeni J, Loud K. A review of spine injuries and return to play. *Clin J Sport Med.* 2005;15(6):453–458.

Schmitt H, Gerner HJ. Paralysis from sport and diving accidents. *Clin J Sport Med.* 2001;11(1):17–22.

Tator CH. Recognition and management of spinal cord injuries in sports and recreation. *Neurol Clin.* 2008;26(1):79–88.

Whiteside JW. Management of head and neck injuries by the sideline physician. *Am Fam Physician.* 2006;74(8):1357–1362.

SPLENIC INJURY

Although the liver is the most frequently injured abdominal organ, the spleen is the most frequently injured organ in sports and the most common cause of death due to abdominal trauma in athletic activity.

Epidemiology and Biomechanics

Injuries to the spleen can result from a direct force to the abdomen, especially the left upper quadrant; from a sudden deceleration when the hilum is torn; or by displacement of lower left rib fractures. Any of these mechanisms are possible in high-speed or contact sports. The mechanism of splenic injury was explored in one study of downhill skiers. In high-velocity or high-impact collisions, for example, with a tree, a chairlift pole, or a snow fence, multiple trauma was always present (fractures or damage to multiple organs). Skiers were unable to move at the scene, and splenectomy resulted in 5 out of 6 cases (83%). With low-velocity or low-impact collisions, often just a single organ was involved. Such injuries resulted from falls on ski trails, on moguls, or on tree stumps or rocks. Presentation in these cases was often delayed for hours while the individual continued skiing. Splenectomy was necessary in 5 of 12 cases (42%). An investigation by Machida and colleagues reported in their 1999 article, published in *Injury*, showed a significantly higher abdominal injury rate in snowboarders than in skiers. Injuries to the kidney, liver, and spleen were seen in both. In snowboarders, riding mistakes after jumping and subsequent falls were responsible for 31.6% of the abdominal traumas. Skiers were more likely to have a collision as the mechanism for their abdominal injury.

Clinical Presentation

Initially, the pain of splenic injury is sharp, followed by a continued dull, left-sided ache. The patient may complain of radiating pain to the left or right shoulder secondary to free intraperitoneal blood irritating the diaphragm. Splenic rupture is associated with abdominal pain, left shoulder pain (the Kehr sign), or periscapular pain.

Physical exam is neither sensitive nor specific for splenic injury. Because the spleen's capsule can contain bleeding, the signs of splenic injury are often delayed, thereby rendering physical examination unreliable and subsequently hindering diagnosis. The abdomen may be distended. Left-upper-quadrant abdominal tenderness may or may not be accompanied by peritoneal signs, such as generalized tenderness, guarding, and rebound tenderness. There may also be tenderness over the left 10th, 11th, and 12th ribs. Indicators of hypovolemia, such as tachycardia and hypotension, are worrisome signs.

Imaging

Patients with an appropriate mechanism or pain should have a computed tomography (CT) scan taken. CT staging of splenic injury does not predict the need for laparotomy, nor does it correlate with clinical outcome; however, it remains the most accurate method of diagnosing initial injury.

Management

The most important determinant of nonoperative management of splenic rupture is hemodynamic stability, including determination of hematocrit.

Exploratory laparotomy is indicated if the individual is hemodynamically unstable, and splenectomy is performed if the injury is extensive or the hemorrhage is otherwise uncontrollable.

Nonoperative management of splenic injuries consists of careful hemodynamic monitoring, frequent physical and laboratory examination, and, most important, strict bed rest.

In many ways, the management of splenic injury parallels that of the liver. Hemoglobin and hematocrit from a complete blood count can indicate the extent of any blood loss. An elevated leukocyte count may be present if a subcapsular hematoma has developed. Diagnostic peritoneal lavage (DPL) classically is positive if any significant bleeding has occurred from injury to the spleen or other abdominal organ.

Given a stable course, the CT scan should be repeated after 5 to 7 days and should show stabilization or improvement of the injury. Avoidance of contact sports is recommended for up to 4 months after injury. This is determined largely by the severity of the injury seen on a CT scan and its resolution (Figure 1). Most authors recommend at least a 3-month period of physical activity restriction, with the first 3 weeks after hospital discharge spent as "quiet" activity at home. Nonoperative splenic management seems to be more successful in children (90%) than in adults (70%).

Epstein-Barr Virus, Infectious Mononucleosis, and Splenomegaly

By age 30, 90% of the population has been exposed to the Epstein-Barr virus, which causes infectious mononucleosis. This may frequently be unrecognized, particularly in children. From 1% to 3% of college students are affected each year. The peak incidence is in 15- to 24-year-olds. A recent study using physical exam alone reported splenomegaly in 8% of patients with infectious mononucleosis. In comparison, a study using ultrasonography demonstrated that 100% of patients with infectious mononucleosis had an enlarged spleen; physical examination detected the abnormality in less than 20% of the same cases. These studies indicate that physical exam alone is an insensitive tool to diagnose splenomegaly in the setting of infectious mononucleosis.

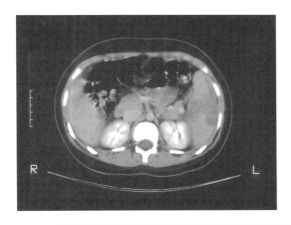

CT scan illustrating heterogeneous signal indicating splenic fracture. A transverse section is shown at the thoracic level, viewed from below. The spleen is located to the right side, adjacent to the ribcage.

Source: Courtesy of David Mooney, M.D., Children's Hospital Boston.

Infectious mononucleosis causes the splenic architecture to become distorted, making the spleen susceptible to rupture from any increased abdominal pressure, even from sneezing or coughing. Splenic rupture in infectious mononucleosis occurs in 0.1% to 0.2% of cases, with the highest estimate being 0.5%. The timing of this complication is predictable, being noted in the first 3 weeks of the illness. Splenic rupture is unusual beyond 3 weeks from the onset of symptoms (headache, sore throat, and fever). The prodromal period is not considered when determining the onset of the illness.

This complication fortunately is often not fatal. Splenectomy is necessary in some instances, although nonoperative management is often successful. Treatment should be individualized. There is no evidence to suggest that corticosteroids reduce spleen size or shorten the duration of the illness.

Return to Sports

The appropriate time to allow an athlete with infectious mononucleosis to resume his or her activity is determined by the duration of the symptoms, as well as the presence of splenomegaly and the risk of splenic rupture. There is concern that contact trauma may precipitate splenic rupture. In a 1976 survey of college team physicians, the respondents identified 22 cases of splenic rupture.

At the time of the trauma, 41% of these were diagnosed with infectious mononucleosis. Seventeen of the student athletes were participating in football. Most splenic ruptures in the setting of infectious mononucleosis, however, are spontaneous and not the result of contact.

Return-to-play recommendations in the literature have been varied. To protect the enlarged spleen, which should probably be assumed to be present in all cases, all strenuous activity should be avoided for the first 21 days. At this point, the athlete may start a graded aerobic program, avoiding contact, if the athlete is asymptomatic, afebrile, and does not have a palpable spleen. At 4 weeks, if the signs are equivocal or the athlete is at a high risk for collision, an imaging study such as an ultrasound should be considered. It should also be noted that normal spleen size has been directly correlated with athlete size; hence, a large athlete with an appropriately sized spleen may be mistakenly diagnosed with splenomegaly if the splenic volume/body mass is not considered.

Hamish A. Kerr

See also Epstein-Barr Virus, Infectious Mononucleosis, and Splenomegaly; Liver Conditions, Hepatitis, Hepatomegaly

Further Readings

Asgari MM, Begos DG. Spontaneous splenic rupture in infectious mononucleosis: a review. *Yale J Biol Med.* 1997;70(2):175–182.

Brodsky AL, Heath CW Jr. Infectious mononucleosis epidemiological patterns at United States colleges and universities. *Am J Epidemiol.* 1972;96(2):87–93.

Burroughs KE. Athletes resuming activity after infectious mononucleosis. *Arch Fam Med.* 2000;9(10): 1122–1123.

Dommerby H, Stangerup SE, Stangerup M, Hancke S. Hepatosplenomegaly in infectious mononucleosis, assessed by ultrasonic scanning. *J Laryngol Otol.* 1986;100(5):573–579.

Esposito JT, Gamelli RL. Injury to the spleen. In: Feliciano DV, Moore EE, Mattox KL, eds. *Trauma.* 3rd ed. Stamford, CT: Appleton & Lange; 1996: 525–550.

Frelinger DP. The ruptured spleen in college athletes: a preliminary report. *J Am Coll Health Assoc.* 1978;26(4):217.

Kaye KM, Kieff E. Epstein–Barr virus infection and infectious mononucleosis. In: Gorbach SL, Bartlett JG, Blacklow NR, eds. *Infectious Diseases.* Philadelphia, PA: WB Saunders; 1992:1646–1654.

Kerr HA, Curtis C, d'Hemecourt PA. Thoracoabdominal injuries. In: Micheli LJ, Powell L, eds. *The Adolescent Athlete: A Practical Approach.* New York, NY: Springer Science + Business Media; 2007: 141–164.

Kinderknecht JJ. Infectious mononucleosis and the spleen. *Curr Sports Med Rep.* 2002;1(2):116–120.

Machida T, Hanazaki K, Ishizaka K, et al. Snowboarding injuries of the abdomen: comparison with skiing injuries. *Injury.* 1999;30(1):47–49.

Maki DG, Reich RM. Infectious mononucleosis in the athlete: diagnosis, complications, and management. *Am J Sports Med.* 1982;10(3):162–173.

Rea TD, Russo JE, Katon W, Ashley RL, Buchwald DS. Prospective study of the natural history of infectious mononucleosis caused by Epstein-Barr virus. *J Am Board Fam Pract.* 2001;14(4):234–242.

Sartorelli KH, Pilcher DB, Rogers FB. Patterns of splenic injuries seen in skiers. *Injury.* 1995;26(1):43–46.

Spielmann AL, DeLong DM, Kliewer MA. Sonographic evaluation of spleen size in tall healthy athletes. *AJR Am J Roentgenol.* 2005;184(1):45–49.

Waninger KN, Harcke HT. Determination of safe return to play for athletes recovering from infectious mononucleosis. A literature review. *Clin J Sport Med.* 2005;15(6):410–416.

SPONDYLOLYSIS AND SPONDYLOLISTHESIS

Spondylolysis is a type of stress fracture in the spine. The fracture occurs in the back of the bone, in an area called the pars interarticularis. The condition is the most common cause of low back pain in adolescent athletes and thought to be an overuse injury that results from repetitive microtrauma to the bone. The term *spondylolysis* originates from the Greek words *spondylo,* meaning "vertebrae" (or bone of the spine), and *lysis,* meaning "to dissolve."

A fracture of the pars interarticularis may become unstable, allowing the vertebrae to slip out of position. This slippage is called *spondylolisthesis.* Typically, the fifth vertebrae shifts forward in relation to the sacrum.

Anatomy

The spinal column consists of 24 bones arranged on top of each other. These bones, separated by fibrocartilaginous disks for cushioning, are called *vertebrae.* The vertebrae provide support and stability for the spinal column and are important for posture and movement.

Facet joints connect the vertebrae and allow them to move freely, resulting in flexibility and movement of the spine. Two other bones—the pedicle and laminae—form the bony ring that surrounds each vertebra. The area of bone that joins the upper and lower facet joints is called the *pars interarticularis.* It is often the weakest link between the pedicle and lamina.

The spinal column consists of three segments, which include 7 cervical vertebrae (in the neck), 12 thoracic vertebrae (in the upper back), and 5 lumbar vertebrae (in the lower back). The lumbar vertebrae are the thickest. The lumbar spine is connected to the pelvis.

Spondylolysis most commonly occurs in the lumbar spine, at the lowest lumbar (L5) vertebral level. Most fractures occur on both sides of the spine and are bilateral; however, they may be unilateral as well.

Causes

Spondylolysis in sports is caused by overtraining and overuse of the spine. Athletes who play sports that involve repetitive hyperextension (bending backward) and rotation of the back have a higher risk of developing spondylolysis than those who do not. Examples of these sports include ballet, gymnastics, diving, and figure skating.

Repetitive hyperextension puts a great deal of stress on the spine. When the spine is overextended, the pars interarticularis is especially vulnerable to these forces, and microtrauma in the bone can result. The body tries to repair these repeated small injuries, but sometimes the repair mechanism is overwhelmed by ongoing damage, leading to a stress fracture (Figure 1).

Sometimes repetitive hyperextension from sports weakens the bone so much that it results in spondylolisthesis. In children and young adults, the most common cause of spondylolisthesis is spondylolysis. Age is a significant risk factor in the development of spondylolysis due to spondylolisthesis.

Symptoms

The most common symptom of spondylolysis in athletes is low back pain that worsens with extension, especially while playing sport(s). Pain may be in one location or spread throughout other areas of the back. It is typically dull and aching, similar to a muscle strain. Symptoms are gradual in onset. Hamstring tightness is often present. Initial rest from sports and medication with nonsteroidal anti-inflammatory drugs (NSAIDs) temporarily reduce pain.

Patients with spondylolisthesis complain of muscle spasms and tightness resulting in difficulty with posture and walking. Muscle weakness, leg pain, and sphincter (a circular muscle that helps maintain constriction of a passage in the body) weakness; loss of feeling in the buttocks; and radiating pain from the spine down the legs may also occur.

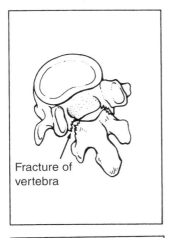

Fracture of vertebra

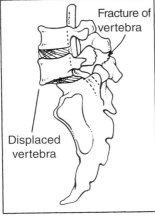

Fracture of vertebra

Displaced vertebra

Figure I   Spondylolysis and Spondylolisthesis

Diagnosis

History

A complete history and physical examination are the first steps in making a diagnosis. A history of the present illness should include the duration of the pain, whether the onset is gradual or sudden, the factors that improve or worsen pain, changes in muscle function, or difficulty with bowel or bladder functions. The presence of night pain may indicate a more serious underlying condition and should be excluded.

It is important to obtain a sport-specific history from the athlete. This includes the maneuvers required for the sport, how long the athlete has been experiencing symptoms, the intensity of the sport, and the level of involvement. Associated factors, such as increased training or growth spurt, should also be considered.

Physical Examination

The spine should be palpated for areas of tenderness, which may indicate the location of the fracture. Tenderness can occur in a part of or throughout the back. It is important to note that an injured athlete's postflexibility should be compared with his or her preinjury flexibility. Range of motion, such as bending forward (flexion) and bending backward (extension), should be tested. In athletes with spondylolysis, this is usually more limited and painful in extension. When the patient stands on one leg and bends backward, the opposite side may be painful. The weight-bearing side is consistent with the painful injured side. Hamstrings are generally tight. An exaggerated curve of the lumbar spine, referred to as *hyperlordosis*, is typical.

Diagnostic Imaging

When the history and physical examination suggest spondylolysis, X-rays are often the first step in imaging. This includes anterior-posterior (AP), oblique (angled), and lateral (side) views. Lateral views show the degree of slip and the angle of slip in spondylolisthesis.

Plain radiographs reveal how the vertebrae are positioned. These are useful in detecting fractures and slippage of the vertebrae. However, X-rays do not always show stress fractures, and more subtle fractures may be missed. In these instances, more advanced diagnostic imaging is necessary. A diagnostic test called a bone scan indicates increased areas of metabolic activity and bone turnover associated with stress fractures. The addition of single-photon emission computed tomography (SPECT) offers an even more sensitive test to detect bone stress. Early fractures not detected on plain radiographs are often shown on SPECT bone scans. When increased areas of bone turnover are present, computed tomography (CT) can be used.

CT identifies bone form and structure. It is used to determine the extent of the fracture as well as its healing potential. Fractures are classified or "staged" as early, progressive, and terminal. Early-stage fractures have the most healing potential.

Magnetic resonance imaging (MRI) offers the advantage of minimizing exposure to radiation while evaluating bony structure and edema (inflammation) in one test. It can also be used to rule out other causes of back pain, including disk problems.

Treatment

The main goal of treatment is complete healing of the fracture and a safe return to sports. Many athletes return to sports with a fibrous union, meaning that although they are asymptomatic, the fracture has not completely healed. This outcome has a favorable short-term prognosis; however, a bilateral bony union is more preferable.

Nonsurgical Treatment

Most athletes with spondylolysis are treated conservatively. Conservative measures include rest from sports, bracing, and physical therapy. It is important to encourage the athlete to be compliant with the treatment plan, particularly rest from sports.

Antilordotic bracing, physical therapy, and modification of activities are often prescribed. Bracing in general remains controversial among practitioners. The purpose of the brace is to reduce the forces on the posterior elements of the spine. Different types of braces are available. Physical therapy includes abdominal strengthening exercises, as well as stretching of the back and hamstring muscles. These exercises strengthen the back and core muscles and help improve lordosis/ swayback.

NSAIDs may initially reduce pain. Nonimpact activities such as swimming and the elliptical should be encouraged in the initial treatment

phase, as long as the patient does not have discomfort with these activities.

As symptoms improve, activity can be slowly increased. Caution should be taken not to return the athlete to sports too early as this could exacerbate the symptoms and delay fracture healing. The athlete can be slowly weaned from the brace if there is no pain with return to sports or provocative extension maneuvers during clinical follow-up.

In instances where conservative treatment has failed (the fracture has not healed and the athlete is still experiencing pain), electrical stimulation may be prescribed. It is thought that the electrical current stimulates bone cells to grow and divide, which accelerates fracture healing.

At periodical follow-up appointments, the health care professional should ensure that symptoms are improving and that the fracture is healing. The athlete should be painfree by history and with provocative extension maneuvers during the clinical evaluation. Computed tomography (CT) may be used to assess healing of the fracture.

Surgical Treatment

The decision to perform surgery is based on the failure of conservative treatment and the severity of the athlete's symptoms. Surgery is necessary if slippage continues to progress and the pain is so severe that it interferes with activities of daily living.

A spinal fusion is used for surgical stabilization. Bones are surgically fused, allowing them to grow together. This ensures that the bones and joints do not move or slip further. In this procedure, a bony bridge is created between the sacrum at the lower part of the spine and the area of slippage.

Surgery may also be performed to remove bone or other tissue. This takes pressure off the spinal cord or spinal nerve roots and is called *decompression*. A fusion and decompression may be performed together depending on the athlete's symptoms and slippage. After surgery, a brace is used and physical therapy prescribed to strengthen the core muscles. As with conservative treatment, caution should be taken to return the athlete to sports gradually and slowly.

Christine Curtis

Further Readings

Bono CM. Low back pain in athletes. *J Bone Joint Surg Am.* 2004;86(2):382–396.

D'Hemecourt PA, Donahue M, Curtis C, Micheli LJ. Active patients turn spondylolysis care into sports medicine. *Biomechanics*. 2004;11(10):55–58.

Hu SS, Tribus CB, Diab M, Ghanayem AJ. Spondylolisthesis and spondylolysis. *J Bone Joint Surg Am*. 2008;90(3):656–671.

Micheli LJ, Curtis C. Stress fractures in the spine and sacrum. *Clin Sports Med*. 2006;25(1):75–88.

Standaert CJ, Herring SA. Spondylolysis: a critical review. *Br J Sports Med*. 2000;34(6):415–422.

SPORT AND EXERCISE PSYCHOLOGY

In the past 30 years, sport psychology has been recognized as a distinct area of study in human behavior. Sport psychology is concerned with the psychological and emotional factors that influence both participation in sports and performance activities and the psychological effects derived from them. There are many dimensions to participation in sports, exercise, and performance activity that are influenced by psychological factors. Sport psychologists study motivation, personality, leadership, team building and cohesion, coaching styles, athletic identity, the psychology of injury rehabilitation, and variables related to achieving optimal performance. Sport psychologists work with individuals, teams, parenting organizations, coaches, and health care providers. The field has grown and has become integrated into the overall development of athletes and performers. Psychological factors are considered to be critical in achieving optimal performance after the talent playing field is leveled. Psychologists also contribute to understanding the effects that participating in physical activity has on psychological development, health, and well-being. While some sport psychologists work exclusively with athletic performance, many focus on the psychological factors involved in exercise—developing strategies to encourage sedentary people to exercise or evaluating the effectiveness of exercise as a treatment for depression. The field has been broadened and is now called *sport and exercise psychology*.

Sport psychology has two primary specialties: (1) clinical sport psychology and (2) educational sport psychology. A significant distinction is made in the field between the two. Clinical sport psychologists have extensive training in clinical and/or counseling psychology and have developed their skills to detect and treat individuals with emotional disorders. Clinical sport psychologists are typically licensed by state boards to practice and have augmented their training to include the subspecialty of sport and exercise psychology and the sports sciences. Educational sport psychology consultants have extensive training in sport and exercise science, physical education, and kinesiology. They also understand the psychology of human movement as it manifests in sport and exercise environments. Educational sport psychology consultants often provide "mental coaching" and psychological skills training. They are often called on to work with teams and individual athletes to teach anxiety management strategies, improve athletic confidence, improve coach-athlete communication, and build team cohesion.

History of Sport Psychology

The first known sport psychology laboratory was established in Germany in 1920. Coleman Griffith has been recognized as the father of this science in the United States. In 1925, he established the first ever sport psychology facility in the nation, the Athletic Research Laboratory. Griffith focused his research on various sport science and psychology issues in 1918, and he introduced the first university-level courses in sport psychology at the University of Illinois in 1923. Coaches showed interest in the psychological aspects of athletic performance in competition even before there was a science called sport psychology. The "pep talk" was highlighted by Knute Rockne—the football coach of the fighting Irish of Notre Dame—in the 1920s. Academic sport psychology was established by the mid-1960s. Physical education had become an academic discipline (now called kinesiology or exercise and sport science), and sport psychology had become a separate component within this discipline. Sport psychologists had also developed the applied side of their field and started to work with athletes and teams.

The field is thriving and vibrant, with many applications in sports, exercise, physical health, and sports medicine. Applied sport psychologists find their skills and application of knowledge helpful in many domains. In coach-training programs, the sport psychologist can help coaches understand the complex relationship between thought, emotions, motivational factors, and behaviors when an athlete is both acquiring a specific sport skill and applying it in athletic situations (with teammates, opponents, officials, and their coaches). Education is provided to help the coach understand the differences between using positive and aversive approaches to influencing behavior—as well as helping coaches use tools to assess their own effectiveness.

In sports medicine, the clinical sport psychologist is called on to treat injured or physically challenged athletes (those with overtraining, eating disorders, burnout, or overuse injuries or on postsurgical rehab) with emotional disorders. In addition, the sport psychologist assists athletes with the psychological process that goes alongside physical rehabilitation from acute and chronic sports injuries. The psychologist assists with the intricate recovery from sports concussions—both in the psychological assessment and in the counseling process. In addition, athletes often face challenges to their athletic identity when confronted with injuries and career-ending situations. The overall adjustment of the athlete is often improved by the specific skill set of a psychologist trained to work with athletes and high performers.

Sport psychology specialists provide consultation, education, and counseling to youth sports organizations. In the United States alone, an estimated 45 million children younger than 18 years are involved in school and extracurricular physical activity programs. Many children are intensively involved in organized sports. On average, youth sports activities require 11 hours weekly in the specific sport for about an 18-week season. Children are offered the opportunity through sports to participate actively in an activity that has meaningful consequences for themselves, their peers, their family, and the community around them. Most children peak in sports around age 12. Developmental psychology has provided the research to help us understand the critical periods for children that have important consequences on their self-esteem, body image, and social development. Hence, the youth sports experience can have important lifelong effects on the personality and psychological development of children. There are few hotter topics in parenting arenas than those surrounding the current challenges and opportunities facing youth sports. The professionalization and early specialization of young athletes have raised important questions about the developmental appropriateness of competition, sports selection, overuse injuries, overscheduled children, and the overzealous coach or parent.

Violence and Aggression in Sports

Another headlining topic that brings in the sport psychology consultant is violence and aggression in sports. Psychologists use the working definition of aggression as "any form of behavior directed toward the goal of harming or injuring another living being who is motivated to avoid such treatment." Psychologists further divide the term into two types of aggression. *Hostile aggression* has as its primary goal the infliction of harm or injury (physically or emotionally). *Instrumental aggression*, on the other hand, occurs as part of a nonharmful goal. A hockey check and a boxer's solid blow to an opponent's head are examples of instrumental aggression. Anger and violence often erupt in sporting situations because the line between instrumental and hostile aggression becomes blurry. Deaths have occurred when a player or spectator has not been able to regulate the aggressive arousal often stirred by high-contact play. The sport psychology consultant provides opportunities for coaches and players to address how to maintain the fine line between instrumental and hostile aggression and develop strategies for dealing with impulsive actions if an athlete, coach, or spectator feels out of control.

College Athletics and Sport Psychology

Many college athletic departments have begun to use and integrate the services of sport psychology consultants. College students and most student-athletes find themselves in a flux of emotionally taxing life transitions—some of which are predictable and result from the athletic commitments made and others that are developmental in nature. Student-athletes are a diverse group of individuals often trying to find their way in a more complex world than that of their predecessors. The commercialization of college athletics has brought new stressors to these athletes and their coaches. Navigating through the complicated National Collegiate Athletic Association (NCAA) rules and contractual obligations of scholarship monies leaves the student-athlete often unprepared for the stressful fallout from such a relished position. The NCAA has come to recognize the significance of counseling and mental health issues in the lives of student-athletes. The sport psychologist is available to assist with performance-based issues in the sports or game situation. He or she is also available to help the athlete balance academic demands, injury, time management, drug and alcohol use, and postcareer planning and transitions.

Professional sports and high-profile competitions such as the Olympics draw attention to the mental side of sports and have made it a "no-brainer" that the mind is often the defining factor in winning and losing. Specific mental skills are honed over time by well-trained and highly competitive athletes—including performing optimally under pressure, with optimal regulation of mood, anxiety, and thought—so that their performance is at a peak. When needed, the sport psychology consultant teaches a range of psychological skills to improve the mental side of the athlete's performance. These skills usually include goal setting, arousal control, self-talk, visualization, imagery, concentration and attention control training, and communication. These skills are used to address and improve performance issues. Sport psychology consultants also help athletes distinguish between performance enhancement and more problematic emotional issues. Depression, anxiety, adjustment disorders, and other mental health issues often affect athletic performance and can be disguised by the athlete or coach's perception that the struggle is performance based.

Exercise and Rehabilitation Psychology

Exercise psychology is an emerging field that separates itself somewhat from applied sport psychology but often shares many of the same underlying principles and tools. Exercise psychology is concerned with the application of psychological principles to the promotion and maintenance of exercise and physical activity and the psychological and emotional consequences of recreational physical activity. A field closely related to exercise psychology is rehabilitation psychology, which deals with the relationship between psychological factors and the physical rehabilitation process.

Exercise rehabilitation is broader than recovery from sports injuries. It includes exercise rehabilitation from cardiac events, Type I and Type II diabetes, obesity, spinal cord injuries, and other medical events requiring exercise as a part of rehabilitation. Rehabilitation psychology also addresses the role of physical activity as a complementary strategy for treating disease and disability.

Some of the critical concepts in exercise psychology include studying the psychological antecedents of exercise behavior. While the American College of Sports Medicine recommends being physically active "most" days per week, the rate of exercise adoption and adherence is sluggish. They report that only 20% of adults engage in the minimal recommended amount of activity. Health care professionals frequently recommend exercise regimens as they relate to physical and mental health. However, compliance rates are often low, and adherence is primarily seen as related to psychological factors. In view of the alarming rates of inactivity in most industrialized nations, exercise psychology provides research and intervention strategies to address this epidemic. The U.S. Centers for Disease Control and Prevention have reported that lack of physical activity, along with poor diet, is responsible for at least 300,000 "preventable" deaths per year.

Exercise psychology relies on several theories and models to build understanding and interventions of physical activity behavior. At the core of the predominantly used exercise psychology theories is a common core construct—self-referenced thought. For example, self-determination theory begins with the basic assumption that individuals possess three primary psychosocial needs: (1) the need for self-determination (autonomy, self-dependent behavior), (2) the need to demonstrate competence, and (3) the need for relatedness. They hypothesize that individuals who exercise for reasons related to low self-determination (e.g., improving appearance) would be less likely to adhere to exercise interventions than someone who exercises for the pure pleasure of it. This theory predicts that improvements in intrinsic motivation to exercise would be aimed at enhancing an individual's sense of competence and autonomy in an environment that is supportive of satisfying social interactions. The systematic identification of the relevant psychological variables allows physical educators, trainers, and rehabilitation specialists to design a program making the best use of the strategies that should lead to long-term adoption of and adherence to exercise.

Practitioners and researchers in exercise psychology have extensively addressed questions related to mental health and physical activity. Considerable research has been done on the prevalence of depression, anxiety, and stress and the role that exercise can play in the alleviation of symptoms. Exercise is also studied for its self-esteem benefits and the overall contribution it makes to emotional well-being. Of course, the physical correlates of positive emotional well-being have been documented for decades and extend the value of this field well beyond the mental domain.

Sport Psychology in Sports Medicine

Only very recently has the sport psychologist also become part of an interdisciplinary orthopedic or sports medicine practice. There is a growing interest and need among sports medicine professionals to include the emotional component of the patient in rehabilitation from acute and chronic sports injuries. The sport psychologist works in coordination with sports medicine physicians, orthopedic surgeons, physical therapists, athletic trainers, nutritionists, fellows, and interns in training. Many sports injuries—both acute and overuse—respond well to a sport psychology counseling consultation. Acute injuries that are rather straightforward—broken bones, fractures, sprains, and strains—do not often even make it to the psychologist's office. Patients with recurrent or chronic injuries (e.g., multiple anterior cruciate ligament [ACL] injuries, which require long periods of rehabilitation; chronic back pain; regional pain syndrome) often suffer long periods of frustration, loss, and at times career-ending consequences. Counseling targeting the physical and emotional rehabilitation process often helps with injury recovery and overall adjustment. Children and adults who strongly identify with their sport/performance domain have difficulties making the transition to other activities while injured. As noted earlier, where an ACL repair can take up to 9 months before return to play is possible, athletes find it difficult to manage the unstructured time that is often consistent with being injured.

Coordinating care around concussion management is particularly useful, as return-to-play decisions are often based on very subtle symptom recovery, requiring care and supervision from the treating physician or athletic trainer. In families with young athletes with concussions that last more than a few weeks, the psychologist can facilitate the implementation of physician recommendations for brain rest, academic accommodations, and modified physical activity. Based on anecdotal report, many young athletes recover more quickly from concussion symptoms when the treatment includes a psychological consultation.

Many athletes find the line between maintaining a healthy body weight and a strong performance weight to be a challenge. Sports medicine patients who are identified as possibly having nutritional, body image, or eating disorder issues are frequently referred for both nutritional and psychological counseling. The importance of maintaining a healthy body weight is significant for long-term performance issues in both men and women. Female athlete triad is a well-known condition for women who push the line in their athletic pursuits, creating conditions that prevent them from enjoying full physiological health. In many cases, these athletes do not resemble the psychological profile of the clinical eating disorder. In other cases, sports performance–based eating issues can become full-blown cases of anorexia and bulimia and need to be treated as such.

It is not always clear to the medical professional, athletic trainer, or coach as to when an athlete should be referred for counseling or psychotherapy. In much of the performance enhancement literature, most problems in performance are related to competition anxiety, motivational problems, and poor self-talk and concentration. However, sometimes athletes are struggling for reasons related to longer-term emotional issues that need to be identified. As noted at the beginning of this entry, there are sport psychologists who treat performance issues only and others with clinical/counseling training who can facilitate the care of athletes with emotionally based issues. When anxiety generalizes beyond the performance domain, it is usually indicative of issues that extend beyond athletic performance. Other kinds of issues facing athletes who benefit from counseling are identity issues, sexual orientation and homophobia, sexuality and human immunodeficiency virus (HIV)-related issues, eating disorders, alcohol and substance abuse issues, anger and aggression control, and relationship issues.

Sharon A. Chirban

See also Anger and Violence in Sports; Imagery and Visualization; Psychological Aspects of Injury and Rehabilitation; Psychological Assessment in Sports; Psychology of the Young Athlete

Further Readings

Abrams M. *Anger Management in Sport: Understanding and Controlling Violence in Athletes*. Champaign, IL: Human Kinetics; 2010.

Lox C, Martin K, Petruzzello S. *The Psychology of Exercise: Integrating Theory and Practice*. Scottsdale, AZ: Holcomb Hathaway; 2003.

Williams J, ed. *Applied Sport Psychology: Personal Growth to Peak Performance*. Mountain View, CA: Mayfield; 1998.

Winberg R, Gould D. *Foundations of Sport and Exercise Psychology*. Champaign, IL: Human Kinetics; 2003.

Sports Biomechanist

This entry provides a brief overview of sports biomechanics and explains the role of the biomechanist in improving performance and understanding sports injuries. Specific examples highlight the importance of integrating sports medicine, biomechanics, and coaching.

Sports Biomechanics

Emerging as a subdiscipline of human movement biomechanics, the evolution of sports biomechanics has been driven by a desire to understand technique in sports performance. Interestingly, some early enquires were related to humans and animals and were based on how these groups organize their biological systems to produce successful performance. These investigations drove the development of theory and technology commonly used today. A famous example comes from the latter part of the 19th century, when the horse racing enthusiast Leland Stanford of California wanted to know if during a trot a horse had a flight phase. Eadweard Muybridge (1830–1904) used early photographic technology to address this question.

In general, the sports biomechanist considers technique from two interrelated perspectives: injury and performance. In the former, scientifically grounded methods are employed to understand and explain the biological responses to load and movement patterns that occur during sports and exercise; this type of biomechanics leads naturally to the clinical applications discussed in the entry Biomechanics in Sports Medicine. Using the same scientifically valid methodologies, the performance perspective presents a number of challenges; including identifying the underlying biomechanical determinants of successful performance, explaining effective and efficient techniques, and ultimately optimizing performance. The research challenge is often complicated by the need to maintain a high level of ecological validity.

In his keynote address at the International Society of Biomechanics in Sports (ISBS) conference in Salzburg, in 2006, former ISBS president Bruce Elliot highlighted the need for biomechanists to conduct research in a "real-world" meaningful environment. Collecting data during training and competition across a diverse range of activities requires flexibility in the methodology used. Fixed-volume analyses maybe used in sports such as gymnastics, where the performance occurs in a small volume, compared with sports such as ski jumping, skiing, and track-and-field events, where panning cameras maybe required. These factors complicate the research design and emphasize the need for innovation while maintaining internal validity, accuracy, and reliability. One result of this is that research has focused on certain sports that lend themselves to fewer complications (e.g., gait analysis compared with kayaking).

The principal ways in which sports biomechanics can help improve performance, develop the coaching process, and explain the most effective ways to train fall into a number of interrelated categories.

Mindset Development

Sports biomechanics can provide coaches with an accurate conceptual understanding of what constitutes successful technique, highlighting the key movement patterns, timings, and phases of the skill. This conceptual model allows the coach to effectively develop technique, strength, and conditioning exercise and preparatory activities. The development of a mindset is the first step in providing an effective coaching-biomechanics interface.

Coach Support

Working alongside the athlete and the coach, the sports biomechanist can provide direct feedback to the coach and/or performer. The feedback can range from basic timings—for example, in sprinting, split times at 5- or 10-meter (m) intervals are very useful—to the more complex kinematic (movement patterns) or kinetic (forces, joint forces) analyses. The important aspect of this feedback is that it is based on key performance variables that are directly related to successful performance. Issues can arise from the use of commercially available qualitative video analysis systems in terms of accuracy and reliability.

Feedback Enhancement

Another topical role that sports biomechanists may play is in the development of innovative technologies, athlete-worn sensors, and motion analysis system technologies that aim to provide meaningful biomechanical feedback to coaches and or performers. These systems are more scientifically grounded than the commercial qualitative video systems and provide precise and relevant information about performance; in addition, the information is presented in a sport-specific effective fashion.

Models of Performance

One important aspect of sports biomechanics is the development of performance or hierarchical models; these were first published by the late James Hay, who was also the former president of both ISBS and ISB (International Society of Biomechanics). These models are based on the underlying laws of human movement and aim to identify the key variables that have a causative effect on success. The models help explain the biomechanical requirements of skill and prevent the arbitrary selection of variables. Different levels of

analysis are used within the development of these models, including:

- single-joint analyses,
- intersegmental coordination analyses, and
- joint kinetic analyses (moments, powers, work, energy).

Optimization of Performance

Another approach to understanding and explaining technique is through the use of forward dynamic analyses. Forward dynamics or computer simulation modeling provides a strong and useful tool that allows sports biomechanist to address questions in a completely controlled environment. This approach allows optimal technique to be determined and also predicts what may be possible to perform. Theoretically adapting performance to achieve specific performance criteria allows subject-specific optimal performance to be determined.

Conclusion

The future progression of sports biomechanics, specifically from the performance perspective, rests with the development of the coaching-biomechanics interface (CBI). Increases in effective technology and ecologically valid scientific enquiry will promote the development of the CBI. The integration of sports biomechanics, sports medicine, and sports coaching represents an evolution from a mono- to multidisciplinary research perspective and ultimately to an interdisciplinary approach.

Gareth Irwin

Further Readings

Elliott B. Biomechanics: an integral part of sport science and sport medicine. *J Sci Med Sport*. 1999;2(4): 299–310.

Hay JG. *Biomechanics of Sports Techniques*. 4th ed. Redwood City, CA: Benjamin Cimmings; 1993.

Robertson G, Caldwell G, Hamill J, Kamen G, Whittlesey S. *Research Methods in Biomechanics*. 1st ed. Champaign, IL: Human Kinetics; 2004.

Wilmore JH, Costill D, Kenney WL. *Physiology of Sport and Exercise*. 4th ed. Champaign, IL: Human Kinetics; 2007.

SPORTS DRINKS

Sports drinks are part of a giant multibillion-dollar industry whose products are marketed to the active athletic population. They are a varied group of noncarbonated beverages now widely used to provide energy, to avert fatigue, to enhance concentration, and, most important, to replenish exercise-related fluid, carbohydrate, and electrolyte losses associated with dehydration. The ultimate goal is to optimize athletic and academic performance through the use of sports beverages. However, sports drinks are not universally indicated or needed during exercise, particularly for short-duration, low- to moderate-intensity exercises. The energy derived from sports drink ingestion does provide a nutritive substrate for longer-duration exercise and aids in recovery from high-intensity workouts. Sports drinks must be differentiated from "energy drinks," which typically include nonnutritive stimulants such as caffeine, guarana, taurine, ginseng, carnitine, creatine, and/or glucuoronolactone, with varying amounts of carbohydrate, protein, amino acids, vitamins, sodium, and other minerals.

How Sports Drinks Provide Energy for Exercise

Sports drinks derive their "energy" primarily from carbohydrates, which fuel the metabolic pathways used during exercise, particularly by muscle and brain. Caloric energy comes from sugars such as glucose or fructose. After approximately 20 minutes of aerobic exercise, as the glycogen stores are depleted, blood glucose becomes an increasingly important energy source. Calories (cal; 1 cal = 4.2 joules) in sports drinks range from 10 to 70 per serving (14 grams [g] average per 240 milliliters [ml] or 8 ounces [oz]). There is much greater variability in the caloric content of energy drinks, ranging from 10 to 270 cal per serving. Sports drinks are designed to restore the fluids, carbohydrates, and electrolytes lost during intense physical activity. A carbohydrate sports drink of no more than 6% to 8% is needed to supply the requirements for this nutrient during moderate, prolonged, or strenuous exercise provided that adequate hydration is maintained. A slight rise in insulin is a natural response to ingestion of carbohydrate-containing foods or beverages. The insulin release that follows sports drink ingestion during exercise helps increase the rate of glucose uptake and use by working muscles to prolong the intensity and duration of exercise.

Appropriate Use

Copious ingestion of sports drinks can result in unnecessary or excessive ingestion of carbohydrates. High doses of simple carbohydrates can evoke the greatest insulin responses. For exercise of less than 1-hour duration, most of the energy is readily obtained from the glycogen stores and the metabolic breakdown of protein and fat. Therefore, the primary goal of fluid intake during exercise is to maintain adequate hydration. This should be easily achieved with water ingestion only. Furthermore, sports drinks should not be used during lunch or snacks as a replacement for low-fat milk or water. In this setting, the higher-calorie sports drinks contribute to excessive caloric intake as well as insufficient intake of other essential nutrients, increasing the risk for overweight and obesity in children and adults, not unlike soda ingestion. Low-calorie sports drinks will not contribute to the risk of overweight or obesity and yet do not provide adequate carbohydrates for intense exercise; therefore, their role, if any, in the athlete's diet is yet to be determined.

During prolonged and intense exercise, the body can experience fatigue and impaired sports performance without adequate energy substrates available. A switch from hydration with water only to a carbohydrate-electrolyte beverage after the initial hour of vigorous exercise is appropriate to replenish the calories and electrolytes lost while rehydrating and to maintain exercise intensity. Continued exercise with water intake alone can have negative consequences on the body due to the depletion of the essential nutrients required to maintain the body's energy balance and function. Athletes often prepare for intense exercise by eating a diet high in carbohydrates. But during exercise, eating solid food is usually not an option. Sports drinks provide an easily digested carbohydrate source for the body, thus allowing the athlete to maintain optimum energy levels. Table 1 provides a recipe to prepare your own custom sports drink.

Table I Make Your Own Custom Sports Drink

Ingredients

¼ cup sugar
¼ tsp salt
¼ cup water
¼ cup orange juice (not concentrate) or a
    combination of 100% fruit juices
2 tbsp lemon juice
3½ cups cold water

Directions

1. Dissolve the sugar and salt in the water.
2. Add the juices and the remaining water; chill.
    Makes four servings.

Caloric Content

Per 8-ounce serving: 50 calories; 12 grams
    carbohydrate; 110 milligrams sodium

Note: 1 ounce (oz) = 28.35 grams (g); 1 calorie (cal) = 4.2 joules.

Sports Drinks Versus Water

Water is an essential part of our daily diet. During exercise, water is the appropriate choice for hydration for 60 minutes or less of exercise and does not need to be ingested in the form of a sports drink or other beverage. Clothes, diet, medications, illnesses or chronic conditions, fitness level, and acclimatization influence the body's sweat rate and risk of dehydration. Sweat rates vary greatly among individuals but can reach 1 to 3 liters (L)/hour. Environmental conditions such as heat, humidity, intensity, and duration of exercise all affect the quantity of water needed to maintain a euvolemic state. Exercise-induced dehydration is caused by a mismatch of fluid lost in sweat and adequate fluid replacement. Excessive dehydration is associated with premature fatigue, impaired sports performance, and an increased risk of heat-associated illness. Sports drinks offer advantages to promote fluid intake because their flavor, color, and sodium and carbohydrate content all increase the natural tendency to drink during exercise. Offering fluids that are slightly cooled (59–72 °F or 15–22 °C) to athletes also appears to improve their overall fluid intake.

Electrolytes

Sodium and potassium are essential nutrients in our diet. Sodium maintains blood volume and helps preserve the balance of water in the cells. Athletes with low sodium levels may feel nauseated, experience painful muscle cramps, or feel disoriented or confused. Potassium helps regulate muscle control, nerve function, and blood pressure. Potassium works with sodium to keep the body's water in balance. Sweating causes blood sodium levels to rise, which prompts thirst. However, thirst is not generally a sufficient stimulus to maintain fluid balance during exercise in the heat. Therefore, thirst should not be relied on solely as a warning to prevent excessive body water deficits. Athletes should be taught to drink water before, during, and after exercise without waiting for thirst to prompt them; this would reduce the risk of significant dehydration and related heat illness.

For strenuous and endurance activities where large sweat losses are seen, sports drinks are helpful for electrolyte replacement and the prevention of hyponatremia or other electrolyte abnormalities. Several electrolytes, including sodium and potassium, are ingredients of both sports and energy drinks. Sodium content varies from 100 to 200 milligrams (mg) per 240 ml (8 oz), while potassium content ranges from 30 to 90 mg. Too much sodium can cause an excessive feeling of thirst, leading to overdrinking while still overloading the body with salt. Athletes may need as little as 50 mg of sodium per 8 oz. When choosing a beverage, it is important to know its electrolyte content.

Protein, Amino Acids, Vitamins, and Minerals

Many sports and energy drinks contain B vitamins as well as vitamin C. There is no advantage in consuming these vitamins in these drinks as they can be obtained in a well-balanced diet. Protein is an essential part of an athlete's diet. Protein intake should be spread throughout the day. This allows the body opportunity to use the necessary amino acids (AA) throughout the day rather than convert them to fat. Protein ingested shortly before workouts may lead to gastric upset in some individuals. It also may serve as exercise fuel and in small amounts may have a muscle sparing effect preexercise when added to carbohydrates (CHO) in small amounts.

Protein does appear to have an important role in postexercise recovery when combined with carbohydrate. Protein intake provides the necessary amino acids to rebuild muscle broken down during intense exercise and improves muscle hydration. Consumption of CHO + AA (4:1 ratio) after exercising improved postexercise recovery, thus preventing declines in endurance performance in consecutive-day heavy exercise bouts. What research has failed to demonstrate is an actual improvement in exercise performance in endurance athletes following protein or CHO + AA supplementation. Thus, the optimal intake of carbohydrates/protein quantities is likely individual and is influenced by personal tolerance, dietary practices, metabolism, and exercise type as well as duration. Further research is needed to establish optimal carbohydrate/protein types, amounts, and timings of intake with regard to specific types of exercise. Sports drinks containing protein and amino acids can be used for postexercise recovery and rehydration; low-fat milk is another popular option.

Conclusion

Sports drinks have an important but limited role in an athlete's diet. Sports drinks have no significant daily nutritive value in the diet. Their use should be limited to hydration and CHO-E (carbohydrates + electrolytes) supplementation during prolonged, vigorous exercise or CHO-E (±AA) during the immediate postexercise period for rehydration and muscle recovery. Overdrinking can contribute to excessive carbohydrate intake and can contribute to the overweight obesity epidemic in the United States. Sports drinks often contain substances such as vitamins that are better obtained from other dietary sources. The optimal balance of carbohydrates, electrolytes, and water for athletes varies greatly depending on environmental conditions, sweat rates, and the duration and intensity of exercise; therefore, it is difficult to determine the ideal content of a sports drink. Commercially available sports drinks vary greatly in content of carbohydrates, electrolytes, and other substances. An athlete using a sports drink should familiarize himself or herself with the contents of the beverage of his or her choice. It is important to distinguish sports drinks from energy drinks. Energy drinks containing stimulant substances are not recommended for use in children or adolescents and should be avoided in athletes in general. For low to moderate exercise of less than 1-hour duration, water remains the beverage of choice for maintaining an athlete's hydration. Ongoing research continues to add to our knowledge regarding the need for carbohydrates, electrolytes, and protein/amino acids in the athletic population and will likely influence the commercial sports drink industry.

Holly J. Benjamin

Further Readings

Casa DJ, Yeargin SW. Avoiding dehydration among young athletes. *Health Fitness J.* 2005;9(3):20–23.

Committed on Sports Medicine and Fitness. Climatic heat stress and the exercising child and adolescent. *Pediatrics.* 2000;106(1):158–159.

Ellison RC, Singer MR, Moore LL. Current caffeine intake of young children; amount and sources. *J Am Diet Assoc.* 1995;95(7):802–803.

Froiland K, Koszewski W, Hingst J, Kopecky L. Nutritional supplement use among college athletes and their sources of information. *Int J Sport Nutr Exerc Metab.* 2004;14(1):104–120.

Ganio MS, Casa DJ, Armstrong LE, Maresh CM. Evidence-based approach to lingering hydration questions. *Clin Sport Med.* 2007;26(1):1–16.

Horswill CA, Horn MK, Stofan JR, Passe DH, Murray R. Adequacy of fluid ingestion in adolescents and adults during exercise. *Pediatr Exerc Sci.* 2002;15:104.

Minehan MR, Riley MD, Burke LM. Effect of flavor and awareness of kilojoule content of drinks on preference and fluid balance in team sports. *Int J Sports Nutr Exerc Metab.* 2002;12(1):81–92.

Rivera-Brown A, Gutierrez R, Gutierrez JC, Frontera W, Bar-Or O. Drink composition, voluntary drinking, and fluid balance in exercising, trained heat-acclimatized boys. *J Appl Physiol.* 1999;86(1):78–84.

Winnick JJ, Davis JM, Welsh RS, Carmichael MD, Murphy EA, Blackmon JA. Carbohydrate feedings during team sport exercise preserve physical and CNS function. *Med Sci Sports Exerc.* 2005;37(2):306–315.

SPORTS INJURIES, ACUTE

Injuries can be divided into two categories—*acute* and *chronic*. In acute injury, a specific event causes direct trauma to the body and subsequent injury to the tissues involved. Acute injury can vary greatly, from an ankle sprain to a corneal (eye) abrasion and almost everything in between. Acute injury can occur to soft tissue, bone, organs, or nerves. Treatments and duration of healing of acute injuries depend on the severity of trauma and the type of injury. In contrast, chronic injuries are problems that develop over time, often in a predictable manner, and may be the result of repetitive overuse of a region of the body. In sports, the musculoskeletal system, which includes ligaments, tendons, muscles, and bones, represents the primary tissues affected by chronic injury. The treatment of chronic injury also varies based on the type of injury; however, stopping the noxious, repetitive actions is generally required for healing.

Clinical Evaluation

Acute injuries vary in their level of severity. The most common acute injuries involve bruises, sprains, and strains. A mild ankle sprain may require little or no intervention to allow immediate return to play. In contrast, a high-velocity hit to an athlete's abdomen has the potential to cause internal bleeding; a similar blow to the extremities or the spine may cause a fracture. All these can be serious situations that require timely on-site evaluation, stabilization, and transportation to a health care facility. These variations in severity make the clinical evaluation of an acute injury extremely important. Timely assessment is necessary to obtain the most accurate information and exam. Serial exams can reveal clues to a developing serious condition—for example, an intracranial bleed or visceral laceration. Serial exams may also provide reassurance regarding a less worrisome condition that is clinically improving, such as a mild concussion or upper extremity "stinger."

History

The history for an acute injury should be focused and pertinent. The examiner needs to determine when the injury occurred and during what type of movement and what derangements occurred. The timing, character, progression, or improvement of pain and the aggravating or alleviating factors can give helpful clues to the type of injury. Accompanying symptoms of swelling, locking, catching, bruising, bleeding, and neurologic complaints are important for diagnosis. It is also important to know whether the athlete has had any prior injuries, problems, or surgeries, as well as to learn the patient's medical history, for example, chronic illness, medications, and allergies. A thorough, pertinent history can often provide all the clues necessary to make the diagnosis and will at least significantly narrow the differential of diagnosis. The medical history will help determine if the individual has a severe and potentially life-threatening problem that will require more emergent interventions and an escalated level of assistance.

Physical Exam

Physical exams in the setting of acute injury should always follow the American Heart Association guidelines for Basic Life Support. The exam should begin with assessing the athlete's airway, breathing, and circulation (ABCs) and treating problems with these systems before moving to examination of any other body systems or parts, no matter how severe or distracting the injury may appear. Special care and attention needs to be given to any athlete who may have a head or spine injury, and further exam maneuvers need to be done in a way that prevents further injury. For an alert athlete, the exam can focus on the area of injury and first visualize the area of injury, checking for swelling, ecchymosis or bruising, deformity, or skin trauma. Then the area of injury is palpated for tenderness, crepitance, edema (swelling), and, in the case of an abdominal injury, rebound or guarding. More specific exam maneuvers to help better pinpoint the type of injury are then carried out. In the case of a patient with a head injury, who is alert and awake, one would attempt a more complete neurologic exam to include memory, recall, balance, strength, sensation, and coordination. Often, the most accurate physical exam can be obtained immediately following the injury. Serial exams done over the first few minutes to hours after an injury may determine if a condition is deteriorating or improving.

The physical exam may be done at different stages, depending on the nature of the injury and the type of setting in which it is being evaluated. An on-field injury during the course of competition may require a triaged history and focused exam to determine whether the athlete can be safely removed from the field of play. On removal, a more thorough history and physical exam can be performed, either on the sideline or in the locker room. Any athlete, whose injury is deemed to be more severe than can be adequately stabilized and treated on-site should be immediately transported by ambulance to the appropriate health care facility, such as the local emergency room.

Diagnostic Tests

Diagnostic testing may provide helpful clues to the type of injury. Specific tests used and their utility vary. Many injuries require no diagnostic testing at all. Depending on the circumstances, helpful information can be gathered from a variety of diagnostic sources. Computed tomography (CT), magnetic resonance imaging (MRI), and neuropsychological testing may provide information about a head injury. Bone scans, X-rays, ultrasound, compartmental pressure testing, CT scans, and MRI scans can be helpful in musculoskeletal injuries. Laboratory tests, including blood tests and urine tests, as well as some imaging modalities, such as ultrasound or CT scan, can be helpful in chest and abdominal injuries. The type and severity of injury often dictate the need for further diagnostic testing.

Treatment

Treatment of acute injuries varies as widely as the types of acute injuries. Minor scrapes and bruises may require no interventions at all. Intracranial bleeds or abdominal visceral lacerations may require emergency surgeries. Treatment always begins with addressing the basic life support ABCs and when the athlete is stable from a cardiopulmonary standpoint. When the clinician is fully cognizant of any potential spine injuries, further interventions can be done.

A common mnemonic for the treatment of simple, acute musculoskeletal injuries is RICE: *r*est, *i*ce, *c*ompression, and *e*levation. Analgesics may be necessary to control pain in acute injury and rehabilitation settings. Certain injuries may also require casting, bracing, or other form of support or immobilization, and may require nonemergent surgical interventions as well. Physical therapy

or other forms of rehabilitation are often used to help an athlete recover from an injury. Occasionally, modalities such as ultrasound, iontophoresis, electrical stimulation, and others can be helpful in getting an injured athlete back to play.

Prevention

The area of injury prevention has become a very important focus of most sports and their governing bodies. It is the reason why protective equipment has been instituted and mandated in many sports. Helmets were introduced into the National Football League and have successfully decreased concussions and head trauma. Mouthguards are now a mainstay in many sports to minimize dental injuries. Contact sports such as lacrosse, field and ice hockey, and football require pads and helmets. People in positions of high risk for contact and injury, such as the catcher in baseball or the goalie in hockey, may be required to wear different safety equipment from others in the same sport at lower risk. Modifications have also been made to playing surfaces in an attempt to minimize injuries, such as the increasingly common synthetic turf in replacement of grass fields or the breakaway bases found on many baseball and softball diamonds. Rules have also been instituted to minimize injuries. For example, head-to-head contact in football is penalized due to safety concerns in allowing this type of collision. Injury prevention will continue to be a focus of all sports, and new equipment, gear, and rules will continue to figure in sports.

Return to Sports

Many acute injuries require little or no intervention and do not prevent athletes from missing any time from their sport. Return to sports is usually dictated by the athletes' ability to recover to the extent that they can function at a level high enough to be productive in their sport and be able to protect themselves from further injury. This means that they must recover full range of motion, sensation, and enough strength to participate without placing themselves or others at higher risk of additional injury. Some acute injuries can be career ending, as many spinal cord–injured athletes have tragically discovered. Other injuries, such as fractures and ligament tears, can have a prolonged recovery period, often with a surgical and postoperative phase with extended rehabilitation, before one can get back to competitive sports. On return, some injuries require further preventive measures, such as bracing or equipment changes, for the athlete to continue to participate.

Benjamin Phipps

See also Ankle Sprain; Contusions (Bruises); Elbow Sprain; Hamstring Strain; Knee Ligament Sprain, Medial and Lateral Collateral Ligaments; Strains, Muscle; Wrist Sprain

Further Readings

Griffin LY, Greene, WB, eds. *Essentials of Musculoskeletal Care.* 3rd ed. Rosemont, IL: American Academy of Orthopaedic Surgeons; 2006.

McKeag DB, Moeller JL, eds. *ACSM's Primary Care Sports Medicine.* 2nd ed. Philadelphia, PA: Lippincott Williams & Wilkins; 2007.

Sports Injuries, Overuse

Injuries can be broadly divided into two categories: chronic and acute. Chronic injuries are problems that develop over time, often in a predictable manner, and may be the result of repetitive overuse of a region of the body.

The human body is remarkably adaptable to physical stresses. Force loads on tissues cause microtrauma and tears of those tissues. The body reacts to this by rebuilding, reinforcing, and strengthening those tissues as it heals them. An increase in the stress on a bone, such as with initiating a new running program, causes a reactive increase in bone matrix, stability, strength, and integrity. Increases in tensile or shear forces of tendons, ligaments, and muscles cause the body to adapt and strengthen these structures as well. When the balance of microtrauma and repair is disrupted, the tissues are unable to heal adequately because tissue breakdown occurs at a rate greater than healing. Over time, the result is development of pathologic tissue that becomes painful and weak. This can occur from excessive loads placed on normal tissues, normal loads applied abnormally to tissues, or normal loads applied to abnormal tissue. Chronic injuries, such as stress fractures, shin splints, exertional compartment syndromes, and tendinopathies, can then result.

Clinical Evaluation

The number of chronic injuries is on the rise in many of our young athletes as we have seen a transition from the multisport athlete to the year-round, single-sport athlete. This has taken away the variety of physical experiences from participation in multiple sports as well as the relative rest that athletes undergo with the change in sports seasons. The clinical evaluation of chronic injuries is imperative to the diagnosis and the treatment of the injury. Chronic, or overuse, injuries represent a significant portion of injuries in many sports. Early and accurate diagnosis can allow for early intervention and breaking of the overuse cycle. The earlier the diagnosis, the more likely the athlete can return to sports in a timely fashion.

History

History is the most important component to helping an athlete with an injury. The history provides the clues to an accurate diagnosis and can give the clues to why the chronic injury developed in the first place. The history should be approached with two outcomes in mind: First, by determining the type of injury present as accurately as possible; and, second, by determining why this injury has occurred. The primary symptom of an overuse injury is pain. It is important to determine when the pain began initially, as well as the descriptive properties of the pain—sharp, dull, ache, burn, and so on. Associated mechanical symptoms such as locking, clicking, or popping should also be noted. Accompanying symptoms of swelling, bruising, and neurovascular problems are also important. The timing of the pain in relation to the athlete's activities may give clues to the extent of the injury. Most chronic injuries follow a typical pain pattern. Initially, they are often noted as a vague ache or discomfort in the few hours to days after a workout. This may evolve in severity and duration of discomfort as the injury progresses, and limitations begin to occur with minimal activity or even at rest. The timing and quality of the discomfort, as well as any change in these factors especially as they relate to specific activities, can give important clues as to the severity of the chronic injury. A history of similar injuries in the past in the same or different locations can aid one in assessing the risk of injury recurrence.

To answer the question "why" an injury developed requires more of an investigative approach. These injuries can have multiple causes. Repetitive overuse may be from training errors, poor mechanics, strength and flexibility imbalances, nutritional deficiencies, poor or inadequate equipment, underlying systemic disease, poor nutrition, or anatomical malalignments and can all lead to chronic tissue injury.

Physical Exam

The physical exam for a chronic injury should initially focuses on the area of pain or concern. Observe for swelling, bruising, deformity, or other obvious abnormality. Gentle palpation can help localize tenderness, the anatomical structures involved, and any accompanying edema. The affected joint or limb should then be put through its usual passive and ultimately active range of motion for evaluation of limitations of movements and painful movements. Resisted testing of isolated muscles, ligaments, and tendons, as well as provocative maneuvers such as the test for shoulder rotator cuff impingement, may further specify the type of injury and the structures involved. A thorough neurovascular exam of the area should be included, and one should always evaluate the joint above and below a possible injury.

Once the diagnosis has been established by history and exam, the examiner should again change the focus of the exam to the question of "why" the injury developed and, more specifically, the intrinsic causes of the chronic injury. These can include anatomical malalignments and subsequent abnormal tension and stresses across structures. There may also be underlying strength or flexibility imbalances of the affected extremity or of the athlete's core musculature. In the case of adolescent or growing athletes, growth alone can cause increased stress on structures incapable of handling the loads placed on them, such as that found in the pain from Osgood-Schlatter disease of the knee or Little League shoulder or elbow. A thorough physical exam for a chronic injury should include a psychological assessment. Fatigue, depression, and psychological stress can all predispose an athlete to injury, causing an overtraining syndrome, which results in physical and psychological inability to exert at an otherwise normal level, much less a highly competitive level.

A dynamic exam reproducing the repetitive movement may be very revealing. This may help discern an abnormal gait, throwing pattern, or technique.

Diagnostic Tests

With chronic injury, diagnostic tests may help confirm the diagnosis suspected based on the history and physical exam. Radiography (X-ray), magnetic resonance imaging (MRI), computed tomography (CT), or bone scan may confirm a suspected stress fracture or bone problem. Musculoskeletal ultrasound or an MRI scan helps evaluate soft tissue injury such as tendinopathies, bursal problems, or ligamentous injury. Video analysis of an athlete's form can be helpful with the dynamic physical exam to better note the details of the motions and more easily discern potential problems. Diagnostic tests are not required to make most chronic injury diagnoses but can be helpful in the cases where there is a doubt.

Treatment

The ultimate treatment for any chronic, overuse injury is stopping the repetitive movements causing the pathology. These injuries require rest. This allows the time for the body to prepare the injured tissue in the cycle of tissue breakdown and healing to adapt to stress. The time required for this to occur is variable; healing can take weeks to months. The rest is relative, only the excessive stressors to the damaged tissue need to be removed. Not all chronic injuries require immobilization or complete removal from all activity. A marathon runner who develops a fibular stress fracture from overtraining may have to discontinue running for several weeks to allow the fracture to heal; however, he or she may be able to maintain his or her cardiovascular fitness and overall endurance by cross-training with a bike or an elliptical trainer or by swimming.

Additional treatments—such as analgesics to control pain, frequent icing, and occasionally topical, oral, or injected steroids—in a chronic injury may be helpful. It is also imperative to correct the underlying problems that led to the injury in the first place. Clinicians should counsel about appropriate training and escalation of activity when applicable.

Prevention

Chronic injuries develop over a long period of time and have underlying causes that are treatable. Therefore, theoretically these injuries are all preventable. Counseling is the most important component of prevention. Preventing overuse injuries requires appropriate warm-up, stretching, and strengthening, as well as a well-rounded training program that includes aerobic, anaerobic, strength, flexibility, agility, and proprioceptive conditioning, all of which help prevent injury. Equally important is knowing the body's capabilities and limitations and allowing adequate rest for the athletes in the preseason and during the season and an adequate period of complete rest annually. For most athletes, it is recommended that they have 2 to 3 months per year of complete rest from the repetitive physical demands of their sport as well as psychological rest. Teaching and coaching proper technique, and appropriate equipment selection cannot be overemphasized. Worn-out or inappropriately sized equipment can be the causative factor in many chronic injuries.

Return to Sports

The athlete is able to return to sports from a chronic injury when the pain has subsided, full range of motion has been regained, and adequate strength has returned. He or she should not return before the underlying cause of his or her injury is addressed, so as not to cause recurrence. Additionally, the return requires a slow progression because resting the affected tissues causes a relative deconditioning. Not allowing appropriate rest for healing to occur will cause recurrence of the initial injury.

Benjamin Phipps

See also Apophysitis; Bursitis; Compartment Syndrome, Anterior; Sports Injuries, Acute; Stress Fractures; Tendinopathy

Further Readings

Griffin LY, Greene, WB, eds. *Essentials of Musculoskeletal Care.* 3rd ed. Rosemont, IL: American Academy of Orthopaedic Surgeons; 2006.

McKeag DB, Moeller JL, eds. *ACSM's Primary Care Sports Medicine.* 2nd ed. Philadelphia, PA: Lippincott Williams & Wilkins; 2007.

SPORTS INJURIES, SURGERY FOR

With participation in competitive sports increasing throughout society, the number of sports injuries has increased as well. Most sports injuries are treated nonsurgically, with the use of rest, bracing, physical therapy, and rehabilitation. Today, however, more and more sports injuries are being treated with surgery instead. There are many reasons for this. Over time, our knowledge and experience in sports medicine have evolved. Studies have shown that certain injuries, such as anterior cruciate ligament (ACL) tears, recover better if they are treated surgically. In addition, the invention of newer imaging techniques such as magnetic resonance imaging (MRI) has allowed sports medicine physicians to more precisely diagnose torn structures. Advances in surgical instrumentation and technique have made it possible to surgically repair ligaments, tendons, and cartilage and restore native anatomy without damaging the surrounding tissue. Specifically, the advent of arthroscopy, which allows joint surgery to be performed through tiny incisions using miniature instruments, has been the major surgical innovation in the field of sports medicine.

The rapid increase in the number of sports injuries combined with the growing interest among health care professionals to optimize treatment has led to an explosion in the field of sports medicine. This dedication to perfecting the repair and rehabilitation of sports-related injuries is manifested by two prominent professional sports medicine societies.

Professional Sports Medicine Societies

The American Orthopaedic Society for Sports Medicine (AOSSM) is made up of more than 2,000 orthopedic surgeons who are dedicated to the field of sports medicine. Most members are team physicians whose research has advanced our knowledge of sports injuries. The society was founded in 1972 and often works directly with physical therapists, athletic trainers, and other health professionals interested in sports medicine. Each year, an annual meeting is held in which members meet to discuss and present new ideas and techniques in the field. New recommendations for the treatment of various sports injuries and guidelines for prevention are episodically published by the society.

The American College of Sports Medicine (ACSM) includes all health professionals interested in sports medicine. It has more than 20,000 national and international members, including physicians, surgeons, physical therapists, athletic trainers, and other health professionals who are dedicated to the field of sports medicine. Founded in 1954, the stated purpose of this college is to advance health through science, education, and medicine. Presently, it is headquartered in Indianapolis, Indiana. Each year, the college holds meetings, exhibitions, conferences, and team physician courses that educate and integrate scientific research in exercise science and sports medicine.

Sports Injuries

Each individual sport places distinct stresses on specific joints and muscle groups. Injury rates vary between sports, depending on which structures are at risk. Sports in which the athlete constantly uses his or her arms to throw, shoot, block, or bear weight place high demands on the shoulder, elbow, and wrist. Sports in which the athlete has to move quickly and change direction have a high incidence of lower extremity injuries in the hip, knee, and ankle. Baseball pitchers, swimmers, and tennis players have a high rate of shoulder and elbow injuries. Gymnasts often use their arms to walk or push off and have a high incidence of elbow and wrist injuries. Soccer, basketball, and field hockey athletes need to pivot and often get knee and ankle injuries. Hip injuries are common in kicking sports, such as soccer, and also in dancing. Not surprisingly, foot injuries also occur frequently in dancers.

Most sports injuries do not require surgery. Sprains or strains occur when the muscles or ligaments around the joint are stretched more than they can withstand and suffer tiny tears. These injuries usually heal well over time. Tendons and bursae can become irritated and inflamed, leading to tendinitis or bursitis. These are generally overuse injuries and also heal well over time. These sports injuries are commonly treated with a combination of rest, anti-inflammatory medications (e.g., ibuprofen), and physical therapy aimed at stretching and strengthening the appropriate muscle groups.

Certain injuries do not heal well with rest and rehabilitation and generally require surgery. There are various reasons why some injuries require surgery while others do not. In some cases, the injured structure is located in a joint, where its blood supply and capacity to heal on its own is limited. In others cases, repetitive injuries have stretched the structure too thin and compromised its function. Common sports injuries that require surgery in the shoulder joint include tears of the rotator cuff and labrum and a stretched shoulder capsule resulting from multiple shoulder dislocations. In the knee, ACL tears, meniscal tears, cartilage injuries, and loose bodies are common sports injuries best treated with surgery. In the ankle and elbow, stretched ligaments from repetitive sprains may require repair or reconstruction.

Terminology

An understanding of surgery in sports medicine necessitates a familiarity with the terminology of sports medicine procedures. The following is a list of commonly used terms.

Diagnostic Arthroscopy

Arthroscopy is a minimally invasive surgical technique that uses an arthroscope or small camera inserted into a joint. This will be discussed in more detail below. A diagnostic arthroscopy is that part of the procedure where the surgeon examines the entire joint to look for any sources of pain.

Meniscectomy Versus Meniscus Repair

The *meniscus* is a rubbery cushion inside the knee between the thigh and leg bones. A twisting knee injury can cause a tear in the meniscus. *Meniscectomy* is a common knee arthroscopic surgery in which a small tear in the meniscus is removed. The remainder of the meniscus is left alone. *Meniscectomy* differs from *meniscus repair* in which the tear is not removed but is instead sutured back together.

Repair Versus Reconstruction of Tendons and Ligaments

Repair involves using sutures to tighten an injured structure that has stretched. A repair is usually done for injured ligaments or tendons that have a good capacity to heal but are too lax in their present state. Examples include repair of torn ankle ligaments and patellar tendon repair. *Reconstruction* involves replacing an injured tendon or ligament with a separate structure that can perform the function of the injured structure. Reconstruction is usually performed on injured tendons or ligaments that will not heal properly over time. For example, ACL tears in the knee are usually treated with ACL reconstruction, using a hamstring or patellar tendon to replace the function of the torn ACL.

Loose Body

A free-floating piece of bone or cartilage that has broken away and is moving around a joint is referred to as a *loose body.*

Excision

Excision means removal. For example, a loose body in the knee joint is often treated with excision.

Debridement

Debridement is the cutting out of unstable, frayed pieces of a torn structure. The process of debridement smooths the roughened surfaces of the injured structure so that it does not get caught in places during joint motion. For example, a tear in the labrum of the shoulder or hip is often treated with debridement.

Chondroplasty

Chondroplasty is the smoothing of torn cartilage on the joint surface. Chondroplasty is usually done with the aid of an arthroscopic shaver that levels out the cartilage surface by selectively removing torn and unstable fragments.

Microfracture

In *microfracture,* tiny holes are made in the exposed bone in an area of the joint where the full thickness of the cartilage has been completely damaged. Microfracture uses a miniature awl to perforate the exposed bone in a joint. The goal of microfracture is to stimulate the bone to bleed and form a blood clot over itself. Over time, this blood clot can help form a new type of cartilage, called fibrocartilage, over the area of exposed bone.

Arthroscopy

Arthroscopic surgery uses multiple small incisions (1.5 inches [in.; 1 in. = 2.54 cm]) placed around the joint, called *arthroscopic portals.* A long, thin, pencil-sized rotating video camera called an arthroscope is inserted through one of these portals and into the joint in question. The arthroscope is connected to a monitor, and the image obtained by the camera at the end of the arthroscope appears on the monitor. The joint requiring surgery is filled with a saline solution, and the surgery is done within this solution. The surgeon manipulates the camera with one hand while watching the video image of the joint on the monitor. The surgeon's other hand is used to manipulate the arthroscopic instruments to perform the surgery. Alternatively, a surgical assistant may be used to operate the camera or assist with other instrument manipulation.

Arthroscopy is a minimally invasive alternative to many open surgeries, with advantages including less pain, smaller incisions, and faster rehabilitation. Arthroscopy can be performed on many joints, but it is most commonly used in the knee, shoulder, elbow, hip, and ankle. The types of surgeries that can be performed arthroscopically and the joints in which they can be used are constantly expanding. The requirement for arthroscopic treatment is that the structure in question must be within the joint space and in an area that is accessible using arthroscopic tools. One of the primary indications for arthroscopy is diagnosis. In cases where the diagnosis is unclear after physical exam and imaging, some surgeons may opt to perform an arthroscopy to visualize the injured joint and find the problem.

Arthroscopy is done under sterile conditions in the operating room, as with any other surgery. Many surgeons will use specific positioning devices to allow the limb or joint to be in the ideal position for the procedure. Every arthroscopic procedure begins with a diagnostic arthroscopy, which entails looking around the entire joint to either confirm or determine the causes of the patient's symptoms. The joint surface and the ligaments and cartilage in the joint are thoroughly inspected for tears or abnormalities. The recesses, or pockets, of the joint are checked for fragments of bone or cartilage that may also indicate previous injury.

During the arthroscopy, the surgeon may use a variety of instruments. All instruments are long and thin, with a handle that the surgeon manipulates on one end and the active part of the instrument on the other end. A probe, or a small metal hook, is used to feel and move the cartilage and ligaments seen on the camera. An arthroscopic shaver is a tiny motorized instrument that is used to remove torn and injured tissue inside the joint in a controlled manner. The shaver is connected to a suction device that brings loose and torn tissue into the mouth of the shaver. The tissue is cut by the rotation of the cutter blade. By controlling the amount of suction and varying the types of cutter blades used, the surgeon can control how much tissue is removed. Other small instruments that fit through arthroscopic portals act as scissors, graspers, and cutters, to debride or excise loose pieces of cartilage or tears in the meniscus (knee) or labrum (shoulder and hip).

Commonly performed arthroscopic procedures include debridement, repair, excision, chondroplasty, and microfracture. With arthroscopic debridement, the surgeon can smooth the roughened surfaces that may be causing pain or excise any tissues that may be catching on other joint structures and causing painful symptoms. Ligament and tendon repair and cartilage injuries can also be treated with the aid of arthroscopy. Common arthroscopic procedures done in the shoulder include repair of rotator cuff tears, repair or debridement of labral tears, and tightening of a loose shoulder capsule. Knee problems such as ACL tears, meniscus tears, and cartilage injuries can be treated with meniscus repair or meniscectomy, ACL reconstruction, chondroplasty, or microfracture. Smaller joints such as the elbow, wrist, and ankle often require smaller arthroscopic equipment. Cartilage injuries and loose bodies of the ankle and elbow are often treated with arthroscopy.

Arthroscopic surgery has many benefits. When compared with open surgery, in which the joint is opened through a larger incision and the procedure is done under direct visualization, arthroscopy offers a minimally invasive approach. As noted earlier, the arthroscopic procedures use multiple tiny incisions, which result in a better cosmetic appearance. There is less disruption of the tissues under the skin and in the joint, which causes less scarring and stiffness. The smaller incisions also allow a smaller area of the joint to be exposed to the air, decreasing the risk of infection. Because patients have less pain after arthroscopy, they are able to participate in rehabilitation sooner.

Not all diseases or conditions involving a joint can be treated with arthroscopy. Some surgeries require large exposures of the joint, which arthroscopy cannot offer. Complicated arthroscopic cases may require the surgeon to repair the joint under direct visualization, with an open procedure. This most often happens if a structure that needs to be repaired cannot be reached through the small incision without causing injury to other structures or if there is poor visualization within the joint due to bleeding or other factors.

Most arthroscopic surgeries are done as outpatient cases, meaning that the athlete is able to go home on the day of the surgery. The incisions are small and can often be covered with an adhesive bandage strip. Depending on the type and location of the surgery, the surgeon will make recommendations regarding activity limitations. Some procedures will have strict restrictions on how one can use the operative site (e.g., crutches or lifting restrictions), while others may have no restrictions.

Recovery Time and Rehabilitation

Nearly all athletes who undergo arthroscopic surgery will need physical therapy before they can resume their normal sporting activities. Recovery time varies depending on the nature of the procedure. To return to sports, the patient must demonstrate full range of motion and full strength in the affected joint. The initial goal of physical therapy focuses on *regaining full motion* in the affected joint. After motion is gained and the surgical repair has healed sufficiently, the physical therapists will concentrate on *regaining strength*.

For complicated procedures such as knee ACL reconstructions, shoulder rotator cuff repairs, and shoulder labral repairs, full recovery takes 6 months to 1 year after surgery. For knee meniscal repairs and chondroplasty for cartilage injuries, return to sports generally occurs at about 3 months after surgery. For smaller procedures such as diagnostic arthroscopy, joint debridement, and meniscectomy, return to sports takes about 6 to 8 weeks.

Miho J. Tanaka and Dennis E. Kramer

See also Arthroscopy; Knee Injuries, Surgery for; Principles of Rehabilitation and Physical Therapy; Shoulder Injuries, Surgery for

Further Readings

Abboud JA, Ricchetti ET, Tjoumakaris F, Ramsey ML. Elbow arthroscopy: basic setup and portal placement. *J Am Acad Orthop Surg.* 2006;14(5):312–318.

DeBerardino TM, Arciero RA, Taylor DC, Uhorchak JM. Prospective evaluation of arthroscopic stabilization of acute, initial anterior shoulder dislocations in young athletes. Two- to five-year follow-up. *Am J Sports Med.* 2001;29(5):586–592.

Kelly BT, Williams RJ 3rd, Philippon MJ. Hip arthroscopy: current indications, treatment options, and management issues. *Am J Sports Med.* 2003;31(6):1020–1037.

Mintzer CM, Richmond JC, Taylor J. Meniscal repair in the young athlete. *Am J Sports Med.* 1998;26(5):630–633.

Nam EK, Snyder SJ. The diagnosis and treatment of superior labrum, anterior and posterior (SLAP) lesions. *Am J Sports Med.* 2003;31(5):798–810.

Stetson WB, Ferkel RD. Ankle arthroscopy: II. Indications and results. *J Am Acad Orthop Surg.* 1996;4(1):24–34.

SPORTS MASSAGE THERAPIST

Sports massage therapy, a specialized branch of traditional massage, is a burgeoning profession worldwide, due to the growing need for it as an adjunct to traditional medical treatment. A 20% increase in demand has been projected over the next decade.

Manual massage (initially called "friction") is performed to improve muscle function and blood circulation via manipulation of the body's soft tissue. Based on the patient's needs and characteristics (e.g., athlete, elderly, pregnant, child), any of several massage treatment techniques or modalities may be used. Each therapist may develop his or her own unique style and may specialize in treating patients with certain diagnoses or conditions.

Sports massage therapy (also known as *manual medicine*) was developed to help athletes recover from an event or workout and to prepare them for top performance. It can be used before, during, and after an event. It is estimated that Americans spend more than $4 billion annually on massage therapy for a variety of reasons, including work, sports, rehabilitation from a motor vehicle accident, and also as a luxurious treat.

In the past few years, referrals for manual medicine have increased significantly and have been integrated into a permanent component of the athlete's training protocol, at all levels—from high school to professional athletic programs. It is a medical preemptive intervention based on the belief that a regimen of massage provides a competitive edge to the athlete. Sports massages are used for athletes as well as for those recovering from an injury. Sports massage is promoted by athletic trainers, team physicians, and sports medicine doctors to assist athletes to prepare their bodies to achieve optimal performance. In a field where a matter of seconds can mean the difference between victory and defeat and where the latest technologies are used to provide an edge over the opponent, sports massage is growing to be an important adjunct.

The reasons to incorporate manual medicine modalities on a regular basis range from aiming to win the gold medal in an Olympic event to assisting in the recovery process of a person with restricted range of motion due to injury. Sports massage is a logical choice, especially if the injury was caused after a sporting event such as a marathon. Preemptive intervention is crucial to prevent injuries. Massage can help promote symmetry and stability of the muscles and joints in the body, thereby avoiding the potential for injury due to abnormal movement or functioning of muscles or fascia.

Massage therapy has become a standard and integral component of athletic training in most sports clinics all over the world. The ultimate goal of a massage therapist is to improve emotional and physical health. The techniques and time spent for each session and the number of sessions may vary based on the physician's massage therapy prescription and goals, as well as the patient's expectations. Massage therapists can specialize in one or more particular techniques based on their interests, community needs, and the market. Currently, there are more than 50 common massage techniques used to promote a healthy mind and body. Each therapist will select a modality that is based on his or her previous experience as well as the needs of the patient.

Some common manual medicine modalities include Swedish massage, deep tissue massage, acupressure, and sports massage. In addition, doctors of osteopathic medicine (DOs) are fully licensed physicians who use various manual medicine techniques, known as *osteopathic manipulative treatment* (OMT), to assist patients toward a return to health. Typically, a massage therapist works along with a physician or athletic team. Most patients seek a massage therapist based on a referral and the specialty of the therapist. There is a wide range in the hours worked per week as well as income earned by massage therapists. One therapist may work 80 hours/week and another in the same area only 15 hours weekly. Income may vary from $30 to $200/hour, based on where the therapist is employed. Variations that may help explain the wide range of salaries include differences in training, which range from 500 to 1,000 hours; knowledge of basic anatomy, physiology, and kinesiology (study of human movement); and practical demonstration of skills. Other factors include interpersonal skills, which affect referrals by other clients, moral character, professionalism, referrals from physicians, attitude, empathy toward the patient, and the ability to engage the patient in a trusting and therapeutic relationship. Prerequisites to become a certified massage therapist include, at the minimum, completion of high school and a desire to assist others. Most massage therapy schools require attendance for at least 6 months and sometimes up to or beyond 12 months, depending on the particular modality specialized in.

In addition to didactic coursework and reading, it is mandatory to obtain experience in the various manual medicine modalities and techniques. It is worth noting that many allopathic medical schools are incorporating several related manual medicine techniques into their curriculum to give their graduates exposure to all forms of manual medicine.

Osteopathic manual therapy is a hands-on form of care. Osteopathic physicians use their hands to diagnose as well as treat injuries and musculoskeletal problems. The first osteopathic medical school was begun in 1892 by Dr. Andrew Taylor Still. Dr. Still was an allopathic physician who was frustrated with aspects of medical care in his time and sought to devise a better way of treating patients.

Most people enjoy getting a massage, and for patients who have been injured during a sporting event and for those who are competitive athletes, seeking the services of a specialist in sports massage therapy may promote speedy recovery, help maintain body shape and symmetry, decrease stiffness and soreness, and reduce the potential for injury.

George Kolo and Daniel Kandah

See also Complementary Treatment; Manual Medicine

Further Readings

Clay JH, Pounds DM. *Basic Clinical Massage Therapy: Integrating Anatomy and Treatment*. Baltimore, MD: Lippincott Williams & Wilkins; 2002.
Werner, Ruth. *A Massage Therapist's Guide to Pathology*. Philadelphia, PA Lippincott, Williams & Wilkins; 1998.

Sports Socialization

Participation in recreational and competitive sports is widespread in Western cultures. The physical and psychological benefits of physical activity are well known, and most experts agree that everyone should engage in physical activity on a regular basis. Sports participation, including planned physical training and competition, has both positive and negative developmental consequences for participants. Positive benefits from participation include discipline, loyalty, physical development, improved self-esteem, teamwork, sportsmanship, time management, and lifetime patterns of fitness. Conversely, sports participation can also be related to stress, stereotyping, and risk-taking patterns. Sports socialization is the process by which individuals are introduced to sports, taught the physical and behavioral standards, and incorporated into the culture of sports. Parents, coaches, peers, and society all influence the process of socialization into sport.

Process of Socialization

There are numerous theories on the process of sports socialization. Common to most theories is that there is an initial introductory phase where knowledge, cultural norms, and skills of the sports are acquired. Children and adolescents often begin playing the sports that their siblings, friends, and parents find interesting and in which they participate. Depending on individual interests and innate skills, youth self-select the sports in which they would like to continue to participate. Following the introductory phase, individuals further develop their skills, associate with other participants, begin to view themselves as athletes, and are recognized by others as athletes.

Parents have the greatest influence on the sports socialization of their children and adolescents. With the goal of teaching their children positive values and traits, parents introduce their children to sports through game play, television, discussion, and watching as spectators. Parent interaction during sports can also offer opportunities to teach their children lessons regarding desirable morals and social behavior such as sportsmanship, loyalty, teamwork, and determination. It has been shown that children whose parents communicate the importance of sports and foster their training in them find greater enjoyment in sports participation. Surprisingly, parental pressure to succeed has not always been associated with decreased enjoyment.

Sports Goals/Beliefs

Individual motivation and definition of success are personal attributes taught through the socialization process. Two distinct goal orientations have been described: *task* and *ego*. The task-oriented individual describes success in terms of effort and self-improvement, while the ego-oriented individual describes success in terms of comparison with others and demonstrating superiority. Parents and coaches directly influence these two orientations by their actions and their focus on effort, hard work, and collaboration (task) or their focus on winning at all costs, impressing others, and demonstrating superior skills (ego). Similarly, the belief patterns of young athletes can affect their motivation to participate and work hard. Teaching youth that effort should be the focus during participation will foster a pattern of hard work and determination.

Gender Issues in Socialization

The athletic experience is often very different between boys and girls. Competitive males are seen as leaders and deemed role models. Classically male qualities and traits such as intimidation, dominance, insensitivity, and lack of emotional display are often fostered in the realm of sports. These qualities are vastly different from the traits that are often fostered in females during social development (nurturing, sensitivity, and emotionality). Over the past century, women's involvement in competitive sports has become socially accepted and supported. Despite the great strides in equality, female athletes are still expected to possess these dual and often discordant sets of traits.

Burnout and Discontinuation of Sport

A tenet of physical education educators has been to socialize children to sports as a means of beginning a life of physical activity. The idea that involvement in sports as a youth will continue into physical activity as an adult is a common belief; however, it is well documented that individuals tend to discontinue sports participation with increasing age. Research has demonstrated that a pattern of physical activity as a youth can lead to a lifelong engagement in physical activity, but even more consistent is the observation that a pattern of inactivity as a youth leads to inactivity as an adult. Athletes decide to discontinue sports for many reasons, including burnout, changing interests, and changing life situations (work, school, and parenthood).

Burnout among athletes is a phenomenon seen in youth who have been very involved in sports suddenly losing interest in continuing participation and competition. This is seen more often in individual-sport athletes whose lives are consumed by participation in their sports. These athletes often describe a lack of social interaction and a sense of being a one-dimensional individual. Focusing on developing skills outside the sports arena and being involved in more than one sport may decrease the likelihood of burnout and desocialization from sports.

Jason Diehl

See also Burnout in Sports; Mental Health Benefits of Sports and Exercise; Psychology of the Young Athlete; Sports Socialization

Further Readings

Barnett NP, Wright P. Psychological considerations for women in sports. *Clin Sports Med.* 1994;13(2): 297–313.

Coakley J. Sport and socialization. *Exerc Sport Sci Rev.* 1993;21:169–200.

Larson RW, Hansen DM. Differing profiles of developmental experiences across types of organized youth activities. *Dev Psycol.* 2006;42(5):849–863.

Vanreusel B, Renson R, Beunen G, et al. A longitudinal study of youth sport participation and adherence to sport in adulthood. *Int Rev Sociol Sport.* 1997;32(4):373–387.

White SA, Kavussanu M, Tank KM, Wingate JM. Perceived parental beliefs about the causes of success in sport. *Scand J Med Sci Sports.* 2004;14(1):57–66.

Static Stretching

Static stretching is a form of stretching that slowly elongates the muscle. This can be done actively or passively. In the active form, the person stretches the desired muscle or muscle group to the point of discomfort and holds this for a period of time. The passive form involves a second person (usually a physical therapist or athletic trainer) who assists in stretching the desired muscle or muscle group. Whether active or passive, the goal of the static stretch is to desensitize tension sensors in muscles. Once this occurs, the muscle is able to take on more force before it becomes damaged. A long-standing belief is that this leads to a reduction of injuries as the muscle is more compliant.

Uses

Static stretching has been used as a treatment modality in injury rehabilitation. After a muscle injury, the torn muscle fibers heal in a contracted pattern. Therapists can use static stretching to restore the muscle to its normal length. This helps improve the range of motion in the affected body area. This is usually done in the subacute phase of injury recovery. It can also be used for rehabilitation of certain joint injuries. A common example is stretching the shoulder capsule. Improper mobility following a shoulder injury may result in a frozen shoulder or adhesive capsulitis. The therapist may use static stretches (both active and passive) to improve the shoulder range of motion.

Static stretching has long been used in "warm-up" routines by those engaging in sports activity. The common thought is that loose muscles are less likely to be injured. Multiple studies show that static stretching before an athletic contest may cause small tears in the muscle and make the muscle more prone to injury.

A recent critical review of the literature showed that after a single bout of static stretching, muscle force and torque as well as jump height were diminished. However, when the static stretching was repeated over days to weeks, there seemed to be an increase in muscle force and torque. There was a positive effect of a single bout of static stretching on running economy but not on running speed. Based on these results, it is considered beneficial to perform regular static stretching but not immediately before an athletic contest. Muscles should be warmed by other types of stretching—mainly dynamic stretching.

Examples

An example of a static stretch is the *seated hamstring stretch*. This is performed by sitting on the floor with one leg straight out while the other is bent at the knee with the foot touching the opposite thigh. Then, while keeping the back straight, reach forward with the arms by bending at the waist. A slight stretch should be felt in the hamstring. This is held for 15 to 30 seconds. It may be repeated two to three times.

Another example of a static stretch is the *butterfly stretch*. In the seated position, the knees are bent with the soles of the feet touching. The elbows are used to direct a downward force on the legs. This should cause a slight stretch in the adductor muscles (groin). This is held for 10 to 30 seconds. It may be repeated two to three times.

Richard A. Okragly

See also Exercise Physiologist; Preventing Sports Injuries; Strains, Muscle; Stretching and Warming Up

Further Readings

Fyfe S. Stretching: what's the point? http://www .sportsinjurybulletin.com/archive/stretching.htm. Accessed January 24, 2010.

Kovacs MS. Is static stretching for tennis beneficial? A brief review. *Med Sci Tennis.* 2006;11(2):14–16.

Shrier I. Does stretching improve performance? A systematic and critical review of the literature. *Clin J Sport Med.* 2004;14(5):267–273.

Walker B. *The Stretching Handbook.* 3rd ed. Sydney, Australia: Walkerbout Health; 2007.

STERNAL FRACTURE

Sternal fractures are rare yet potentially serious injuries in athletes. Few sports have a high risk of blunt trauma to the anterior chest wall, the main cause of most sternal fractures. Rapid deceleration injuries fall into this category, often resulting from motor vehicle accidents with the patient restrained. Such injuries are primarily seen in the trauma and emergency department setting, but the sports medicine physician should be aware of suspicious patient complaints associated with chest trauma. Awareness concerning sternal injuries may prevent missed diagnoses, unnecessary and expensive work-ups, and frustration for the athlete.

Sternal and stress fractures have been reported in golfers, weight lifters, and athletes involved in other contact and noncontact sports. Injuries have been reported in repetitive hyperflexion of the torso, such as in exercises that involve sit-up postures. Athletes involved in high-speed sports, high-altitude sports, and high-energy contact sports are theoretically at risk. Other patients at risk are those with osteoporosis or osteopenia, those with severe thoracic kyphosis, and any patient subjected to cardiopulmonary resuscitation.

Anatomy

With direct chest wall trauma, the sternum may fracture at any point. The sternum consists of three parts: (1) the manubrium; (2) the body, or corpus; and (3) the xiphoid process. The xiphoid process forms the distal tip of the sternum. The joint between the manubrium and the body, the manubriosternal joint, forms the sternal angle at the second rib. The manubrium is found at the third and fourth thoracic vertebrae. The superior border is formed by the suprasternal notch. The clavicle and first rib articulate with the manubrium. The sternal head of the sternocleidomastoid muscle inserts at the anterior of the manubrium, along with the sternocostal head of the pectoralis major. The sternohyoid and sternothyroid muscles attach to the posterior surface of the manubrium. The rectus abdominus attaches to the distal xiphoid process.

Symptoms

The patient's history may reveal an abrupt stop or direct chest wall trauma during an athletic event. Initial symptoms of a sternal fracture include acute sternal pain and tenderness with palpation directly over the sternum. There may be soft tissue swelling and bruising but usually not a palpable deformity as most fractures will be nondisplaced. The examining physician should keep in mind the cause of the injury, should influence the acuity of the assessment, and should plan for the patient. For example, sternal fractures related to motor vehicle seat belt injuries are not associated with thoracic vascular injuries or spinal cord injuries and are, therefore, not associated with a significant mortality risk. With more serious traumatic injuries, there may be signs of respiratory compromise, including retractions, tachypnea, and cyanosis. Other conditions associated with direct trauma include rib fractures, pulmonary and cardiac contusion, and intrathoracic vascular trauma, including aortic rupture, cardiac tamponade, flail chest, pneumothorax, hemothorax, spine fractures, spinal cord injuries, diaphragmatic rupture, tracheobronchial rupture, and esophageal rupture.

Diagnosis

The American College of Surgeons provided guidelines in the Advanced Trauma and Life Support algorithms for the management of chest trauma (see the list of recommended readings). Any patient seen initially who has sustained blunt thoracic trauma should have a primary survey for potentially life-threatening conditions, including a complete history and physical exam. Initial studies and labs may include complete blood count, electrolytes, coagulation panel, type and screen, arterial blood gas, and electrocardiogram (EKG). Initial radiographs of the sternum should include a lateral view and a frontal view, with the patient prone and slightly rotated away from the midline. These views have a reported sensitivity of greater than 90%. X-ray (radiographs) may also diagnose other potentially serious injuries, including rib fractures, hemothorax, pneumothorax, and pulmonary contusion.

Radiographs remain the initial gold standard for the evaluation of sternal injury. A frontal view and a lateral view should be obtained, as any displacement usually occurs in the sagittal plane. Any evidence of more serious diagnoses such as arrhythmias, hemodynamic instability, or a widened mediastinum should be evaluated with echocardiography and, possibly, computed tomography scans. The body, or corpus, of the sternum is the area most frequently injured. Ultrasound may be slightly more sensitive in diagnosing fractures, but most experts still consider radiographs to be the first initial choice.

Treatment

After the initial work-up, and after potentially life-threatening injuries have been excluded, further course of treatment involves pain management, usually with oral analgesics. There should be a period of relative rest, especially from contact sports or the offending activity. The patient should be encouraged to perform deep-breathing exercises, as with rib fractures, to prevent atelectasis and pneumonia.

Rehabilitation and Return to Sports

The athlete should be encouraged to maintain cardiovascular fitness if unable to participate in practice or contact drills. Otherwise, the decision to return to play should be made on the basis of whether the athlete can compete painfree in his or her event. The literature on rehabilitation is scanty, but therapy for similar injuries includes early rest and lower extremity exercises, followed by range-of-motion exercises,

and eventually chest- and core-strengthening exercises. The time required for complete resolution of pain varies; pain can persist from a few months up to a year or longer.

Christopher McGrew and Edward Dubois Smith

See also Chest and Chest Wall Injuries; Football, Injuries in; Rugby Union, Injuries in

Further Readings

ACS Committee on Trauma. *Advanced Trauma Life Support for Doctors.* 6th ed. Chicago, IL: American College of Surgeons; 1997.

Athanassiadi K, Gerazounis M, Moustardas M, Metaxas S. Sternal fractures: retrospective analysis of 100 cases. *World J Surg.* 2002;26(10):1243–1246.

Brookes JG, Dunn RJ, Rogers IR. Sternal fractures: a retrospective analysis of 272 cases. *J Trauma.* 1993;35(1):46–54.

Chiu WC, D'Amelio LF, Hammond JS. Sternal fractures in blunt chest trauma: a practical algorithm for management. *Am J Emerg Med.* 1997;15(3):252–256.

Engin G, Yekeler E, Guloglu R, Acunas B, Acunas G. US versus conventional radiography in the diagnosis of sternal fractures. *Acta Radiol.* 2000;41(3):296–299.

Gregory PL, Biswas AC, Batt ME. Musculoskeletal problems of the chest wall in athletes. *Sports Med.* 2002;32(4):235–250.

Habib PA, Huang GS, Mendiola JA, Yu JS. Anterior chest pain: musculoskeletal considerations. *Emerg Radiol.* 2004;11(1):37–45.

Howell NJ, Ranasinghe A, Graham T. Management of rib and sternal fractures. *Trauma.* 2005;7(1):47–54.

Keating TM. Stress fracture of the sternum in a wrestler. *Am J Sports Med.* 1987;15(1):92–93.

Perron AD. Chest pain in athletes. *Clin Sports Med.* 2003;22(1):37–50.

Pidcoe PE, Burnet EN. Rehabilitation of an elite gymnast with a type 2 manubriosternal dislocation. *Phys Ther.* 2007;87(4):468–475.

Roy-Shapira A, Levi I, Khoda J. Sternal fractures: a red flag or a red herring? *J Trauma.* 1994;37(1):59–61.

STERNOCLAVICULAR (SC) JOINT, SEPARATION OF

The *sternoclavicular joint* (SCJ) is located on the anterior chest where the clavicle (collarbone)

meets with the sternum (breastbone). Separation of the SCJ is relatively uncommon in athletes and is usually caused by significant trauma to the area resulting from high-velocity injuries, such as those incurred in contact sports or motor vehicle accidents. Separation of the SCJ may be life threatening because of the large blood vessels that run just underneath the clavicle. The practitioner must have a high level of suspicion for these injuries to recognize them when they occur.

Anatomy

The SCJ is a two-sided joint and provides the only true joint connection between the trunk and the upper extremity. The SCJ has an inherent instability, with less than one half of the inner clavicle bone articulating with the upper angle of the sternum. This bony articulation of the joint is inherently unstable. Several ligaments help stabilize the bony anatomy of the joint. These include the weaker anterior and the stronger posterior sternoclavicular and interclavicular ligaments, as well as the costoclavicular ligament. Because of the bony instability, the ligaments are at increased stress and are more susceptible to injury (sprain or disruption) (Figure 1).

Important structures lie in direct proximity to the SCJ. Major vascular structures such as the internal thoracic artery and vein, and the brachiocephalic and subclavian veins travel just underneath the clavicle. Deeper important structures in the SCJ and clavicle include the subclavian and brachiocephalic arteries, the trachea (wind pipe), the esophagus, and the brachial plexus (a major group of nerves that innervate the upper extremity). Injuries to these structures are the main concern following an SCJ separation.

Causes

The most common cause of SCJ separation is vehicular accidents; the second is an injury sustained during participation in sports. This usually involves an athlete falling on one side with an opposing force to the top of the opposite shoulder, such as a pile-up in football or rugby.

The most common mechanism of injury is a blow to the outer aspect of the shoulder, such as a fall on the shoulder. This most commonly levers the medial clavicle (the portion of the clavicle closest to

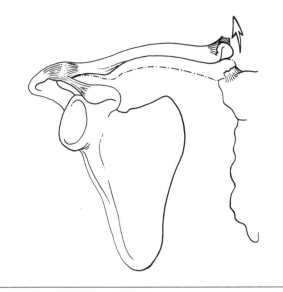

Figure 1   Sternoclavicular Joint Separation

Note: Sternoclavicular joint (SCJ) separation is a sprain of the ligaments of the SCJ, which connects the sternum, or breastbone, with the clavicle (collarbone).

the sternum) anteriorly, increasing the strain on the supporting ligaments and potentially leading to separation of the SCJ. Less commonly, the injury may be caused by a direct blow to the clavicle at its junction with the sternum.

Injuries to the SCJ ligaments fall into three categories. Grades I and II are mild or moderate sprains with minimal displacement of the bony elements of the joint. Grade III injuries are severe and involve complete ligament disruption and significant joint displacement. SCJ separations can occur in both anterior and posterior directions. Anterior SCJ dislocations are more common and less threatening than posterior dislocations. Posterior SCJ dislocations may be life threatening due to the potential damage to vascular structures deep to the SCJ and clavicle. Prompt diagnosis is paramount with posterior dislocations to avoid these serious potential complications.

Diagnosis

Patients generally present with pain and swelling in the area of the SCJ following a history of an acute injury. However, as a result of the significant force needed to cause injury to the SCJ, the patient may have other traumatic injuries that distract both the patient and the examiner from the SCJ injury. The patient may have other life-threatening injuries that warrant immediate attention. A high index of suspicion is required in trauma situations to detect SCJ injuries. Conversely, when an SCJ injury is suspected (especially a posterior dislocation), patient stability should take priority by first assessing the patient's airway, breathing, and circulatory status.

The patient with an injury to the SCJ often has severe pain at the joint that is increased with any movement of the arm, particularly when the shoulders are pressed together by a lateral force. The patient usually supports the injured arm across the trunk with the unaffected arm. The affected shoulder appears to be shortened and thrust forward when compared with the normal shoulder. The head may be tilted toward the side of the dislocated joint. The patient's discomfort increases when he or she is placed in the supine position, at which time the involved shoulder will not lie back flat on the table.

Any injury to the SCJ is difficult to assess with standard X-ray films; however, there are several specialized views, such as the *Heinig view* and *Hobbs axial or serendipity view,* that can make assessment easier. Many experts agree that computed tomography (CT) is the ideal method to image the SCJ. CT is much better at distinguishing separation of the joint from fracture. Additionally, a chest CT with contrast material can also assess the major important structures that run underneath the SCJ.

Based on the degree of injury to the SCJ, injuries are classified as Grades I, II, and III. With Grade I sprains, there is stretching and partial tearing of the SC ligaments. The costoclavicular ligament is usually not involved. With Grade II SC sprains, there is complete tear of the SC ligaments and the SC capsule. The costoclavicular ligament may be stretched or have partial tearing. Instability of the SCJ is present with possible subluxation. Grade III sprains involve a dislocation of the SCJ either anteriorly or posteriorly, with complete tearing of the SC and costoclavicular ligaments.

Treatment

Treatment of SCJ separation depends on the severity of injury. Mild ligamentous sprains (Grade I) are stable and are always treated conservatively.

Ice is recommended initially to reduce the inflammation. The involved extremity is immobilized in a sling for 1 to 2 weeks, followed by early range-of-motion exercises.

Grade II sprains differ from Grade I sprains in that a joint subluxation has occurred. The capsule, intraarticular disk, and costoclavicular ligaments may be partially disrupted. The sprained SCJ is stable and can be painful. These injuries can usually be reduced satisfactorily by drawing the shoulders backward as if reducing and holding a fracture of the clavicle. A clavicle strap can be used to hold the reduction. A sling and swath is used to hold up the shoulder and to prevent motion of the arm. The patient should be protected from further injury for 4 to 6 weeks.

SCJ dislocations (Grade III sprain) are the most severe in the continuum of SCJ injuries. This is considered an unstable injury, and if posterior dislocation occurs, the underlying structures can become compressed and may be life threatening. The treatment of choice is a closed reduction restoring the normal bony anatomy of the joint. Techniques for this type of reduction depend on the type of dislocation and should be performed as quickly as possible. If an anterior dislocation has occurred, the patient should be informed that these injuries have a high incidence of recurrent instability but that the symptoms rarely limit normal activities. This avoids misunderstandings later in the treatment course.

Return to Sports

The return-to-play decision must be made with the athlete's well-being as the single most important deciding factor. Consideration should be given to the athlete's ability to move the arm through a full range of motion. Strength is vitally important so that athletes can both protect themselves and be effective in their sport. Special custom padding (or shoulder pads) can be worn to protect the top of the shoulder or the front of the sternum. Even after return to play, it is not unusual for the athlete to experience periods of discomfort for up to several months.

Chad Asplund and James Borchers

See also Acromioclavicular (AC) Joint, Separation of; Football, Injuries in; Musculoskeletal Tests, Shoulder; Rugby Union, Injuries in; Shoulder Dislocation; Shoulder Injuries

Further Readings

Bicos J, Nicholson GP. Treatment and results of sternoclavicular joint injuries. *Clin Sports Med.* 2003;22(2):359–370.

Wirth MA, Rockwood CA. Acute and chronic traumatic injuries of the sternoclavicular joint. *J Am Acad Orthop Surg.* 1996;4(5):268–278.

STIMULANTS

Athletes have been known to use stimulants in and out of competition. Most stimulants are banned by the World Anti-Doping Agency (WADA), but a few stimulants, such as caffeine, are monitored and allowed up to certain levels in the urine.

Stimulants are substances that activate the sympathetic nervous system. This is the part of human physiology that gives us the "fright, fight, or flight" response. The sympathetic nervous system is what gives a person the burst of energy, power, and alertness to deal effectively with a threat or stressor. In the wild, it is the response we would have if we were threatened by a hungry predator. Similarly, it is the response we feel with the stress of public speaking or the excitement of competition. Physiologic effects include increased heart and breathing rates, dilation of the pupils, and sweating. A person would also feel a burst of energy, a heightened state of alertness, and possibly improved concentration or even euphoria. Stimulation of the sympathetic nervous system also inhibits gastric motility (activity in the intestine), stimulates piloerection (goose bumps, or hair standing on end), and liberates nutrients in the body for muscle action.

There are many different types of stimulants, and they come in different forms and strengths. Amphetamines, nicotine, and even cocaine all fall into the category of stimulants. The most commonly used stimulant is caffeine. This is found in different concentrations in *coffee,* tea, soft drinks, and energy drinks. A typical cup of coffee (8 ounces [oz; 1 oz = 28.34 grams]) generally has approximately 100 milligrams (mg) of caffeine (although larger sizes of stronger brewed coffee may have up to 150 mg). Tea usually has around 50 mg per cup (8 oz), and soft drinks have between 50 and 65 mg per 12-oz serving. Energy drinks may have up to 150 mg of caffeine per serving. Soft drinks are required by the Food and Drug Administration (FDA) to keep caffeine levels below 65 mg per 12-oz serving. This rule does not apply to energy drinks, and they often come in serving sizes larger than 12 oz. Some energy drinks containing more than 300 mg of caffeine have been marketed. In addition, energy drinks or dietary supplements may also contain other ingredients that have benign- or exotic-sounding names but still have stimulant properties. Common examples of these lesser-known stimulants include guarana, ma huang, and yohimbe.

Caffeine is also available in a concentrated tablet form, and it is used to increase alertness, energy, and mood. Stimulants such as caffeine also have an appetite-suppressive effect, and they have been used to aid in weight loss. Stimulants do have a performance-enhancing effect in some sports. They have been used by athletes to increase the utilization of body fat for energy and to decrease perceived effort, particularly during intense endurance training.

Caffeine in particular has an interesting history when it comes to sports. In the 1980s and 1990s, caffeine was a banned substance, and several athletes were banned for positive tests. Before January 2004, caffeine levels over 12 micrograms/milliliter (μg/ml) in the urine were unacceptable. Since that time, caffeine has been removed from the list of banned substances by WADA. It is still considered a restricted substance with the National Collegiate Athletic Association (NCAA; the governing body for college sports). If the concentration of caffeine in the urine exceeds 15 μg/ml, the athlete can be disqualified. Urine concentration levels vary per individual, but, in general, to exceed this level, an athlete would have to ingest around 500 mg of caffeine 2 to 3 hours prior to the test.

Cathine and ephedrine are still restricted by WADA. Cathine is a stimulant related to amphetamines and is found in the khat plant. It is a Schedule IV drug in the United States (prescription medication) and is used as an appetite suppressant and decongestant. Cathine is prohibited by WADA when its concentration in urine exceeds 5 μg/ml. Ephedrine is commonly found in over-the-counter cold remedies, antihistamine products, energy drinks, and dietary supplements. Ephedrine and methylephedrine are prohibited by WADA when their concentration in urine exceeds 10 μg/ml. Athletes are responsible for knowing all the contents, effects, and consequences of any product that they ingest, and they are responsible for the product's effect on their test results.

The stimulant epinephrine (adrenaline) is included with some local injectable or transdermal anesthetic agents such as lidocaine or novocaine. Use of small amounts of epinephrine in this form is not prohibited.

The stimulants amphetamine and dextroamphetamine have been used as a treatment for attention deficit disorder (ADD). Increase in the concentration of these medications makes them beneficial.

Anyone who takes stimulants should be aware of their potential side effects. Because there is an increase in heart rate and blood pressure, heart attack or stroke is possible. They can temporarily raise blood sugar levels in patients with diabetes and contribute to insomnia. Overdose or long-term abuse of stimulants can cause paranoia, depression, and psychosis. Stimulants such as caffeine can cause stomach cramps, dizziness, or tremor. Athletes ingesting stimulants such as caffeine must take this into account before training or competing, particularly in endurance events or events that require a steady hand such as archery. Possession of certain outlawed stimulants such as cocaine, ephedra, or MDMA (3,4-methylenedioxy-N-methamphetamine; found, among other chemicals, in the recreational drug of abuse ecstasy) also has legal consequences.

Michael O'Brien

See also Doping and Performance Enhancement: A New Definition; Performance Enhancement, Doping, Therapeutic Use Exemptions

Further Readings

Bramstedt KA. Caffeine use by children: the quest for enhancement. *Subst Use Misuse.* 2007;42(8): 1237–1251.

Docherty JR. Pharmacology of stimulants prohibited by the World Anti-Doping Agency (WADA). *Br J Pharmacol.* 2008;154(3):606–622.

Goldstein ER, Ziegenfuss T, Kalman, D, et al. International society of sports nutrition position stand: caffeine and performance. *J Int Soc Sports Nutr.* 2010;7(1):5.

Greydanus DE, Patel DR. Sports doping in the adolescent: the Faustian conundrum of hors de combat. *Pediatr Clin North Am.* 2010;57(3):729–750.

Websites

National Institute on Drug Abuse (NIDA), Drugs of Abuse: http://www.drugabuse.gov/drugpages.html

NIDA for Teens: http://teens.drugabuse.gov

UpToDate: http://www.uptodate.com/patients

World Anti-Doping Agency (WADA): http://www.wada-ama.org

STRAINS, MUSCLE

Strains often occur in muscles that move two joints, for example, the hamstring muscles that flex the knee and extend the hip joint. These are caused by overstretching or eccentric overload and are located in the muscle-tendon junction. These ruptures occur as a result of the intrinsic force generated in the athlete's muscles, often in the change between eccentric and concentric traction, which is common in high-speed sports and accounts for 10% to 40% of injuries in soccer, Australian Rules football, and American football. When the demand made on a muscle exceeds its innate strength, rupture may occur—for example, in overload during eccentric muscle traction.

Muscle and tendon strains are caused by an abnormally high tensile force that causes rupturing of the tissue and subsequent hemorrhage and swelling. The likelihood of injury depends on the magnitude of the force acting and the structure's cross-sectional area. The greater the cross-sectional area of muscle, the greater its strength, meaning the more force it can produce and the more force that is translated to the attached tendon. The muscle portion of the musculotendinous unit usually ruptures first because tendons, by virtue of their collagenous composition, are about twice as strong as the muscles to which they attach. Muscle strains are rated according to the extent to which associated motion is impaired.

Strains can be classified by the degree of rupture: First- and second-degree strains are partial ruptures, and third-degree strains are complete ruptures or disruptions. A first-degree, or mild, strain describes an overstretching of the muscle with a rupture of less than 5% of the muscle fibers. A second-degree moderate strain involves a more significant but less than complete tear of the muscle. The pain will be worsened by contracting the muscle. A third-degree, or severe, strain involves complete disruption of the muscle.

Abdominal Muscle Strains

Muscular strains are caused by direct trauma, sudden twisting or extension of the spine, or the Valsalva maneuver during weight lifting. The rectus abdominis is the most commonly affected muscle. Pain and spasm in the injured muscle may evoke muscle pain, and any attempt to do a sit-up, straight leg raise, or hyperextension of the back significantly increases muscle pain.

Elbow Strains

Injury of the elbow flexors will result in point tenderness on the anterior distal arm. Pain increases with resisted elbow flexion. With a triceps strain, resisted elbow extension produces discomfort. Strains to the common wrist flexor group result in pain on resisted wrist flexion, whereas strains to the wrist extensors produce pain with wrist extension.

Wrist and Finger Strains

In the hand, muscle strains involving the finger flexors or extensors tend to be more serious. These injuries may involve avulsing the tendon from the bone.

Jersey finger: A jersey finger typically occurs when an individual grips an opponent who simultaneously twists and turns to get away. The ring finger is more commonly involved.

Mallet finger: Mallet finger occurs when an object hits the end of the finger while the extensor tendon is taut, such as when catching a ball.

Cervical Strains

Usually, the sternocleidomastoid or upper trapezius is involved. Strains typically occur at the extremes of motion or in association with a strenuous muscle contraction, an external force, or weakness caused by poor posture.

Pectoralis Major Muscle Strains

The strain may be caused by sudden violent deceleration movements. The frequent underlying reason is abuse of anabolic steroid. The mechanism for this strain may be inappropriate muscle hypertrophy and an increase in power without a concomitant increase in tendon size.

Strains of the Hip and Thigh

Strains of the hip and thigh are encountered in many sports or exercise activities with repetitive motions. Signs and symptoms include a local sharp pain, edema, weakness, and difficulties to contract against resistance.

Hamstring Strain

Ballistic action or a violent stretch may cause this injury. Risk factors are poor flexibility and posture, muscle imbalance, improper preparation, muscle fatigue, lack of neuromuscular control, previous injury, overuse, and improper training technique.

Chronic Muscle Strains

A chronic muscle injury can be defined as an injury that is characterized by disruption of muscle fibers that results in muscle dysfunction. Chronic muscle strain injuries account for 10% to 20% of all muscle strain injuries. These injuries are frequently not recognized and can cause considerable disability, particularly in athletes without any preparedness. Aggressive rehabilitation aiming to restore muscle strength, flexibility, and neuromuscular control is a treatment of choice. Deep transverse friction, stretching of the fibrotic muscle area, and conditioning of the affected muscle with concentric isotonic or isokinetic exercises to eccentric exercises is recommended. Muscle endurance exercises must also be added early in the program.

Repetitive Strain Injuries

These injuries develop following repetitive or sustained submaximal work of the soft tissue structures (i.e., muscles, tendons, ligaments, and nerves). The number of repetitions, duration and intensity of the exercise, and ergonomics of the activity contribute to this damage. Management should include careful review of the exercise program and modification of the inciting repetitive loads. Surgery is reserved for those with no response to conservative therapy.

A history of muscle strain and muscle weakness is a risk factor for muscle strains. Muscle-strengthening programs with an eccentric loading to specific muscle groups create a risk for injuries. Injury-prone athletes should be addressed with appropriate interventions to reduce the incidence of muscle strains.

Şirin Topçu

See also Calf Strain; Gluteal Strain; Groin Strain; Hamstring Strain; Hip Flexor Strain

Further Readings

Abdulaliyev Z, Çelik Ö, Göller G, Kayalı S. Investigation of forces and stresses acting on a shoulder-hand system considering strains in muscles. *Turkish J Eng Env Sci.* 2007;31:1–8.

Anderson MK. *Fundamentals of Sport Injury Management.* 2nd ed. Philadelphia, PA: Lippincott Williams & Wilkins; 2003.

Bradley PS, Portas MD. The relationship between preseason range of motion and muscle strain injury in elite soccer players. *J Strength Cond Res.* 2007;21(4):1155–1159.

McHugh MP. The prevention of muscle strains in sport: effective pre-season interventions? *Int Sportmed J.* 2004;5(3):177–187.

O'Neil BA, Forsythe ME, Stanish WD. Chronic occupational repetitive strain injury. *Can Fam Physician.* 2001;47:311–316.

Peterson L, Renstrom P. *Verletzungen im Sport. Handbuch der Sportverletzungen und Sportschaeden für Sportler, Übungsleiter und Aerzte.* 2 Auflage. Köln, Germany: Deutscher Aerzte-Verlag; 1987.

Peterson L, Renström P. *Sport Injures: Their Prevention and Treatment.* London, UK: Martin Dunitz; 2002.

Schwellnus MP. Chronic muscle strain injuries in sport: a brief review. *Int Sportmed J.* 2004;5(3):238–243.

Volpi P, Melegati G, Tornese D, Bandi M. Muscle strains in soccer: a five-year survey of an Italian major league team. *Knee Surg Sports Traumatol Arthrosc.* 2004;12(5):482–485.

STRENGTH TRAINING FOR THE FEMALE ATHLETE

Since the inception of Title IX of the Educational Amendments of 1972, female participation in sports activities has increased dramatically. The desire to become stronger and thereby improve performance has also risen. Women who use strength training to improve performance range from high school athletes, to the postmenopausal age-group, to those pursuing strength training sports such as bodybuilding and power lifting. Strength training is defined as the use of barbells, dumbbells, machines, and other resistive methods to increase one's ability to exert or resist a force. *Strength training* and *resistance training* are often used synonymously. Strength training has many known benefits, including cardiovascular fitness, good body composition, better bone health, lowering of cholesterol, and better mental health. The female athlete may also benefit from the improved attitude and body image that strength training often provides.

The Gender Difference

It is well documented that the response of muscle tissue to strength training by both males and females is similar. Anatomic differences, however, influence the absolute changes females are able to make in their physique with strength training. Males have a longer growth period than females, resulting in the average adult man being larger than the average adult woman. For women, this results in a lower center of gravity and better balance compared with men. Men also weigh about 11 kilograms (kg) more than women but have about 11% less fat than women. Women have narrower shoulders and wider hips. Females have less muscle mass compared with an equally trained male. This accounts for a male's ability to jump higher, run faster, and lift heavier weights compared with an equally trained female. Hormonal differences (lower levels of testosterone) in females will prevent them from becoming too bulky or large. These differences still allow males and females to strength train the same way. However, a training program should be tailored to the individual.

Nutritional Aspects

While males and females may strength train the same way, their nutritional needs are different. Males tend to use glycogen (stored glucose) for energy during exercise, whereas females tend to use more intramuscular (within the muscle) fat. The popular idea of a higher–carbohydrate, low-fat diet for a female who is strength training may not yield the strength gains that a diet higher in healthy fats would. The common practice of females withholding calories to lose weight will further impair the benefits of strength training. The diet of a strength-training female athlete should still consist of carbohydrates, protein, and fat. Carbohydrates should have a low glycemic index (produce small fluctuations in blood glucose levels) and include fruits, vegetables, brown rice, enriched whole-grain breads, whole-grain prepared cereals, rolled oats, beans, legumes, and sweet potatoes. Protein consumption should be 1.4 to 1.8 grams (g)/kg daily. The optimal anabolic (muscle growth) environment would be one of several portions of high-quality, rapidly digested protein with carbohydrate throughout the course of a day. Appropriate sources of protein would include lean pork and beef, poultry, fish, eggs, and low-fat dairy products. These are also excellent sources of micronutrients such as vitamin B_{12} and D, thiamine, riboflavin, calcium, phosphorus, iron, and zinc. Vegetarianism limits the amount of protein in the diet, and these females are at risk for iron-deficiency anemia.

Healthy fat intake is often a difficult concept for females using strength training to improve their physique. Fat has more readily available energy per gram than any other food source. It is necessary for the production of endogenous (made by the body) hormones such as estrogen and testosterone. When fat is withheld from the diet, menstrual disturbances and compromises to bone health may occur. Healthy fat sources include nuts, seeds, nut butters, fatty fish (salmon and trout), fish oil supplements, flaxseed oil, sunflower oil, canola oil, avocados, and egg yolks.

The Preadolescent and Adolescent Female

Controversy has surrounded strength training by children. For many years, children and adolescents have been discouraged from strength training because of concerns about damage to the growth plate from shear forces. However, it is now accepted that strength training is a viable method of improving performance and decreasing risk of injury in young athletes.

The age at which strength training should begin has not been determined. It has been found though that strength training of sufficient intensity and duration can enhance strength beyond what is considered normal for a particular age. A child or adolescent is likely ready for strength training when he or she is emotionally mature, follows instructions, and understands the risks and benefits. The American College of Sports Medicine recommends that children strength train two to three times weekly on nonconsecutive days. By allowing for adequate recovery time, overuse injuries should be prevented. In this population of athletes, greater strength gains have been found in moderate-weight, higher-repetition exercises than vice versa.

The mode of training can be a challenge for this population. Adult-sized machines may be too large, and child-sized weight machines are expensive and difficult to find. Free weights are a good option, because they are readily available and inexpensive. It is imperative that proper supervision is provided. Barbells are often preferred over dumbbells as they promote better form. In children and adolescents, much of the emphasis during strength training should be on core (low back, abdomen, and hips) strength.

A strength program should consider the goals, level of experience, and sports activity both current and past. Training should not take up more than 20 hours a week. A session should include warm-up (5–10 minutes of aerobic activity and stretching), aerobic activity, and then resistance training. One to three sets of 13 to 15 repetitions of many different exercises would be ideal.

The Older Female

The older female strength trains for slightly different reasons from younger females. The cardiovascular, bone, and cholesterol benefits are still attained. The difference is that strength training in the older female aims at increasing muscle mass and avoiding disability. In large part, the goal of strength training in this population is to maintain independence. A fall inducing a hip fracture is most serious for older women, due to the resultant permanent alterations in activity and long hospitals stays. Prevention of hip fracture has an obviously huge impact on the feasibility of independence in older women. The normal process of aging leads to a tremendous amount of atrophy and weakness that can be avoided with strength training. High-intensity training has been found to be more beneficial than low-intensity training in the older female.

Conclusion

Strength training is an excellent way to promote long-term health and increase muscle mass for females. While males and females have many anatomical differences, the effect or strength training on muscle tissue is quite similar. Special dietary considerations with adequate amounts of fat, protein, and carbohydrate should be included. The continued increase of females in athletics will most likely coincide with a continued increase in strength training by females. As noted earlier, strength training programs should be tailored to each individual. The goals of the female should dictate the choice of exercises, intensity, repetitions, and rest period combinations. This individual approach will likely result in long-term benefits from strength training.

Michelle Wilson and Jeffrey Guy

See also Core Strength; Female Athlete; Resistance Training; Running a Strength Training and Conditioning Facility

Further Readings

Ahmed C, Hilton W, Pituch KJ. Relations of strength training to body image among a sample of female university students. *J Strength Cond Res.* 2002;16(4):645–648.

Guy JA, Micheli LJ. Strength training for children and adolescents. *J Am Acad Orthop Surg.* 2001;9(1):29–36.

Holloway JB, Baechle TR. Strength training for female athletes. A review of selected aspects. *Sports Med.* 1990;9(4):216–228.

McCambridge TM, Stricker PR. Strength training by children and adolescents. *Pediatrics.* 2008;121(4): 835–840.

Porter MM. Power training for older adults. *Appl Physiol Nutr Metab.* 2006;31(2):87–94.

Volek JS. Nutritional aspects of women strength athletes. *Br J Sports Med.* 2006;40(9):742–748.

Volek JS. The relationship between physical activity and mental health in a national sample of college females. *Women's Health.* 2007;45(1):69–85.

STRENGTH TRAINING FOR THE YOUNG ATHLETE

Strength training refers to a specialized method of physical conditioning that involves the progressive use of a wide range of resistive loads and a variety of training modalities designed to enhance or maintain muscular fitness. Despite the traditional concern that strength training is potentially injurious to the developing musculoskeletal system of children and adolescents, research studies and clinical observations indicate that participation in strength-building activities can be safe, effective, and enjoyable for children and adolescents. Because muscular fitness is required for success in most sports, a growing number of young athletes now strength train in school-based programs and sports training centers.

Potential Benefits of Youth Strength Training

Well-designed youth strength training programs may offer observable health and fitness value to children and adolescents. In addition to increasing muscular strength, muscular power, and local muscular endurance, regular participation in a youth strength training program has the potential to positively influence aerobic fitness, body composition, bone mineral density, and selected psychological measures. Moreover, carefully planned youth strength training programs may enhance motor performance skills, such as jumping and sprinting, and improve sports performance.

Another important benefit of youth strength training is its ability to improve the preparedness of young athletes for the demands of sports practice and competition. A growing number of aspiring young athletes are ill-prepared for the demands of sports training due to their sedentary lifestyle. While factors such as growth, improper footwear, and hard playing surfaces have been implicated as risk factors for overuse injuries in young athletes, the background physical activity level of boys and girls must also be considered. A significant number of injuries sustained by youth while playing sports could be prevented if more emphasis was placed on enhancing musculoskeletal strength and improving skill-related fitness abilities such as agility, balance, and coordination prior to sports participation. Preseason conditioning programs that included strength training have resulted in decreased injury rates in adolescent athletes, and it seems likely that this type of conditioning could offer a similar protective effect in children.

Risks and Concerns

The belief that strength training is unsafe for young athletes is not consistent with the needs of children and adolescents and the documented risks associated with this type of training. While the unsupervised and improper use of strength training equipment may be injurious, there is no scientific evidence to suggest that the risks and concerns associated with supervised and sensibly progressed youth strength training programs are greater than those arising from other sports and recreational activities in which children and adolescents regularly participate.

A long-established concern associated with youth strength training involves the potential for injury to the epiphyseal plate or growth cartilage. Although young athletes are susceptible to epiphyseal plate fractures, this type of injury has not been reported in any prospective youth strength training study. Furthermore, strength training will not negatively affect growth or maturation during childhood and adolescence. It appears that the greatest concern for young athletes who strength train is the risk of overuse soft tissue injuries, particularly to the lower back.

To reduce the risk of injury, youth strength training programs must be well designed and supervised by qualified professionals who should be careful to match the strength training program to the needs, interests, and abilities of each child. This is particularly important for untrained youth, who often overestimate their physical abilities and

may not be aware of the inherent risks associated with strength training equipment. Special care is also needed when children and adolescents use exercise equipment at home, where they may be more likely to strength train without supervision or engage in unsafe behavior. Professionals must be aware of the inherent risk associated with strength training and should attempt to decrease this risk by following established training guidelines. Youth should not strength train on their own without guidance from qualified professionals.

Program Design Considerations

Although there is no minimum age for participating in a youth strength training program, children should have the emotional maturity to accept and follow directions and should appreciate the benefits and concerns associated with this mode of exercise. If a child is ready for participation in some type of sports activity (generally at age 7 or 8), then he or she may be ready to strength train. It is important that young athletes begin strength training at a level that is commensurate with their physical and cognitive abilities. Prescribing a program that exceeds a child's capabilities not only increases the risk of injury but may also undermine the enjoyment of the strength training experience. While the long-term goals of youth and adult strength training programs may be the same, the focus of youth programs should be on skill development and having fun.

A variety of strength training programs have been developed and recommended for children and adolescents. Various combination sets and repetitions and different types of equipment, including weight machines, free weights (barbells and dumbbells), medicine balls, elastic tubing, and body weight exercises, have proven to be safe and effective. Factors such as cost, proper fit, weight stack increments, and quality of instruction should be considered when evaluating strength training equipment for youth. Since most children are too small for adult-sized weight machines, child-size weight machines or other less expensive types of equipment can be used. If equipment is not available, a circuit of body weight exercises can be developed.

In general, it has been recommended that children and adolescents strength train 2 or 3 days per week on nonconsecutive days and perform one to three sets of 6 to 15 repetitions on 8 to 12 exercises that focus on the upper body, lower body, and midsection. It is reasonable to begin strength training with one or two sets of 10 to 15 repetitions with a light to moderate weight of basic exercises. As youths gain confidence in their abilities to perform these exercises with proper technique, heavier weights and more advanced multijoint movements can be incorporated into the strength training program. However, when learning any new exercise, youths must first learn how to perform each exercise correctly with a light weight and then gradually increase the training weight without compromising on exercise technique. This approach will not only allow for positive changes in muscle function but also provide an opportunity for participants to gain confidence in their abilities to perform strength exercise.

Over time, continual gains can be made by changing the exercise choice, exercise order, training weight, number of repetitions, number of sets, or training frequency. On average, a 5% to 10% increase in training weight is appropriate for most exercises. Since training-induced strength gains are impermanent and tend to regress toward the pretraining values once the training stops, program variation is needed to optimize training adaptations, reduce boredom, and promote exercise adherence. Planned variation in the strength training program can also help prevent training plateaus, which are not uncommon after the first 2 to 3 months of strength training.

Basic education on proper exercise technique, fitness training, and realistic outcomes should be part of all youth strength training programs. Professionals who work with youth need to listen to each child's concerns and monitor progress. Some youths with poor levels of fitness may not be able to tolerate the same amount of exercise as some of their peers in the same training program. This is where the art and science of developing a strength training program come into play, because the principles of training specificity and progressive overload need to be balanced with individual needs, goals, and abilities.

Youth strength training requires qualified supervision, appropriate overload, gradual progression, and adequate recovery between exercise sessions. When designing strength training programs for young athletes, the goal of the program should not be limited to increasing muscular fitness. Teaching youth about their bodies, promoting safe training procedures, and providing a stimulating program that gives participants a more positive attitude toward strength training and physical activity are equally important. Strength training should be recommended to young athletes as part of a total fitness program that should include a variety of physical activities and sports pursuits.

Avery Faigenbaum

See also Conditioning; Resistance Training; Young Athlete

Further Readings

Behm D, Faigenbaum A, Falk B, Klentrou P. Canadian Society for Exercise Physiology position paper: resistance training in children and adolescents. *J Appl Physiol Nutr Metab.* 2008;33(3):547–561.

Faigenbaum AD. Resistance training for children and adolescents: are there health outcomes? *Am J Lifestyle Med.* 2007;1:190–200.

Faigenbaum AD, Westcott WL. *Strength and Power for Young Athletes.* Champaign, IL: Human Kinetics; 2000.

Malina R. Weight training in youth-growth, maturation and safety: an evidenced-based review. *Clin J Sports Med.* 2006;16(6):478–487.

Vaughn J, Micheli, L. Strength training recommendations for the young athlete. *Phys Med Rehabil Clin N Am.* 2008;19(2):235–245.

Stress Fractures

Stress fractures are overuse injuries of bones. They are common in both competitive and recreational athletes who participate in repetitive activities such as running, jumping, marching, and skating. Stress fractures were first described as "march fractures" in military recruits who had recently increased their level of impact activities. These injuries are true overuse injuries that result from an accumulation of microdamage during exercise, exceeding the body's natural ability to repair this damage. This accumulation of microdamage can cause pain, weaken the bone, and lead to stress fracture. The majority (95%) of stress fractures occur in the lower extremity and most commonly involve the tibia, fibula, metatarsals, or navicular bone. Treatment of stress fractures depends on both the site and the severity of injury.

Etiology

During repetitive loading cycles, bones are exposed to mechanical stresses that can lead to microdamage or microscopic cracks. Fortunately, when given adequate time for recovery, the body has the ability to heal and further strengthen bones through remodeling and repair mechanisms. These healing mechanisms depend on many factors, including hormonal, nutritional, and genetic factors. Unfortunately, under certain conditions, such as starting a new training program or increasing the volume of a current program, the damage to bones is enough to overwhelm the body's ability to repair. In these circumstances, there can be an accumulation of cracks and inflammation that leaves the bones at risk of fatiguing and fracturing. This fatigue failure event is termed the stress fracture. The severity of the injury is determined by the location of the stress fracture and the extent to which the fracture propagates across the involved bone.

Diagnosis

History and physical examination are fundamental for the practitioner in making the diagnosis promptly. Patients typically present with an insidious onset of localized pain at or around the site of the injury. Initially, the pain from a stress fracture is only experienced during strenuous activities such as running and jumping. However, as the injury worsens, pain may be present during activities of daily living, such as walking or even sitting. Physical examination classically reveals a focal area of bony tenderness at the site of the fracture. Soreness in the surrounding joint and muscle is common, and in severe cases, palpable changes to the bone at the site of injury may be present.

Multiple modalities of imaging are routinely used in diagnosing stress fractures. Plain radiography (X-rays) is the most commonly used test to diagnose a stress fracture, but within the first few weeks of injury, X-rays often will not reveal the presence of the fracture. Bone scans, a nuclear-enhanced image modality, have classically been used in the evaluation of stress fracture and have proven to be very sensitive. In recent years, magnetic resonance imaging (MRI) has become the diagnostic test of choice for many physicians because of its superior availability, shorter exam time, earlier fracture detection, and image quality and because it can show damage to other structures such as muscles or ligaments, which conventional X-rays do not.

Classification

Stress fractures can be classified as high- or low-risk injuries based on their location. This classification allows a practitioner to quickly implement treatment for each stress fracture. Low-risk sites include the medial tibias (shin), femoral shafts (thigh), first four metatarsals (foot), and ribs. These locations tend to heal and have a lower likelihood of recurrence, progression to nonunion (not healing), or completion (worsening) of the fracture. Conversely, high-risk stress fracture sites have a higher complication rate and require prolonged recovery or surgery before the athlete can return to participation. Common high-risk sites include the femoral neck (hip), anterior tibia, medial malleolus (ankle), patella (kneecap), navicular (ankle), sesamoids (foot), and proximal fifth metatarsal.

Treatment

The treatment of stress fractures will vary with the location of the injury, severity of injury, and treatment goals. Low-risk stress fractures generally heal faster and with a lower incidence of poor outcomes than high-risk stress fractures. Depending on the particular injury, treatment may include discontinuation of the precipitating activity only, discontinuing all training activities, or, for more serious injuries, crutches or surgery. For minor injuries, healing may take as little as 3 to 6 weeks of avoiding the precipitating activity with continued cross-training followed by a gradual return to the pre-injury level of participation. More severe injuries often take 2 to 3 months or more of aggressive treatment. While treating the stress fracture, it is important to evaluate and modify risk factors that may predispose the athlete to future injuries, including anatomic abnormalities, biomechanical forces, hormonal imbalances, and nutritional deficiencies. Returning to play after a stress fracture usually is granted once the athlete is painfree with activities, is nontender to palpation, and, for high-risk sites, shows evidence of healing on imaging.

Jason Diehl

See also Femoral Neck Stress Fracture; Foot Stress Fracture; Groin Strain; Hip Stress Fracture; Olecranon Stress Injury; Pelvic Stress Fracture; Rib Stress Fracture; Spondylolysis and Spondylolisthesis; Stress Fractures; Tibia and Fibula Stress Fractures

Further Readings

Bennell KL, Malcolm SA, Wark JD, Brukner PD. Models for the pathogenesis of stress fractures in athletes. *Br J Sports Med.* 1996;30:200–204.

Boden BP, Osbahr DC. High-risk stress fractures: evaluation and treatment. *J Am Acad Orthop Surg.* 2000;8(6):344–353.

Boden BP, Osbahr DC, Jimenez C. Low-risk stress fractures. *Am J Sports Med.* 2001;29(1):100–111.

Brukner P, Bradshaw C, Bennell K. Managing common stress fractures: let risk level guide treatment. *Phys Sportsmed.* 1998;26(8):39–47.

Jones BH, Thacker SB, Gilchrist J, Kimsey CD, Sosin DM. Prevention of lower extremity stress fractures in athletes and soldiers: a systematic review. *Epidemiol Rev.* 2002;24(2):228–247.

STRETCHING AND WARMING UP

From time immemorial, stretching and warm-ups have been a part of athletic training and competition. These routines are purported to improve performance and to reduce injury and postexercise soreness. Perhaps surprisingly, although research supports the position that warming up is critical, the evidence is tenuous that stretching itself is beneficial. In fact, some stretching evidently predisposes to injury and reduces performance. A long-term program of stretching after exercise probably reduces injuries or postexercise soreness, but this is also controversial. Thus, there is a major shift occurring in the practice of stretching. This entry describes what, why, and how we should stretch and then reviews what role stretching should play in warm-ups.

What to Stretch

Stretching affects the ligaments that provide joint stability, the tendons that connect muscle to bone, and/or the muscle that produces power. Stretching has been discovered to induce changes in the nervous system as well. Ligament stretching is generally not desirable, as described below. Tendon stretching is difficult and of limited benefit. It is in the muscle that most stretching occurs.

Muscles have elastic properties, which means that if stretched, they will tend to return to their original length. They also have viscous and plastic properties, which means that if stretched for long enough (repeatedly for about 30 seconds), they tend to remain lengthened and only slowly return to their original length. The viscoelastic changes that occur with stretching have been considered the reason why the muscle lengthens. But some of the changes turn out to be the result of decreased pain thresholds or decreased muscle strength, which have as many detrimental effects as good ones.

Why Stretch?

The traditional reasons to stretch are to increase range of motion (ROM) around a joint, to increase flexibility of the muscle, and to warm up the body in preparation for intense exercise. We will deal with each of these putative attributes in turn.

Range of Motion

ROM is the arc through which a joint can move. Some sports such as gymnastics require large ROM. But simply increasing ROM around a joint is not necessarily useful. An increased range must be accompanied by sufficient muscle strength to protect the ligaments, tendons, and muscles from injury. This muscle strength is also necessary to allow use of the body in that new ROM, or it has little purpose. For instance, the ability of a backstroke swimmer to externally rotate the arm so that the hand is above and behind the head is only useful if the ROM is also accompanied by strength and power of the muscles to produce faster swimming. Much of the stretching we have traditionally done produces increased ROM by stretching the ligaments, which may already be too loose, and actually decreases the power of the muscles for a short time.

For example, a stretching exercise sometimes used by swimmers to increase shoulder external rotation is having a partner pull the arms back as far as possible. The anterior ligaments of the shoulder that limit this motion are rarely tight because most swimming motions stretch them daily. Stretching these ligaments may adversely affect joint stability. Tightness in the front of the shoulder arises when muscles such as the pectoralis get short. If we are to increase ROM, it must be done under control, preferably with the athlete's own muscles, so that strength and power increase in coordination with flexibility of all the related muscles.

Ligaments hold joints in precise positions throughout the ROM, and usually they are best left alone to do what they were marvelously designed to do. But occasionally they do need stretching. One example is the ligaments in the posterior part of the shoulder, which often *are* tight, but the muscles are long and weak. Here, it is important to stretch the ligaments but not the muscles. An exercise intended to stretch these tight posterior ligaments is where the upper arm is forced across the chest. But more often it actually only stretches the scapular stabilizer muscles, which may already be too long. An athletic trainer or physical therapist will need to ensure that the athlete does stretches very precisely to stretch the right thing without damaging something else.

Flexibility

Flexibility is the ability of a muscle to work over a full ROM—in a short length and a long one. What has been perhaps better appreciated in recent years is that flexibility cannot be created in an isolated muscle. A related property is stiffness, which is the amount of force needed to elongate a muscle. Stiffness is not necessarily bad, but muscle stiffness must be balanced. Often, it is a balance of the flexibility and stiffness of opposing muscles that needs to be corrected, not just a change of one muscle group. We have come to realize that there is such a thing as too much flexibility.

Using the above shoulder example, even if the pectoralis muscle is carefully stretched without damaging the ligaments (i.e., it becomes more flexible), this new elongated status may only last a few minutes. One common reason is that many athletes have a rounded shoulder posture from hours of computer keyboarding, which is what really caused the pectoralis to become short in the first place. Unless the long and weak posterior rotator cuff muscles and scapular stabilizers are corrected, it will be virtually impossible to maintain an elongated pectoralis. The longer-term solution is to stretch the pectoralis by stiffening (strengthening and shortening) the posterior muscles. When your mother told you to sit up straight with your shoulders back, this is what she was intuitively trying to accomplish.

Warm-Up

Studies have clearly shown that warming up muscles before exercise improves performance and prevents injuries. Stretching has been an important part of "warming up" for exercise, but the benefits of warming up have been inappropriately attributed to stretching. Research is showing that traditional stretching is not the best way to warm up. The actual temperature of the muscle is probably the most important factor, and so sitting in a hot tub is almost as effective; warming muscles with moderate dynamic activity is the best. Dynamic movements effectively prepare the muscles for powerful action throughout the needed ROM.

Therefore, we need to reassess how to stretch to get the benefits of a useful increase in balanced ROM, flexibility, and warm-up, without the potential drawbacks or wasted time.

How to Stretch

Stretching can be *static,* where an athlete assumes the stretching position using his or her own opposing muscles. Stretching can also be *passive,* where the force for achieving the stretching position is provided by a partner. In both cases, we seek to stretch to a point of mild discomfort in a muscle for about 30 seconds. While these actions do elongate the muscle, there is increasing evidence that they actually decrease power and speed, at least for several minutes. One study showed that the time for a 600-meter (m) run was improved by 2.4% if athletes had routinely done dynamic exercises, whereas it worsened by 2.5% in the athletes who had done a static stretching routine. Ballistic stretching, which involves swinging a body part to force the joint into an extreme ROM, overactivates some neurological reflexes and may increase the risk of muscle damage.

Dynamic stretching is the currently recommended technique. This involves dynamic movements as opposed to static positions and thus may not appear to be stretching in the former sense. Overload movements such as jumping with weights show even more promise. This activates the nervous system, while static stretching inhibits it. As mentioned above, ballistic stretching also activates the nervous system but probably in a deleterious way. Passive stretching usually stretches more ligaments than muscles and must be used very carefully, if at all.

To show how these various kinds of stretching might be used, let's see how we might approach tight hamstrings. An example of passive stretching would be to have the athlete sit with legs extended and have a partner push on that athlete's back. There is a danger that this will increase ROM, but by stretching back the ligaments, which increases predisposition to back pain, there is little improvement of tight hamstrings. An example of passive stretching would be to have the athlete sit in the same legs-extended position and hold his or her head on the knees. If done correctly, this will result in increased hamstring length but at the cost of short-term decreased strength and power of the hamstrings. Standing on one leg and swinging the other one to the limit of ROM would be ballistic stretching. This may cause tears, again without significantly increasing flexibility of the muscle. Dynamic stretching would involve active movements such as striding, lunging, or whole-body movements similar to the sport itself, all the while maintaining a stable lower back and pelvis. Tai chi, yoga, and pilates often include this type of movement. It is also the essence of "core" training that is critical to all musculoskeletal health.

Dynamic stretching results in a durable rebalancing of muscle strength, flexibility, and stiffness and does not damage the ligaments.

An example of how stretching is related to core strength is what one well-known physical therapist calls the "tail wagging the dog." Athletes with strong legs may produce undesired motions and pain in the back and pelvis, because the back and pelvis (core) are not strong enough to stabilize the leg motion. In this situation, the core muscles are less stiff (more flexible) than the leg muscles. The

long-term solution to stretch the "tight" leg muscles is to "stiffen" the core muscles. Doing such rebalancing with isolated stretching of the leg muscles is virtually impossible, while real-world movements of dynamic stretching done with proper form will create a practical balance of flexibility.

Conclusion

In summary, warming up before exercise continues to be very important, but stretching, at least passive or static stretching, has little to no function in a pre-exercise routine. It may have limited benefit after exercise, where at least it has little deleterious effect. Warming up should be done with moderate activity similar to the sport to be undertaken. Muscle flexibility and ROM are best improved with a careful long-term training program. Muscle strength and power, working from a strong core, are developed gradually over the needed ROM. This usually entails sportlike activities done with more attention to form than force.

Ronald P. Olson

See also Preventing Sports Injuries; Static Stretching; Strains, Muscle

Further Readings

Da Costa BR, Vieira ER. Stretching to reduce work-related musculoskeletal disorders: a systematic review. *J Rehabil Med.* 2008;40(5):321–328.

Herman SL, Smith DT. Four-week dynamic stretching warm-up intervention elicits longer term performance benefits. *J Strength Cond Res.* 2008;22(4):1286–1297.

Holt BW, Lambourne K. The impact of different warm-up protocols on vertical jump performance in male collegiate athletes. *J Strength Cond Res.* 2008;22(1):226–229.

Winchester JB, Nelson AG, Landin D, Young MA, Schexnayder IC. Static stretching impairs sprint performance in collegiate track field athletes. *J Strength Cond Res.* 2008;22(1):13–18.

Subarachnoid Hemorrhage

Subarachnoid hemorrhage occurs when there is bleeding into the space between the two innermost protective coverings surrounding the brain, the pia mater and the arachnoid mater. A subarachnoid hemorrhage most often occurs as the result of significant head trauma and is usually seen in the setting of skull fractures or injuries to the brain itself. In this setting, the presence of a subarachnoid hemorrhage has been linked to significantly worse outcomes, although it is unclear whether the presence of the blood in the subarachnoid space is directly responsible or whether it is just a marker for a very serious injury. In either case, a subarachnoid hemorrhage is typically symptomatic, with headache and an alteration of consciousness being common. Once identified, the subarachnoid hemorrhage requires immediate medical attention, and quick intervention is necessary to improve the chance of a positive outcome.

Anatomy

The brain is protected inside the skull by three separate layers of tissue (meninges). The innermost layer, the *pia mater*, is a thin and delicate membrane that lies on the surface of the brain. The second layer, the *arachnoid mater*, covers the brain and pia mater but does not follow the contour of the involutions of the brain. The outermost layer, the *dura mater*, provides a thicker and tougher layer of protection.

These layers define three potential spaces for blood to collect. The *epidural space*, between the skull and the dura; the *subdural space*, between the dura and the arachnoid layer; and the *subarachnoid space*, between the arachnoid and pia layers—each having their own potential sources of hemorrhage. The pia mater is too closely adhered to the brain and too fragile to act as a barrier for blood, and therefore, there is no potential space between the pia and the brain for a hemorrhage to form. A subarachnoid hemorrhage is simply defined as the presence of blood in the subarachnoid space.

Mechanism of Injury

The subarachnoid space is prone to blood collection whenever there is damage to any of the cerebral blood vessels that travel beneath the arachnoid layer, in close proximity to the surface of the brain. Subarachnoid hemorrhage can also occur when there is a substantial injury to the brain tissue itself.

In either case, this type of hemorrhage is most often the result of a significant mechanical force applied to the skull. Accompanying skull fractures are common, as are other types of bleeding such as epidural and intracerebral hematomas. This mechanism is relatively rare in sports, especially in those that require the use of a helmet, as long as the helmet is used properly. It is still possible in any sport, however, and more likely when there has been a significant force applied directly to the skull.

Subarachnoid hemorrhages can also occur spontaneously. In these cases, approximately 85% of the hemorrhages are the result of a ruptured cerebral aneurysm. Other causes of spontaneous subarachnoid hemorrhage include arteriovenous malformations, anticoagulation therapy such as coumadin, and the use of certain illicit drugs such as cocaine.

Risk Factors

In the case of the subarachnoid hemorrhage that is caused by an athletic injury, the baseline risk is primarily a function of the type of sport being played, the equipment being used, and the playing technique of the athlete. Additional risk, although hard to quantify, likely exists for athletes who have abnormal vascular anatomy, such as an aneurysm or arteriovenous malformation. Otherwise, the risk of developing a subarachnoid hemorrhage is defined by the nature of the injury and the severity of the impact. Certain sports that involve high velocities and little, if any, protective equipment, such as soccer and field hockey, may also pose additional risk.

In the case of most spontaneous subarachnoid hemorrhages, the risk is determined mainly by the size and location of any vascular abnormality. Although it can be difficult to accurately define the risk of any one aneurysm rupturing, a general rule is to take a conservative approach of repeat neuroimaging for any aneurysm 10 millimeters (mm) in diameter or less. The size and location of aneurysms larger than 10 mm should be carefully considered before undergoing a procedure designed to prevent rupture in the future.

Signs and Symptoms

When a subarachnoid hemorrhage is secondary to head trauma, there is typically a constellation of symptoms similar to that seen in all serious head injuries that includes confusion or loss of consciousness, memory loss, dizziness or unsteadiness, lack of coordination, nausea and/or vomiting, or sleepiness. If the patient is lucid enough to describe symptoms, he or she will typically describe an extremely severe headache. While the subarachnoid hemorrhage may not be directly responsible for neurological deficits such as numbness or weakness on one side of the body, these signs may be present as a result of concurrent injury to the brain.

In the setting of a spontaneous subarachnoid hemorrhage, the hallmark symptom is known as the "thunderclap headache." This headache occurs quite suddenly and is severe. It is often described by patients as feeling like somebody hit them on the head with a blunt object. The sudden nature and severity of this headache are distinct and should always warrant consideration of a subarachnoid hemorrhage as the cause.

Clinical Evaluation

With any athletic head injury, care should be taken on the field to first assess the "ABCs" (airway-breathing-circulation) and evaluate the possibility of cervical spine trauma, instituting cervical immobilization when appropriate. The level of consciousness should then be noted using the Glasgow Coma Scale. Any language, memory, or orientation abnormalities should also be noted. A physical examination should then be performed to evaluate for skull fracture or any focal neurologic abnormality, including pupillary, visual field, and funduscopic examinations, followed by a careful assessment of strength, sensation, reflexes, coordination, and gait. Any evidence of fracture or focal neurologic abnormality warrants activation of emergency medical services.

Following the on-field assessment, appropriate monitoring and serial examinations should be performed to document any changes in signs or symptoms. If the situation gets worse, the patient should be further evaluated in a hospital setting. Care should be taken to establish an accurate timeline of events, and the accurate documentation of findings will help clarify the athlete's postinjury course.

Diagnostic Tests

The presence of a subarachnoid hemorrhage is usually confirmed with a computed tomography (CT) scan of the head. Magnetic resonance imaging (MRI) of the brain can also be used. While MRI may provide more information regarding damage to the brain itself, it is more expensive, requires more time, and is not available at every medical facility. The initial diagnosis, therefore, is typically made with a CT scan. If the clinical suspicion is high enough but the CT of the head is normal, a lumbar puncture can be performed as an alternative method to establish the diagnosis. If a subarachnoid hemorrhage is present, the cerebrospinal fluid that is obtained via the spinal tap will almost always have evidence of blood or blood products. In the case of spontaneous subarachnoid hemorrhages, an intravenous, catheter-based procedure, a cerebral angiogram, is the most useful test for establishing the source of the bleed.

Management

Once the "ABCs" have been addressed, the patient is in the appropriate medical facility, and the patient is medically stable, the next step should be to establish the source of the hemorrhage. Further management depends on the identified cause. In the setting of sports trauma, the cause is likely known (a direct force to the skull). In these cases, there are likely concurrent injuries that need attention, such as a skull fracture. Neurosurgical consultation is required to determine the next steps in management, which could include a catheter-based procedure, surgery, or the placement of a device to monitor the pressure inside the skull. Blood in the subarachnoid space can cause the surrounding arteries to spasm, increasing the chances of further damage to the brain. Medicines can be used to help prevent this phenomenon, and further diagnostic tests can help monitor the cerebral vasculature.

Prevention

As with the prevention of other head injuries in athletics, proper technique, well-fitted and certified equipment, and adherence to the rules of play are paramount. The prevention of spontaneous subarachnoid hemorrhages is applicable only in very specific situations. If an athlete has two or more first-degree relatives (father, mother, siblings), some studies have shown that screening for aneurysms is warranted. If an aneurysm is identified, it may then be evaluated further for the possibility of performing a procedure to reduce the risk of rupture in the future. These decisions are best made carefully and after direct consultation with a vascular neurosurgeon.

Return to Sports

No athlete should return to participation in contact sports as long as he or she is still symptomatic from any head injury. In the case of a subarachnoid hemorrhage, the decision to return to sporting activity should be made very carefully and with the mechanism of the hemorrhage in mind.

Jeffrey S. Kutcher

See also Concussion; Epidural Hematoma; Head Injuries; Intracranial Hemorrhage; Neurologic Disorders Affecting Sports Participation; Subdural Hematoma

Further Readings

Durand P Jr, Adamson GJ. On-the-field management of athletic head injuries. *J Am Acad Orthop Surg.* 2004;12(3):191–195.

Ghiselli G, Schaadt G, McAllister DR. On-the-field evaluation of an athlete with a head or neck injury. *Clin Sports Med.* 2003;22(3):445–465.

Goetz C. *Textbook of Clinical Neurology.* 3rd ed. Philadelphia, PA: Saunders; 2007.

Marx JA, ed. *Rosen's Emergency Medicine: Concepts and Clinical Practice.* 6th ed. Philadelphia, PA: Mosby; 2006.

Subdural Hematoma

Subdural hematomas are a type of head injury that involves bleeding into the space between the brain and its outermost protective covering, the dura. They typically result when a traumatic force applied to the head creates significant fast-changing velocities of the contents inside the skull. The expanding hemorrhage can increase the pressure inside the skull and compress the underlying brain tissue. While subdural hematomas are relatively uncommon in sports, they are very serious injuries that can lead to significant disability or death. Early

recognition of the warning signs and quick medical attention are paramount to a good outcome.

Anatomy

The brain is protected inside the skull by three separate layers of tissue (meninges). The innermost layer, the *pia mater*, is a thin and delicate membrane that lies on the surface of the brain. The second layer, the *arachnoid mater*, covers the brain and pia mater but does not follow the contour of the involutions of the brain. The outermost layer, the *dura mater*, provides a thicker and tougher layer of protection.

These layers define three potential spaces for blood to collect. The *epidural space*, between the skull and the dura; the *subdural space*, between the dura and the arachnoid layer; and the *subarachnoid space*, between the arachnoid and pia layers— each with their own potential sources of hemorrhage. The pia mater is too closely adhered to the brain and too fragile to act as a barrier for blood, and therefore, there is no potential space between the pia and the brain for a hemorrhage to form.

Mechanism of Injury

A network of veins traverses the space between the surface of the brain and the dura. These veins, the *bridging veins,* can tear if the contents of the skull experience sudden changes in velocity. Blood leaking from the bridging veins then collects in the subdural space, creating a hematoma. The size of the hematoma and the speed with which it expands depend primarily on the number and size of the tears in the bridging veins. Given that the blood in the bridging veins is coming from the venous side of the circulatory system and is therefore under less pressure, subdural hematomas typically expand at a much lower rate than hematomas that are formed from arterial blood, such as epidural hematomas. The expanding subdural hematoma increases the intracranial pressure and can lead to damage of the underlying brain.

Subtypes

Subdural hematomas are often classified based on their acuity into *acute, subacute,* and *chronic* subtypes. Acute subdural hematomas are extremely dangerous and frequently lethal without quick surgical intervention. Symptoms develop quickly, and mortality rates are estimated between 60% and 80%. Subacute subdural hematomas become symptomatic over several hours to days and carry a better prognosis. Chronic subdural hematomas develop over days to several weeks and are common in elderly individuals. Frequently, they are only mildly symptomatic or without symptoms completely. In these cases, the bleeding is self-limited, and no surgery or acute intervention is required. In the athletic population, a subdural hematoma caused by a physical impact is more likely to present as an acute or subacute subtype.

Risk Factors

Any process that increases the distance that the bridging veins must travel to cross the subdural space increases the risk of tearing and, therefore, of hematoma formation. Brain atrophy is probably the biggest contributor of increased risk. Subdural hematomas, therefore, become more common as people age and the brain undergoes the natural process of age-related atrophy. Processes that increase brain atrophy, such as Alzheimer disease or chronic alcohol exposure, can increase the risk even further.

While brain atrophy increases the risk of developing a subdural hematoma, it also decreases the speed and severity of the related symptoms. This is due to the fact that brain atrophy provides more space for the hematoma to expand before it begins to increase intracranial pressure and interfere with brain function. Conversely, younger patients, without atrophy, will typically develop symptoms over a shorter period of time.

Signs and Symptoms

As mentioned above, the signs and symptoms of subdural hematoma typically have a slower onset than those seen in epidural hematomas. Depending on the particular subtype, symptoms can develop within the first 24 hours or may be delayed in onset by several days or weeks. The speed with which the majority of symptoms develop depends mainly on the degree of tearing of the bridging veins and the amount of space available for the hematoma to occupy before intracranial pressures begin to

increase. Headache, either constant or fluctuating, can certainly occur during any stage of the process. Other common signs or symptoms that may occur as the result of a subdural hematoma include, but are not limited to, the following:

- Loss of consciousness
- Numbness
- Decrease in consciousness
- Seizure
- Amnesia
- Lethargy
- Disorientation
- Slurred speech
- Blurry vision
- Dizziness
- Nausea or vomiting
- Weakness
- Balance difficulty
- Personality changes

It should be noted that the presenting signs and symptoms of subdural hematoma are similar to those of other head injuries, including concussion. Oftentimes, the main difference is in the time course of symptoms. If any athlete develops new symptoms several minutes after a witnessed impact or if there is any perceived clinical worsening, emergency medical services should be notified.

Clinical Evaluation

As with any athletic head injury, care should be taken on the field to first assess the "ABCs" (airway-breathing-circulation) and evaluate the possibility of cervical spine trauma, instituting cervical immobilization when appropriate. The level of consciousness should then be noted using the Glasgow Coma Scale. Any language, memory, or orientation abnormalities should also be noted. A physical examination should then be performed to evaluate for any focal neurologic abnormality, including pupillary, visual field, and funduscopic examinations, followed by a careful assessment of strength, sensation, reflexes, coordination, and gait. Any focal neurologic abnormality warrants activation of emergency medical services.

Following the on-field assessment, appropriate monitoring and serial examinations should be established to document any changes in signs or symptoms. If the situation gets worse, the patient should be further evaluated in a hospital setting. Care should be taken to establish an accurate timeline of events, and accurate documentation of findings will help clarify the athlete's postinjury course.

Diagnostic Tests

The presence of a subdural hematoma is usually confirmed with a computed tomography (CT) scan of the head. Magnetic resonance imaging (MRI) of the brain can also be used. While the MRI scan may provide more information regarding damage to the brain itself, it requires more time for image acquisition and is not available at every medical facility. The initial diagnosis, therefore, is typically made with a CT scan.

Management

The management of a patient with a subdural hematoma will depend greatly on the extent of the bleed, its location, and the overall clinical status. Small, asymptomatic subdural hematomas can be managed conservatively with serial CT scans of the head to assess for any interval change in hemorrhage size. Larger hemorrhages, or those that are producing a more significant clinical compromise, should be emergently evaluated for surgical decompression.

Prevention

As with other head injuries in athletics, proper technique, well-fitted and certified equipment, and adherence to the rules of play are paramount in preventing a subdural hematoma.

Return to Sports

No athlete should return to participation in contact sports as long as he or she is still symptomatic from any head injury. In the case of a subdural hematoma, if surgical intervention was required, contact sports should be avoided indefinitely. For smaller, less complicated hemorrhages, there are no clear return-to-play guidelines, but a conservative approach is encouraged.

Eric E. Adelman and Jeffrey S. Kutcher

See also Concussion; Epidural Hematoma; Head Injuries; Intracranial Hemorrhage; Neurologic Disorders Affecting Sports Participation; Subarachnoid Hemorrhage

Further Readings

Cantu RC. Head injuries in sport. *Br J Sports Med.* 1996;30(4):289–296.
Cooper PR. *Head Injury.* 4th ed. New York, NY: McGraw-Hill; 2000.
Durand P Jr, Adamson GJ. On-the-field management of athletic head injuries. *J Am Acad Orthop Surg.* 2004;12(3):191–195.
Ghiselli G, Schaadt G, McAllister DR. On-the-field evaluation of an athlete with a head or neck injury. *Clin Sports Med.* 2003;22(3):445–465.

Sudden Cardiac Death

Sudden cardiac death (SCD) in athletes has recently generated much discussion as well as some controversy in the field of sport and exercise medicine. The possibility that an athlete who epitomizes health and longevity could suddenly die in the midst of athletic competition or practice is highly unnerving and unsettling. It is difficult for all of us, health professionals and the lay public alike, to fathom this apparent paradox, often leading to increased scrutiny and attention when a tragic death does occur within a community and to question whether something more can or should be done to prevent this from occurring in the first place.

It is important to remember that sports activity itself is not lethal, but rather it may be the trigger for sudden cardiac arrest (SCA) in an athlete whose susceptibility is increased due to an underlying, silent cardiac condition. It is not unusual for the athlete to not have any symptoms, or perhaps not have recognized them, before the actual episode leading to SCA and death.

Causes

Fundamentally, the heart is a muscle, and its function is to contract and pump blood, carrying oxygen to the body. Unlike other muscles, the heart has an elaborate electrical conduction system that regulates or signals its own activity.

The most common cause of sudden cardiac death in the United States in those above 35 years of age is hypertrophic cardiomyopathy (HCM). In adults above 35 years of age, the number one cause of SCD is atherosclerotic coronary artery disease.

Hypertrophic Cardiomyopathy

In HCM, the heart is thickened abnormally, and usually asymmetrically, and is at risk for abnormal function. There is a genetic basis for this condition; however, the physical expression of the condition is variable. There are much fewer cases of diagnosed HCM than people with the genetic defect, which is believed to be about 1 in 500 people. It is not clear what other factors contribute to an athlete actually being diagnosed with HCM.

Diagnosing HCM, as with other cardiac conditions that cause SCD, starts with having a low threshold of suspicion for findings in the athlete's history, physical exam, and electrocardiogram (EKG; a tracing of the electrical activity of the heart). Listening to the heart with a stethoscope (cardiac auscultation), a certain type of heart murmur consistent with turbulent blood flow within the heart may be detected in an athlete with HCM. There are, however, a number of types of heart murmurs, and the presence of a murmur can be normal or benign. An echocardiogram may be obtained to help confirm the presence of HCM.

It is worth noting that there are normal physiologic adaptations of the heart in response to exercise. The condition of "athlete's heart" encompasses normal cardiac responses to exercise, including heart muscle hypertrophy and electrical changes as evidenced on an EKG. Because of the clinical overlap in findings between an athletic heart and one with HCM, the diagnosis of one versus the other can sometimes be challenging.

Coronary Atherosclerotic Disease

In adults above 35 years of age, coronary atherosclerotic disease (CAD) can lead to sudden death in exercising individuals. Over time, susceptible individuals will build up fatty plaque within the arteries, which causes significant narrowing. As exertion increases, as during exercise, the heart requires more oxygen; the narrowed artery can limit the amount of blood flow that can get to the heart. The oxygen demand can outpace the supply, causing heart muscle ischemia; this in turn can disrupt the electrical signal, throwing the heart into a lethal rhythm, as in ventricular fibrillation. The atherosclerotic plaques may also break off, especially during times of high demand or stress on the heart; the plaque can then limit or cut off blood flow distal to the blockage, causing heart muscle ischemia and tissue death. Diagnosis of CAD can be supported indirectly with a variety of cardiac stress tests and directly with invasive cardiac catheterization. Of note, changes of CAD have been found in people in their 20s and younger and so may contribute to some cases of SCD in this age-group as well.

Other Causes

Other, less common causes of SCD in young people include structural and electrical abnormalities such as, but not limited to, congenital anomalies of the coronary arteries, arrhythmogenic right ventricular dysplasia (ARVD), myocarditis, and conduction abnormalities such as long QT syndrome.

Congenital coronary artery anomalies are normal anatomic variants. In certain alternate locations, the coronary artery can pass between structures such as the back of the heart and aorta, which can in turn cause the compression of the artery and thereby limit flow, especially during exercise. The consequence is similar to what occurs in coronary artery disease in that the decreased flow leads to myocardial ischemia, heart muscle death, and fatal arrhythmia. Diagnosis is difficult, and this condition is typically diagnosed at the autopsy after an SCD event; a cardiac CT (computed tomography) angiogram or cardiac catheterization may be helpful if clinically suspected.

In ARVD, the heart muscle is affected, undergoing changes that replace the normal healthy cardiac muscle tissue in the right ventricle with abnormal, irregular, disorganized, nonfunctioning fibrofatty connective tissue. Fibrofatty tissue can be thought of as scar tissue except that unlike with typical scar tissue formation, there is no precipitating injury or damage to the muscle in patients with ARVD. Family history, and thus a genetic component, may be contributing factors. The mechanism that leads to SCD is likely the result of arrhythmia that occurs as the conduction system tries and fails to work properly in tissue that is abnormal and in disarray. An EKG may raise clinical suspicion, and further imaging with echocardiogram or possibly cardiac MRI may be indicated for confirmation.

Myocarditis is an acute illness that causes inflammation of the heart muscle as a result of infection with a virus or bacteria. The athlete may experience chest pain, palpitations, and shortness of breath, along with associated systemic signs of fever, myalgia, and fatigue. While there is considerable overlap in the symptoms of myocarditis with severe viral illness such as the "flu," a rapid pulse out of proportion to other features should alert the physician to this possibility. Consider holding the athlete from return to play for several months after the acute illness resolves as the heart muscle may continue to be at risk for a period of time during recovery.

Prolonged QT syndrome describes a certain electrical conduction abnormality within the heart that predisposes the athlete to SCD. There may be a family history of SCA or SCD, and there are at least six genetic variants that have been identified thus far. Diagnosis is confirmed by EKG. There is no cure per se for this, though the risk for SCD may be reduced with appropriate risk stratification and medical management.

Management

Acute

The mechanism by which most cardiac conditions are thought to cause sudden death during exercise pertains to structural changes in the heart that disrupt normal electrical conduction or rhythm. Typically, in SCD, the final lethal heart rhythm resulting in an irregular, chaotic rhythm is due to *ventricular fibrillation.*

Once ventricular fibrillation occurs, an electrical shock delivered by a defibrillator (e.g., an automated electronic defibrillator, or AED, which can be used by a lay person with little to no prior training) must be provided quickly; otherwise, this rhythm is usually fatal. The success of defibrillation declines rapidly by the minute once the heart is in ventricular fibrillation. If successful, the defibrillator shock will restore a normal electrical rhythm to the heart and restore normal blood flow through the body. At the very least, basic resuscitation efforts including calling for help and beginning CPR (cardiopulmonary resuscitation) with regular breaths and chest compressions should be initiated immediately for the fallen athlete with no detectable pulse.

Follow-Up

If an athlete is found to have any of these conditions, he or she may be disqualified from competing in most, but not necessarily all, sports for some period of time. Some conditions are amenable to medical management, including medications, activity modification, and possibly an implanted defibrillator. Treatment may depend on whether the athletes have previously had an event of SCA and survived, whether they have any symptoms related to their cardiac condition, or whether they have any close family members with the same condition who have had an SCA event. None of the medical interventions, however, guarantees the athlete a return to the same low level of risk for SCD that an athlete without any of these conditions has. All these heart conditions place the athlete at increased risk for SCD, and all these athletes need close medical follow-up and monitoring.

Regardless of management, careful consideration should still be given to the athlete's diagnosis, condition, and expected level of function and sports, and the risks and benefits of sports participation should be carefully weighed on an individual or a case-by-case basis.

Prevention

Though SCD is fortunately rare (annual incidence is 1 in 200,000), prevention of SCA and SCD events is the best and optimal approach. Many physicians currently rely on the sports preparticipation screening history and examination to help identify at-risk athletes. (For all 12 elements of the American Heart Association–recommended preparticipation cardiovascular screening steps in athletes, refer to the 2007 article by B. J. Maron et al., published in *Circulation.*) Some of the essential questions that should be asked at all preparticipation physicals include the following:

1. Have you ever passed out while exercising?

2. Have you ever had chest pain, palpitations (rapid or irregular heartbeats), or shortness of breath while exercising?

3. Has there been a sudden, possibly unexplained, death in an apparently healthy, otherwise young relative?

Utilization of the screening EKG in preventing SCA and SCD is currently controversial. The discussion on whether to perform screening EKGs for all athletes is complicated to say the least, and it is beyond the scope of this entry. Factors to consider in the controversy involving EKG screening are the accuracy of the EKGs, the potentially significant number of false-positives (i.e., normal hearts that would look abnormal on EKG), and the effectiveness and financial impact of large-scale mandatory EKG screening (as well as the impact of further testing and subspecialty consultations that the EKG screening would necessitate). This could be very burdensome to an already strained health care system, not to mention the individual athlete and his or her family having to undergo further mandated evaluation prior to participating in sports.

Eugene S. Hong and Laura Anderson

See also Athlete's Heart Syndrome; Cardiac Injuries (Commotio Cordis, Myocardial Contusion); Preparticipation Cardiovascular Screening; Pulmonary and Cardiac Infections in Athletes

Further Readings

36th Bethesda Conference: Eligibility recommendations for competitive athletes with cardiovascular abnormalities. *J Am Coll Cardiol.* 2005;45(8):1317–1375.

Basso C, Corrado D, Marcus FI, Nava A, Thiene G. Arrhythmogenic right ventricular cardiomyopathy. *Lancet.* 2009;373(9671):1289–1300.

Maron BJ. Sudden death in young athletes. *New Engl J Med.* 2003;349(11):1064–1075.

Maron BJ, Thompson PD, Ackerman MJ, et al. Recommendations and considerations related to preparticipation screening for cardiovascular abnormalities in competitive athletes: 2007 update. *Circulation.* 2007;115(2):1643–1655.

Pigozzi F, Rizzo M. Sudden death in competitive athletes. *Clin Sports Med.* 2008;27(1):153–181.

Seto CK. Preparticipation cardiovascular screening. *Clin Sports Med.* 2003;22(1):23–35.

The Physician and Sportsmedicine. *Preparticipation Physical Evaluation.* 3rd ed. New York, NY: McGraw-Hill Healthcare; 2005.

Sunburn

Sunburn is characterized by skin redness, swelling, tenderness, and blistering in response to sunlight exposure. Given the number of athletes who play outdoor sports, prevention of the negative short- and long-term health effects of sunburn is important.

Sunlight

Sunlight is divided into visible light, infrared radiation, and ultraviolet radiation (UVR). UVR is categorized further into UVA (320- to 400-nanometer [nm] wavelength), UVB (290–320 nm), and UVC (<290 nm) radiation. UVB radiation can lead to the acute skin changes seen in sunburn. It has the ability to directly damage DNA, causing genetic mutations and cancer. UVA radiation is associated with skin wrinkling and may also contribute to some skin cancers. UVC does not contribute to sunburns.

Environmental factors play a role in determining UVR exposure. The stratosphere contains ozone, which absorbs all UVC, high amounts of UVB, and a small amount of UVA radiation. Ozone concentrations vary with temperature, weather, altitude, and latitude. UVB radiation increases by 3% per degree of latitude, and UVR intensity has been found to increase by 4% for every 300 meters (m) of elevation. Midday sunlight passes through less of the atmosphere than at any other point in the day, leading to more UVR exposure during midday hours. Clouds, fog, and haze can decrease UVR by 10% to 90% but never fully block it out. Snow and sand can reflect up to 90% of UVR. Even under water, UVR can penetrate to a depth of 1 m.

Skin Changes

The *epidermis* forms the protective, outermost layer of the skin. The deepest layer of the epidermis is constantly repopulated by new keratinocytes (cells composed of keratin), which migrate superficially, replacing the older keratinocytes and turning over the entire epidermal layer in approximately 28 days. *Melanocytes* (cells that produce melanin) are located in the deepest layer of the epidermis. The melanin is stored in melanosomes, which can be transferred to the keratinocytes. Skin color is influenced by the number and size of melanosomes, the type of melanin they contain, and the rate at which melanin is broken down.

Sunburn occurs as the skin tries to protect itself by absorbing UVR. UVA radiation is partially absorbed by melanin, which produces a darkening of the skin as the melanin is transferred to the keratinocytes. The resulting tan appears immediately after exposure and lasts for a few hours but does not protect the skin against future damage from sun exposure. UVB radiation is responsible for the redness, swelling, tenderness, and blistering that appears 6 to 12 hours after exposure and peaks in effect around 24 hours. These changes are caused by the release of inflammatory mediators, leading to dilation of the blood vessels and increased vascular permeability. In response to the damage, melanocytes accelerate the production of melanin and its transfer to keratinocytes. This results in a darkening of the skin that appears 2 to 3 days after sunlight exposure, persists for days to weeks, and reduces the skin's sensitivity to UVR by two- to threefold.

Risk Factors

Athletes with more melanin, and darker skin, are at lower risk for sunburn, while fair-skinned athletes are more likely to sunburn. But UVR still penetrates the skin and causes damage in people with dark skin. People living at higher altitudes or locations with predominantly sunny climates have an increased risk due to more exposure to sunlight. Sweating has also been found to increase the photosensitivity of the skin and to increase the risk of sunburn.

Signs and Symptoms of Sunburn

Sunburn is characterized by skin that feels hot or warm to the touch along with the development of red or pink skin after exposure to even a brief period of sunlight or other source of UVR. There will likely be discomfort in the affected area and possibly swelling. Fluid-filled blisters may develop on the skin. Headache, fever, and fatigue may also go along with sunburn. Sunburned eyes have a gritty, painful feeling. A few days after sunburn appears, the skin will begin to become flaky and peel.

Most sunburns do not require assessment by a medical provider. However, the following findings with sunburn require evaluation:

- High fever, intense pain, vomiting, diarrhea, or confusion
- Blistering that covers a large part of the body
- Signs of a skin infection (drainage of yellow pus from the area or increased pain or swelling in an affected area)
- Pain that is not adequately controlled with home treatments

Long-Term Complications

Skin photoaging, actinic keratoses (rough, scaly patches of skin), and skin cancer are some of the long-term effects of sun exposure. Over time, sun exposure causes the connective tissues of the skin to weaken, leading to dryer, rougher skin with deep wrinkling. Large brown macules, called solar lentigines (liver spots), can appear on sun-exposed areas. Actinic keratoses are usually white, pink, flesh-colored, or brown patches that commonly develop on the face, ears, lower arms, and backs of the hands. Actinic keratoses occur mainly in fair-skinned individuals who have had a large amount of sun exposure. They are considered precancerous, and they can develop into squamous cell skin cancer. Exposure to UVR, especially UVB radiation, is thought to be the main determinant in the development of basal and squamous cell skin cancers and is also thought to play a role in the development of cutaneous malignant melanoma. An increased prevalence of either precancerous or cancerous skin lesions has been found in professional mountaineers, surfers, marathon runners, and other athletes who practice outdoors.

Prevention

Avoidance of the sun's rays when they are the strongest, generally between 10 a.m. and 4 p.m., is the best recommendation to avoid sunburn. As this is not always possible, protection in the form of clothing, sunglasses, hats, and sunscreen should be used. The sun protection factor (SPF) is a ratio used to indicate the amount of protection against UVB radiation afforded by a given skin protectant compared with unprotected, sun-exposed skin. An SPF of 15 indicates that a person who normally has skin redness after 10 minutes of sun exposure could go in the sun with sunscreen for up to 150 minutes without experiencing the same skin effect.

There are many different agents used in sunscreens. These chemicals protect the skin by both reflecting and dispersing UVR (zinc oxide, titanium dioxide) or absorbing UVR (benzophenones, cinnamates, salicylates, and numerous other compounds). All types of sunscreen should be applied 30 minutes prior to sun exposure and reapplied at least every 2 hours for best protection. Clothing is also an important part of skin protection. Clothes that are tightly woven, loose fitting, dry, unbleached, and made of thicker fabrics increase the UVR protection. Light-colored, cotton, wet, or loosely woven fabrics all offer lower levels of protection. It is also important to wear a broad-brimmed hat and sunglasses that fit close to the face and block out UVR.

Treatment

Once sunburn occurs, skin damage is already present. Treatments are targeted toward symptom relief but do not decrease any of the long-term risks associated with sunlight exposure. It is very important to rule out heat illness in an athlete with acute sunburn. Cool compresses or baths can provide immediate relief. Skin-moisturizing creams, aloe vera lotion, and other over-the-counter emollients containing combinations of menthol, camphor,

pramoxine, calamine, or lidocaine can be used to keep the sunburned skin moist and ease some of the tenderness. Oral pain medication such as ibuprofen or other nonsteroidal anti-inflammatory drugs (NSAIDs) have been found to be most beneficial if taken immediately after the signs of sunburn begin to appear. Oral and topical corticosteroids have been found to have minimal impact on sunburn. If blistering appears, it is best to leave the blisters intact to decrease the risk of skin infection. Eventually, the skin will begin to peel as the body removes the damaged cells from its top layers. Moisturizing creams are recommended during this process.

Ryan N. Hatchell and Kevin D. Walter

See also Cholinergic Urticaria; Dermatology in Sports; Head Injuries; Heat Illness; Skin Disorders Affecting Sports Participation; Sunburn and Skin Cancers

Further Readings

American Academy of Pediatrics Committee on Environmental Health. Ultraviolet light: a hazard to children. *Pediatrics.* 1999;104(2):328–333.
Han A, Maibach HI. Management of acute sunburn. *Am J Clin Dermatol.* 2004;5(1):39–47.
Lautenschlager S, Wulf HC, Pittelkow MR. Photoprotection. *Lancet.* 2007;370(9586):528–537.
Meurer LN, Jamieson B, Thurman C. Clinical inquiries. What is the appropriate use of sunscreen for infants and children? *J Fam Pract.* 2006;55(5):437, 440, 444.
Morelli JG. Photosensitivity. In: Kliegman RM, Behrman RE, Jenson HB, Stanton BF, eds. *Nelson Textbook of Pediatrics.* Philadelphia, PA: Saunders; 2007: 2697–2702.

SUNBURN AND SKIN CANCERS

The incidence of skin cancer has been increasing in the general population for the past several years, and the amount of sun exposure remains the most important risk factor. Athletes should be taught basic prevention measures, such as avoiding sunburn by using sunscreen and protective clothing as well as avoiding sun exposure during peak ultraviolet B (UVB) hours. Sunburn is the painful, erythematous reaction of the skin in response to excessive sun exposure that often afflicts athletes who spend many hours training outdoors. In the United States, 30% to 40% of adults and 70% to 85% of children and adolescents have reported at least one occurrence of sunburn in the previous year. Sunburns not only cause acute discomfort after sun exposure but may ultimately lead to skin cancer.

Anatomy

The skin is the body's largest organ, covering the entire outside of the body and weighing about 6 pounds (lb; 1 lb = 0.45 kilogram). In addition to serving as a protective shield against infection, the skin also regulates body temperature and stores water, fat, and vitamin D. The skin is made up of three layers, each of which has a specific function: (1) the *epidermis*, which provides a barrier to infection; (2) the *dermis*, which is made of connective tissue that cushions the body from stress and strain; and (3) the *hypodermis* layer, which is mainly for fat storage.

Causes

Sunburn is a burn on the skin caused by UV radiation. The damaging effects of UV radiation can occur after as few as 15 minutes of sun exposure for light-skinned persons. The symptoms of sunburn do not begin until 2 to 4 hours after the damage has occurred. Minor sunburn is a first-degree burn that turns the skin pink or red. Prolonged sun exposure can cause blistering and is described as a second-degree burn. Sunburn never causes a third-degree burn or scarring.

Frequent sun exposure and suntans can also cause premature aging of the skin (wrinkling, sagging, and brown sunspots). Also, repeated sunburns increase the risk of skin cancer in the damaged areas. Each episode of blistering sunburn doubles the risk of developing *malignant melanoma,* which is the most serious type of skin cancer.

Symptoms

Mild and uncomplicated cases of sunburn usually result in minor skin redness and irritation. Initially, the skin turns red between 2 to 4 hours after exposure and feels irritated. The peak effects are noted at 12 to 24 hours. Other common symptoms of sunburn involve flulike symptoms, including fever, chills, nausea, and vomiting. More severe cases have complications such as severe skin burning and blistering, massive fluid loss, electrolyte imbalance, and infection.

Symptoms of skin cancer may vary from a melanocytic lesion that is completely asymptomatic to a painful bleeding erosion characteristic of squamous cell carcinoma. Routine skin evaluation by a medical provider has been recommended, because most skin cancers are asymptomatic and are found on routine screening examinations.

Diagnosis

Diagnosis of sunburn is usually not difficult and could be made based on symptomatology and a recent history of sun exposure. The appearance of a characteristic reaction on sun-exposed skin with sparing of skin that was covered or shaded is usually sufficient to diagnose sunburn.

The first step in detecting skin cancer begins with each individual. It is recommended that each person examine his or her skin once a month for any suspicious changes, such as moles that have changed in color, size, and/or surface texture. Also, sores that do not heal may also indicate cancerous or precancerous conditions of the skin that need attention.

Actinic keratoses are precancerous conditions that typically occur in individuals with a long history of sun-damaged skin. Lesions appear as rough, crusty bumps on the back of the hands, lips, face, scalp, or neck that may itch or feel tender. If untreated, these bumps may develop into skin cancer.

Basal cell carcinomas show up as flat, firm, pale areas or as small raised pink or red pearly bumps that may appear anywhere on the body that is regularly exposed to the sun, such as the head and neck. They grow slowly and rarely spread to other parts of the body.

Squamous cell carcinomas appear as nodules or as red, scaly patches, typically on the ear, face, lips, and mouth. These patches eventually develop into large masses. This type of skin cancer is more likely to spread to other parts of the body than basal cell carcinoma. Squamous cell carcinomas are highly treatable, with a 95% cure rate.

Melanoma can develop from a preexisting mole or on clear, smooth skin. Unlike a noncancerous mole, melanoma is irregularly shaped or has irregular borders and is black, brown, or tan. The leg is the most common site where melanoma is found in women, and the trunk is the most common site in men. Early diagnosis is the most important factor to improve the prognosis in this potentially fatal disease.

Treatment

A number of treatments aimed at altering the course of sunburn have been prescribed, but none will immediately reverse the damage from sunburn. These treatments include nonsteroidal anti-inflammatory drugs (both topical and oral), cold compresses, aloe vera gel, and topical anesthetics such as benzocaine. Currently, treatment of sunburn is only symptomatic, and athletes should avoid further sun exposure until the symptoms resolve.

There are many treatments for skin cancer, which vary depending on the type of skin lesion. Cryotherapy is commonly used on actinic keratosis. This treatment includes applying liquid nitrogen to the lesion for 3 to 5 seconds, which causes the lesion to slough off within a few days. Another common method for treating all other skin cancers is surgical excision of the affected area of skin. The physician cuts out or excises the cancerous tissue and a surrounding margin of healthy skin. A wide excision of skin is often used to ensure that no malignant cells remain.

Laser therapy may be used to produce a precise, intense beam of light to vaporize growths. Generally, this will cause little damage to the surrounding tissue and minimal bleeding, swelling, and scarring. Mohs surgery is a procedure for large, recurring, or difficult-to-treat skin cancers, which may include both basal and squamous cell carcinomas. The surgeon removes the skin growth layer by layer, examining each layer under the microscope until no abnormal cells remain. This procedure allows cancerous cells to be removed while leaving as much surrounding healthy skin as possible.

Curettage and electrodesiccation are a procedure in which, after removing most of the growth, the doctor scrapes away layers of cancer cells using a circular blade called a *curet*. An electric needle destroys any remaining cancer cells. This procedure is common in treating small or thin basal cell cancers and leaves only a small, flat, white scar.

Radiation therapy may be used to destroy basal and squamous cell carcinomas if surgery is not an option. Systemic chemotherapy can be used to treat skin cancers that have spread to other parts of the body. Photodynamic therapy (PDT) is a treatment that destroys skin cancer cells with a combination of laser light and drugs that makes cancer cells sensitive to light. Photodynamic therapy for precancerous skin lesions is currently available by prescription.

Prevention

Limiting sun exposure is the most important part of preventing sunburn; when avoiding exposure is not possible, proper use of sunscreen and protective clothing is vital. Routine self-examination followed by regular skin checks by your health care provider is the best way to detect any skin abnormalities that could be diagnosed as skin cancer. The American Academy of Dermatology has developed an easy-to-use method to evaluate your skin for melanoma, titled the "ABCDs of melanoma." Look for the following:

Asymmetry: One half of the spot is not shaped like the other half.

Border irregularity: The border is poorly defined, ragged, blurred, notched, or "scalloped."

Color: Across the mole, there are various shades of tan, brown, black, and sometimes red, white, and blue.

Diameter: The mole is greater than 6 millimeters.

Blake R. Boggess and Cameron Howes

Further Readings

Gloster HM, Brodland DG. The epidemiology of skin cancer. *Dermatol Surg.* 1996;22(3):217–226.
Habif TP. *Clinical Dermatology: A Color Guide to Diagnosis and Therapy.* 3rd ed. St Louis, MO: Mosby; 1996:714–715.
Katsambas A, Nicolaidou E. Cutaneous malignant melanoma and sun exposure. Recent developments in epidemiology. *Arch Dermatol.* 1996;132(4):444–450.

Kopf AW, Salopek TG, Slade J, Marghoob AA, Bart RS. Techniques of cutaneous examination of the skin. *Cancer.* 1995;75(2):684–690.

Marks R. The epidemiology of non-melanoma skin cancer: who, why and what can we do about it. *J Dermatol.*1995;22(11):853–857.

Marks R. An overview of skin cancers. Incidence and causation. *Cancer.* 1995;75(2):607–612.

Tucker MA, Halpern A, Holly EA, et al. Clinically recognized dysplastic nevi. A central risk factor for cutaneous melanoma. *JAMA.* 1997;277(18): 1439–1444.

Whited JD, Grichnik JM. The rational clinical examination. Does this patient have a mole or a melanoma? *JAMA.* 1998;279(9):696–701.

SUPERFICIAL HEAT

Application of superficial heat is an adjunct to a therapeutic treatment program in the rehabilitation of an injury. Superficial heat is a modality that provides pain control, promotes muscle relaxation, and increases blood flow to the area. Types of superficial heat include fluidotherapy, hot packs, and paraffin. Indications for use are joint stiffness, muscle spasm, pain, and weakness. The normal responses to application of superficial heat are decreased pain, swelling, and muscle spasm; an increase in circulation; and mild redness of the skin. The abnormal responses to superficial heat are increased pain, fainting, bleeding, and prolonged skin redness and/or blistering.

Fluidotherapy

Fluidotherapy is a modality that uses air-fluidized solids called Cellex (particles made from corn cobs), which are placed into a container. Heated air is then blown into the enclosure, causing the Cellex to circulate. An arm or leg can be inserted into the container, and the warmed, moving Cellex flows around the injured arm or leg. Fluidotherapy provides localized heat while the patient completes active or passive range-of-motion exercises.

Contraindications include respiratory distress, skin disorder, corn allergy, circulatory obstruction, arterial occlusion, blood clots, lymph occlusion, acquired immune deficiency syndrome (AIDS), poor sensation, hepatitis, chicken pox, typhoid, paratyphoid, sepsis, and/or other infectious diseases.

Precautions should be taken in the case of an open wound or poor mental status.

Hot Packs

Hot packs provide superficial moist heat via conduction. They are applied to the injured area for 15 to 20 minutes. Hot packs are usually made of canvas covers filled with bentonite, hydrophilic silicate, and other heat-retaining substances. Some hot packs are stored in water with a controlled temperature of approximately 160 °F (71.1 °C). Contraindications include fever, acute inflammatory conditions, active bleeding, long-term steroid therapy, blood clots, and malignancy. Precautions are necessary in case of pregnancy, sensory or circulatory impairments, older age, and the inability to stay still for 15 to 20 minutes. A thick protective barrier must be placed between the hot pack and the skin to avoid burning.

Paraffin

Paraffin application is a method of applying superficial heat that uses conduction through a mixture of paraffin wax and mineral oil in a 6:1 or 7:1 ratio. The heating container should maintain the temperature of the paraffin at 118 to 130 °F (47–54.4 °C).

Contraindications include open wounds, skin lesions, fever, acute inflammatory conditions, active bleeding, long-term steroid therapy, and blood clots. Precautions should be taken in case of poor mental status, age, sensory loss, and newly healed skin.

Rachel K. Tombeno, Kathleen Richards, and Michelina Cassella

See also Cryotherapy; Electrotherapy; Hydrotherapy and Aquatic Therapy; Principles of Rehabilitation/Physical Therapy

Further Readings

Cameron MH. Thermal agents: physical principles, cold and superficial heat. In: *Physical Agents in Rehabilitation: From Research to Practice.* Philadelphia, PA: Saunders; 1999:125–173.

Michlovitz SL. Biophysical principles of heating and superficial heat agents. In: *Thermal Agents in Rehabilitation*. Philadelphia, PA: FA Davis; 1990: 88–106.

Starkey C. *Therapeutic Modalities for Athletic Trainers.* Philadelphia, PA: FA Davis; 1993.

SUPERIOR LABRUM FROM ANTERIOR TO POSTERIOR (SLAP) LESIONS

A *SLAP* (superior labrum from anterior to posterior) *lesion* is a tear in the superior part of the shoulder joint lining (glenoid labrum) in an anterior-posterior direction. Typical causes of this tear include, but are not limited to, the following:

1. Sports: particularly activities that induce compressive forces on the shoulder, such as baseball, volleyball, and tennis

2. Overuse: doing too much at one time (e.g., overhead activity) coupled with severe tension on the biceps muscle tendon

3. A sudden increase in activity, such as lifting a very heavy barbell

4. A fall onto an outstretched arm.

5. An imbalance between the muscles and ligaments that provide stability to the shoulder joint

To understand the mechanism of the injury, a basic understanding of the anatomy of the involved structures is necessary.

Basic Anatomy

The shoulder is a ball-and-socket joint; the glenoid fossa (cavity) of the scapula (shoulder blade) is the socket and is composed of bone at the base and lined with cartilage. It is surrounded with additional lining at the circular rim by the *glenoid labrum* (from the Latin meaning "upper lip"), which is composed of cartilage, providing a cushion. It also makes the socket deeper and provides more stability to the joint, permitting easier

movement with minimal friction. The ball of the joint is the proximal part of the humerus (upper arm bone) that is embedded in the glenoid fossa and surrounded by the glenoid labrum.

Several muscles and ligaments help with movement by initiating, maintaining, and balancing the forces that enable the ball to remain in the joint. The major muscles involved include the deltoid, biceps, and supraspinatus. The glenohumeral ligaments attach to the lesser tubercle of the humerus and the lateral part of the scapula. The semicircular ligament runs side to side, which is very important for stability. Synchronous motion of the ligaments and muscles provides stability and strength to the shoulder. Major motions include abduction (motion away from the body), adduction (motion toward the body), and internal and external rotation.

The main muscles are as follows:

- The *deltoid muscle* covers the shoulder joint and provides a smooth contour of the shoulder. It acts as abductor of the arm and is innervated by the axillary nerve. Any injury to this nerve will affect this function of the deltoid muscle. It originates from the humerus and inserts into the shoulder joint, covering the joint from three surfaces.
- The *biceps muscle* acts to flex and supinate (turn up) the arm. It originates at the elbow and inserts into the glenoid labrum superiorly by its tendon (a band of dense fibrous tissue that unites muscle to bone). The muscle is innervated by musculocutaneous nerve.

The word *tendon* comes from the Latin word meaning "to stretch." The tendon transmits force when the muscles contract. Ligaments are similar, but they originate in bone and insert to bone.

Injuries can occur in a variety of ways—if a patient tries to lift a heavy weight, a lot of force will be exerted on the tendon and its area of insertion (in this case, the glenoid labrum). Two possible injuries could occur. The tendon could get inflamed and begin to tear from the area of insertion or, in the worst case, avulse (snap off), possibly taking a part of the glenoid labrum (cartilage) as well, causing a SLAP tear.

The supraspinatus is part of the rotator cuff muscles, which also include the infraspinatus, teres minor, and subscapularis. The supraspinatus originates at the scapula, or wing bone, passing under the acromion and inserting into the ball of the humerus, and is innervated by the suprascapular nerve. It causes abduction of the arms and is the most commonly injured among the rotator cuff muscles, especially with eccentric repetitive load applied to the muscle.

The infraspinatus originates at the shoulder blade and inserts at the humeral head, which is encapsulated under the coracoacromial arch. It laterally rotates the arm and is innervated by the suprascapular nerve.

Because the muscle tendons pass through a very narrow area, they are very susceptible to injuries. In addition, any buildup of calcification (bone spurs) may also cause problems.

The shoulder has two sets of muscles and ligaments, both with differing functions. Some hold the joint in place, whereas the others permit free motion of the shoulder and upper arm in all directions with ease and without any limitation.

Many factors come into play to ensure good shoulder movement.

The mechanism of injury is not fully understood; however, one scenario is that a sudden contraction of the biceps muscle causes stress on the tendon that is attached to the labrum, and to prevent dislocation of the shoulder, the labrum will tear.

As an example, throwing a ball in a sport such as baseball can cause shoulder injury. The technique of throwing has six phases, each of which can induce certain stresses on the shoulder. In the SLAP tear injury, the late cocking and deceleration phases are the primary contributors of injury in baseball players.

Phase 1: Wind-up is the phase during which there is minimal stress to the shoulder.

Phase 2: Early cocking is a slight-load phase, where the shoulder moves into abduction (away from the center of the body).

Phase 3: Late cocking begins with the stride leg being planted and ends with the shoulder in maximum external rotation, up to 180°. Muscle activity reaches its maximal stress in this phase.

Phase 4: Acceleration rotates the shoulder to the ball release point of 90° rotation, maintaining shoulder abduction.

Phase 5: Deceleration is the most harmful phase of the throwing cycle, where maximal eccentric contractions occur in several muscles to prevent rotation of the arm.

Phase 6: The follow-through is the phase where the body is rebalancing, and the body moves forward until the motion stops and returns to resting levels.

The entire throwing motion, through all six phases, will take less than 2 seconds.

Diagnosis

The patient's history is the key to the diagnosis, and a typical patient may present with complaints that include the following:

- General weakness
- Anterior-lateral sharp pain that gets worse with lifting items
- A perception of the shoulder being unstable
- Diminished arm range of motion
- Feeling as if the joint needs lubrication, due to the consciousness of internal friction
- An increase in pain when trying to do activities that require the arm to be up and behind
- A history of overuse and repetitive activities
- Trauma such as falling on an outstretched arm, which may force the biceps and other shoulder muscles to contract or stretch in unsynchronized actions that may cause a tear

The patient may often be an athlete, especially one involved in sports that require contraction of the biceps, such as swimming, racquetball, football, and so on.

Diagnosis of a SLAP Lesion

Physical Exam

The patient's history is the primary key to the diagnosis, along with the physical exam. The physical exam should include the following:

- Observe the patient for any swelling, deformity, or color changes.

- Evaluate active range of motion: The patient moves his or her shoulder and arms in all directions without assistance from the examiner.
- Evaluate passive range of motion: The examiner moves the shoulder and arms in all directions without the patient's help.
- Evaluate for isometric resistance and muscle strength of the shoulder joint: The patient moves the shoulder or the arm while the examiner tries to prevent the movement by applying force.
- Palpate the joint of the patient for tenderness.
- Evaluate the shoulder and upper arm for sensory deficit.
- Evaluate the blood flow by palpating the pulse at the biceps area.
- Evaluate for osteopathic somatic dysfunction, incorporating manual medicine to evaluate the joint for any restrictions of movement.
- Incorporate special tests that primarily stress the shoulder joint, muscles, and tendons:
  - *Speed test:* The patient flexes the forearm against resistance from the examiner. Pain will increase at the area where the biceps tendon passes to the joint.
  - *Yergason test:* The patient flexes the forearm toward the body while the examiner resists, leading to an increase in pain.

Radiologic studies are not always helpful as an X-ray will not help establish a diagnosis.

For a clinically suspected tear, the orthopedic surgeon can obtain an arthrogram by injecting dye into the joint and obtaining an X-ray to make the lesion more visible. Arthroscopy may also be done, which involves using a small fiber-optic camera to evaluate the lesion.

There is no single physical exam test to diagnose a SLAP lesion. The aforementioned special tests aid, along with the patient's history, in establishing the diagnosis.

Nonsurgical Interventions

Some nonsurgical interventions are listed below:

- The patient has to decrease those activities that cause the symptoms.
- Anti-inflammatory medication as tolerated is administered.

- Physical therapy to regain range of motion is advised.
- Surgical repair is suggested if all the above fail.

Surgical Intervention

Based on the extent of the injury, the surgeon will either reattach or possibly trim the excess tissue.

Postsurgical Intervention

Ensure that physical therapy (shoulder rehabilitation exercises) is initiated as soon as possible, based on the type of injury sustained. Typically, patients need to rest for a month and then increase activities as tolerated.

In summary, this lesion is not very common, but once it occurs, it can be very debilitating, affecting activities of daily living and participation in sports. Prevention is the key. The athlete is advised to start slowly and increase the activity level gradually as tolerated. At the first sign of the symptoms discussed, a visit to the physician is recommended.

Athletes with this shoulder injury should refrain from participation in sports pending clearance from their physician to prevent further damage to the shoulder.

George Kolo

See also Musculoskeletal Tests, Shoulder; Shoulder Injuries; Shoulder Injuries, Surgery for

Further Readings

Bergert N, Harmon B, Yocum L. Shoulder injuries. In: Starkey C, Johnson G, eds. *Athletic Training and Sports Medicine.* Sudbury, MA: Jones & Bartlett; 2006:267–336.

Karageanes SJ. The shoulder. In: *Principles of Manual Sports Medicine.* Philadelphia, PA: Lippincott Williams & Wilkins; 2005:159–200.

Kinderknecht JJ. Shoulder pain. In: Puffer JC, ed. *Twenty Common Problems in Sports Medicine.* New York, NY: McGraw-Hill; 2002:3–28.

Petron DJ, Khan U. The shoulder and upper extremity. In: McKeag DB, Moeller JL, eds. *ACSM's Primary Care Sports Medicine.* 2nd ed. Philadelphia, PA: Lippincott Williams & Wilkins; 2007:359–386.

Scuderi GR, McCann PD. *Sports Medicine: A Comprehensive Approach.* 2nd ed. St Louis, MO: Mosby; 2004: Chapter 18.

SURFING, INJURIES IN

Surfboard riding (surfing) is a sport practiced in coastal areas around the world. For the purposes of this entry, surfing will describe the sport whereby the participant engages waves in the water while standing on a surfboard. This is in contradistinction to many other wave and board sports, ranging from bodysurfing to boogie boarding to kite boarding and other activities.

Surfing is a sport that is practiced in increasing numbers: It is estimated that 1.7 million people in the United States and more than 18 million people worldwide participate in this sport.

Overview of the Sport

The sport began centuries ago in the South Pacific. Westerners first encountered surfing in the 18th century when exploring the Pacific islands. In Hawaii, for instance, it was considered the sport of the royalty. It is reported that missionaries actively suppressed the practice in the European settlements, and the sport continued to decline until the 20th century.

The resurgence of the sport in the 20th century began with Duke Kahanamoku, a Hawaiian Olympic swimmer who performed surfing exhibitions in America and Australia. In the mid 20th century, a nexus of factors contributed to the rise in the popularity of surfing: Advances in surfboard design allowed for mass production of lighter-weight boards using materials such as balsa wood, foam, and fiberglass, and cultural changes, including increased emigration to the warm coastal zones and the rise of a "beach culture," saw markedly increased numbers of people take up the sport. By the turn of the millennia, surfing had grown into a worldwide participatory sport and a big business: 195 million surfboards were sold worldwide in 1995.

Surfing is primarily a recreational sport, though worldwide there are increasing numbers of competitions and attempts at forming surfing associations.

The Association of Surfing Professionals (ASP) organizes regular competitions at the professional level. On the local level, there are an ever-increasing number of amateur and school-based competitions. There are contests also that center on "big-wave" riding, with its inherently higher risk of injury; "Mavericks" in Northern California is perhaps the most famous.

The vast majority of participants, however, will mostly take to the water to have fun and will be under no formal regulations or requirements. On some level, all that is needed to participate in the sport is a board and access to waves. Surfers can be of all ages and both genders, though many authors have noted a preponderance of male surfers: In many studies, the ratio of male to female surfers is on the order of 9:1. This too, as in many sports, appears to be changing, and increasing numbers of women are taking up the sport.

A final note should be made about the distinct difference between *longboards* and *shortboards,* which represent the two principal types of boards a surfer might use. Each uses a slightly different style. Longboards are typically greater than 2.2 meters (m) in length and are characterized by a rounded nose with one to three fins. They are marked by being more buoyant, more stable, and less maneuverable than shortboards. Shortboards are 2.2 m or less in length, typically have a pointed nose and three fins, and are very light. Shortboard riders often aim to perform more dynamic moves on the waves, including cutbacks, 360° rotations, and "aerials" (launching into the air off a wave). Neophyte surfers typically learn on longboards; more expert surfers may choose either type of board, depending on the wave conditions and the goals for any particular surf session.

Most boards also include a leash attached to the surfer's ankle, enabling the surfer and his or her board to be in somewhat close proximity after the inevitable wipeout. Using a leash can also prevent one's board from flying into a neighbor on the water, but the device is not without risk, as will be discussed subsequently.

Demands of the Sport

Real-time analysis has found that surfing is an intermittent sport in which paddling accounts for

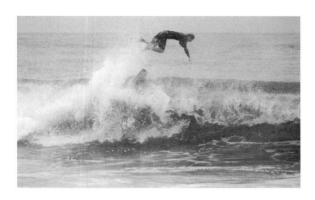

A surfer wiping out on Hawaii's Bonzai Pipeline. Surfers are prone to injuries related to environmental exposure as well as acute and repetitive stress injuries.

Source: Jan Tyler/iStockphoto.

50% of the activity and waiting for suitable waves while on the board accounts for another 40%; only 5% to 10% of a surf session is actually spent riding a wave. A large amount of the time in the water, then, a surfer will be paddling prone, with his or her back in hyperextension. When "catching a wave," the surfer will then pop up from a prone to a standing position as he or she descends the face of the wave. Executing subsequent maneuvers, ranging from turning at the bottom of the wave to cutting back up the face of the wave to still more (see www.riptionary.com), will require an extraordinary amount of balance and lower body strength.

The unique demands of the sport require that the surfer possess a decent amount of both aerobic and anaerobic fitness. Paddling out to a surf break and negotiating obstacles (ranging from waves to other surfers) requires high levels of upper body strength, especially in the shoulders, and a good deal of upper body fitness. Studies have shown that elite surfers will have peak oxygen uptake characteristics similar to other elite upper body athletes (e.g., kayakers) and anaerobic power capacities similar to rugby players.

Injuries

Surfers are prone to *acute* injuries; chronic, repetitive motion injuries; and injuries related to environmental exposure. The reported injury rate has been 4 per 1,000 hours of play (comparatively, the injury rate among National Collegiate Athletic Association [NCAA] male soccer players is 18 per 1,000 hours of play). Some caution should be used, however, in interpreting these numbers, as the novice participation rate in the sport is ever increasing and it is likely that the studies reflect some underreporting in injury rates. Likewise, injuries are thought to be on the rise with increased crowding in the water leading to more likely collisions between surfers and other people and objects in the water. Overall, however, surfing appears to be a relatively safe activity.

Soft tissue injuries such as contusions and abrasions are among the most frequent injuries a surfer will sustain, with lacerations being the most common, representing 42% of all acute injuries. Injury surveillance studies note that the surfer's face is the most common area for lacerations, and the culprit is typically the surfer's own board. The board leash is implicated in many of these injuries, as the board can easily recoil into the surfer after a wipeout. Minor wounds are typically treated in the usual manner, with particular attention to thorough irrigation and exploration to remove retained foreign bodies. Major wounds oftentimes require consideration of delayed primary closure and/or prophylaxis against infection from common marine pathogens, including *Vibrio* species—fluoroquinolones or third-generation cephalosporins. Ruling out an associated open fracture is also important, and consideration should be given to appropriate imaging if indicated.

There are a great number of musculoskeletal conditions that can plague the surfer. Given the great amount of paddling a surfer will do, it is not surprising that shoulder problems are common. Overuse injuries such as impingement, rotator cuff tendinitis, and acquired acromioclavicular (AC) joint arthropathies are seen. Acute injuries, such as shoulder dislocations, can give rise to acquired instability and labral pathology. The back knee of the surfer (farthest away from the board's nose) is another joint at risk, as many maneuvers will require the surfer to put this knee into acute valgus position, courting potential disaster to the medial collateral ligament and meniscus as well as the anterior cruciate ligament (ACL). The front knee, conversely, is oftentimes at risk of hyperextension injuries, including hamstring strains.

Paddling requires the surfer to be in a hyperextended position for prolonged periods of time, and this leads to some special injury patterns. Simple low back strain is common. The typical surfer needs to pay special attention to core and abdominal strength, as well as flexibility of the back, hamstrings, and hip flexors. Over time, isometric hyperextension, repetitive torquing of the lower spine from various maneuvers, and acquired trauma from waves and the like can give rise to spondylolysis and spondylolisthesis. Older surfers often develop degenerative disk disease of the lumbosacral spine.

A unique condition is being increasingly reported in novice surfers: *surfer's myelopathy*. A nontraumatic, usually temporary, paraplegia can develop and appears to be the result of ischemia to the lower thoracic spinal cord caused by the prolonged hyperextension seen when board paddling. Signs and symptoms include lower extremity sensory changes and weakness, new-onset mid to low back pain, and urinary retention. Treatment protocols are still being developed.

Cervical spine trauma is a possibility, as waves can break on reefs, on sand bars, and near fixed objects such as jetties. Aging surfers with preexisting, acquired spondylolysis are at particular risk of catastrophic injury from forced neck hyperextension.

Head, eyes, ears, nose, and throat (HEENT) issues are seen frequently in surfers. Recoil of a board, for instance, can cause much more damage than lacerations. Concussions, oral and maxillofacial injuries, orbital fractures, ruptured globes, and a detached retina have all been seen as a result of trauma sustained during surfing. There is an increasing awareness of the danger to the eye courted by surfers, and there are increasing attempts to encourage use of eye protection when in the surf.

Less severe, but oftentimes more troubling to the surfers because of their frequency and ability to keep them out of the water, are acute conditions such as otitis externa, ruptured tympanic membrane, and the chronic condition known as "surfer's ear." Otitis externa should be treated in the usual manner. Prophylaxis can be achieved by using ear plugs and after a surf session instilling a 50:50 mix of white vinegar and alcohol. A ruptured tympanic membrane will usually spontaneously heal after approximately 2 weeks, and the surfer should not be allowed to enter the water until that time. Close follow-up is indicated.

Surfer's ear is a term applied to external auditory exostoses that develop over years of participation in the sport. The external ear canal develops a reactive hyperemia on exposure to water, particularly cold water; chronically, the reaction can proceed to development of exostoses in the canal. These growths can cause a progressive, albeit reversible, obstructive hearing loss and can also predispose the surfer to recurrent external ear infections. Studies have demonstrated that the longer one surfs and the more the surfer exposes himself or herself to cold water, the higher the chance of developing this condition: A male surfer who has surfed regularly for more than 20 years has a one in two chance of developing this condition. Treatment is surgical, but this is an eminently preventable condition with regular use of ear plugs.

Finally, this is a sport in which the environment affects the participant in a much more direct and significant way than seen in many other sports. Surfers are at high risk for acute and chronic sun damage to the skin and eyes: Sunburns, skin cancers, actinic conjunctivitis, and pterygiums are seen frequently in the surfing population. As ever, prevention can play a significant role here. Regular and frequent use of a waterproof sunblock is encouraged. There are also commercial eye protection devices that can provide ultraviolet protection as well as protection against trauma; it remains to be seen how often a surfer might use these.

The "big risks" of being in marine environments, such as shark attacks, get a lot of media attention but are very rare. More common are marine envenomations from coelenterates (jellyfish and related organisms), stingrays, sea urchins, and coral reef lacerations. Treatment for these injuries can be found in the recommended readings. Drowning, as in all water sports, is a risk every surfer takes. The best prevention of this catastrophe is prudence. At all times, the surfer should be aware of environmental conditions, avoid concomitant use of mind-altering substances, surf with a "buddy," and avoid surfing if conditions exceed one's ability.

James Patrick Macdonald

See also Ear Injuries; Friction Injuries to the Skin; Outdoor Athlete; Sunburn and Skin Cancers

Further Readings

Avilés-Hernández I, García-Zozaya I, DeVillasante JM. Nontraumatic myelopathy associated with surfing. *J Spinal Cord Med.* 2007;30(3):288–293.

Kroon DF, Lawson ML, Derkay CS, Hoffmann K, McCook J. Surfer's ear: external auditory exostoses are more prevalent in cold water surfers. *Otolaryngol Head Neck Surg.* 2002;126(5):499–504.

Mendez-Villaneuva A, Bishop D. Physiological aspects of surfboard riding performance. *Sports Med.* 2005;35(1):55-70.

Nathanson A, Bird S, Dao L, Tam-Sing K. Competitive surfing injuries: a prospective study of surfing-related injuries among contest surfers. *Am J Sports Med.* 2007;35(1):113–117.

Nathanson A, Haynes P, Galanis D. Surfing injuries. *Am J Emerg Med.* 2002;20(3):155–160.

Renneker M, Starr K, Booth G. *Sick Surfers Ask the Surf Docs and Dr. Geoff.* Boulder, CO: Bull Publishing; 1993.

Sunshine S. Surfing injuries. *Curr Sports Med Rep.* 2003;2(3):136–141.

Taylor KS, Zoltan TB, Achar SA. Medical illnesses and injuries encountered during surfing. *Curr Sports Med Rep.* 2006;5(5):262–267.

Websites

Riptionary—Surf Lingo Lexicon: http://www.riptionary.com

SWIMMING, INJURIES IN

Swimming is a highly popular sport involving participants of all ages, various body types, and both genders. People take up the sport for leisure and cardiovascular exercise as well as competition. Swimming can be broadly defined as nearly any movement an individual can do in the water. For the purposes of this entry, the concept of *swimming* will be restricted to what is generally considered supervised lap swimming, using defined stroke techniques. There will also be some discussion of open-water swimming, which is a sport pursued in its own right as well as one component of the triathlon event. (Serious and catastrophic cervical spine injuries that may occur when diving into a pool or open water are not discussed in this entry.)

Most swimmers will train in pools, which are typically set up as "short course" (25 meters [m] in length) or "long course" (50 m in length). Open-water swimming refers to swimming in lakes, ocean, or other bodies of water; the distances involved here sometimes are measured in miles.

The four principal competitive strokes are the front crawl, breaststroke, backstroke, and butterfly. Over the years, there have been some modifications in the forms, techniques, and regulations pertaining to each stroke. The recommended reading section gives a fuller treatment of each stroke. The term *freestyle* is sometimes used synonymously with the front crawl but more accurately means *any style* for individual distances and *any style but breaststroke, butterfly, and backstroke* for the medley events.

Some authors have argued that swimming possibly provides the most balanced form of exercise. Use of different strokes and variation in technique emphasize at different times the upper extremities and the lower extremities. The swimmer can develop endurance, power, agility, and coordination in the entire body. Swimmers attest to the psychological benefits of the sport. In competition, the athlete can perform both as an individual and as a team member, especially in relay events. The sport can, therefore, appeal both to the loner and to those who socialize. Equipment is minimal. Perhaps, the only drawbacks are the obvious need for access to water and the fact that swimming does not involve full-body weight-bearing impact on the skeleton and hence does not enhance bone density.

Swimming is particularly suited to the developing athlete. Acquiring good fundamentals as a youth can lead to mastering an activity that can be carried forth through one's geriatric years. Studies have demonstrated an exceptionally low acute injury rate. Compared with age-matched nonathlete controls of ages 13 to 19, young swimmers have been found to demonstrate enhanced physical, cardiovascular, mental, and social skills.

A final note should be made about equipment. At the most basic level, a swimsuit is all that is needed. Goggles are typically worn to prevent irritation to the eyes from the chlorine often used to clean pools. There are many different devices used by coaches and athletes for stroke work or overload training. The most common are fins, kickboards, pull buoys (a flotation device put between the legs of the swimmer to move without the use of the legs), and hand paddles. At times, these devices can be involved both in the development and in the treatment of injuries, as is discussed below.

Injury Patterns

General Principles

From an orthopedic perspective, overuse conditions predominate as the type of injuries that swimmers will encounter. It is estimated that the average collegiate swimmer performs 1 to 2 million strokes annually with each arm. Periodicity is sometimes less than ideal: Swimming for many participants is a year-round activity, often involving two practice sessions daily. During these sessions, the athlete may swim extraordinary distances: 10,000 to 15,000 m/day of training is not uncommon at the college level. Additionally, the swimmer may engage in "dry-land" weight training and stretching activities, some of which may actually increase the risk of injury.

Besides overuse, technique can also expose the swimmer to injury. Poor stroke mechanics applied in the front crawl are frequently implicated in the development of shoulder problems. The arm pull in the butterfly stroke and breaststroke, and less frequently the freestyle, can cause stress syndromes of the elbow. The breaststroke, with its specialized kick, can cause a similar stress injury to the knee. Though swimming, especially the front crawl, is often an exercise prescribed for the treatment of back pain, the unique movements of some strokes expose the back to some risk. The breaststroke can induce an exaggerated lordotic posture of the lower back, causing extension-based back problems. The butterfly stroke has been implicated in the development and exacerbation of Scheuermann kyphosis.

Given this involvement of overuse and technique, most orthopedic issues seen in swimmers, after an accurate diagnosis has been made, will respond to rest, targeted physical therapy, and attention to appropriate modification of technique.

As a final note, though management of most swimming injuries will require rest, it is important to minimize the swimmer's time out of the water not only to avoid deconditioning but also to enhance compliance. Intelligent use of other strokes and/or equipment can often allow the swimmer to rest the affected body part while still being in the pool.

Shoulder

The upper extremity is frequently injured as a result of overuse in the competitive swimmer, and of the involved joints, the shoulder is, far and away, the most frequently implicated: It has been reported that 90% of the complaints by swimmers that bring them to a doctor are related to shoulder problems.

Swimmer's shoulder is the most common injury seen. This is an inflammatory condition of the supraspinatus and biceps tendons, resulting from overuse, glenohumeral instability, and, at times, improper stroke technique. All three contributory causes should be addressed in the diagnosis and treatment of the condition.

The glenohumeral instability seen in this condition is often acquired. Many elite swimmers have inherent ligamentous laxity and often will have multidirectional shoulder instability. However, all swimmers will overdevelop the adductor and internal rotator muscles of the shoulder simply by performing their stroke. The relative weakness of the external rotators and scapular stabilizers of the shoulder results in a humeral head that can migrate anteriorly and superiorly during the front crawl and also the butterfly stroke. Related to overuse, technique, training style (e.g., pull buoys, paddles), and acquired muscular imbalances, the adductors and internal rotators become overdeveloped and the anterior capsule more lax.

The patient will typically present with diffuse shoulder pain and aching that have gradually increased with training. At times, the pain will be localized to the posterior or anterior shoulder, corresponding to the location of the supraspinatus and the biceps tendon. Physical examination generally reveals weakness of the rotator cuff muscles. Maneuvers designed to assess impingement, including the Neer and Hawkins tests, will oftentimes be positive. So too, maneuvers assessing the biceps tendon, such as the Speed and Yergason tests, can be positive. The patient will oftentimes have generalized ligamentous laxity, and the shoulder will often be found to be exceptionally lax or even unstable; occasionally, anterior apprehension and anterior subluxation of the shoulder can be seen on exam.

Imaging is usually not indicated in swimmer's shoulder and should be reserved for recalcitrant cases, atypical presentations, or at times initially for the older swimmer.

Treatment will begin with relative rest. Typically, the front crawl will need to be avoided. If the patient's symptoms are unilateral, they may be allowed to do the one-armed butterfly stroke. Breaststroke and backstrokes are often forgiving. Kick drills can be done, but kick boards (which tend to forward flex the shoulder and aggravate impingement) should be avoided. Paddles and pull buoys, which often contribute to the problem in the first place, should be entirely avoided.

A coach should look at the swimmer's mechanics. In a properly performed front crawl technique, the elbow remains well above the hand when the arm is out of the water, during the recovery phase of the stroke, and as the hand enters the water, during the "catch" phase. Swimmers who allow their elbows to drop may irritate the rotator cuff muscles.

Rehabilitation should focus on stretching the posterior capsule; strengthening the scapular stabilizers as well as the rotator cuff muscles, especially the infraspinatus and teres minor; and occasionally addressing core stability weakness. Exercises in the initial phase should exclude movements that abduct or flex the shoulder beyond 90°.

True rotator cuff tendinitis and bicipital tendinitis can be seen and should be treated accordingly. Degenerative diseases of the shoulder are typically seen in masters-level swimmers. Acromioclavicular and glenohumeral joint arthritis are found in this population, as well as true bony impingement. The geriatric patient may present with a frank, degenerative tear of the rotator cuff tendon. The clinician should have a low threshold for obtaining plain-film radiography, and possibly advanced imaging, in swimmers above the age of 35 years. Treatment would initially be similar to that described above for swimmer's shoulder, but in degenerative cases, more aggressive treatment, including referral to orthopedic surgery, is often indicated. The details of this treatment are beyond the scope of this entry and are found elsewhere in this encyclopedia.

Knee

Knee injuries in swimmers are almost exclusively seen in breaststrokers and are related to the use of the whip kick in that stroke. A study reviewing knee pain in breaststrokers demonstrated an association between more frequent knee pain and higher age of the swimmer, increasing years of competition, increase in training distance, and decrease in warm-up. Nevertheless, the very biomechanics of the stroke can put any breaststroker at risk.

The whip kick itself does not use the flexion and extension patterns seen in the flutter and butterfly kicks, which are natural motions for the knee joint. Rather, the motion applies a significant valgus strain to the joint, resulting in three recognized injury patterns: (1) medial collateral ligament (MCL) stress syndrome, (2) patellofemoral syndrome (PTFS), and (3) medial synovial plica syndrome.

The clinician can diagnose MCL stress syndrome by taking a careful history. Pain is typically activity related, insidious in onset, and localized at the medial aspect of the knee. Palpation over the course of the MCL, from the adductor tubercle of the femur to the insertion on the medial tibia, typically reveals tenderness. Applying a valgus stress to the knee with the leg in external rotation causes pain. The clinical findings of PTFS present no differently in the swimmer than in other athletes. Medial synovial plica syndrome typically presents with complaints of pain experienced at the extension phase of the whip kick. The medial synovial plica is a fold of synovium, which can become irritated; physical examination can frequently reveal a tender, thickened plica crossing the medial femoral condyle. There is typically no pain with a valgus stress.

Treatment for these conditions is typically one of relative rest and the use of anti-inflammatory medications. Occasionally, training can continue by performing strokes other than the breaststroke but only if the swimmer is painfree. Ice and nonsteroidal anti-inflammatory drugs (NSAIDs) are helpful in controlling the inflammation. Addressing stroke mechanics is imperative for all three conditions.

MCL stress syndrome by its nature can persist and can be difficult to treat; it occasionally necessitates changing over to other strokes indefinitely. PTFS is amenable to classic physical therapy techniques addressing patellar tracking. Medial plicae can cause persistent trouble and may require steroid injections or surgical excision.

Foot and Ankle

The most common injury seen in swimmers is tendinitis of the extensor tendons at the extensor retinaculum of the dorsal foot. In this area, the tendons of the extrinsic foot dorsiflexors are encased in their tendon sheaths and are prone to irritation.

In both the flutter kick of the front crawl and the dolphin kick of the butterfly stroke, the foot and ankle are carried through extreme plantarflexion back to neutral position, setting up a situation where the extensor tendons can become inflamed.

Diagnosis is usually straightforward. There can be swelling and tenderness over the extensor retinaculum. Passive range of motion of the ankle typically elicits crepitus in the tendons; having the patient dorsiflex the foot against resistance can evoke pain.

Treatment involves the use of modalities such as ice and ultrasound; NSAIDs may be used to help decrease the inflammation as well. Relative rest is indicated. The patient may swim using a pull buoy to avoid kicking. A program of gentle, pre-exercise stretching of the extensor tendons should commence. Return to full swimming with normal kicking should progress in a graduated fashion.

Elbow

Stress syndromes of the elbow are seen in the arm pull, particularly in the butterfly strokes and breaststrokes. Occasionally, lateral epicondylitis can be seen. Treatment would include relative rest, attention to stroke mechanics, and eccentric strengthening of the wrist extensors.

Wrist and Hand

Less commonly, de Quervain tenosynovitis can be seen, especially in the older swimmer. Frequently, the inciting cause is poor technique. Diagnosis and treatment are the same as in other athletes with these symptoms. Thoracic outlet syndrome, discussed elsewhere in this text, is occasionally seen in swimmers as well. Presenting complaints include paresthesias radiating down the shoulder and arm into the hand, especially over the small finger, complaints of weakness and aching of the arm, and weakness of the hand grip.

Back

As discussed previously, extension-based back pain, including mechanical low back stress, spondylolysis, and spondylolisthesis, can be seen in the breaststroke and, occasionally, the butterfly stroke, especially when the latter stroke is poorly executed. Scheuermann kyphosis can be seen in the butterfly stroke specialist. Degenerative disease of the cervical spine is occasionally seen in the masters-level swimmer. The clinician should attempt to make a precise and accurate diagnosis and treat accordingly. The specifics of treatment for each condition are elaborated elsewhere in this encyclopedia.

Medical (Nonorthopedic) Issues

Asthma is not infrequently seen in swimmers. Some of those suffering from asthma have positively embraced swimming and have noticed that the warm, humid environment of an indoor pool makes their breathing easier. Others will find that an enclosed environment with chlorine fumes may exacerbate the problem. Clinicians caring for swimmers should be conversant with the management of asthma.

Skin and hair problems are seen in swimmers. Viruses and fungi can be transmitted from pool decks and locker room floors, giving rise to plantar warts and athlete's foot. As ever, prevention (including in this case the use of sandals) beats treatment, which would be done in the usual fashion. Swimmers occasionally will shave their bodies prior to meets, giving rise to folliculitis. Pseudomonas as well as *Staphylococcus* infections are often implicated. Topical antibiotics may be used, but occasionally, oral antibiotics will be required for severe or resistant cases. Chlorine and other chemicals used in the treatment of pool water can affect a swimmer's hair, giving rise to color changes. The most effective treatment is, again, prevention: the use of swim caps and frequent shampooing.

Not surprisingly, otitis externa is seen commonly in swimmers. Prevention is best achieved by wearing a tight-fitting swim cap that covers the ears. Alternatively, commercial products containing vinegar and alcohol can be instilled in the ears after swimming to "dry" the ear canal out. If the patient becomes symptomatic, the use of prescription antibiotic/antifungal/anti-inflammatory eardrops and a period of scrupulous avoidance of water are recommended. Out-of-pool time can last as long as 7 days, but if the patient is asymptomatic after 2 to 3 days, he or she may be allowed back in the pool while continuing treatment.

Eating Disorders

Though more definite data are needed, swimming is recognized, along with cross-country running, gymnastics, and diving, as one of the sports in which female athletes especially will have higher rates of eating disorders, including bulimia, anorexia, and other disordered eating behaviors. In one study, 15% of college female athletes had some form of subclinical eating disorder; this is a higher rate than is seen in the general population. Olympic swimmer Dara Torres has publicly shared her struggle with bulimia as a young swimmer. Swimmers often will pursue disordered eating behaviors in the misguided belief that they will help them swim faster or in pursuit of a more idealized body image. Since a principal hallmark of these illnesses is denial, it is incumbent on coaches, trainers, clinicians, and parents to have a high degree of suspicion when addressing the problem in their athletes.

Drowning

As with any event associated with water, swimming exposes the athlete to the risks of drowning. The danger is greater for the open-water swimmer. It is recommended that an athlete always train in a supervised pool setting (i.e., with a coach or lifeguard) or train with a "buddy," either in the pool or in the open water.

James Patrick Macdonald

See also Asthma; Female Athlete Triad; Fungal Skin Infections and Parasitic Infestations; Scheuermann Kyphosis; Shoulder Instability

Further Readings

Fowler PJ, Regan WD. Swimming injuries of the knee, foot and ankle, elbow, and back. *Clin Sports Med.* 1986;5(1):139–148.

Kammer CS, Young CC, Niedfeldt MW. Swimming injuries and illnesses. *Phys Sportsmed.* 1999;27(4):51–60.

LATTC. Video clips of various swimming strokes. http://wellness.lattc.edu/real/strokes.html. Accessed June 14, 2010.

McMaster WC. Swimming injuries. An overview. *Sports Med.* 1996;22(5):332–336.

Weldon EJ, Richardson AB. Upper extremity overuse injuries in swimming. A discussion of swimmer's shoulder. *Clin Sports Med.* 2001;20(3):423–438.

Wikipedia. Backstroke. http://en.wikipedia.org/wiki/Backstroke. Accessed June 14, 2010.

Wikipedia. Breaststroke. http://en.wikipedia.org/wiki/Breaststroke. Accessed June 14, 2010.

Wikipedia. Butterfly stroke. http://en.wikipedia.org/wiki/Butterfly_stroke. Accessed June 14, 2010.

Wikipedia. Front crawl. http://en.wikipedia.org/wiki/Front_crawl. Accessed June 14, 2010.

Websites

USA Swimming: http://www.usaswimming.org

T

TAILBONE (COCCYX) INJURIES

The tailbone, or *coccyx*, projects below the pelvic bone, first curving backward and then curving forward at the tip. There are three to five segments dividing the coccyx. Between these segments are joints, much like those seen between the bones of the spine. However, these may be fused in the coccyx. Injuries to the region of the coccyx can result when the fused joints are repeatedly forced out of their normal positions with regular activities, causing inflammation of the tissues surrounding it.

When a person is sitting, the coccyx, along with the two prominent regions of the pelvic bone, called the *ischial tuberosities*, bears the weight. When a person leans back in a seated position, the weight load on the coccyx increases. The birth canal in women is defined posteriorly by the coccyx. The muscles responsible for the voluntary control of bowel movement attach onto the coccyx.

Mechanisms of Injury

The coccyx is easily exposed to blunt trauma. A fall backward into a seated position is the most common cause of injury. Direct trauma can occur from a kick, using a trampoline, falling from a horse, or a skiing mishap, causing the coccyx to be bruised, broken, or dislocated. Poor posture while sitting for a prolonged period of time, such as while traveling in a car or plane, or sitting on a hard surface can result in trauma as well. Injuries can be encountered as a result of repetitive pressure on the coccyx, as in cycling and rowing. Prolonged sitting, even on a soft seat (i.e., office workers and students), has been documented on patient history as a reason for coccyx tenderness. Anal intercourse has been implicated in injury to the coccyx.

Because the birth canal is bounded by the coccyx at the back, pressure exerted during childbirth can instigate injury. The coccyx is literally "in the way" during childbirth. The resulting pain can involve the muscles used in bowel movement as well as the muscles of the buttocks.

Signs and Symptoms

The coccyx will be painful and often markedly tender, especially while sitting in a leaning-back position. Pain may also be felt on standing from a seated position, with bowel movements, and during sexual intercourse. The adjacent structures may not be tender.

It is important that spinal and pelvic conditions are ruled out, as these may cause pain over the coccyx area. Disk disease may be misinterpreted as injury to the coccyx. However, the coccyx will usually not be tender if only the spine is involved, and the examiner should consider other diagnoses.

Other possible causes of pain that may be misinterpreted as injury to the coccyx include the following:

- Pain of the pyriformis muscles
- Injury to the pudendal nerve, especially in bikers who sit for prolonged periods of time
- Pilonidal cysts, Tarlov cysts, or meningeal cysts

- Obesity, which leads to excess pressure on the coccyx when sitting
- A bursitis-like condition in slim people, who have little fat padding in their buttocks, causing the tip of the coccyx to constantly rub against the subcutaneous tissues

A rectal and pelvic examination may also be performed to rule out other conditions.

Imaging

Management of the condition often does not change with findings on X-rays, so there is often no need to obtain them, unless the examiner finds the results of a physical examination to be inconclusive. X-rays usually include a lateral view of the coccyx. Lateral views may be taken while standing and sitting to measure coccygeal mobility. X-rays of the coccyx reveal four different types. Most people have a Type I coccyx, which curves slightly forward. The Type II coccyx curves forward, with its tip almost pointing straight forward. The Type III coccyx sharply angles to the front. The Type IV coccyx shows movement of the usually fixed joints within the sacrum or within the coccyx itself. The coccyx can move up to 22° when a person repositions from standing to sitting. Subtle backward movement of the coccyx can be noted by taking a sitting lateral X-ray and comparing it with a standing film to check the amount of translation. Mild displacement is defined as more than 25% movement of the coccyx from the standing to the sitting view. In dynamic X-ray imaging, abnormally increased movement of the coccyx is defined as more than 25° of forward movement on a lateral X-ray. Measurement of the angle formed between the first and last segments of the coccyx can provide an objective measurement of forward movement of the coccyx. Computed tomography (CT) scans and magnetic resonance imaging (MRI) scans often do not add significant information to standing and sitting dynamic views. However, an MRI can be helpful if a tumor or infection is suspected.

Repetitive stretching of the surrounding ligaments and muscles attached to the coccyx may result in inflammation of these tissues, causing pain and soreness when sitting or with straining. Continued movement may prevent healing of this injury, resulting in further damage and perpetuation

of the cycle. In such cases, X-rays and MRI scans may be required. Abnormal movement of the coccyx may be due to partial dislocation, and this may be noted on patient X-rays taken in the standing and sitting positions.

Treatment

Relief from pain caused by coccyx injuries may take weeks or even months. Pain in the coccyx after an injury may become chronic in some patients. Referral to a specialist is usually unnecessary; however, referral to pain specialists, medication, rehabilitation, anesthesiology, or orthopedic surgery may be needed for patients who develop chronic pain in the coccyx. Pain due to trauma to the coccyx usually resolves on its own with protection of the bone from further injury. Pain medications, heat, or ice can bring relief. Leaning forward while sitting protects the coccyx, as weight is mainly borne on the ischial tuberosities with this position. Weight may be distributed away from the coccyx by using "doughnut" cushions or pillows with a central hole. "Wedge" cushions or pillows with a wedge-shaped section cut out of the back may also be used. These may be purchased or made quite easily. Hot or cold compresses appear to work in selective cases. Pain relief may be obtained with nonsteroidal anti-inflammatory medications. Narcotic painkillers should be avoided unless the pain is severe.

Specialists may inject a local anesthetic, with or without corticosteroids, using X-rays for guidance. Positive results have been noted in some studies with this treatment, although pain relief has been shown to last only for a few weeks.

Specialists are able to manipulate the coccyx through the rectum. The purposes of this treatment are to massage the muscles attached to the coccyx, as they are often spasmodic, or to mobilize the fascia surrounding the coccyx. Several studies have shown modest improvement with these manipulation techniques.

In chronic cases, antidepressants or antiepileptic medications may be helpful. Acupuncture may be a reasonable option, although it is not known whether modalities such as ultrasound or transcutaneous nerve stimulation actually work to relieve pain due to coccyx injury.

Surgical removal of the coccyx is the last resort. Pain relief obtained after this procedure has been studied, with varied results, mostly leading to the conclusion that surgery does provide pain relief for most patients. However, it is important to note that complications such as infection, injury to the rectum, and problems with bowel movement may occur following this procedure.

George Guntur Pujalte

See also Hip, Pelvis, and Groin Injuries; Lower Back Contusion; Sports Injuries, Acute

Further Readings

Hodges SD, Eck JC, Humphreys SC. A treatment and outcomes analysis of patients with coccydynia. *Spine J.* 2004;4(2):138–140.

Howorth B. The painful coccyx. *Clin Orthop.* 1959;14:145–160.

Maigne JY, Doursounian L, Chatellier G. Causes and mechanisms of common coccydynia: role of body mass index and coccygeal trauma. *Spine.* 2000;25(23):3072–3076.

Traycoff RB, Crayton H, Dodson R. Sacrococcygeal pain syndromes: diagnosis and treatment. *Orthopedics.* 1989;12(10):1373–1377.

Wray CC, Easom S, Hoskinson J. Coccydynia. Aetiology and treatment. *J Bone Joint Surg Br.* 1991;73(2): 335–338.

TAPING

The application of tape in sports plays a significant role in today's athletic performance arena. In professional or collegiate sports, the Olympic Games, or local youth league games, a wide array of taping as well as bracing applications are used to enable athletes to enhance their performance, correct minor functional abnormalities, and participate in sports while recovering from injury.

In 1895, what is now known as the *closed basket weave* was described by V. P. Gibney. This original ankle taping was first known by the name "Gibney boot" and was an imitation of a procedure performed by army medics in England. Since that first taping application, not only has the practice of taping expanded dramatically, but also the taping and bracing industry has undergone considerable growth; currently, there are more than 10 major tape manufacturers, providing a wide variety of padding, braces, adhesives, and tapes for use by practitioners.

In the field of sports medicine, taping techniques are currently taught in a variety of courses for specialists. For Certified Athletic Trainers, taping and bracing is a curriculum requirement mandated by the Board of Certification. Although it is not a mandatory class for those seeking certification as a Licensed Physical Therapist, there are various continuing education and undergraduate elective courses that candidates can take to gain this knowledge and skill. A sound understanding of the mechanisms of injury, detailed knowledge of anatomy, and continuous practice of effective methods are the keys to learning how to tape and brace correctly. Once the basic skills are learned, they can then be adapted to a variety of real-life situations and applications.

Appendix A provides detailed information on the materials and clear, step-by-step explanations, accompanied by photographs, of the taping and wrapping methods and techniques most commonly used by specialists.

Arthur Horne and Cheryl Blauth

See also Ankle Instability; Ankle Instability, Chronic; Athletic Trainers; Bracing; Knee Injuries

Further Readings

Beam JW. *Orthopedic Taping, Wrapping, Bracing and Padding.* Philadelphia, PA: FA Davis; 2006.

Firer P. Effectiveness of taping for the prevention of ankle ligament sprains. *Br J Sports Med.* 1990;24(1):47–50.

Herrington L. The effect of corrective taping of the patella on patella position as defined by MRI. *Res Sports Med.* 2006;14(3):215–223.

Perrin DH. *Athletic Taping and Bracing.* Champaign, IL: Human Kinetics; 1995.

Ubell M, Boylan J, Ashton-Miller J, Wojtys E. The effect of ankle braces on the prevention of dynamic forced ankle inversion. *Am J Sports Med.* 2003;31(6):935–940.

TARGET HEART RATE

The premise of aerobic exercise is to exercise at an intensity that will challenge the aerobic energy system while minimizing the risks of adverse health consequences. One way of remaining cognizant of the intensity at which one is exercising is to monitor the heart rate. Heart rate increases in a predictable fashion as exercise intensity increases from light to moderate to vigorous. There is a linear relationship between the heart rate and exercise intensity, and the heart rate is generally accepted as an accurate means of assessing and monitoring relative exercise intensity.

This relationship is a function of the heart's greater demand to pump blood and oxygen to skeletal muscle at higher intensities. The other parameter that increases the heart's ability to pump blood is an increase in "stroke volume," or the volume of blood pumped during each heartbeat. The extent to which these parameters increase is primarily determined by training status: Untrained individuals rely more on increasing the heart rate, whereas trained athletes have a greater ability to increase stroke volume and thus rely less on heart rate at the same exercise intensity.

Individual athletes have a maximum heart rate often predicted by the simple equation "220 minus age," which reflects the physiological ceiling below which the system operates. Younger athletes tend to have higher maximum heart rates; this maximum declines with age. There is also a difference between the sexes; the equation described above has an error of ±10 beats/minute.

Exercising at intensities close to maximum heart rate has theoretical risks. There is slightly increased incidence of adverse coronary events when the heart is maximally challenged, likely a consequence of relative ischemia (or lack of oxygen supply) to areas of heart muscle, particularly in male athletes younger than 35 years. This ischemia can result in a myocardial infarction or an abnormal heart rhythm, such as ventricular tachycardia, both of which can result in sudden death. This risk is multifactorial and slight and does not preclude athletes around the world from competing at intensities close to the maximum. However, when developing guidelines for the general population to perform aerobic exercise, attention has been focused on encouraging exercise at intensities <85% of the maximum.

Determining the exercise intensity, and hence heart rate, most effective for achieving one's exercise goals depends on what those goals are. Aerobic exercise at lower (light) intensities tends to rely on the oxidation of fatty acids for fuel and hence is a suitable intensity for those attempting to achieve weight loss by "burning" adipose tissue or fat stores.

Athletes hoping to improve aerobic performance seek to optimally challenge the aerobic system at vigorous intensities close to a zone termed the *anaerobic threshold* or *lactate threshold*. This is the intensity of exercise during which the skeletal muscle involved in the activity transitions from mostly aerobic energy production (using oxygen) to energy production incorporating *anaerobic* systems, which do not need oxygen. Stimulation of the anaerobic system results in lactate production and a rise in blood lactate that can be detected at this threshold. Athletes exercising above the anaerobic threshold develop fatigue more rapidly than when solely relying on their aerobic system. Different strategies can be used to account for this, such as exercising just below the anaerobic threshold or exercising using *interval training*, where an athlete raises his or her exercise intensity above the anaerobic threshold for a short period of time, then dips back below the threshold and continues exercising.

Monitoring the heart rate is easily accomplished by counting the pulse rate, either at the wrist (radial pulse) or at the neck (carotid pulse). Typically, counting the pulse for 15 seconds (and multiplying the total by 4) or 30 seconds (and multiplying the result by 2) is sufficient to obtain an accurate representation of the frequency of beats per minute. The exercise industry also now markets heart rate monitors, usually incorporating a strap that is worn around the chest and a monitor that can be worn at the wrist like a watch.

The ease and low cost of monitoring the heart rate has led to its widespread use as a gauge of relative exercise intensity. Nonetheless, there is some concern regarding the use of heart rate to monitor exercise intensity due to a phenomenon known as *cardiovascular drift*. This phenomenon describes an increase in heart rate with prolonged exercise (greater than 10 minutes) despite the exercise continuing at the same intensity. Cardiovascular drift is likely to be related to the sympathetic nervous system and catecholamine control of the sinus node, where the heartbeat originates. It should be noted that factors other than exercise intensity also affect the heart rate, such as ambient temperature and caffeine intake.

Research has recently focused more on heart rate variability (HRV). Evidence suggests that trained individuals have higher HRV than untrained individuals. Most research shows that during graded exercise, HRV decreases progressively up to moderate intensities, after which it stabilizes. HRV could potentially play a role in the prevention and detection of overtraining. This is currently an area of great research interest, with mixed results reported in the scientific literature. Measuring HRV overnight, in supine sleeping athletes during training camps, has been the most widely reported method. High HRV is associated with high $\dot{V}o_2$max (peak oxygen uptake) values, while it has been found that low HRV is associated with increased mortality, the incidence of new cardiac events, and the risk of sudden cardiac death in asymptomatic patients.

Hamish A. Kerr

See also Overtraining

Further Readings

Achten J, Jeukendrup AE. Heart rate monitoring: applications and limitations. *Sports Med.* 2003;33(7):517–538.

American College of Sports Medicine. *ACSM's Guidelines for Exercise Testing and Prescription.* Philadelphia, PA: Lippincott Williams & Wilkins; 2007:143–147.

American College of Sports Medicine Position Stand, The recommended quantity and quality of exercise for developing and maintaining cardiorespiratory and muscular fitness, and flexibility in healthy adults. *Med Sci Sports Exerc.* 1998;30(6):975–991.

Astrand PO, Astrand I. Heart rate during muscular work in man exposed to prolonged hypoxia. *J Appl Physiol.* 1958;13(1):75–80.

Team and Group Dynamics in Sports

Shortly before the 2008 Olympic Games, Mike Krzyzewski, coach of the U.S. men's basketball team, remarked:

> From Athens [where the team finished third] we learned we need time to develop camaraderie. We have to be committed to one another before we can be committed to the team. We're developing a program, not "selecting a team." No one ever "selects a team"; you select people and hope they become a team.

Several weeks later, the U.S. basketball team went on to win the gold medal in Beijing and were noted for the high level of cohesion displayed by the team members during both training and tournament play. Indeed, this example illustrates that while it is clearly important to select the right personnel when creating a team, hard work is required to forge a collection of players into a highly integrated, cohesive, and effective team.

Group Dynamics

The study of *group dynamics* is concerned with understanding the various psychological processes that occur within and between groups. The term *group dynamics* can be traced back to the prominent social and organizational psychologist Kurt Lewin (1890–1947). In the context of group dynamics in sports, considerable attention has been given to identifying the factors that influence team functioning. Among these factors, *cohesion* represents one of the most extensively studied psychological constructs. Cohesion can be thought of as the glue that acts to attract and retain members within groups. The attention given to cohesion among sport psychology researchers is perhaps not surprising given that cohesion has consistently been found to predict team performance, across both highly *interactive* (e.g., soccer) as well as *coacting* (e.g., golf) team sports settings. According to the prominent Canadian sport psychologist Albert Carron, cohesion is multidimensional in nature, consisting of task as well as social dimensions, plus individual-level and group-level orientations. Specifically, cohesion involves the extent to which team members are attracted to the team's task and social activities, as well as the extent to which members perceive the group as a whole to be integrated around these task and social activities. Although research evidence suggests that increasing a team's level of cohesion will lead to increased performance, it is worthy of note that the relationship between cohesion and performance is actually bidirectional in nature. That is, teams also tend to become more cohesive when they perform well.

Role Conflict, Role Ambiguity, and Performance

Beyond performance, cohesion is also influenced by a variety of other factors, such as the types of roles that are performed by team members, the group norms and goals that members establish, the behaviors of those in leadership positions, as well as members' perceptions of their team's capabilities. From the perspective of team roles, athletes are typically expected to perform a range of responsibilities with the team's task-related objectives in mind. When athletes are unclear about their various role responsibilities, they are said to experience role ambiguity. This can lead to greater precompetition anxiety, less satisfaction, and diminished levels of performance. While reducing role ambiguity is vital within sports teams, it is also important to curtail any role conflict that athletes might experience. Role conflict occurs when athletes receive conflicting information and/or expectations about what is required of them. When athletes experience role conflict, they tend to perceive greater role ambiguity and report reduced role-related confidence. Although minimizing role ambiguity and conflict has many benefits for member and team functioning, one must also consider the degree of role acceptance among team members when attempting to maximize performance. Sir Clive Woodward, coach of the 2003 World Cup winning English rugby team, was known to emphasize the importance of selecting and developing a team of "energizers," who bought into the team concept, accepted their prescribed roles, and contributed to team cohesion. If some athletes, who he described as "energy sappers," did not accept their roles and could not be turned into energizers, his recommended strategy was to remove them from the team before they destabilized team chemistry and debilitated the team's level of cohesion.

Team Norms and Group Cohesion

Norms correspond to the accepted standards of behavior that exist for members within teams. Team norms are usually unconnected from the position-specific roles prescribed by a team's coach. These norms are often unwritten and evolve through the course of ongoing group development. While those responsible for developing teams, such as coaches, can allow team norms to evolve naturally, several benefits are associated with formalizing appropriate team norms. This can be accomplished by encouraging team members to contribute to and decide on their own set of expectations for off-field and/or on-field interpersonal engagement (i.e., in the form of an athlete "charter"). Such an approach can foster athlete autonomy and is more likely to result in athletes committing to these rules than if the rules are directly prescribed by a coach or a manager. This, in turn, can facilitate a sense of cohesion among team members. The use of goal-setting strategies has also been found to positively influence team cohesion. In particular, when athletes are involved in setting out their own process- and performance-oriented goals (rather than having these goals prescribed to them), they tend to be more committed to the group's endeavors, thus resulting in improved group integration.

While team cohesion, to a large extent, depends on the quality of interpersonal relations among athletes within a team, the coach can also play a prominent role in fostering group cohesion and a healthy team culture. For example, a growing body of evidence from various organizational settings has found that when leaders display transformational behaviors (see the entry Leadership in Sports), their teams tend to be more cohesive. Transformational leaders motivate followers to go beyond their self-interests for the good of the group and give group members the confidence to exceed minimally accepted standards. In sports teams, when coaches display transformational leadership behaviors, their athletes have been found to display more self-determined forms of motivation (e.g., intrinsic motivation) and also tend to perform better than athletes who are coached by nontransformational leaders.

In the field of sport psychology, a vast amount of research attention has been directed at understanding the determinants and consequences of athletes' self-efficacy beliefs. Self-efficacy refers to a situation-specific form of self-confidence and has been found to be positively related to outcomes such as athlete persistence, effort, and task performance.

While numerous studies have examined the factors that contribute to athletes becoming more efficacious in their *own* abilities to perform specific skills, researchers have also sought to examine the role of collective efficacy beliefs in sports teams. Collective efficacy refers to members' perceptions about their team's conjoint tasks, and in a variety of team sports settings, these beliefs have been found to influence team functioning. Interestingly, collective efficacy has also been found to be both predictive of and predicted by team cohesion. That is, the relationship is reciprocal, whereby team members can become more confident in each other when the team is more cohesive and, conversely, the team can also become more cohesive when members develop confidence in each other.

In light of the various correlates of group cohesion in sports, a burgeoning area of enquiry has centered on developing and testing effective team-building interventions. *Team building* is the umbrella term given to the process of developing cohesion within groups. As the research described above would suggest, team building does not represent a singular unitary process and may involve a range of processes that can be applied to meet the team's specific needs. Team-building interventions in sports tend to be either *direct* or *indirect* in nature. With direct interventions, the interventionist (e.g., the sport psychology consultant) intervenes directly with the target population. In comparison, indirect interventions involve the psychologist working with a proxy agent (i.e., a third party), such as a coach, who then leads the intervention with his or her athletes. Although the direct approach has been found to be effective in a variety of team sports settings, one of the benefits of the indirect approach is that coaches are given the requisite skills and are empowered to attend to the team's needs on a day-to-day basis and are not reliant on external personnel in facilitating behavioral change.

In summary, a considerable amount of human behavior in sports settings occurs within groups of one kind or another, and in light of the fact that the psychological processes that occur within groups have been found to predict important personal and group-level outcomes, the study of group dynamics in sports continues to represent a vibrant area of enquiry.

Mark R. Beauchamp and William L. Dunlop

See also Exercise Addiction/Overactivity Disorders; Imagery and Visualization; Psychological Aspects of Injury and Rehabilitation; Psychological Assessment in Sports; Psychology of the Young Athlete

Further Readings

Bandura A. Exercise of human agency through collective efficacy. *Curr Dir Psychol Sci.* 2000;9(3):75–78.

Carron AV, Colman MM, Wheeler J, Stevens D. Cohesion and performance in sport: a meta-analysis. *J Sport Exerc Psychol.* 2002;24(2):168–188.

Carron AV, Shapcott KM, Burke SM. Group cohesion in sport and exercise: past, present and future. In: Beauchamp MR, Eys MA, eds. *Group Dynamics in Exercise and Sport Psychology: Contemporary Themes.* London, UK: Routledge; 2008:117–139.

TEAM PHYSICIAN

The team physician occupies an important position in the public consciousness. News reports about injuries to specific players on sports teams inevitably include interviews with or references to the team physician. In fact, sports physicians—and then team physicians—have enjoyed a high-profile role throughout history.

Historical Perspective

Historians note that battle physicians in ancient times were deemed a necessity. Galen (131–201 CE), a Roman physician of Greek origin, is considered by many to be the epitome of sports medicine practitioners. His voluminous writings reveal that he performed anatomical research and studied physiology, neurology, and wound care. He was appointed physician to the gladiators and was a teacher and a private surgical practitioner. Galen's qualifications to care for athletes and nobles need to be emulated.

Even though there was a marked increase in basic scientific and biological knowledge over the next centuries, there does not appear to have been a similar increase in athletic care and injury reduction in the United States. One possible exception was Edward Hitchcock, MD, who as a school physician at Amherst College in 1854 introduced swimming and gymnastics, emphasized baseball and basketball, and penned a book on athletes and medicine. With the increased popularity of sports participation, the injury rate also escalated. Because severe and often career-ending injuries were occurring so numerously, Harvard University appointed an orthopedic team surgeon in 1890. Other large eastern schools soon followed with similar appointments.

In 1904, the Germans were the first to use the term *sports physician,* and then they proceeded to hold a sports physicians' congress in 1912. This impetus evolved into the Fédération Internationale de Médecine Sportive (FIMS; International Federation of Sports Medicine) in 1933, with the primary goal being to facilitate clinical and scientific research in cooperation with Olympic federations. In 1938, Augustus Thorndike, MD, published a monograph depicting his experiences and knowledge as a team surgeon. His writings, which included much of the scientific knowledge in sports medicine, served as a primary source of pertinent sports medicine information in the 1960s.

A distinct change in sports medicine care of the high school and college athlete occurred when Dr. Jack Hughston (1917–2004) developed team coverage in the early 1950s. He and his orthopedic group and trainers began to "cover" high school football games on Friday night and college games on Saturday. During the week, his crew visited colleges and schools, noted injuries, arranged rehabilitation, and helped decide return to practice and refer, if necessary, back to clinic. This entire program was enacted with the cooperation of the local physician, who was a specialist or generalist, to maintain rapport. This program was not readily accepted until approved by the Georgia State High School Coaches Association. Adjacent states quickly followed this system of sideline and midweek team coverage that persists nationwide to this writing.

In the period after World War II in the United States, there was an exuberance expressed in physical activity and the formation of team sports. Physicians returning home from active duty restarting or starting up a practice often were ushered into a position as a team physician. Most had no sports medical experience, but used good medical knowledge quite successfully. Predominantly, these physicians were generalists in the high school and junior college settings. In contrast, the larger colleges,

universities, and professional teams tended to select an orthopedist as the primary team physician. While this selection arrangement was transpiring, research and teaching organizations came on the scene such as the American College of Sports Medicine (ACSM), American Orthopaedic Society for Sports Medicine (AOSSM), American Medical Society for Sports Medicine (AMSSM), and the National Athletic Trainers' Association (NATA). Of even greater significance to the practice of sports medicine was the establishment of orthopedic and general sports medicine fellowships. These board-eligible candidates were elected to take an additional year of specialized, sport-centered training under qualified individuals. These mentors used current therapy and ancillary techniques, the most salient of which was the development of the Watanabe arthroscope. This instrument revolutionized the practice of orthopedics and initiated visual understanding of injuries to the knee, shoulder, and elbow.

Even after a fellowship at an accredited institution and after the formal academic process is completed, there are major concerns that must be addressed prior to undertaking the position of a sports medicine physician. No less than for Galen in the ancient world, the essence of practice for Dr. Don O'Donoghue (1917–2004), often referred to as the father of modern sports medicine, was the skillful restoration of the injured patient back to participation status as expeditiously as possible. Times, therapy techniques, and teachings have changed, and certain personal and professional criteria have evolved for both orthopedic and medical sports physicians to contemplate and emulate.

General Criteria

Optimally, to embark successfully into the field of sports medicine as a physician, certain attributes are mandatory. Personal integrity, the athlete's welfare, and the sanctity of the doctor-patient relationship are paramount. Love of sports necessitates considerable time spent at games, practices, and examinations and in the consulting room, so family interaction needs to be facilitated. To function well, the team doctor must possess a working knowledge of a broad range of medical and orthopedic topics and the confidence to make accurate decisions. The measure of a solid team physician is being adept at diagnosing accurately a case of appendicitis as well as an anterior cruciate ligament (ACL) deficiency.

It is imperative that the team physician formulate a program to maintain official standings in state and local academic boards and societies. The physician should join and participate in scientific organizations, cooperate in research protocols, keep abreast of current literature and techniques, and attend sports medicine–related courses and seminars. Since the implementation of Title IX (1974), the team physician must become proficient in caring for the female athlete. Another one of the many important relationships that need to be fostered by the doctor is camaraderie with the head trainer and the staff. Mutual trust and true friendships are to be cultivated.

Another important entity in forming a sound musculoskeletal performance base is the experienced physical therapist. This person needs to be trained in rehabilitation techniques, should be compliant with the wishes of the head trainer and medical personnel, and yet be skilled enough to judge the capacity of the athlete to return to full activity.

The role of the strength coach is integral to this functional group. This person is responsible for personal and team strength improvement and must be certified in the profession. He or she, therefore, knows sports and is capable of enhancing effective playing strength and reducing the risk of injury in the athletes. Strength coaches must respond to the position team coaches and develop programs accordingly.

The head coach of each sport and the subordinates constitute the foundational element in the operational unit that is responsible for caring for the athlete. In addition to mental and physical preparation of the athletes, the head coach determines each athlete's ability, judges what areas need to be improved, and integrates all within the practice schedule. His or her interaction with the players is as important as daily meetings with the other members of the foundational unit (team doctor, trainer, physical therapist, strength coach, and coaches). The coach must communicate freely with the athlete, set a mutual goal, and care for the well-being of the athlete. Additional members of this foundational unit may become involved as the level or caliber of the sport necessitates.

Sports Medicine Physician

Level I

Having complied with state and national stipulations of licensure and satisfactorily completed a sanctioned sports medicine fellowship as an MD or DO in orthopedic or general sports medicine, the team doctor enters into private practice alone or in a small multispecialty group and is legally advertised as a sports medicine physician. In the office, the physician cares for the injuries and illnesses of all caliber of athletes and gratefully accepts insurance. Soon, his or her positive successes bring in parents and then others. The local middle school seeks the doctor's services for all of its sports. When the high school officially recognizes this doctor, then truly he or she is a team physician. The new stipulation requires the team physician to become aligned with radiological, surgical, and medical specialists. To maintain an office practice, a nonwritten agreement with the school officials is mandatory. This official arrangement, which indicates the team physician's scheduled coverage of sports, preparticipation physical examinations, and relationship with high school personnel, is sealed with a handshake. At this stage of the doctor's career, he or she has become the team physician not only of that school but also of the entire area and its active population.

Level II

Officially, the doctor is offered the position of team physician to a fully accredited Division II college in his or her general area with at least 12 different teams. The verbal agreement, witnessed by notables, will allow the doctor to maintain his or her office sports medicine practice, and the school will provide a certified athletic trainer and an office in the school for his or her half-day doctor's visit. It is agreed that the trainer would prepare the athletic field and sidelines and have emergency equipment available. As the sports medicine physician, the doctor would carry a personal sideline kit that contains emergency paraphernalia, oral and injectable medications, the medical history of the players participating, and necessary home and emergency phone numbers. Also, he or she would provide sideline coverage for home football games. For away games, the physician would call his or her counterpart at the other school and secure backup coverage and obtain a hospital contact. The physician would reciprocate when that team plays at his or her school. This new relationship demands more commitment on the sports medicine physician's part. Procedures, routine and pre- and postgame schedules, handling of injuries, and explicit review of emergency protocols and documentation in keeping with National Collegiate Athletic Association (NCAA) rules and regulations are an absolute necessity. It behooves the physician to become a friend, companion, and confidant of the trainer in order to outline rehabilitation and help determine return to play, as well as to be the liaison between coaches, school officials, and parents. When friendship is firmly established, the trainer knows the athletes, their personalities, and their demeanor and is more apt to be aware of abnormal behavior or activity. As noted previously in Level I, establishing consultants in many specialties is deemed necessary in referrals, for preparticipation examinations, and especially with drug testing screening. Any specific problem that is beyond the physician's orthopedic or general medical expertise often requires the athlete, with his or her records, to be examined off campus. Hence, it is an absolute necessity to establish contacts with specialists early in the practice of sports medicine.

Level III

The sports medicine physician accepts a salaried appointment to the state university that holds a membership in a Division I conference. There are eight men's and women's teams with a playoff in each to determine the bowl candidate. Academically, the physician's rank equals that of a full professor and entails comparable perks, including health insurance and prestige, but his or her take-home pay is noticeably less than in office practice. Yet he or she does not have any office expenses since the university provides a fully supplied office, medicines, and travel expenses and allows for state and national license fees. Personal malpractice insurance premiums may be covered in the universities' umbrella policy. Athletic trainers function efficiently as office nurses. Computer and record-keeping facilities are provided and maintained. Since the physician has gratefully experienced and pleasantly succeeded in a sports medicine practice

and upheld its qualifications and definitions, this change of venue appears quite inviting to him or her and his or her family.

As in any successful office practice, many functional details persist. An amicable relationship between the trainer, student trainers, physical therapists, and the athlete is mandatory. Duties allocated to the staff with regard to equipment and supplies must be supervised. As in routine office practice, the well-being of the athlete is paramount and requires perfected communication with the individual, parents, and coaches. Previous experience in severe musculoskeletal injuries, surgical cases, diabetic problems, infections, and rashes needs to be supplemented by referrals to competent physicians. On the other hand, newer obligations are to be undertaken. The proper techniques, rules and regulations, and probable injury patterns in each sport must become firsthand knowledge. Why don't women lacrosse players wear masks as men lacrosse players are required to wear? Is the skin eruption on the wrestler similar to that seen on the women gymnast from a floor mat? These and similar problems provoke serious contemplation and research.

The sports medicine physician is indeed fortunate to have an accredited curriculum of athletic training at this university, where athletic training fundamentals are taught and meshed with practiced applications. After the senior year, the student athletic trainer is properly prepared to pass the written, practical, and now computer examinations of the NATA. He or she is obligated to teach this curriculum and partner with the designated department head to determine the course content. These endeavors supplement the one-on-one demonstrations of the diagnostic maneuvers used in musculoskeletal injuries.

A typical week begins with sick call for those athletes who are unable to attend class or those in for recheck to determine their level of function. The history is obtained and documented in the chart by the head trainer. The sports medicine physician's physical examination clarifies the diagnosis and determines the disposition, such as to continue medications and return to class, to arrange for care in the infirmary, or to send to the hospital. In each instance, coaches and parents need to be informed. Parental permission is previously obtained and signed with the athletic department's full documentation on the NCAA identification of eligibility.

Follow-up evaluation of postsurgical care and games/practice injuries is conducted with input from the head trainer, physical therapists, and surgeons. The progress of the rehabilitation protocol is documented, and the coaches are informed. The ultimate outcome of the athlete's situation must be determined— whether he or she is able to return to sports or is to be disqualified for the season, or possibly to file for a "red-shirt" exemption. Orthopedic consultation is obligatory and is welcomed in musculoskeletal problems.

Before the hospital rounds, in consultation with the hospital-based physicians and nurses, the X-rays, computed tomography scans, electrocardiograms, and magnetic resonance imaging scans are reviewed and discussed as a teaching element with the trainers, physical therapist, and staff. This endeavor requires maintaining high-level expertise in radiological disciplines.

Afternoons in season are spent at football practice with the head trainer and his or her staff. The sideline material necessary for routine care of injuries is evaluated, the emergency setup with transportation is alerted and kept in readiness, cell phones are charged, and pertinent numbers are placed in the pockets of trainers. Personnel assignments for the practice are dispensed in concert with the published itinerary for the sanctioned practice. While conversing with the coaches, athletes are scrutinized as to characteristic walk and run, the knowledge of which will be profitable later when returning from injury or surgery. Dehydration, fatigue, and cramps should be urgently treated. Injuries are triaged as to disposition— either to the training room or to the hospital. Those not needing special procedures or consultation are evaluated and tested, and rehabilitation is instituted on the sideline.

Travel with the football team to all away games and to the championships of other sports, when requested by the president of the university, requires considerable preparation with the coaches, trainers, and staff. Consultation and cooperation with the home institution, its facility staff, their physicians, and the hospital for referrals when necessary is the obligation of the team physician. Travel sideline preparations are under the domain of the head trainer but are ratified by the team physician. There is close contact with the players, staff, and medical personnel, so that potential problems can be alleviated early. Team meetings, dining, recreational activities, and bedtime checks all are included in the team physician's itinerary. Occasionally, a member of the traveling academic staff, the athlete's parent, or an eminent supporter may require a visit from the team physician at an inopportune time.

Pregame or practice at home and away involves consideration of each player for play ability, proper taping and protective gear, dehydration prevention, and the issue of medication orally or by injection.

Before spring practice, coordination of and participation in preparticipation screening examinations are absolutely necessary. Usually performed at multiple stations, these screening examinations require many physicians, nurses, trainers, and secretary personnel to record basic information and to review parental signed history forms, as well as technicians to perform blood pressure, visual acuity, and special blood and urine tests. The NCAA manual requires an initial thorough history and an examination that includes cardiovascular and orthopedic evaluations and referral when deemed necessary. Annually, an appraisal of the athletes' records is made, a pertinent history is obtained, and new problems are addressed. A yearly, formal, complete physical exam is not required by the NCAA. Some programs in Division I do obtain more elaborate yearly evaluations.

Recently, it has become a policy for universities to perform an exit evaluation of all athletes, which elaborates the significant medical and surgical history and the final appraisal by the medical and orthopedic team physicians. In the form of a legal document, the head trainer, the team physicians, and the athlete sign a statement indicating the condition of the athlete at the completion of eligibility. Such documentation relieves the university of inappropriate and costly future repercussions.

It is quite common for universities to have high school outreach programs in which trainers and physicians actually attend games of contact sports, as well as hold intraweek injury evaluations. A group of these high schools with established relationships with the university often request assistance in their preparticipation evaluations. As with the university preparticipation examination, a convenient time and location at the university are used. At a scheduled time, a busload of high school athletes with previously signed permission and histories are processed in compliance with the university protocol. The aim of the examination is to enhance medical awareness, determine cardiovascular or medically abnormal conditions, and initiate solutions so that the young athlete can safely continue in the program. Significant findings that require disqualification are documented, the teacher/coach and the patient are informed immediately, and written suggestions are given for a physician's follow-up.

Unfortunately, the perils of narcotics and other banned substances in society permeate into athletics in the university setting. In-house testing of each team is done under the supervision of the team physician. Positive results require evaluation by a certified counselor. In an attempt to obviate this dangerous situation, the NCAA requires each student-athlete to attend talks concerning drug education and the pitfalls of using illegal and forbidden substances.

An ancillary, but extremely important, role for the team physician is related to the weight of the individual athlete. Certain sports require maintaining bulk and strength, while others demand a trim physique. Each athlete needs to be monitored in keeping with the position coach's and the athlete's personal goals. Unauthorized supplements of unknown content taken to gain weight may lead to abnormal symptoms. Excessive weight loss may be indicative of anorexia nervosa or bulimia and may result in myriad physical and mental complications. Initially, private consultation with the athlete may be helpful, but often referrals are indicated. The physician needs to eat in the student cafeteria or its equivalent frequently and notice the display, kind, and array of foods, as well as what foods are usually eaten by the athletes. A working friendship with the school dietitian or the food supervisor may facilitate alteration in the menu and variety. Control of eating problems, as suggested by the team physician and enforced by the head coach's orders, is partially enhanced by making breakfast mandatory for the teams in season.

In the university setting, the woman athlete presents a diverse array of circumstances for the team physician to contemplate. By nature, a woman is hyperelastic in essentially all her joints. With regard to the glenohumeral joint, she may subluxate and spontaneously relocate with minimal labral pathology. Unfortunately, her shoulder subluxation may become recurrent just with walking down the stairs. Rehabilitation may not be completely successful, and subsequently, either open or arthroscopically assisted tightening, because of the texture of the rotator cuff, may be less than optimal even with an appropriate surgical technique.

Hyperelasticity allows women gymnasts to perform outstanding maneuvers that are enjoyed by spectators. However, their popularity leads them to attempt more difficult routines. School and conference competitions encourage more recklessness and higher pyramids. Falls produce bizarre injuries, fractures, and central nervous system mishaps.

The woman athlete, because of a lower center of gravity, anteversion of the hips, and a large quadriceps angle while being quadriceps dominant and with tibial torsion, tends to land after jumping with knees adducted and the trunk upright. This sequence of events may produce patellofemoral symptoms, shin splints, or avulsion of the ACL from its attachment to the femur. Research has shown that with torso (core) strengthening, learning to land bent forward, and better leg muscle control, the incidence of ACL tears can be reduced significantly. It is the team physician's obligation to institute these preventative methods into the training program.

In the era of the resurgence of good health through fitness and sports activity, the team physician must be acutely aware that extremes invariably tend to be manifest and moderation becomes socially unacceptable. The philosophy of being the best in any endeavor and winning at any cost becomes a way of life, initially brought about by the use of performance-enhancing drugs. Drug testing has partially alleviated this problem, but even more sinister elements prevail. The ideology of perfection permeates players, coaches, administrators, and almost all parents. To gain an edge, youngsters are started at a young age to excel in one sport year-round. This methodology is encouraged by specialty coaches, tournament administrators, camps, and television and newspaper coverage. A family vacation may consist of watching one of their youngsters in a competition in another state. Emotionally, family life can suffer, as can musculoskeletal growth and maturation. There is a harmful fallacy that exists that to be bigger, stronger, and faster, as adult athletes are today, the young athlete must become one-dimensional. Forgotten are the facts of heritage, supervised good health, and medical care in infancy and childhood on which organized sports is grounded. Young teenage girls are also involved in this push to excel at a very tender age. The phenomenon is especially noted in gymnastics, cheerleading, racquet sports, swimming/diving, and ball sports. In young girls, overuse or abuse often results in shoulder pathology after repeatedly pitching windmill style for four games in a weekend tournament. Preteen boys who throw excessively at home and in games, even under recent guidelines, are at jeopardy, especially when trying to throw a curve ball instead of developing consistency and a changeup. Orthopedic sports medicine centers are evaluating more and more young boys with medial elbow pathology—formerly seen only in seasoned adult pitchers—that requires surgical intervention. Biomechanical studies have found that faulty mechanics with overpitching and throwing curves in the muscularly immature athlete favors the development of ulnar collateral ligament (UCL) weakness, followed by tearing. Reducing total pitch count in an inning, per game week, or at home is a significant measure in the prevention of painful elbow symptoms and UCL pathology.

Published guidelines for parents and coaches are standards to be adhered to with regard to pitch count totals for fast balls and changeups. Whether to use the skeletal or the clinical age to determine when to learn to throw the curve balls is a matter of controversy. One sage orthopedic team physician stated that optimally the best age for throwing the curve balls is when the athlete is old enough to shave. It behooves the sports medicine physician to vigorously encourage an educational program directed at parents, coaches, and school administrators that outlines the factors that must be ameliorated to reduce the incidences of premature medial elbow pathology.

Level IV

The orthopedic team physician, who has served as the primary orthopedic surgeon, director, and consultant to a Division I athletic department, maintains a specialty practice in a metropolitan setting, either in a multicentered hospital or in a building on the campus of the medical school. Because of clinical success, surgical prowess, and skill in treating professional athletes, recreational sports enthusiasts,

and others with shoulder, elbow, and knee musculoskeletal pathology, the surgeon's renown in sports circles has escalated. Continued success is due to the orthopedic team physician's proficiency in using the arthroscope and the greatly improved, accurate diagnostic capabilities with radiological interpretation. Intra-operative local and general anesthesia, control of postoperative pain, early mobilization, and a proficient rehabilitation unit are salient features of a successful orthopedic sports medicine practice. This entire entity is now delineated as a center. Soon the sports medicine center becomes identified in that geographic area with the principal orthopedist. In time, another center comes up, and competition for fellows and for identification with a prominent athletic program ensues.

Although the sports orthopedist has been trained by prominent orthopedists and is perfectly capable of performing essentially all musculoskeletal operations, he or she soon realizes the need for other specialists in the group whose interests are primarily hand, neck-back, foot-ankle, and general trauma.

Along with the rapid growth and popularity of sports activity in all ages, there evolved the need to determine the etiology of many of these musculoskeletal injuries. Hence, biomechanical facilities came of age. Initially, characteristic motions of elite athletes were filmed—for example, pitching, passing, and hitting a golf ball. From this information, angles, vectors, and acceleration of joint motions were determined and used as basic information on which other athletes were judged for form variations that may need to be altered. The biomechanics laboratory plays a diagnostic role for the sports orthopedist as a marker to strive for in alteration of motion, if possible, or the level to attain after definitive surgery and rehabilitation.

In the United States, about the time orthopedic fellowships became operational, there was a spirited movement also to create general sports medical fellowships. These selected individuals were board-eligible from essentially all nonsurgical medical residency programs. Characteristically, each man or woman had a keen interest in sports, accepted the guidelines of conduct and regulations imposed by state and national organizations, and demonstrated practice of his or her basic specialty successfully.

Within the orthopedic sports medicine group, these generalists would continue to have a formal practice in their specialty in order to satisfy their board requirements while rotating in the clinic in association with orthopedic fellows who are under the supervision of the team orthopedists or the medical sports–trained counterpart. Orthopedic and general sports medicine fellows tend to complement each other socially and share each others' views, experiences, and knowledge.

In addition, while the orthopedic fellows are in the operating room, the medical sports fellows triage new patients, provide care to others who do not need to be seen orthopedically, follow those in rehabilitation, and make scheduled visits to assigned high schools or colleges. In most established orthopedic team physicians' offices, the preadmission physical examination is performed by outside internal medicine sources, so that the general sports medicine fellow usually is not primarily responsible for that duty.

Both orthopedic and general medicine fellows are given research projects to be completed, if possible, within the year. A formal presentation by each fellow is made to the entire staff and families, and monetary awards are given for excellence and merit. The completed research manuscripts must be designed to comply with the criteria outlined by the referred journals. Ancillary services provided by the orthopedic medical center for the fellows include a staffed library, available secretarial assistance, patients' history files, and available sports-oriented biomechanics. Each fellow is expected to report accurately and succinctly every patient contact, as well as the formal medical opinions expressed by the attending staff member.

Biweekly scientific seminars on assigned topics are delivered initially by fellows' clinical mentors and later by the fellows on specific subjects and on their research progress. Attendance is essential. Usually, monthly journal clubs are convened at a staff member's home or a comparable facility, where discussion of the assigned articles is led by the fellows' clinical mentors.

The fundamental aims of each fellow are to endeavor to increase general knowledge and to develop skills. Also, each must generate an awareness of sport injuries and their diagnoses, treatment, rehabilitation, and prevention. Learning and applying this information mutually results in confidence and accuracy of diagnosis.

Each sports medicine orthopedist or medical center develops a relationship with a school or university to cover that school's sports program. All fellows participate in preparticipation examinations. In addition, each fellow is assigned to a high school and a college team to visit weekly and attend football games. Because of the operating duties of the orthopedist fellows, much of this coverage falls on the general sports medicine fellows. Another practical learning session occurs in the special emergency room area for injury coverage on Friday nights after football games in the orthopedic center's locality. In season, players, cheerleaders, coaches, and officials are brought to a portion of the emergency room and initially examined by the team physician and the general sports medicine fellow, along with backup from the orthopedic fellow. Decisions are made, treatment is instituted, and rehabilitation is begun by the centers' assigned trainers, and office visits are scheduled.

The continued success of an orthopedic center potentially depends on referrals from schools that have established a sideline and midweek coverage relationship. Other noncovered schools and junior colleges in the surrounding area served by the orthopedic center may request preparticipation physical examinations. The general sports medicine fellows will use this experience profitably by suggesting care, treatment, and rehabilitation and arranging orthopedic consultations.

The orthopedic fellows, while in the operating room under expert tutelage, must avail themselves of the opportunities to improve their operative techniques, to visualize new surgical procedures, and to observe the proper postoperative care designed for that particular operation. Rounds of postsurgical patients are characterized by a blend of the previous experience of the fellows and that of the staff orthopedist. Absorption of this experience plus that gained on outpatient follow-up evaluation is essential. Initially, the fellow checks the chart, obtains the history, examines the surgical site, and then presents the information to the staff orthopedist. General sports medicine fellows who are rotating through the orthopedic service are often included in postsurgical, outpatient rounds. This exposure is priceless, fundamentally, but the interplay of both categories of fellows is bilaterally profitable at that time and also in the future when in practice.

Toward the end of this fellowship, the fellows prepare to make significant future plans. Some plans were begun back in residency and some after contacts when attending professional organizational meetings. A few are referred by staff personnel and pertain to specific situations. A very few fellows will sign a contract to go to a foreign country for a lucrative fee to help pay their education bills. It is noteworthy that most fellows going out into practice have not considered a short-term medical or orthopedic missionary trip. The vast majority of fellows already have engaged a lawyer to include certain aspects of insurance, coverage, promotions to partners, percentage of profits and overhead, and area of noncompetition. Family input into decisions is desired, and when this is lacking, it may lead to unhappiness and separation.

Level V

It is extremely rare for a fellow who has recently completed his or her fellowship to step into the position of head team physician of a professional team. Should the new partner be fortunate to come on board and learn that the senior orthopedic partner currently is firmly entrenched as team physician of a professional American football team, a wonderful opportunity ensues to learn what the senior partner has seen and experienced over the years! Equipment has improved, research has brought about rule changes, treatment is now scientifically based, and surgical procedures are more advanced. In recent years, the National Football League (NFL) has instituted a pre-affiliation screening of recently graduated college players for athletic ability, as well as for identifying orthopedic or medical problems. This evaluation process is called a "combine" because all the professional football teams' orthopedic team physicians are eligible to participate. Also, other team physician specialists' services are used when expert opinions are needed for unusual cardiac, pulmonary, psychological, hematological, neurological, and radiological situations.

By now, the professional team physician, the orthopedist, and the generalist have gained a broad base of experience outside their primary specialty. After a specific plan of action is determined for a specific entity, the player, the team, coaches, and agents must be informed and an agreement reached. The action must be recognized by code number for insurance purposes. The effectiveness of rehabilitation has to be determined to accurately predict

return to play. History of the players' dependability, substance participation, and psychological makeup may determine long-range surgical success. Follow-up arrangements with trainers and physiotherapists to use published protocols are mandatory.

It would be wise for the team physicians who aspire to a professional association to visit the U.S. Olympic training center in Colorado Springs, Colorado. Essentially, every Olympic sports federation trains there, so that contacts can be established and training facilities and methods critiqued. Each federation, although somewhat political in nature, benefits by engaging an enthusiastic and knowledgeable team physician. The experiences are rewarding and mutually beneficial.

In addition to the examples of the NFL and Olympic teams, there is an abundance of professional and semiprofessional sports teams in the United States and Europe whose longevity depends on the competence of their team physicians in routine preparticipation evaluations, treatment of orthopedic and medical situations, and preventative care. Also, professional companies of performers, such as the circus or a theatrical group, or entertainment troops depend on orthopedic and sports medicine coverage to maintain a rigorous schedule. In these instances, the orthopedist is the primary physician with a sports medical backup. In others, the reverse may be noted. Cooperation is paramount to successful interplay.

Industry uses fellowship-trained sports physicians to evaluate workers' abilities to perform certain physical tasks as well as to ascertain the merit of worker's compensation cases. Many large manufacturers provide the doctor with an office and staff support within the plant to determine applicants' capabilities with regard to job requirements, introduce new safety features, treat injuries and illnesses, determine the percentage of disability, and promote good health habits among employees. Problems do occur with lawyers and union officials when employment termination is needed.

Sports physicians, both orthopedists and medical generalists, at times are openly solicited by pharmaceutical corporations. These recruited physicians are extremely valuable in evaluating clinical trials, especially those related to musculoskeletal effects. Writing a prospectus or a protocol and developing clinical results for publication often reflect fellowship training and personal inclinations. Being engulfed in medicine and clinical outcomes is exciting and an adjunct to clinical practice. To those scientifically inclined, the application of stem cells in the treatment of ligamentous and tendinous pathology would be intriguing.

There are qualified sports physicians employed by international steamship lines not only to examine and care for the crew, but also to hold sick call in order to determine the extent of illness or injury and ascertain the need for removal from ship. Paramedical personnel are provided, and the ports of call are very interesting.

In summer, coaches tend to schedule sports camps for high school and college students at their own university or at a convenient site that is easily accessible. The camps may vary depending on the sport, level of expertise, and position. A full complement of coaches, therapists, trainers, and emergency personnel are housed on campus or at a hotel for a 7- to 10-day period. The qualified sports medicine physician, orthopedist, or generalist signs up or volunteers for previous or future gratuities and enjoys the change of venue and a vacation.

Before entering into a professional relationship as a qualified sport physician to an entity, group, or physical situation, considerable investigation, contemplation, and consultation with an attorney who is knowledgeable in that particular environment are required for the subsequent contract to be mutually gratifying.

James A. Whiteside

See also Fieldside Assessment and Triage; History of Sports Medicine; Legal Aspects of Sports Medicine; Running a Sports Medicine Practice

Further Readings

Appelboom T, Rouffin C, Fierens E. Sports and medicine in ancient Greece. *Am J Sports Med.* 1988;16(6): 594–596.

Dunn WR, George MS, Churchill L, Spindler KP. Ethics in sports medicine. *Am J Sports Med.* 2007;35(5): 840–844.

Jacobson KE. Jack C. Hughston, MD: orthopedist and pioneer of sports medicine. *Am J Sports Med.* 2004;32(8):1816–1817.

Jobe FW, Pink MM. The process of progress in medicine, in sports medicine, and in baseball medicine. *Am J Orthop.* 2007;36(6):298–302.

McBryde A, Barfield B. Sports medicine: the last 100 years. *South Med J.* 2006;99(7):790–791.

McKeag DB. Sports medicine: the times, they are a-changin.' *J Fam Pract.* 1991;33(6):573–574.

Peltier LF. The lineage of sports medicine. *Clin Orthop Relat Res.* 1987;(216):4–12.

Puffer JC. Sports medicine: the primary care perspective. *South Med J.* 2004;97(9):873–874.

Rich BS. "All physicians are not created equal." Understanding the educational background of the sports medicine physician. *J Athl Train.* 1993;28(2):177–179.

Silverstein CE. The profession sports team physician. *Md Med J.* 1996;45(8):683–685.

Smodlaka VN. Sports medicine in the world today. *JAMA.* 1968;205(11):762–763.

Snook GA. The father of sports medicine. *Am J Sports Med.* 1978;6(3):128–131.

Snook GA. The history of sports medicine: part 1. *Am J Sports Med.* 1984;12(4):252–254.

Steiner ME, Quigley DB, Wang F, Balint CR, Boland AL Jr. Team physicians in college athletes. *Am J Sports Med.* 2000;33(10):1545–1551.

Team physician consensus statement. *Am J Sports Med.* 2000;28(3):440–441.

Tipton CM. Sports medicine: a century of progress. *J Nutr.* 1997;127(5 suppl):878S–885S.

Warren RF. The professional team physician, 1984–present. *Pediatr Ann.* 2002;31(1):71–72.

Temperature and Humidity, Effects on Exercise

Different environmental conditions, such as temperature and humidity, affect exercise tolerance and capacity in many ways. It is important for athletes to maintain their body temperature at or near 98.6 °F. Environmental conditions, in particular air temperature and humidity, determine the rate at which heat is lost or gained for the exercising athlete.

The body is able to regulate core temperature within a narrow range and must be able to manage heat transfer by convection, conduction, or evaporation. When the outside temperature is cooler than an athlete's body temperature, heat will be lost from the skin to the environment through conduction. The rate at which this heat is lost will be determined by the temperature difference between the environment and the athlete's body. Continual replacement of the warmer air near the body by cooler air from the environment causes loss of heat from the body by means of convection. Convective heat loss is determined by the speed at which air flows across the body. Evaporation is the most effective way in which the body loses heat. However, with high humidity, sweat loss by evaporation is reduced.

At rest, athletes regulate their body temperature around 98.6 °F. Muscles produce more heat during exercise than at rest. The thermoregulation system of the body must compensate for this increase in heat production, and inability to do so could lead to hyperthermia. External factors such as extreme temperatures and humidity also contribute to the development of both hyperthermia and hypothermia.

Hypothermia

When environmental conditions are particularly cold, there is a risk that the athlete will lose heat faster than he or she can produce it. Under these conditions, the body may be unable to maintain a safe temperature, leading to *hypothermia*. Swimmers are particularly at risk because cold water is an excellent conductor of heat, approximately 30 times more effective than air, and the body may be unable to produce heat as rapidly as it is lost by conduction to the surrounding water.

Hypothermia Prevention

There is a high rate of heat production during exercise, but once an athlete stops exercising, this rate falls sharply, and the risk of hypothermia rises significantly. Wearing proper clothing and gear is important in preventing hypothermia. Air is a poor conductor of heat but makes a good insulator. In contrast, water is a very poor insulator but a great conductor; therefore, a thin layer of air trapped next to the skin by specialized clothing creates a layer of insulation, thereby lessening the likelihood of developing hypothermia.

Hypothermia Diagnosis and Treatment

Hypothermia can be diagnosed when an athlete has been exercising in a cold environment, his or her core temperature is low, and he or she has fatigue, disorientation, muscle weakness, or loss of coordination. The treatment of hypothermia begins with removal of the athlete from the cold environment and applying dry clothing and external heating methods, such as convective heat, hot water bottles in the groin and axilla, or heated intravenous fluids.

Hyperthermia

Hyperthermia is described as an increase in body temperature above the normal resting upper limit. Elevated body temperatures occur with exercise because athletes produce heat when exercising, and this exceeds the capacity of the hot environment to absorb that heat. The humidity of the air determines the extent to which heat can be transferred from the body to the environment in the form of sweat. Sweat evaporates from the skin surface, involving a phase change from liquid to gas, which cools the surface of the skin. However, as the humidity of the air rises, the efficiency of heat loss by evaporation falls, and the body may be unable to balance heat production and heat loss.

Hyperthermia Diagnosis and Treatment

The most important aspect of diagnosing heat illness is to recognize the early signs, before the athlete has progressed to the later stages of the illness. Evaluate the athlete's core temperature, amount of sweating, and thirst. If heat illness is suspected, a thorough musculoskeletal and neurologic examination should be performed, noting any confusion, dizziness, or nausea, as well as noting core temperature, all of which could lead to early diagnosis, treatment, and prevention of the progression of heat illness.

Heat cramps can be treated on the field, and once cramping has ceased, return to play is allowed after ensuring proper hydration and electrolyte supplementation. With heat exhaustion and heat stroke, the primary goal should be to return the athlete's core temperature to normal. Cooling the athlete should be the first and most important action taken. Different facilities will have different methods available, including immersion in cool water, misting fans, and cooling vests.

Hyperthermia Prevention

There are many steps that can be taken to reduce the chances of heat illness. Avoid exercising in the middle of the day, when temperature and humidity are at their highest; ensure appropriate fluid and electrolyte replacement; be aware of the signs and symptoms of heat illness; and act according to the limitations of one's body. Have sufficient cooling methods and appropriate fluids on the sidelines of games to ensure that if athletes begin to struggle with heat illness, proper treatments are available. It is also important to note that once an athlete has suffered from heat exhaustion or heat stroke, he or she is at risk for recurrence. Heat illnesses are avoidable if the proper precautions are taken and if the signs and symptoms of the earlier stages are recognized and treated appropriately.

Blake R. Boggess and Cameron Howes

See also Cramping; Heat Illness

Further Readings

Armstrong LE, Casa DJ, Millard-Stafford M, Moran DS, Pyne SW, Roberts WO. American College of Sports Medicine position stand. Exertional heat illness during training and competition. *Med Sci Sports Exerc.* 2007;39(3):556–572.

Binkley HM, Beckett J, Casa DJ, Kleiner DM, Plummer PE. National Athletic Trainers' Association Position Statement: exertional heat illnesses. *J Athl Train.* 2002;37(3):329–343.

Cheung SS, McLellan TM, Tenaglia S. The thermophysiology of uncompensable heat stress. Physiological manipulations and individual characteristics. *Sports Med.* 2000;29(5):329–359.

Smith JE. Cooling methods used in the treatment of exertional heat illness. *Br J Sports Med.* 2005;39(8):503–507.

Wexler RK. Evaluation and treatment of heat-related illnesses. *Am Fam Physician.* 2002;65(11):2307–2314.

TENDINITIS, TENDINOSIS

Tendons are vital components of the musculoskeletal system as they serve to attach the contractile units of the body (muscles) to the levers (bones). They are thereby responsible for the transmission of the forces required to produce movement. The cross-sectional areas of tendons are small in relation to their attached muscles, and therefore, the stress (force per unit area) they are exposed to is substantial during activity. It is perhaps no surprise, therefore, that they are subject to inflammatory and degenerative pathology. Tendon injuries are reported to account for up to 30% of all running-related injuries and can result in considerable morbidity lasting several months despite appropriate management.

Tendon Structure

Macroscopically healthy tendons are white in color and are found in a variety of forms, from rounded cords to flattened ribbons, depending on their function and anatomical site. Normal adult tendon fibers are composed predominantly of large Type I collagen fibrils (65–80% of the dry mass) arranged in a ropelike configuration with smaller amounts of Type III collagen, proteoglycans, and elastic fibers (2%). The predominant cells found within the tendon structure are tenocytes and tenoblasts (immature tenocytes), which account for 90% to 95% of the cell population. These cells lie between the collagen fibers along the long axis of the tendon. The remaining cells include chondrocytes at the tendon insertion sites, the synovial cells of the tendon sheath, and vascular cells. The endotenon, a thin retinacular structure, invests each tendon fiber. The epitenon surrounds the tendon and contains the vascular, lymphatic, and nerve supply and is in turn surrounded superficially by the paratenon. Synovial tendon sheaths, consisting of an outer fibrotic sheath and an inner synovial sheath, may be found in areas subject to increased mechanical stress, where efficient lubrication is required. The inner sheath produces synovial fluid by a process of ultrafiltration. At the myotendinous junction, the weakest point of the musculotendinous unit, collagen fibrils of the tendon insert into deep recesses formed by the myocytes of the associated muscle. The osteotendinous junction is composed of four zones (dense tendon zone, fibrocartilage, mineralized fibrocartilage, and bone). The blood supply of tendons originates from intrinsic systems at the myotendinous and osseotendinous junctions and an extrinsic system through the paratenon or synovial sheath.

Contrary to traditional beliefs, tendons are metabolically active. Tenocytes have a low metabolic rate and a well-developed anaerobic energy generation capacity that allows them to resist load and maintain tension for prolonged periods. Animal studies suggest that the physical properties of tendons (tensile strength, stiffness, collagen content, and cross-sectional area) are all enhanced with physical activity. Type I collagen synthesis in particular depends on overall protein synthesis and on tensile loading and is thought to occur in a nonuniform way throughout the tendon structure.

Pathophysiology

The relationship between *tendinosis* (degeneration without inflammation) and *tendinitis* (inflammation) is unclear. The terms are often used interchangeably, leading to confusion. The best generic descriptive term for clinical conditions arising in and around tendons is *tendinopathy*. The low metabolic rate that makes the cells of the tendon suitably adapted for their role in load bearing also, however, results in delayed healing following injury. Tendinopathies tend to occur with greater frequency in the older athlete, and it is perhaps not surprising that with increasing age the metabolic pathways of tenocytes shift from aerobic to more anaerobic energy production. In addition, tendon vascularity is compromised at the junctional zones between the intrinsic and extrinsic systems or where there is localized torsion, friction, or compression. A good example of this is seen in the Achilles tendon, where there is a zone of hypovascularity 2 to 7 centimeters (cm) proximal to the tendon insertion, a common site of rupture. It is important to note that tendon blood flow also decreases with increasing age and mechanical loading.

Tendinopathy

Despite the relative frequency of tendon overuse injuries in sports medicine practice, the etiology of tendinosis and tendinitis remain unclear. The processes are multifactorial but on a local level are thought to be one of accumulated trauma as a result of repetitive mechanical loading. Tenocyte damage may occur as a result of localized hypoxia or as a result of free radicals produced during reperfusion after relaxation, which may be compounded by hyperthermia within the tendon produced by repeated or prolonged bouts of exercise. On a macroscopic level, there may be a combination of intrinsic factors such as malalignment, inflexibility, and muscle weakness or imbalance. Biomechanical faults, in particular hyperpronation of the foot, are reported to play a causative role in two thirds of Achilles tendon disorders in athletes. These may be exacerbated by age-related degeneration and diminished vascular supply. Tendons loaded beyond their physiological threshold respond by inflammation of their sheath (synovitis/tendinitis), degeneration of their body (tendinosis), or a combination of the two processes. Macroscopically, the diseased tendons look gray-brown and amorphous, and they may be thickened. Histological examination of tendons in symptomatic patients reveals disordered healing and noninflammatory degeneration. The fibers are thin and disorganized with scattered vascular in-growth. Inflammatory lesions and granulation tissue are infrequent in the chronic situation. Pain may result from a number of mechanical and biomechanical factors. Chemical irritants implicated in the production of pain include glutamate and Substance P.

Sites

Common sites of tendinopathies include the ankle (Achilles tendon/tibialis posterior), knee (patellar tendon), shoulder (supraspinatus tendon/bicipital tendon), and elbow ("tennis" elbow/"golfer's" elbow).

Diagnosis

The diagnosis of tendinopathy or tendinitis depends on the acquisition of a detailed history and a thorough examination. The patient generally complains of pain on loading the affected structure. There has often been a change in the frequency or intensity of activity prior to the onset of symptoms. Examination may reveal localized pain on deep palpation or thickening of the affected structure. Significant loss of function or the presence of a palpable defect should alert the examiner to the possibility of partial or complete tendon rupture. Magnetic resonance imaging (MRI) or ultrasound scanning with Doppler may be useful to identify changes within the tendon substance, including the increased blood flow associated with neovascularization.

Treatment

It is important at the outset to identify whether the problem is an acute episode with an inflammatory component or a chronic condition. Tendinopathies may require lengthy multimodal management, and patients often respond poorly to treatment. The mainstay of treatment is generally conservative. As in most conditions, the keystone of successful treatment lies in the accurate assessment of the factors contributing to the problem. These must then be systematically addressed during the treatment phase. Training patterns and the equipment used by the athlete should be assessed, preferably in conjunction with the coaching staff. Poor technique and "training errors" should be avoided, and where possible, biomechanical factors should be corrected. There is little convincing evidence for the use of nonsteroidal anti-inflammatory drugs (NSAIDs) in chronic tendinopathy, although they may be useful in the acute situation. It is important to recognize that in many sites, there is little evidence of a lasting benefit from the peritendinous injection of corticosteroids. If there is an inflammatory component such as a tenosynovitis or bursitis, these agents may be used to address any associated inflammation, and cautious use of locally applied ice may be helpful in providing pain relief. The degree of tendon loading that should be applied to promote healing is a matter of debate. Prolonged immobilization of tendons is detrimental, leading to tendon atrophy and reduced tensile strength. Controlled stretching is likely to increase collagen synthesis and improve the quality of the regenerate tendon.

Many physical therapies have been proposed for the treatment of tendinopathies, with little good-quality evidence for their efficacy. There is evidence from animal models of the usefulness of extracorporeal shock wave therapy (ESWT) in improving experimentally produced tendinopathy, but the results of clinical trials in humans are conflicting. Other treatments have included the use of pulsed magnetic fields, laser therapy, and radiofrequency coblation, again with variable results. There is good support for the use of an eccentric training program in short-term symptom relief in Achilles and patella tendinopathies. Other modalities used with conflicting evidence include dry needling, the image-guided injection of sclerosants, and the use of glyceryl trinitrate (GTN) patches. Surgical debridement of the macroscopically unhealthy tissue can be considered in cases resistant to other treatment modalities.

Future therapies may involve the use of cytokines and growth factors, gene transfer, or the implantation of mesenchymal stem cells to modify the healing environment.

Conclusion

The assessment and management of tendinopathies is one of the key skills required in the sports medicine practitioner. Further research and scientific evaluation of the available literature are required before evidence-based management protocols can be instituted.

Angus Robertson and William D. Stanish

See also Achilles Tendinitis; Patellar Tendinitis; Peroneal Tendinitis; Tendinopathy

Further Readings

Rompe JD, Furia J, Maffulli N. Eccentric loading compared with shock wave treatment for chronic insertional Achilles tendinopathy. A randomized, controlled trial. *J Bone Joint Surg Am.* 2008;90(1):52–61.

Sharma P, Maffulli N. Tendon injury and tendinopathy: healing and repair. *J Bone Joint Surg Am.* 2005;87(1):187–202.

Stanish WD, Curwin S, Mandel S. *Tendinitis: Its Etiology & Treatment.* Oxford, UK: Oxford University Press; 2000.

Visnes H, Bahr R. The evolution of eccentric training as treatment for patellar tendinopathy (jumper's knee): a critical review of exercise programmes. *Br J Sports Med.* 2007;41(4):217–223.

Woodley BL, Newsham-West RJ, Baxter GD. Chronic tendinopathy: effectiveness of eccentric exercise. *Br J Sports Med.* 2007;41(4):188–199.

TENDINOPATHY

Overuse or exercise-related tendon injuries are common in competitive and recreational athletes, as well as in manual laborers. *Tendinopathy*, the term used to describe an overuse tendon injury or disorder, usually presents as pain in the region of the involved tendon. Tendinopathy usually results from chronic repetitive overuse or subclinical injury rather than a single acute injury. Under the Bonar classification, tendinopathy includes tendinosis (degenerative change of the tendon), tendinitis (inflammation of the tendon) with tendinosis, paratenonitis (inflammation of the tendon outer covering), and tendinosis with paratenonitis (see Table 1). Some examples of common tendinopathies are listed in Table 2.

While there is some overlap in the symptoms and physical findings of patients with different causes of tendon pain, the patient's symptom history provides important clues to help in correctly diagnosing and treating the underlying tendon injury. In addition to guiding appropriate treatment, proper diagnosis also provides the ability to properly educate patients about the expected course of their tendon problem. One important clinical distinction in tendinopathy is between acute, inflammatory conditions (tendinitis, paratenonitis), and chronic, degenerative conditions (tendinosis). While inflammatory tendon conditions are usually self-limited and respond well to anti-inflammatory treatments, degenerative tendon changes, since they are usually chronic, typically require a more robust, long-term treatment plan focused on reversing the degenerative process. Furthermore, because inflammatory and degenerative conditions often coexist, both must be considered in developing an appropriate short- and long-term treatment plan.

Anatomy

Tendons are predominately Type I collagen, which consists of tropocollagen chains grouped in a triple helix arrangement. These triple helices are very closely grouped longitudinally in the tendon, with each level of organization being surrounded by an outer covering. The entire tendon is also surrounded by an external covering called the *paratenon*. In areas where tendons bend at acute angles (e.g., the flexor tendons of the fingers) over bone, the paratenon is usually thicker and lined with synovium, which not only provides mechanical resistance to shearing forces but also produces synovial fluid, lubricating the tendon to decrease frictional injury. This is also commonly referred to as the tendon sheath. It is in these areas that the inflammation can commonly occur, causing synovial fluid production and associated swelling (e.g., intersection syndrome). In the remaining tendon areas, the paratenon is thinner and not lined with synovium.

Causes

As mentioned previously, tendinopathy usually results from chronic overuse microtrauma to a tendon. The precise pathogenesis of tendinopathy is still unknown, but general causative mechanisms

Table I   Classification of Tendinopathies

Tendon Condition	Formerly Used Terms	Macroscopic Appearance/Pathology
Normal tendon		White, glistening, firm
Tendinosis	Tendinitis	Dull, slightly brown, soft; intratendinous degeneration
Tendinitis with tendinosis	Tendinitis	Intratendinous inflammation (repair response) superimposed on tendinosis
Paratenonitis	Tenosynovitis, tenovaginitis, peritendinitis	Inflammation of the outer tendon layer
Paratenonitis with tendinosis	Tendinitis	Combined degenerative changes of paratenonitis with degenerative changes of tendinosis

Table 2   Common Tendinopathies

Tendon	Paratenon Synovial Lining?	Common Tendinopathy
Rotator cuff tendons		
Supraspinatus	No	Supraspinatus tendinosis (due to subacromial impingement)
Infraspinatus	No	Rotator cuff tendinosis
Teres minor	No	Rotator cuff tendinosis
Subscapularis	No	Rotator cuff tendinosis
Biceps brachii	Yes (long head in intertubercular groove)	Biceps paratenonitis (long head), biceps tendinosis (long head) ± paratenonitis
Common wrist extensor	No	Medial epicondylosis
Common wrist flexor	No	Lateral epicondylosis
Flexor digitorum tendons (superficial and deep)	Yes (over carpal bones)	Flexor digitorum paratenonitis, Flexor digitorum tendinosis ± paratenonitis
Abductor pollicis longus (APL), Extensor pollicis brevis (EPB), Extensor carpi radialis longus (ECRL), Extensor carpi radialis brevis (ECRB)	Yes (over carpal bones)	APL/EPB paratenonitis (de Quervain), APL/EPB/ECRL/ECRB paratenonitis (intersection syndrome)
Patella	No	Patellar tendinosis
Achilles	No	Achilles tendinosis
Posterior tibialis	Yes	Posterior tibialis paratenonitis, Posterior tibialis tendinosis ± paratenonitis

are becoming more clearly understood. Other than paratenonitis, all other categories of tendinopathy have a component of tendinosis or degenerative tendon changes. It is now understood that these changes can occur as early as 3 weeks after the start of the overuse injury.

While general aging and tendon underuse can contribute to degenerative tendon changes, most tendinopathy is caused by any combination of excessive repetition, anatomic abnormality (e.g., limb length discrepancy), malalignment (e.g., hyperpronation), muscle imbalance or weakness, improper technique, improper equipment, and

incomplete recovery after overuse. These etiologies hold true for competitive and recreational athletes as well as for recreational and vocational laborers.

Clinical Evaluation

History

While a patient complaint of pain over a tendon clearly causes one to consider tendinopathy, the clinical history is very important in helping distinguish among the types of tendinopathy. A patient with only paratenonitis will usually complain of a recent increase in his or her activity level or intensity, such as a soccer athlete with ankle hyperpronation who complains of posterior tibialis pain and swelling 1 week after starting preseason conditioning. Of note, pain from paratenonitis will usually be constant and proportional to activity level.

A patient with tendinosis will usually have a prior history of overuse, such as playing competitive tennis in a patient with supraspinatus tendinosis or playing competitive basketball in a patient with patellar tendinosis. Furthermore, tendon pain from tendinosis will typically start during the warm-up phase and, in less advanced disease, decrease during activity and increase during the warm-down and recovery phases. Additionally, pain from tendinosis is usually sharp and more intense early and becomes duller and more achy later in the disease process.

In the evaluation of tendon pain, it is also important to rule out other causes of the patient's pain. Most patients with tendinopathy should not have associated paresthesia, weakness, radiation of pain, blunt trauma, fever, and overlying skin changes. Furthermore, pain from tendinopathy should not persist with relative rest and should not cause night symptoms.

Physical Examination

Physical examination is useful to distinguish inflammatory from noninflammatory tendinopathy. Patients with tendinopathy will have pain with palpation of a tendon under strain using manual muscle testing. As with most inflammatory conditions, patients with paratenonitis or tendinitis complicating tendinosis will often have associated swelling and increased temperature over the affected area of the tendon. Additionally, patients with these conditions can have crepitus with passive joint range of motion, moving the tendon back and forth.

Imaging

Clinical assessment is usually sufficient for the diagnosis and classification of tendinopathy. However, magnetic resonance imaging (MRI) and ultrasound can be helpful adjuncts in assessing tendinopathy. Areas of tendinosis will be most visible as hypoechoic regions on an ultrasound scan and increased signal on T2 and STIR (short T1 inversion recovery) sequences on an MRI scan.

However, imaging can also complicate the clinical picture because a high percentage of asymptomatic patients can have evidence of tendinosis on imaging, especially of the rotator cuff in older patients.

Treatment

The mainstay of tendinopathy treatment has been conservative therapy relying on relative rest, ice, and nonsteroidal anti-inflammatory medications (NSAIDs). While modalities to decrease inflammation, such as steroid anti-inflammatory medications (either local or systemic), may be of benefit in proven cases of paratenonitis or tendinitis complicating tendinosis, these medications do not treat the underlying pathology of tendinosis when present. Furthermore, because NSAIDs mostly have analgesic properties, if not coupled with reversal of the causative factors and relative rest, further injury may ensue.

The most widely accepted treatment modality for reforming degenerative tendon has been eccentric muscle strengthening of the affected muscle-tendon unit. There has been some suggestion that eccentric strengthening following soft tissue mobilization has further benefit, but this has not been borne out in the literature. Some other treatment modalities, such as topical nitric oxide and shock wave therapy, have been used but still remain experimental.

In rare cases of tendinosis that do not respond to a prolonged course of conservative treatment options, surgical treatment to remove a section of degenerative tendon may be indicated. Athletes must understand that surgery will not hasten their return to sports and often will guarantee a 6- to 12-month hiatus from full competition.

The most important part of any treatment plan for tendinopathy includes correction of the underlying cause. If the patient has a muscular insufficiency or imbalance, proper identification and physical therapy are essential. If errors in technique or training schedules are identified and corrected as part of the treatment, the patient will often see long-term benefit.

Conclusion

Tendinopathy is a common condition affecting athletes, resulting from overuse injury to the tendon.

Inflammatory conditions of the tendon do occur but predominately involve inflammation of the outer covering of the tendon, or paratenon. More commonly, patients have underlying tendon degeneration, or tendinosis. These patients require a robust treatment plan, including eccentric strengthening exercises and correction of modifiable risk factors, such as muscle imbalances and training errors.

Jeffrey D. Smithers

See also Tendinitis, Tendinosis

Further Readings

Fredberg U, Stengaard-Pedersen K. Chronic tendinopathy tissue pathology, pain mechanisms, and etiology with a special focus on inflammation. *Scand J Med Sci Sports.* 2008;18(1):3–15.

Khan KM, Cook JL. The painful non-ruptured tendon: clinical aspects. *Clin Sports Med.* 2003;22(4): 711–725.

Khan KM, Cook JL, Bonar F, et al. Histopathology of common tendinopathies. Update and implications for clinical management. *Sports Med.* 1999;27(6): 393–408.

Maffulli N, Wong J, Almekinders LC. Types and epidemiology of tendinopathy. *Clin Sports Med.* 2003;22(4):675–692.

Perugia L, Postacchini F, Ippolito E. *The Tendons. Biology, Pathology, Clinical Aspects.* Milan, Italy: Editrice Kurtis; 1986.

Riley G. Tendinopathy—from basic science to treatment. *Nat Clin Pract Rheumatol.* 2008;4(2):82–89.

TENNIS AND RACQUET SPORTS, INJURIES IN

Injuries are common in players of racquet sports. A retrospective analysis of sports injuries in 2000 showed squash injuries to be more frequent than tennis and badminton injuries, with more men injured overall than women and with persons over age 25 more vulnerable to injuries. The higher proportion of squash injuries were attributed to greater physical stress and more contact. Acute traumatic injuries were seen especially in squash players, most often affecting the knee,

lumbar region, and ankle. The most common tennis injuries were lateral epicondylitis, patellofemoral pain, and lumbar disk prolapse. The badminton injury pattern overlapped the others. Lower limb injuries predominated in all racquet sports. Detailed assessment of 106 cases showed many to be new, infrequent, social players. Poor warm-up was a common factor in both new and established players.

Typically, injuries in racquet sports are overuse injuries. These result from repetitive stresses and minor traumatic events, such as the effect on the shoulder of serving thousands of times or the influence on the knee of playing hundreds of points with pivots, twist, and aggressive stops and starts.

Tennis injuries may be categorized as either acute or chronic. *Acute injury* describes a new injury or complaint from the time it occurs and for the short time following the start of injury (e.g., ankle sprain). A *chronic injury* typically recurs or repeats itself due to continued tennis play or lack of proper rehabilitation (e.g., tennis elbow).

Among elite junior tennis players, injuries in descending order of frequency were as follows: back, 24%; shoulder, 21%; foot, 19%; knee, 15%; elbow, 12%; and ankle, 12%.

Head Injury

Although head injuries are uncommon in tennis, they sometimes occur, particularly in doubles play, where the bodies or racquets of two partners may come into contact.

Bruises and Cuts

Bruises are usually caused by being hit by the ball on a smash shot. It's more common in doubles play because the player at the net has less time to react. Being hit by the partner's racquet may also cause a bruise.

Bruises can usually be treated by icing them to reduce swelling and control pain. If the skin is broken, it is cleaned with soap and water, and an antiseptic spray or cream may be applied. Nonsteroidal anti-inflammatory drugs (NSAIDs) may provide pain relief. If a blow causes loss of concussion or memory, or disorientation, the player should be seen promptly by a physician.

Broken Nose

A blow to the nose by a racquet or ball can fracture the nasal bones or injure the cartilage of the septum—the structure that separates the two nostrils.

Any nose suspected to be broken should be iced down to limit swelling and bruising. The athlete should be seen by a physician, and radiographs should be taken. Once fixed, the nose is usually protected with a splint until it heals completely, which can take 4 to 6 weeks.

Eye Injuries

Most eye injuries in racquet sports are caused by being struck in the eye with the ball or, rarely, a blow from a partner's racquet. Eye injuries may cause bleeding into the orbit and surrounding tissues, scratch the cornea, cause bleeding inside the eye, or even cause a detached retina. Any injury to the eye should be examined promptly by an ophthalmologist.

Blowout Fracture

A blow to the eye or cheek from the racquet can fracture the orbital bones surrounding the eyeball. As with any fracture, an athlete who suffers a suspected blowout fracture must see a physician for treatment, which may include surgery.

Neck Injury

Along with the head, the neck area is affected in many racquet sports injuries. The neck is tremendously mobile to allow the head to swivel, so the range of motion between the vertebrae in the neck is greater than in the lower spine.

Pinched Nerve

An injury that initially may seem like a sprain but is actually more complex is a pinched nerve; this happens when a cervical disk ruptures or degenerates.

Tennis players, who may make fairly violent neck motions, are prone to pinched nerves. The problem usually responds to some form of cervical traction (neck brace) for 2 to 6 weeks, with accompanying physical therapy to reduce muscle spasm.

However, if severe symptoms persist, particularly in the arm and the hand, surgery may be required to repair damage to the offending intervertebral disk.

Neck Muscle Injuries

Wryneck, or *spastic torticollis*, is due to a pulled muscle, or muscle spasm. The athlete who looks up and serves or hits an overhead smash may feel pain on one side of the neck, and the neck may be pulled over slightly to that side.

The proper treatment is to apply ice for 20 minutes at a time and gently stretch the neck. If the pain is severe, the athlete may need medication, such as a muscle relaxant or anti-inflammatory agent, and physical therapy.

Perhaps the best way to prevent neck injury is to strengthen the neck muscles. Every tennis player should work on improving neck strength. Basic exercises include applying resistance against oneself or by working with a partner.

Shoulder Injury

The shoulder is one of the most commonly injured joints among tennis players, particularly among junior elite players.

Rotator Cuff Injury

The *rotator cuff* is a group of muscles that work together to provide the shoulder joint with dynamic stability, helping to control the joint during rotation. The rotator cuff muscles include the supraspinatus, infraspinatus, teres minor, and subscapularis.

Due to the function of these muscles, sports that involve a lot of shoulder rotation—for example, tennis—often put the rotator cuff muscles under considerable stress. Rotator cuff injuries may range from an impingement to a complete tear. The impingement causes the nerves under the shoulder to fire and shoot pain down through the tendons of the shoulder into their connecting muscles. Tennis players feel the pain particularly in the long head of the biceps. Tennis players with this injury may be able to hit ground strokes effortlessly, but when they try to hit an overhead or serve, they experience shoulder pain.

Treatment for shoulder impingement may include a series of lifting and stretching exercises to strengthen the rotator cuff muscles and increase range of motion.

Shoulder Muscle Strain

A muscle strain can happen to almost any muscle in the body; the shoulder is particularly subject to such strains, or "pulls," which occur when a sudden, severe force is applied to the muscle and the fibers are stretched beyond their capacity. If only some of the fibers tear, it is called a muscle strain. If most of the fibers tear, it is called a muscle tear.

Common treatment for a muscle strain is a rest period, about 3 to 7 days, followed by stretching and then strengthening exercises.

Tennis Elbow

Lateral epicondylitis, or *tennis elbow*, is probably the most common of all upper extremity injuries in racquet sports. This term refers to the overuse injury resulting from repetitive trauma to the tendons that control wrist and forearm movement. Tennis elbow usually results from improper technique during backhands.

The single biggest factor in preventing tennis elbow is using a proper biomechanical tennis stroke technique. Rubber tubing exercises are used effectively to strengthen these muscles.

Treating tennis elbow requires an exercise program to increase the strength and flexibility of the forearm muscles and tendon.

Players with a history of tennis elbow or the athlete who feels elbow pain after play should wait at least half an hour after a match and then ice the elbow down, keeping the elbow cool for up to 30 to 40 minutes.

Grip size of the tennis racquet is important. The correct grip size is the distance from the proximal transverse palmar crease to the tip of the ring finger. An appropriate brace or splint for the forearm, applied distally to the elbow, is believed to dampen some of the shock that contributes to epicondylitis. Adequate warm-up, muscle stretching, and cooldown are always advisable. A physiological heat retainer may also be very useful and should be worn as often as possible.

Formerly, the standard treatment for tennis elbow was local cortisone injection. This form of therapy is no longer in wide use, especially as long-term treatment, because of reports of cortisone injections causing irreparable damage to the tendon.

Another type of tennis elbow causes pain on the inner side of the elbow (the medial epicondyle). This pain involves inflammation of the muscles and tendon that the palm faces down. Prevention and treatment measures are the same as for the first type of tennis elbow.

Torn Biceps

A sudden, severe movement of the arm can tear the biceps muscle. One head of the biceps can be literally torn in half. This is usually seen in an older tennis player who hits a hard forehand smash.

Treatment involves allowing the torn muscle to rest for 2 or 3 weeks while it heals. This is followed by a training program to strengthen the other head of the biceps so that it can take over the full function of the muscle. Arm curls are the best exercise to strengthen the biceps muscle.

Wrist Injuries

Racquetball and squash especially require a snapping motion of the wrist. Thus, the tendons and ligaments of the wrist are frequently injured.

Sprained Wrist

The most common injury to the wrist is a sprain. Strength and flexibility exercise of the muscles that cross the wrist helps protect the wrist and the ligaments that keep the wrist together.

Broken Wrist

A wrist usually fractures from a fall. Any severe wrist pain following a fall or a blow to wrist should be seen by a physician and X-rayed because of the possibility of fracture.

If the bone does not reknit, it probably will need to be fixed surgically.

Racquet Wrist

Tennis players may develop pain at the base of the hand, below the pinky finger. This usually occurs because the racquet butt is too large for the player's hand.

If the pain is severe, the athlete should see a physician. The little hook of bone at this location might be broken. If it is, then it will need to be treated as a fracture.

Tendinopathy

Overuse of the wrist in sports causes irritation of the finger tendons attached to these forearm muscles. This results in swelling, pain, and limited function in one or more of the fingers.

Treatment involves resting and icing the tendon in the wrist, followed by taking anti-inflammatory agents and immobilizing the thumb and wrist to reduce the inflammation. Appropriate strengthening exercises (e.g., ball squeezing) may be prescribed.

Carpal Tunnel Syndrome

Carpal tunnel syndrome is a painful disorder of the wrist and hand. The carpal tunnel is a narrow structure formed by the bones and other tissues of the wrist. This tunnel protects the median nerve, which gives feeling in the thumb, index, middle, and ring fingers. When surrounding tissues, such as ligaments and tendons, become swollen or inflamed, they press against the median nerve, causing pain or numbness. Anyone who tightly grips something while exercising, such as a tennis racquet, may suffer carpal tunnel syndrome.

The treatment is to rest the affected wrist and apply ice. In some cases, surgery is needed for relief of symptoms. Postoperatively, physical therapy with wrist and finger exercises is important to ensure good recovery and return to full function.

Arm Injuries

How equipment is used can affect the athlete's arm. String tension of the racquet is one important factor. Decreasing the racquet's string tension by a few (2–4) pounds (lb; 1 lb = 0.45 kilograms) is recommended for players who are experiencing shoulder, elbow, or wrist pain.

Research suggests that vibration dampeners have no affect on the arm itself; these dampeners do affect high-frequency vibration, such as that coming off the strings.

Knee Injuries

Knee injuries may occur in any racquet sport, but they are of particular concern in racquetball and squash, in which nearly every type of knee injury can occur.

Patellar pain syndrome may be the most frequently encountered condition in persons playing racquetball or squash. The syndrome usually has an insidious onset and is characterized by dull, aching, poorly localized pain that occasionally radiates to the sides and back of the knee. Initially, patellar pain syndrome occurs after activity; however, it can worsen to the extent that the knee is painful throughout the day. Swelling is rare.

Tennis obviously places a great deal of stress on the knee joint from bending, quick starts and stops, and explosive acceleration. Because tennis is a noncontact sport, the bone-crushing knee injuries we equate with football or skiing are not prevalent. With repeated stress to the legs, such as tennis play, and without sufficient strength and endurance of the thigh muscles, the kneecap can become irritated. This repeated irritation can wear down the back side of the kneecap and produce significant pain.

Preventing knee injuries in tennis focuses on two strategies: Strength and flexibility exercises, with proper biomechanics, form the platform for an injury prevention program.

Ankle and Foot Injuries

Acute ankle sprains are another of the most frequent injuries in racquetball and squash players. Most sprains are first degree and are treated in the usual fashion. Ice and elevation, combined with graded exercises, are recommended. Some trainers recommend extra support for the first 6 weeks after play is resumed.

Achilles tendon problems are also frequently encountered. Chronic Achilles tendinitis is characterized by gradually increasing pain that is aggravated by activity and relieved by rest. Rest is most important in the treatment of acute injury. Once pain subsides, gradual stretching of the tendon, along with calf strengthening, should be done.

Less common, and most dreaded, is rupture of the Achilles tendon. Usually, the player is trying to push back from a drop shot at the front of the court and hears a sudden snap, followed by immediate pain. In the Thompson "squeeze" test, the patient lies prone, and the examiner squeezes the calf muscle. An intact Achilles tendon will cause the foot to plantarflex, representing a negative test. The test is positive if this response is absent, due to a ruptured tendon. A tender, palpable swelling may be detected. Palpable or visible defects can also be found, although they may be obscured by bleeding. The patient walks flatfooted with a limp, not pushing off the toes. Treatment may be operative or nonoperative, and the decision is best left to an orthopedic surgeon.

The most common foot problems are related to blisters and calluses. Traditional treatment of blisters includes releasing the fluid, thereby allowing the underlying skin to harden. Some physicians prefer not to drain blisters, so as to avoid creating a portal for possible infection. If the patient wishes to continue playing while the blister heals, a small, doughnut-shaped dressing can alleviate pressure to allow healing. To prevent underlying blister formation, calluses should be smoothed with an emery board or pumice stone.

Plantar fasciitis is the most commonly seen orthopedic condition of the foot in racquet sports enthusiasts. It is characterized by pain at the medial tubercle of the os calcis, where the plantar fascia attaches. The pain may also radiate distally toward the toes or, more commonly, proximally. Most patients complain of pain that begins as they get out of bed, subsides after walking, and recurs later in the day or during a game. Shortening the amount of time spent playing racquet sports or ceasing play altogether is most helpful. This decrease in activity should be followed by the use of orthotics, heel cups, or corrective athletic shoes with good midfoot support.

Asuman Sahan

See also Achilles Tendinitis; Rotator Cuff Tears, Partial; Rotator Cuff Tendinopathy

Further Readings

Bloomfield J, Fricker PA, Fitch KD, eds. *Science and Medicine in Sport*. Oxford, UK: Blackwell; 1992.
Chard MD, Lachmann SM. Racquet sports—patterns of injury presenting to a sports injury clinic. *Br J Sports Med*. 1987;21(4):150–153.
Frontera WR, Herring SA, Micheli LJ, Silver JK. *Clinical Sports Medicine*. Philadelphia, PA: Saunders Elsevier; 2007.
Levy AM, Fuerst ML. *Tennis Injury Handbook*. New York, NY: John Wiley; 1999.
Roetert P, Ellenbecker TS. *Complete Conditioning for Tennis*. Champaign, IL: Human Kinetics; 1998.
Shultz SJ, Houglum PA, Perrin DH. *Assessment of Athletic Injuries*. Champaign, IL: Human Kinetics; 2000.

TENNIS ELBOW

Tennis elbow, or *lateral epicondylitis*, is characterized by pain at the lateral (outer) aspect of the elbow. The patient may also complain of tenderness on palpation of the area of concern, usually the dominant arm. This entity was first described in a scientific article in 1873, and since that time, the mechanism of injury, pathophysiology, and treatment of this condition have been much debated.

The disorder is due to overuse of the extensor carpi radialis brevis (ECRB) muscle, which originates at the lateral epicondylar region of the distal humerus. Tennis elbow can also be classified as *tendinitis*, indicating inflammation of the tendon, or *tendinosis*, indicating tissue damage to the tendon.

The most common cause of lateral epicondylitis is, as the common name suggests, tennis. It is estimated that tennis elbow occurs in 50% of tennis players. However, this condition is caused not only by tennis but also by any activity associated with repetitive extension (bending back) of the wrist. The activity initiates contraction of the muscles that cause the hand to extend (bend back). There is a significant increased risk of overuse injury if playing for more than 2 hours/week and more than two to four times per week. In players older than 40 years, the risk increases two- to threefold. Significant risk factors have been identified and include improper technique and the size and weight of the racquet.

Anatomy and Mechanism of Injury

To understand the mechanism of injury of this condition, knowledge of some basic anatomy of the elbow is helpful. The elbow is a hinge joint—a junction between two bones primarily connected to each other by ligaments and tendons from the muscles near the humerus. The humerus is a long bone originating from the shoulder and extending to the elbow. It has two bumps called *epicondyles*—one on the medial (closest to the body) side and one on the lateral (farthest from the body) side. The radius and ulna are the bones in the forearm. The tendon (connecting tissue) at the medial epicondyle attaches to a muscle that causes the forearm and wrist to bend forward. Similarly, there is a tendon that attaches to the extensor muscle (ECRB) at the lateral aspect of the elbow, which when contracted, causes the forearm and wrist to bend backward (extend). At this junction at the elbow, inflammation at the area of bone attachment (enthesopathy) can occur with repeated stress, which in turn, causes a biochemical change in the tendon at the lateral epicondyle area. Classically, this is caused by overexertion of the extensor muscle while performing a backhand stroke in a game of tennis or other activity causing repetitive forearm muscle contractions (see Figure 1).

The pathophysiology of the condition involves inflammatory processes of the radial humeral bursa (fluid-filled sac) and nearby ligaments. This is caused by microscopic tearing with formation of scar tissue at the area of origin of the ECRB muscle tendon, so these small tears and subsequent repair in response may lead to larger tearing and eventual structural failure. Nirschl categorized this into four progressive stages:

Stage 1: Reversible inflammatory changes

Stage 2: Nonreversible pathologic changes

Stage 3: Rupture of ECRB muscle tendon origin

Stage 4: Tissue fibrosis or calcification noted as a secondary change

The patient may have one or more of the following complaints:

- A steadily increasing pain on the lateral part of the elbow.
- Pain that worsens with recreational activities such as playing tennis or gardening or with occupational activities such as painting walls.

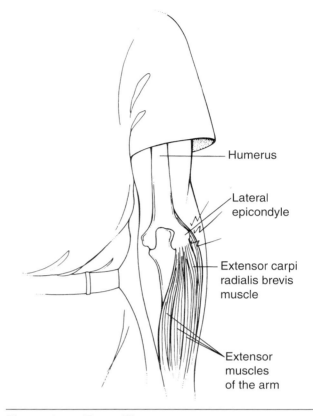

Figure 1   Tennis Elbow

Notes: Among the most common of overuse injuries, tennis elbow is caused by repetitive stress to the forearm muscles. This stress transmits to where the extensor muscle inserts into the lateral epicondyle of the humerus.

- Pain that worsens when strongly squeezing the hand, shaking hands, or turning doorknobs.
- Pain that worsens with moving the wrist against resistance in any direction.
- Pain with handling a knife and fork and opening jars and, at times, even when driving or placing the hands and wrists in an extended position.
- Pain that may begin to occur at night and at rest without any activity.

The physical exam should include the following:

- Inspection of the area for any signs of trauma, swelling, erythema (redness), and deformity, as well as evaluation for asymmetry of the affected side versus the unaffected side.
- Evaluation of range of motion by the patient (actively) and by the examiner (passively).

- Palpation of the affected area to localize the area of tenderness as well as any nodules (bumps). It is worth noting that in some cases the etiology of pain at this location may be related to another condition called bursitis, which is inflammation of the bursa (a fluid-filled sac), which acts like a cushion; this may get irritated as well as infected. Typically, this area will be red, swollen, tender to the touch, and warm. Management could include rest, anti-inflammatory medication, and antibiotics in case of bacterial infection. So proper evaluation is crucial.
- Special stress testing to test whether resistance of the motion initiated by the patient (bending back the wrist while resisted by the examiner) will reproduce or worsen the pain. This would indicate a positive screening test.

Imaging Studies and Electrical Stimulation Study

Radiographs can help in ruling out other disorders or concomitant intraarticular pathology—for example, osteochondral loose body, posterior osteophytes (bone spurs). Calcification in the degenerative tissue of the ECRB muscle origin can be seen in chronic cases.

If indicated, magnetic resonance imaging (MRI) can confirm the presence of degenerative tissue in the ECRB muscle origin and can help diagnose concomitant pathology; however, it is very rarely needed and is usually expensive.

If clinical examination indicates a possible neural involvement with the patient's symptoms, electromyography (EMG) can be used to exclude posterior interosseous nerve compression syndrome (compression of the nerve).

Diagnostic procedures other than the common standards test may include a localized anesthetic injection into the area of concern, which is both diagnostic and therapeutic if the patient experiences relief from his or her symptoms.

Management

Nonsurgical

Generally, early, nonsurgical intervention is sufficient for the management of tennis elbow. Surgical intervention is not readily done due to the potential for scarring and for complications developing during and after the surgery.

Phase 1: Decrease or stop activity for 2 weeks

- Apply ice on the painful area 10 minutes on, 2 hours off for a day.
- Take ibuprofen for 10 days as prescribed, along with topical pain medication.
- Wear a wrist counterforce brace or splint to keep the wrist straight and avoid extension of the wrist or near the elbow to decrease tension on the muscle.

Usually, the symptoms will improve in 2 to 4 weeks.

Phase 2: If the above interventions do not help decrease the symptoms partially or completely, then consider an injection of corticosteroid in combination with a fast-acting anesthetic. These injections are fairly effective; however, chronic and repetitive use (more than two to three times) in the specific area of injection may cause further degeneration of the tendon. Also, a corticosteroid injection may cause wasting of the fatty tissue just below the skin.

Phase 3: Surgery is used only as a last method of intervention, after all other methods of treatment have been tried without improvement for 6 months. Even then, patients should consider surgery only when the symptoms have worsened to the extent of impairing function and activities of daily living due to pain. The surgery can be performed either arthroscopically (using a fiberoptic scope) through a tiny opening in the elbow (which creates a small scar) or by traditional open incision method (which causes a slightly bigger scar). Neither method has an advantage in postsurgical rehabilitation or functionality over the other method; the choice of technique is based on the surgeon's preference and experience, as well as the patient's preference.

Postsurgical Rehabilitation

1. After surgery, the elbow will be placed in a brace and the patient will be sent home with some pain medications as well as a directive to keep the area of incision clean and dry.

2. The patient will return in 5 to 7 days for a follow-up visit, and if the wound is healing well, the sutures will be removed.

3. If everything goes well, the brace will also be removed. Light stretching will be started, along with mild and gentle restoration of range of motion.

4. After 2 months, strength rehabilitation is started lightly and gradually as tolerated.

At this time, the physician will permit resumption of normal and recreational activities as appropriate. About 80% of the time, surgical intervention will be successful; however, one should allocate 4 to 6 months for complete recovery.

Prevention is the key to avoiding progression to surgical treatment. Patients should not delay seeking medical consultation at the earliest onset of symptoms.

George Kolo

See also Elbow and Forearm Injuries; Sports Injuries, Overuse; Tennis and Racquet Sports, Injuries in

Further Readings

Hosey RG. Elbow pain. In: Puffer JC, ed. *Twenty Common Problems in Sports Medicine.* New York, NY: McGraw-Hill; 2002:45–68.

Karageanes SJ. Exercise prescription. In: *Principles of Manual Sports Medicine.* Philadelphia, PA: Lippincott Williams & Wilkins; 2005:77–94.

McCoy RL, Clark CE. The elbow. In: McKeag DB, Moeller JL, eds. *ACSM's Primary Care Sports Medicine.* 2nd ed. Philadelphia, PA: Lippincott Williams & Wilkins; 2007;387–402.

Ryan J, Salvo JP. Elbow injuries. In: Starkey C, Johnson G, eds. *Athletic Training and Sports Medicine.* Sudbury, MA: Jones & Bartlett; 2006:337–384.

Scuderi GR, McCann PD. *Sports Medicine: A Comprehensive Approach.* 2nd ed. St Louis, MO: Mosby; 2004: Chapter 19.

TESTICLE, UNDESCENDED OR SOLITARY

Diseases, congenital anomalies, cryptorchidism (the undescended testicle), trauma, and their treatment may leave a child with a solitary testicle. When these youths come to the office for clearance to play sports, especially contact-collision sports, their reproductive future is at stake. A decision must be made as to whether it is safe to allow them to play.

Evidence from multiple pediatric trauma registries and thousands of contact-collision sports exposures suggests that the risk to the solitary testicle is not significant. In the injury surveillance data gathered from team sports at high school and collegiate levels, there is no evidence showing that these males have a significantly increased risk. For example, the National Pediatric Trauma Registry studied injuries in classic contact-collision sports over a 10-year period. There was only one testicle injury. The testicles are freely mobile, which may protect them from crush injury and disruption. Given a slight hypothetical risk, the recommendation by numerous sports medicine societies, including Medical the American Academy of Pediatrics, is unrestricted full clearance to play in contact-collision sports using a cup, after discussion of the potential risks. In other countries, the clearance-to-play recommendation is not so clear. In Australian rugby, there were 14 injuries, 11 with complete testicle loss, in a group of 15- to 19-year-olds from 1980 to 1993. Finally, the athletes should be given the option of sperm banking, if that is appropriate for their situation.

Cryptorchidism has a prevalence of 2% to 4% in babies weighing more than 2,500 grams (g), which decreases to 0.7% to 1% by the time these children reach 1 year of age. The obvious risk of an undescended testicle is testicular cancer. This risk increases concomitantly with the duration of the cryptorchidism. Most males have already had orchiopexy by the time they reach middle school and have no increased risk of cancer. Unfortunately, undescended testicles are still found in teenagers and in as many as 1% of U.S. military recruits.

The preparticipation exam offers an opportune occasion to find undescended testicles before they pose an increased risk of cancer. Several states now require early periodic screening, diagnosis, and treatment physicals (i.e., well-child exams) at the same time as sports physicals for seventh and ninth graders. This is an excellent time when the physician can perform a comprehensive physical and directly reduce the risk of testicular cancer in individuals found to have cryptorchidism. If an undescended testicle is discovered, the physician should make an immediate referral to a urologist to remove the testicle and repair the inguinal hernia that usually coexists with it.

James Dunlap

See also Abdominal Injuries; Presports Physical Examination

Further Readings

Barthold JS, Gonzalez R. The epidemiology of congenital cryptorchidism, testicular ascent and orchiopexy. *J Urol.* 2003;170(6):2396–2401.

Lawson JS, Rotem T, Wilson SF. Catastrophic injuries to the eyes and testicles in footballers. *Med J Aust.* 1995;163(5):242–244.

Wan J, Corvino TF, Greenfield SP, DiScala C. Contact sports and pediatric kidney and testicle injury: data from the National Pediatric Trauma Registry. *J Urol.* 2003;170(4 pt 2):1525–1527.

THERAPEUTIC EXERCISE

Therapeutic exercise is the systematic application of movement to joints and muscles to assist in the recovery from illness or injury. Therapeutic exercises are usually of a lower intensity and shorter duration than exercises used for conditioning healthy athletes. An individualized therapeutic exercise program is established after a rehabilitation professional obtains a full history and performs a comprehensive evaluation of the athlete.

The overall goal of a therapeutic exercise program in sports medicine is to return the athletes to their baseline level of function in their sport. This process can take a few days to several months depending on the injury. As the athlete advances through the stages of recovery, the exercise program is revised to progressively challenge the neuromusculoskeletal system in a safe manner. The components of a therapeutic exercise program will be discussed in this entry.

Exercise Parameters

Exercise parameters are an integral part of the therapeutic program and should be determined for each exercise. Parameters include frequency, intensity, duration, repetitions, sets, and rest. *Frequency* refers to how often each aspect of the exercise program is performed. *Intensity* refers to the difficulty of the activity. The unit of measurement varies for different types of exercise. *Duration* refers to the length of time an exercise is performed in a given session. *Repetitions* are the number of times an exercise is performed in one set. A *set* is a fixed number of repetitions of an exercise performed without rest. *Rest* refers to the length of time of resting between sets.

Types of Muscle Contraction

Muscles can contract *isometrically* or *isotonically*. Isometric contractions generate muscle force, but no joint movement occurs, such as holding a squat for 10 seconds. Isotonic contractions occur when the muscle contracts and joint movement occurs. There are two types of isotonic contractions. Concentric contractions occur when the muscle fibers shorten as the muscle contracts, such as the lifting phase of a biceps curl. Eccentric contractions occur when the muscle fibers lengthen, such as the lowering phase of a biceps curl.

Position of the Exercise

The body or segment can be positioned in relation to gravity to change the demands of the exercise. Antigravity exercises are performed in an upward direction, or against gravity. Gravity-eliminated exercises are performed in a horizontal plane, which is perpendicular to the force of gravity. Gravity-assisted exercises are performed in a downward direction, or in the same direction as the force of gravity. Exercises can be performed with the affected part in a weight-bearing or closed-chain position or in a non–weight bearing or open-chain position. Push-ups are an example of a closed-chain exercise. Biceps curls are an open-chain exercise.

Types of Exercise

Range-of-Motion Exercises

Passive range of motion involves no active contraction of the muscle. The joint is moved through a range of motion by another person or by an outside force. This type of exercise is often used to increase joint or muscular flexibility or to promote muscle relaxation. Active-assistive range of motion is performed with the assistance of a second person. The athlete uses muscle activity to move the part but is assisted by the practitioner. This type of exercise is often used when the athlete is unable to perform the exercise independently because of an injury or when independent exercise is contraindicated. Active range of motion is performed entirely by the athlete's own muscle power, with no assistance or resistance. This type of exercise can be used to increase the range of motion or for strengthening when resistance is not indicated. Active-resistive range of motion or strengthening is performed against resistance.

Strengthening

Strength is defined as the maximum amount of weight a muscle can move. Strengthening exercises employ resistance to increase the strength. *Resistance* is an outside force applied in a direction opposite to the motion of the body segment being exercised. The amount of resistance can be fixed or varied throughout the range or applied isometrically. Resistance can be applied in a variety of ways. The weight of the body or body segment can be used as resistance in an open- or closed-chain manner. Free weights, dumbbells, bar bells, cuff weights, and medicine balls provide a fixed amount of resistance in small increments. Elastic tubing or bands come in a range of levels of resistance that is somewhat variable through the range as the band is stretched. Manual resistance is provided by the contact of the practitioner's hand against the body segment.

Resistance can be provided by machines or weight stations. Weight increments are often larger than those available with other types of resistance. Weight can be fixed throughout the range of motion, or some systems attempt to vary the resistance throughout the range. *Progressive resistive exercise* (PRE) is a method of strengthening muscles used in rehabilitation settings, in which the resistance is added in selected increments in one session.

Isokinetic exercise is a type of strengthening exercise. Special equipment is required for this. The speed at which the exercise is performed is fixed, and the resistance varies throughout the range of motion.

Plyometrics are activities designed to develop explosive power in muscles, which is a component of strength in athletic activities. The muscle undergoes a repetitive, rapid, eccentric, or lengthening contraction, quickly followed by a rapid, concentric, or shortening contraction, such as jumping in place.

Flexibility

Flexibility refers to the amount of motion allowed by joint structures and the muscle tendon unit. Stretching exercises are usually done passively, with no activity in the muscle or muscle group being stretched. The muscle is placed in a position of stretch or elongation, and the position is maintained. This is called *static stretching*. Thirty seconds is the generally accepted time for holding the stretch to achieve maximum benefit. Bouncing or ballistic stretching is not recommended because it is not effective and may cause further injury. Rehabilitation professionals may employ a technique in which the muscle to be stretched performs an isometric or isotonic contraction first, followed by a stretch of the same muscle or group of muscles to increase flexibility.

Muscular Endurance

Muscular endurance is the ability of a muscle or a group of muscles to perform continuous activity without fatigue. Exercises are directed to specific muscles or muscle groups using low resistance and high repetitions.

Aerobic and Anaerobic Exercise

Cardiovascular endurance can be trained through aerobic activities, such as distance running. Aerobic exercise improves oxygen consumption of the body and typically involves repetitive exercise performed at a moderate intensity for an extended period of time. Guidelines usually suggest a total duration of 30 minutes. Intensity is defined as the target heart rate (THR). A lower THR is used for lower levels of fitness. THR is calculated by the following equations:

$$\text{Maximum heart rate} = 220 - \text{Age of athlete}$$

$$\text{THR} = 60\text{--}85\% \times \text{Maximum heart rate.}$$

The injured athlete can often engage in selected aerobic activities to avoid stress on the injured area and maintain cardiovascular endurance. Anaerobic exercises are performed at a higher intensity but for a much shorter duration than aerobic exercises—up to 2 minutes—and do not improve cardiovascular endurance.

Joint Stability and Balance

Joint stability refers to the ability of the various joint structures and the muscle-tendon unit to resist forces and therefore prevent injury. Proprioceptors are sensory receptors in the muscle-tendon unit and joint structures that provide information to the brain about the position of the limbs and body in space. These receptors, which can become faulty after an athletic injury, provide feedback to the brain, which then controls the response of the muscle to the force.

Balance refers to the static and dynamic components of movement. Many systems are involved with balance, including the proprioceptive, visual, and vestibular systems. Proprioceptive and balance activities include balancing with the eyes open or closed, using a progressively smaller base of support or using an unstable surface. Equipment includes foam surfaces or wobble boards.

Proprioceptive neuromuscular facilitation (PNF) is an example of an exercise technique used to enhance joint stability. PNF uses specific patterns of movement of entire limbs or body segments through a range of motion and may incorporate manual resistance.

Neuromuscular Coordination and Retraining

Neuromuscular training is used at all levels of rehabilitation. The process involves developing correct timing of muscle activation to produce correct execution of sports activities.

Sports-Specific Activities

Sports-specific activities are introduced during the latter stages of the rehabilitation process. Activities include drills that mimic the movements or activities involved in the sport. Gradual return to competition is recommended to allow time to recondition the athlete to the activity and prevent recurrence of the injury.

Christine Ploski and Michelina Cassella

See also Physical and Occupational Therapist; Principles of Rehabilitation and Physical Therapy; Resistance Training; Static Stretching

Further Readings

Kisner C, Colby LA. *Therapeutic Exercise: Foundations and Techniques.* Philadelphia, PA: FA Davis; 2007.

Nyland J. *Clinical Decisions in Therapeutic Exercise: Planning and Implementation.* Upper Saddle River, NJ: Prentice Hall; 2005.

THIGH CONTUSION

An injury to the front part of the thigh, usually from a direct blow to that area, is common in contact sports and should be recognized early. If the muscle trauma is severe enough, it can develop into a compartment syndrome, and if untreated, it can lead to muscle necrosis, fibrosis, and calcification (myositis ossificans). Treatment involves the use of the RICE principles (*rest*, *ice*, *compression*, and *elevation*) and physical therapy. Recovery depends on the severity of the contusion but can take from days to weeks.

Anatomy

The *quadriceps* are a group of muscles on the front part of the thigh. They include four different muscles: (1) rectus femoris, (2) vastus lateralis, (3) vastus medialis, and (4) vastus interomedialis. Their main function is the extension of the knee (straightening of the leg).

History

A quadriceps contusion develops after a direct blow to the thigh. This can be seen in many contact sports (football, rugby, soccer, mixed martial arts). A *contusion* (bruising) is formed by the rupture or breaking of the blood vessels within the muscle

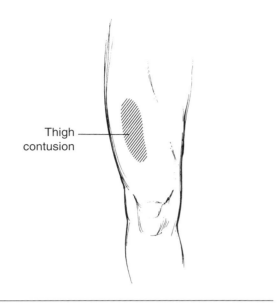

Figure 1   Thigh Contusion

Notes: A thigh contusion is caused by trauma and involves bleeding into the muscle fibers. Unlike strains, which affect the superficial muscles, such contusions occur deep inside the muscle, close to the bone.

(Figure 1). If the bleeding is severe enough, it can cause elevated pressure, which can compress the nerves and other blood vessels within that muscle compartment. This compression of nerves and blood vessels causes tissue death and is otherwise known as *compartment syndrome.* Compartment syndrome is rare in the thigh, but it does occur sometimes, so if this condition is suspected, the patient needs to be examined by a surgeon immediately.

Calcification of the muscle (*myositis ossificans*) can also occur if the athlete tries to rehabilitate a severe contusion too quickly. In this case, the bruised muscle grows bone instead of new muscle cells. Early recognition is the key to preventing this condition.

Symptoms

There will be tenderness at the site of the injury, as well as pain with knee flexion. There may or may not be swelling such that there is an increased circumference of the affected thigh. Sensation should be normal in the lower leg. If this not the case, then compartment syndrome should be considered. Contusions are categorized in three levels: Grade 1, Grade 2, and Grade 3 (most severe). Severity depends mainly on the degree of limited knee flexion (straightening) and on gait abnormalities (limping). Grading of the contusion is important to apply the appropriate treatment.

Imaging

Imaging studies are usually not needed initially for the diagnosis of quadriceps contusions. A diagnosis can usually be made by history and physical exam alone. X-rays are beneficial to look for any fractures of the femur (thighbone) or patella (kneecap), or bone formation in the muscle (myositis ossificans). Ultrasound is a good, inexpensive tool to look for complete muscle tears, but it is not as good for partial tear diagnoses. Magnetic resonance imaging (MRI) is considered the best imaging tool for soft tissue pathology.

Treatment

As soon as a quadriceps contusion is recognized, the athlete should be put into 120° of flexion (knee bent) for at least the first 10 minutes but should not sustain that position for more than 24 hours. This position helps in many ways: It limits the amount of muscle spasm and bleeding into the muscle, decreases the risk of developing bone formation in the muscle, and decreases the amount of pain experienced at that time. Crutches may be necessary early on if walking generates pain. The general RICE principles are applied: *r*est, *i*ce 15 to 20 minutes every 2 to 3 hours, *c*ompression of the thigh with an elastic wrap as needed for swelling, and *e*levation of the leg to decrease swelling. Applying heat should be avoided because this can cause an increase in swelling. Once the pain has been resolved, the athlete should work on stretching, strengthening, and increasing range of motion of the quadriceps and hamstrings (a group of muscles on the back portion of the thigh). Nonsteroidal anti-inflammatory drugs (NSAIDs) such as ibuprofen are often recommended initially for the first few days after onset of injury along with the RICE therapy. They help not only with pain control but also with swelling.

If compartment syndrome does occur, the athlete must be evaluated by a surgeon immediately. A fasciotomy (opening of the compartment) is necessary for treatment. If this is left untreated, the muscle tissue breaks down, which can lead to muscle contractures.

Myositis ossificans can occur in up to 9% of quadriceps contusions. This condition does not develop acutely and usually occurs approximately 3 months after the injury. Initial treatment includes conservative measures such as oral anti-inflammatories, massage, and stretching. If severe pain persists months after this onset, then surgery is recommended.

Prognosis

The athlete's return to play varies depending on the severity of the quadriceps injury. The athlete may resume play once 120° of flexion is achieved painlessly and there is no evidence of quadriceps weakness or atrophy. Protective padding is recommended for the injured area for the rest of the season.

Roberta Kern and Richard A. Okragly

See also Compartment Syndrome, Anterior; Thigh Injuries

Further Readings

Beiner JM, Jokl P. Muscle contusion injuries: current treatment options. *J Am Acad Orthop Surg.* 2001;9(4):227–237.

Beiner JM, Jokl P. Muscle contusion injury and myositis ossificans traumatica. *Clin Orthop Relat Res.* 2002;(403 suppl):S110–S119.

De Berardino TM. Quadriceps injury. http://emedicine .medscape.com/article/91473-overview. Updated January 19, 2010. Accessed June 15, 2010.

Diaz JA, Fischer DA, Rettig AC, Davis TJ, Shelbourne KD. Severe quadriceps muscle contusions in athletes. A report of three cases. *Am J Sports Med.* 2003;31(2):289–293.

THIGH INJURIES

Injuries to the anterior and posterior thigh are fairly common in sports, particularly in running and jumping sports. Particularly common are *muscle strains* and *contusions*. Quadriceps strains are common in running, jumping, and kicking sports, such as track-and-field events, basketball, and soccer. Hamstring strains occur frequently in sports involving high-speed running and kicking, such as sprints, hurdles, long jump, football, and field hockey. In Australian football, hamstring injuries account for 15% of all injuries and are the most common and prevalent injury. Likewise, in British soccer, hamstring injuries constitute 12% of all injuries. These injuries also have the highest recurrence rate (34% in Australian football, 12% in British soccer). Quadriceps contusions, commonly known as a "charley horse," are extremely common in contact sports such as football and basketball and in ball/puck sports such as hockey, lacrosse, and cricket.

Anatomy

The femur is the only bone in the thigh. The quadriceps muscle group in the anterior thigh contains the rectus femoris, vastus lateralis, vastus medialis obliquus, and sartorius. They are the strongest muscles in the anterior thigh and function to extend the knee. The hamstring muscle group in the posterior thigh consists of the biceps femoris, the semimembranosus, and the semitendinosus. The biceps femoris has two heads. The short head acts only on the knee and is innervated by the common peroneal nerve, whereas the long head is innervated by the tibial portion of the sciatic nerve. The hamstrings cross two joints and are responsible for hip extension and knee flexion. The semitendinosus, the semimembranosus, and the long head of the biceps originate on the ischial tuberosity.

The adductor magnus functions in hip extension and adduction and is innervated by the tibial portion of the sciatic nerve, like most of the hamstring muscles. The posterior part of the adductor magnus is sometimes considered functionally to be part of the hamstring group because of its anatomical position.

Evaluation of Injuries

Details of Injury

The exact location of pain and the mechanism of injury in the setting of a thigh injury can help in diagnosis. In the case of contusions (bruises) or muscle strain, the site of pain is usually well localized. Contusions of the anterior thigh are most common in the anterolateral aspect of the thigh or in the vastus medialis obliquus, although they can occur anywhere.

The mechanism of injury can usually differentiate between muscle strains and contusions. Muscle strains usually occur when the athlete is striving for greater speed while running or extra distance while kicking. The athlete usually remembers a specific event that causes pain and some immediate functional limitations. A contusion, however, is usually the result of a direct blow. The athlete's age and skeletal maturity may affect the type of injury seen, as injury patterns in adolescents differ from those in adults, such as avulsion fractures, seen in younger patients with open apophyses.

With severe injuries to the thigh, the athlete may not be able to continue the sporting activity. The athlete may be unable to go back to sports and may be unable to walk or run without pain. There may be swelling and bruising at the site of injury. Injuries to the thigh should initially be treated with the RICE (rest, ice, compression, and elevation) regimen to decrease swelling. Factors such as hot showers/baths, heat rubs, excessive activity, or alcohol ingestion may worsen thigh injuries and prevent healing.

Certain sports make thigh injuries more likely, such as soccer, football, and hockey. Recent changes in the training regimen may contribute to injuries. Previous thigh injuries may predispose an athlete to recurrent injuries. The athlete's age is also important, as during periods of growth, children and adolescents may have muscle inflexibilities and muscle imbalances that may predispose them to thigh injuries.

Anterior or thigh pain that has a gradual onset and is poorly localized may indicate a stress fracture or possible tumor. If anterior or posterior thigh pain is variable, is poorly localized, and lacks specific aggravating factors, the pain may be referred. Bilateral thigh pain is usually referred from the lumbar spine. A high index of suspicion and an understanding of what structures can refer pain to the posterior thigh are essential to make the correct diagnosis. Any "red flag" symptoms, such as night pain, night sweats, weight loss, or neurological symptoms such as numbness or tingling, may indicate infection or cancer as a cause of thigh pain.

Physical Findings

In acute injuries of the thigh, the diagnosis is usually straightforward, and the injury is usually limited to local structures. When pain is more insidious, the cause of the injury may be less straightforward and may be referred from the hip, sacroiliac joint, or lower back.

Thigh injuries may result in bruising, swelling, atrophy, or other deformity to the anterior or posterior thigh. Comparing the injured leg with the uninjured leg can highlight any abnormalities. Athletes with thigh injuries may walk with a limp and be unable to move the leg normally. The range of motion of the hip and knee may be affected. With anterior thigh injuries, stretching of the quadriceps muscle (the athlete lies on his or her stomach and tries to bring the heel of the foot to the buttocks) may be decreased or may cause pain. With posterior thigh injuries, stretching the hamstring muscles (the athlete lies on his or her back and raises the affected leg to the point of pain and then to the end of range) may cause pain.

Thigh muscle strength may be decreased secondary to injury. The athlete may have muscle weakness or pain when trying to resist certain movements. For instance, with quadriceps injuries, the athlete may be unable to extend the knee against resistance when sitting with the hip and knee flexed to 90°. Similarly, the athlete may be unable to flex the hip against resistance. With hamstring injuries, an athlete may be unable to flex the knee against resistance while lying on the stomach. The athlete may be unable to squat, jump, hop, run, or kick secondary to pain or weakness.

Thigh injuries may be accompanied by tenderness, swelling, or defects in the muscle belly. Defects in the muscle belly may be more pronounced when the affected muscle is contracted. The origin of the hamstring at the ischial tuberosity may also be tender with hamstring injuries. In addition, the muscles of the buttocks (gluteal muscles) may be tender to palpation.

A stress fracture of the femur may cause pain in the thigh when a fulcrum test is performed. With the athlete sitting on the edge of the bed and the legs hanging over the edge, the examiner applies pressure over the distal femur. Reproduction of the athlete's pain in the thigh with this maneuver is suggestive of a stress fracture.

Sometimes thigh pain is related to a neurological problem. Certain tests, called *neural tension tests*, can help determine if the thigh pain is caused by damage to the nerves. With anterior thigh pain, a modified Thomas test can be performed with the patient supine and the legs off the end of the bed. The patient flexes the cervical and upper thoracic spine as the examiner passively flexes the patient's knee while extending the other leg. Reproduction of the patient's symptoms indicates nerve involvement. For posterior thigh pain, a slump test can be performed with the patient sitting on the edge of the end of the bed. The examiner flexes the patient's cervical and upper thoracic spine and then extends the patient's leg. Reproduction of symptoms suggests a neural component.

Investigations

In athletes with anterior thigh pain, investigations are usually not necessary. X-rays may indicate myositis ossificans (calcification of the muscle) in a quadriceps contusion that is not getting better. Ultrasound will confirm the presence of a hematoma and may show early calcification. Stress fractures may also be shown on X-rays. If X-rays are negative, bone scan should be performed.

If thigh pain is associated with an abnormal hip examination, hip X-rays should be obtained (Table 1). In adults, there may be evidence of arthritis. In younger patients, Legg-Calvé-Perthes disease or slipped capital femoral epiphysis may be shown.

Prevention of Injury

Many acute thigh injuries can be prevented with appropriate stretching, adequate strengthening, and proper warm-up. The proper safety equipment for the particular sport should be worn and properly maintained. Additionally, playing with athletes at the same skill level can help prevent acute injuries. Prevention of chronic thigh injuries can be achieved by instituting appropriate training programs and avoiding training errors. Common training errors include inappropriate progression of the rate, duration, and intensity of training.

Table I   Common Anterior and Posterior Thigh Injuries

	Common	*Uncommon*	*Must Not Be Missed*
Anterior	Quadriceps contusion	Femoral stress fracture	Legg-Calvé-Perthes disease
	Quadriceps strain	Sartorius/gracilis muscle strain	Slipped capital femoral epiphysis (SCFE)
	Myositis ossificans	Rectus femoris apophysis avulsion	
		Referred pain (lumbar spine, sacroiliac joint, hip joint)	Tumors
Posterior	Hamstring muscle strain	Bursitis	Tumors
	Hamstring muscle contusion	Tendinopathy	
	Referred pain (lumbar spine)	Apophysitis/avulsion fracture of ischial tuberosity	
		Adductor magnus strains	
		Myositis ossificans	
		Nerve entrapments	
		Referred pain (sacroiliac joint)	

Targeting anatomical risk factors such as lower extremity alignment, muscle imbalances, poor conditioning, and inflexibilities can also help decrease thigh injuries. Other risk factors that should be addressed include inappropriate footwear, playing surfaces, and nutrition.

Return to Sports

For most minor injuries of the thigh, such as strains and contusions, a period of rest followed by appropriate therapy emphasizing stretching and strengthening will allow athletes to regain flexibility and strength. Before returning to sports following a thigh injury, strength and flexibility should be back to 80% to 90% of normal to prevent recurrent injury and allow effective movement. Pain should also have resolved. Regular physiotherapy can help monitor progress and determine the athlete's readiness to return to play. Following more serious thigh injuries, such as acute fractures and stress fractures, return to play should be delayed until pain has resolved, there is radiological evidence of healing, and risk factors have been addressed and modified.

Laura Purcell

See also Hamstring Strain; Quadriceps Strain; Slipped Capital Femoral Epiphysis; Thigh Contusion; Thighbone Fracture

Further Readings

Anterior thigh pain. In: Brukner P, Khan K, eds. *Clinical Sport Medicine.* 3rd ed. Sydney, Australia: McGraw-Hill Professional; 2007:427–438.

Nielson JH. Pelvis, hip and thigh injuries. In: Micheli LJ, Purcell LK, eds. *The Adolescent Athlete: A Practical Approach.* New York, NY: Springer; 2007:264–288.

Schache A. Posterior thigh pain. In: Brukner P, Khan K, eds. *Clinical Sport Medicine.* 3rd ed. Sydney, Australia: McGraw-Hill Professional; 2007:439–459.

THIGHBONE FRACTURE

Thighbone fracture refers to fractures of the femur, the sole bone in the thigh. They are caused by high-energy trauma or overuse. This entry reviews the basic types of fractures of the femur, fracture healing, fracture treatment methods, and general outcomes.

Fracture Types

Thighbone (femur) fractures are described by where they are located, how much out of place the bone is, and whether the bone has broken through the skin. In lay terms, it is sometimes assumed that a break is more serious than a fracture; to a physician, both refer to the same thing. A fracture that is incomplete, or not fully through the bone, may be called a *stress fracture.* This can occur in a runner from overuse, for example. A complete fracture, which is fully through the bone, may be described as either *nondisplaced* (hairline crack) or *displaced* (two parts not aligned), ranging from minimally displaced to widely displaced. *Comminuted fracture* refers to a bone being broken in many pieces rather than cleanly. The older term for a broken bone that went through the skin was *compound fracture;* now this is described as an *open fracture.* A fracture that does not pierce the skin is *closed.* Thus, when we say that a person has an open, widely displaced comminuted femur fracture, we mean that the person has a thighbone fracture that is badly out of place and the bone has broken in many pieces and gone through the skin.

In general, most thighbone (femur) fractures are caused by high-energy trauma. Thus, associated injuries in other parts of the body must be looked for too. For example, in a person involved in a high-speed motor vehicle collision, there may be internal bleeding and head injuries along with a thighbone fracture. These need to be managed first.

Fracture Healing

Thighbone fracture healing varies by age of the patient, location and severity of the fracture, and treatment method. In general, children's bones heal much faster than those of adults. In a baby a thighbone may heal in 1 month, while in a 6-year-old the same bone may take 6 weeks and in an adult 6 months to fully heal. When a bone fractures, first a blood clot forms, much like a scab forms on cut skin. Next, the cells in the blood clot recruit bone-forming cells (*osteoblasts*), which begin making new bone. At first, this bone is poorly organized and looks cloudy on an X-ray. This is called *callus*. Usually, the presence of callus allows weight bearing by 6 weeks after the fracture. Over time, this new bone solidifies and reorganizes into strong new bone. This is called *remodeling*. This takes from several months to several years after the injury. In children particularly, bones have wonderful remodeling properties. It is possible for a child to have a bone heal very crookedly at first and then straighten itself out without help over time. Good nutrition, in particular vitamin D (400 international units [IU]/day) and calcium (1,000 milligrams per day), is also very important for fracture healing.

Fracture Treatment Methods

Thighbone fracture treatment varies widely by the age of the patient and the severity of the injury. For a stress fracture (incomplete break in the thighbone), crutches may be all that is needed. For more severe fractures, surgery with rod or plate and screw fixation may be needed. The guidelines for fracture treatment are reviewed below.

Initial Treatment

The initial treatment when someone is injured should be to assess the injury and to stabilize the injured part, straightening it gently if it is bent or twisted. A removable stabilizing device, or splint, is applied. If an open fracture is present, the bone should not be put back through the skin. Instead, a clean dressing should be applied as well as a splint, and urgent transport to a medical center should be arranged. The portion of the leg below the thighbone fracture should be assessed for vascularity and nerve function by checking that the toes can move and are pink and warm. After the initial immobilization, the patient should be assessed by a physician. As thighbone fractures are generally the result of high-energy trauma, transport is generally by ambulance from the accident scene to the emergency room. Generally, X-rays are obtained, and sometimes other studies, such as computed tomography (CT) and magnetic resonance imaging (MRI) scans, are done to determine what kind of fracture is present. Once the fracture has been properly diagnosed, treatment can proceed. If other, more severe injuries are present, these are diagnosed and treated first.

Definitive Treatment

Stress Fractures

These are generally treated nonoperatively with rest, protected weight bearing, and time. For example, a (nondisplaced) stress fracture in the thighbone usually requires the use of crutches and should have no weight on it for 6 weeks. Some stress fractures at the top of the thighbone (hip area/femoral neck) may need screw fixation because of the high risk that they may break all the way through.

Displaced Fractures

Thighbone fractures that are out of place generally need to be straightened (this is called *reduction*) and may need surgery. In babies less than 6 months old, thighbone fractures may be treated in a soft brace called a *Pavlik harness*. In children aged 6 months to 6 years, displaced thighbone fractures can often be treated successfully with reduction and body casting (called a *spica*) for 6 to 12 weeks. In older children and adults, displaced thighbone fractures need surgical fixation for treatment. Fixation may be external fixators (pins that come out through the skin and hold the bone in place by attaching to a bar), plates and screws, or rods put down the hollow middle part (*medulla*) of the thighbone. Most adult thighbone fractures are treated with a strong rod down the middle of the bone. In image (a) on page 1479, a thighbone fracture X-ray is seen. In images (b) and (c), the fracture has been treated with a rod and has healed with a lump of new bone (callus). In severe injuries, the thighbone may be temporarily stabilized with an external fixator; then in a later surgical procedure, a rod or plate and screws may be applied.

Open Fractures

Fractures that come through the skin always need surgery to clean them. This is because they are at high risk of infection. After the surgical cleaning, the bones are fixed using the method most appropriate for the type of fracture.

(a)

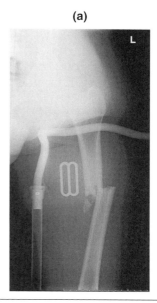

Thighbone fracture.

Source: Photo courtesy of Children's Orthopaedic Surgery Foundation.

(b)

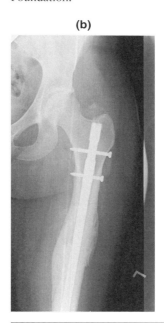

(c)

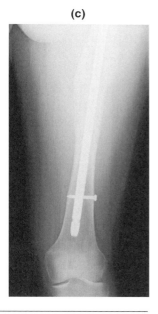

Thighbone fracture with callus formation after treatment with a rod; (b) thighbone fracture after rodding with healing new bone (callus) and (c) lower end of the same thighbone with rod after healing

Source: Photo courtesy of Children's Orthopaedic Surgery Foundation.

Rehabilitation

If a thighbone is treated with a rod, immediate weight bearing with crutches is allowed. Early bone healing is present at 6 weeks, but it may take 4 to 6 months for the bone to fully solidify. Contact sports are not allowed until the bone is solidly healed. Rehabilitating the thigh muscles is equally important and often takes at least as long as the bone healing time. Usually, this involves physical therapy. A physical therapist is someone trained to guide patients through exercising the injured part according to their doctor's orders until return of full strength and function. After a high-energy thighbone fracture, it is often 4 to 6 months before patients can return to any sport. Limping may persist for 6 months to a year as well. In adults, the thighbone rods or other fracture fixation devices are usually left in place permanently unless they are bothersome, in which case they can be surgically removed. In children, some fracture fixation devices may need to be removed, while others may be left in place.

Outcomes

Most patients with thighbone fractures will go through a normal healing process, and the bone will return to a high functional level. Thus, most athletes sustaining a thighbone fracture can expect to return to their sport. However, some permanent quadriceps muscle weakness may be present, especially in severe fractures.

Samantha A. Spencer

See also Football, Injuries in; Rugby Union, Injuries in; Skiing, Injuries in; Sports Injuries, Acute

Further Readings

American Academy of Orthopaedic Surgery. Thighbone (femur) fracture. http://orthoinfo.aaos.org/topic .cfm?topic=A00364. Published August 2008. Accessed June 14, 2010.

Collinge CA, Sanders RW. Percutaneous plating in the lower extremity. *J Am Acad Orthop Surg.* 2000;8(4):211–216.

Dougherty PJ, Silverton C, Yeni Y, Tashman S, Weir R. Conversion from temporary external fixation to definitive fixation: shaft fractures. *J Am Acad Orthop Surg.* 2006;14(10):S124–S127.

Zalavras CG, Patzakis MJ. Open fractures: evaluation and management. *J Am Acad Orthop Surg.* 2003;11(3):212–219.

THUMB SPRAIN

A *thumb sprain* is a stretch or tear of a ligament located at one of the thumb joints. This traumatic injury is common, and athletes in sports such as skiing, football, and wrestling are frequently affected. In fact, in skiers, only the knee is injured more often than the thumb. This condition not only leads to time lost from sports until it is healed, but it also creates the potential for future disability if it is not properly identified and treated.

Thumb sprains can occur at any of the three thumb joints. A thumb sprain however, is synonymous with an injury to the inside ligament (ulnar collateral ligament, UCL) at the middle joint (metacarpophalangeal, MCP) of the thumb. Multiple names are used to describe UCL sprains, including "gamekeeper's thumb" and "skier's thumb." The term *gamekeeper's thumb* was coined after Scottish gamekeepers (ca. 1955) were found to be prone to these particular thumb sprains. Their repetitive practice of breaking the necks of small game by holding the animal in the web space between their thumb and pointer finger would injure the UCL. In recent times, this injury has been more commonly referred to as skier's thumb. Relatively frequent trauma and subsequent falls create a strong correlation between skiers and thumb sprains.

Anatomy

The thumb is composed of three bones and three joints. The bones of the thumb are the metacarpal, proximal phalanx, and distal phalanx. The metacarpal bone is the one closest to the wrist, the distal phalanx is at the tip of the thumb, and the proximal phalanx lies between these two bones. Connecting the thumb bones from the wrist to the tip of the thumb are the carpometacarpal (CMC), MCP, and interphalangeal (IP) joints, in that order. At each joint, there are multiple ligaments that provide stability to the thumb when traumatic or pinching forces are placed on it. They are the collateral ligaments, the volar plate, and the joint capsule. The collateral ligaments are located on the inner and outer sides of each thumb joint and provide side-to-side stability. The UCL is the collateral ligament closest to the little finger, and the radial collateral ligament (RCL) lies on the opposite side of the joint

from the UCL. The volar plate is a ligament located on the palm side of each thumb joint and prevents hyperextension. Finally, the joint capsule is a saclike envelope that encloses the entire joint.

Type of Injury

The majority of thumb sprains occur at the UCL of the MCP joint. The second most common sprain occurs at the RCL of the MCP joint. The IP joint infrequently experiences ligament injury. Rarely are there isolated injuries to the CMC joint. The ligaments at this joint are well protected from trauma. Certainly, fractures and dislocations are associated with ligament sprains, but they are beyond the scope of this entry.

Clinical Evaluation

History

There are numerous traumatic mechanisms that can cause a thumb sprain. All, however, involve a side-to-side force that creates extreme thumb movement either toward or away from the hand. The collateral ligaments are naturally affected as they provide side-to-side stability at the thumb joints. Typical examples of these movements are a fall while holding a ski pole or a fall onto an outstretched and extended thumb.

After a thumb sprain, athletes will experience immediate pain and swelling at the joint. Activities such as pinching and gripping of the thumb will produce pain. If the injury is old and has not been treated, pinching weakness and degenerative arthritis are possible long-term complications. This weakness and instability can be debilitating in those sports that require strong pinching and grasping abilities.

Physical Examination

Swelling and bruising are common findings on physical examination. A finding of localized tenderness over a specific side of the joint is important in isolating the affected collateral ligament. Stress testing is used to assess ligament stability. This involves applying a bending stress to the ligament at 0° and 30° of flexion. When a ligament is completely torn, the joint will significantly "open up" as there is no ligamentous integrity to resist the stress testing. If there is only a partial tear or stretch, the ligament will withstand the applied stress and prevent the joint from moving. It is vital that stress testing is performed on both symptomatic and asymptomatic thumbs to compare results. Patients can have wide variations in their amount of normal joint laxity (looseness).

Diagnostic Tests

Obtaining plain radiographs is a routine part of evaluating a thumb sprain. An avulsion fracture has been found to be associated in 20% of ligament sprains. Some physicians advocate stress X-rays in addition to normal radiographs when the history and physical exam do not reveal a clear diagnosis. Stress X-rays look at the affected joint while a stress is applied similar to the physical exam maneuver above. These views provide additional information as to whether the thumb ligament is partially or completely torn. The benefit and accuracy of magnetic resonance imaging (MRI) in further defining the ligaments of the thumb have not been conclusively determined.

When significant ligamentous laxity is found on physical examination, the joint is said to be unstable, which likely indicates a complete rupture of the ligament. This raises the suspicion that a unique injury to the UCL, called a Stener lesion, is present. A Stener lesion occurs when the UCL tears and the surrounding tissue of an overlying thumb tendon gets lodged between the torn UCL fibers. Subsequently, the UCL is unable to come together and heal due to the interposed soft tissue. In addition to unstable stress testing, a Stener lesion is infrequently identified on physical examination as a mass on the hand side of the MCP joint. Unfortunately, the best way to visualize a Stener lesion is during surgery.

Treatment

The management of thumb sprains is divided according to the stability of the affected ligament. Stable thumb sprains are typically treated nonoperatively, while unstable thumb sprains are treated with surgery. Stener lesions are included in the unstable category and require operative intervention at the UCL.

Nonsurgical Treatment

Initial care of a thumb sprain includes rest, ice, elevation, and over-the-counter pain medication. If available, protection with a splint is helpful to control pain symptoms and reduce motion at the affected thumb joint. When the sprain has been determined to be stable according to the medical evaluation, the athlete is immobilized in a splint or cast that covers the thumb. At periodic follow-ups, the athlete's tenderness to palpation and joint stability are assessed. The thumb is typically immobilized for 4 to 6 weeks until the patient is nontender and the joint is stable. Rehabilitation for the wrist and thumb is often started at approximately 4 weeks with range-of-motion (ROM) and strengthening exercises. This is continued until full ROM and strength are achieved.

Surgery

Surgery of a thumb sprain typically consists of a primary repair. This refers to the reattachment of the two ends of the torn ligaments. A primary repair is most successful soon after the injury. In general, completely torn thumb ligaments can usually be repaired by 6 to 8 weeks after the date of injury. After surgery, the athlete will be immobilized for a period of time and then progressed to a rehabilitation program similar to the one described above.

When operative intervention is delayed or the athlete is not evaluated for a thumb sprain, there is a higher likelihood that the ligament is going to scar and shrink in size. As a result, the ligament ends become very difficult to sew back together beyond the 6-week time period. When this happens, more complicated surgeries are required for successful treatment. They include a reconstruction, where a portion of tendon from another body part is substituted to make a brand new ligament. The other option for delayed treatment is a fusion of the joint. This, however, may be optimally done after the athlete's athletic career is completed.

Return to Sports

Those athletes who are immobilized with a splint or a cast may be able to return to their sport as soon as their symptoms are controlled. In certain sports, athletes are allowed to compete while casted. For example, football players are allowed to participate with a splint or a cast if it is properly padded.

For the athlete who is unable to compete with a splint or a cast, a rehabilitation program is continued after immobilization. When full ROM and strength are achieved, sport-specific drills and a return-to-play progression are begun. For most sports, taping of the MCP joint to the index finger (buddy taping) should continue for up to 12 weeks after the injury.

Samuel Bugbee and Tracy Casault

See also Finger Sprain; Hand and Finger Injuries; Hand and Finger Injuries, Surgery for; Skiing, Injuries in

Further Readings

Campbell CS. Gamekeeper's thumb. *J Bone Joint Surg Br.* 1955;37(1):148–149.

Eiff MP, Hatch RL, Calmbach WL. Fracture management for primary care. 2nd ed. Philadelphia, PA: Saunders; 2003.

Hong E. Hand injuries in sports medicine. *Prim Care.* 2005;32(1):91–103.

Kovacic J, Bergfeld J. Return to play issues in upper extremity injuries. *Clin J Sport Med.* 2005;15(6):448–452.

Peterson JJ, Bancroft LW. Injuries of the fingers and thumb in the athlete. *Clin Sports Med.* 2006;25(3):527–542.

Rettig AC. Athletic injuries of the wrist and hand. *Am J Sports Med.* 2004;32(1):262–273.

TIBIA AND FIBULA FRACTURES

The tibia and fibula, the two long bones of the lower leg, can be fractured during sporting activities. Although isolated fracture of either the tibia or the fibula can occur, most often both bones are fractured in the same injury. Early diagnosis and immediate treatment with splint immobilization are necessary for patient comfort and treatment. Emergent follow-up with an orthopedic surgeon is necessary to evaluate the patient and definitively treat the fracture(s).

Anatomy

The tibia, commonly called the shinbone, is the major weight-bearing bone of the lower leg. The part of the tibia that articulates with the femur at the knee is called the *tibial plateau,* the middle is the *tibial shaft,* and the lower portion, which articulates with the ankle joint, is called the *tibial plafond.* The inner aspect of the ankle bone that can be felt is part of the tibia and is called the *medial malleolus.*

The fibula is the smaller bone on the outer part of the leg. The part near the knee is called the fibular head, the middle is the shaft, and the part that articulates with the ankle is called the *lateral malleolus.*

The tibia and fibula are connected by the interosseous membrane, a broad plane of fibrous connective tissue, and multiple ligaments at the knee and ankle.

There is only a small amount of soft tissue between the tibia and the skin, which is the cause of many open tibia fractures. An *open fracture* occurs when the energy from the injury forces the bone through the skin. The fibula has more soft tissue surrounding it, so a fracture is less likely to be open. The exception to this is at the ankle, where the lateral malleolus is just underneath the skin, with a thin soft tissue layer.

Causes

Sports-related fracture of the tibia and fibula is a relatively low-energy injury. The fracture can occur from a direct blow on either side of the lower leg or by landing hard on the foot of the fractured leg. Additionally, a severe twisting injury can fracture the tibia and fibula.

Symptoms

Pain, swelling, inability to walk, and deformity are common signs and symptoms of tibia and fibula fractures. With an isolated fibula fracture, the athlete is often able to walk or run; therefore, the diagnostic process is much more difficult.

Diagnosis

The diagnosis of a tibia or fibula fracture can often be made based solely on history and physical exam. There is often gross deformity of the lower leg associated with bruising, swelling, tenderness, and occasionally a skin opening or laceration with protruding bone—clearly indicating an open fracture. Palpation along the tibia can reveal crepitance or gross movement of the bony fragments. During the physical exam, it is important to examine the knee for an effusion, and a detailed neurovascular exam of the foot is imperative. The neurovascular exam should include motor (wiggling of the toes) and sensory (testing whether the athlete can feel you touching his or her toes and heel) exams, as well as palpation of the dorsalis pedis and posterior tibial pulse and checking capillary refill. Along with the history and physical examination, radiographs including an anterior-posterior (AP) view and a lateral view can clinch the diagnosis. X-rays of the knee and ankle joint are recommended as well.

There are three types of tibial shaft fractures:

1. *Transverse:* straight perpendicular to the axis of the bone

2. *Spiral:* in a spiral pattern down the bone

3. *Oblique:* at an angle to the axis of the bone

For comminuted (multiple fracture fragments) tibial plateau and tibial plafond fractures (fractures that go into the joint surface of the knee and ankle, respectively), a computed axial tomography (CAT or CT) scan of these areas is often useful to further classify the fracture pattern for preoperative planning.

Treatment

After a thorough history and physical exam, the initial treatment of any tibia or fibula fracture includes reduction (if needed) and immobilization of the lower leg with a splint. Emergent reduction by a trained professional is needed if the athlete has a gross deformity or does not have a pulse in his or her foot or if the foot is discolored. If the athlete sustains an open fracture, a sterile dressing should be applied to the wound, and the leg should then be immobilized. In an appropriate setting (emergency department), the athlete's open wound should be irrigated with sterile saline solution and dressed with a sterile dressing. The athlete should

also receive a tetanus booster, if not up-to-date, and intravenous antibiotics immediately in the emergency department and for several doses. The specific antibiotic(s) to be given should be decided on by the orthopedic surgeon and is determined by the severity of the injury and the contamination within the wound.

After reduction and/or wounds are addressed, the athlete should be placed in a long leg splint (from midthigh to the ends of the toes). There are a variety of splinting materials (prefabricated metal splints, plaster, orthoglass, inflatable plastic splints, etc.) that are available, and any form of immobilization will work in the emergent setting. It is important that the splinting material not wrap all the way around the leg and the leg not be wrapped tightly. Also, access to the foot and calf should be available to frequently check for pulses and check the leg for developing compartment syndrome. Compartment syndrome occurs when swelling increases the pressure in the leg compartments to the point where it exceeds the pressure needed to get blood to the muscles and nerves within the compartment. This leads to nerve and muscle death if not treated emergently with a surgical release of the involved compartments, called a fasciotomy. Compartment syndrome is an orthopedic emergency and is common in the setting of tibia and fibula fractures. Please see the entry Compartment Syndrome, Anterior for signs, symptoms, and treatment.

After immobilization, the athlete should be taken to the emergency department for an orthopedic evaluation and definitive management. Ice application and elevation are extremely important treatment modalities for all fractures and should be implemented immediately and used consistently for the first few days after injury.

Nonoperative Treatment by Fracture Type

Closed fractures of the tibia and fibula may be treated with conservative care and nonsurgical treatment. The question of surgical versus nonsurgical care for a specific fracture is decided by the orthopedic surgeon. The following are some conservative treatment modalities for the different types of tibia and fibula fractures.

Tibial Plateau (Knee Joint Surface of the Tibia). Nondisplaced or minimally displaced fractures (bony pieces touching or very close together in anatomical alignment) can be treated by keeping the athlete non–weight bearing in a knee immobilizer or hinged knee brace. Early ROM exercises and quadriceps muscle strengthening are encouraged. Partial weight bearing (~50% of the athlete's weight) is allowed at 8 to 12 weeks from the injury, with progression to full weight bearing as tolerated.

Tibial Shaft. Nondisplaced or minimally displaced fractures can be treated initially in a long leg splint. The athlete's knee should be flexed from 30° to 60° degrees so that he or she can ambulate with crutches. The athlete will be non–weight bearing for 4 to 6 weeks.

Two weeks after injury, the patient may be transitioned over to a long leg cast if the swelling has subsided. Four to six weeks after injury, transition to a short leg cast (below the knee) is permitted. Weight bearing is progressed in the short leg cast for an additional 4 to 6 weeks. The healing time for tibial shaft fractures is highly variable, with an average time of 16 ± 4 weeks. Fracture braces can be also used to give support while the fracture heals.

Fibular Shaft. Treatment is weight bearing as tolerated. The tibia is the main weight-bearing bone of the lower leg; therefore, a splint, cast, or brace is not necessary for healing. A short period of immobilization (below the knee) may be used to help minimize the pain.

Tibial Plafond (Ankle Joint Surface of the Tibia). Most of these fractures require surgery, even if the fracture is nondisplaced. However, if nonsurgical treatment is elected, the athlete is made non–weight bearing and placed in a long leg splint/cast for 6 weeks. Six weeks after injury, a fracture brace with physical therapy for ROM and strengthening is used, and weight bearing is progressed as tolerated once there is radiographic evidence of healing.

Surgical Treatment by Fracture Type

Open fractures of any type require irrigation and debridement under sterile conditions in the operating room. Irrigation involves washing the fracture and the wound with sterile saline, with or without antibiotics in the solution. *Debridement* is the removal of all debris, such as grass, mud, pebbles, and any dead tissue, from the wound. This should be continued until the wound is cleaned of all possible sources of infection.

Tibial Plateau. Displaced fractures need to be fixed with open reduction and internal fixation, meaning surgical incision, reduction of the fracture, and insertion of plates and screws to hold the pieces of bone together in anatomic alignment. The main goal is to reconstruct the articular surface of the knee. The surgeon may use bone graft or cement to fill any voids and add strength if he or she feels that it is indicated. If the fracture pattern is highly comminuted (lots of small pieces), the surgeon may elect to use an external fixator, which involves placing pins into the bones and bars outside the skin to hold the fracture in anatomic alignment.

Tibial Shaft. Depending on the fracture pattern (transverse or oblique), the amount of comminution, and the fracture location (*proximal*, closer to the knee; middle; or distal, closer to the ankle), the surgeon may choose to use an intramedullary nail, plates and screws, or an external fixator to hold the fracture in anatomic position. An intramedullary nail is a titanium nail introduced through an incision at the knee and placed through the center of the proximal tibia, past the fracture site, and into the distal tibia. Screws are then placed in the proximal and distal tibia so that the nail cannot rotate. External fixation is described above. The fibula fracture is usually not operatively fixed with instrumentation. By fixing the tibia, the fibula is kept in an appropriate position to heal. Since it is not the main weight-bearing bone and it is surrounded by soft tissue, it usually heals without the need for operative fixation.

Fibular Shaft. Isolated fibular shaft fractures rarely need operative intervention. If the fibular shaft fracture is coexisting with an ankle ligament injury (e.g., syndesmosis injury), the surgeon may opt to perform open reduction internal fixation.

Tibial Plafond. The goals of surgery are to maintain fibular length and restore the tibial ankle joint surface. Often, final surgery is delayed for several

(7–14) days to give time for the swelling around the ankle to decrease. The athlete may be placed in a long leg splint and sent home with strict instructions to ice and elevate the ankle at all times until the swelling decreases. Alternatively, the athlete may have staged surgeries with external fixation placement immediately after the injury, with or without open reduction and internal fixation (plates and screws) of the fibula fracture. The athlete then rests with the ankle iced and elevated until swelling is decreased. At that time, the athlete will return to the operating room to have open reduction and internal fixation of the tibial plafond and removal of the external fixator. Bone graft, bone graft substitutes, or cement may be used as necessary. A short leg splint is applied in the operating room after surgery. An external fixator may be used as definitive treatment depending on the fracture type and soft tissue status.

Postoperative Care by Fracture Type

Tibial Plateau. As in nonsurgical treatment, the athlete will be non–weight bearing in a knee immobilizer or hinged knee brace. Early range-of-motion exercises and quadriceps muscle strengthening are encouraged. Partial weight bearing (~50% of the athlete's weight) is allowed at 8 to 12 weeks from the injury, with progression to full weight bearing as tolerated.

Tibial Shaft. No splint/cast is needed; an intramedullary nail or external fixation is used; then a splint/cast may be used after the use of plates and screws. The surgeon will determine the athlete's weight-bearing status based on the fracture pattern and the type of fixation used. Again, average healing time is 16 ± 4 weeks.

Fibular Shaft. This fracture, too, rarely requires an operation, but a splint/cast may be used after the use of plates and screws. The surgeon will determine the athlete's weight-bearing status based on the fracture pattern and fixation type.

Tibial Plafond. The athlete will be non–weight bearing for 12 to 16 weeks. Initially, the athlete will be in a short leg splint and will transition to a short leg cast in 2 weeks. In 4 to 6 weeks, the athlete may be transitioned to a fracture brace/boot, and

physical therapy range-of-motion exercises will be started to decrease the stiffness in the ankle. After 12 to 16 weeks, progression will be made to weight bearing as tolerated once there is radiographic evidence of healing.

It is important to closely monitor the athlete's neurovascular exam status after all types of surgery to avoid the complications of compartment syndrome.

Justin R. Hoover and Jeffrey A. Guy

See also Compartment Syndrome, Anterior; Lower Leg Injuries; Skiing, Injuries in; Sports Injuries, Acute

Further Readings

Berkson EM, Virkus WW. High-energy tibial plateau fractures. *J Am Acad Orthop Surg.* 2006;14(1):20–31.

Cannada LK, Anglen JO, Archdeacon MT, Herscovici D, Ostrum RF. Avoiding complications in the care of fractures of the tibia. *J Bone Joint Surg Am.* 2008;90(8):1760–1768.

Koval KJ, Zuckerman JD. *Handbook of Fractures.* 3rd ed. Philadelphia, PA: Lippincott Williams & Wilkins; 2006.

Mashru RP, Herman MJ, Pizzutillo PD. Tibial shaft fractures in children and adolescents. *J Am Acad Orthop Surg.* 2005;13(5):345–352.

Zalavras CG, Patzakis MJ. Open fractures: evaluation and management. *J Am Acad Orthop Surg.* 2003;11(3):212–219.

TIBIA AND FIBULA STRESS FRACTURES

Stress fractures in the tibia and fibula are common in athletes. It has been reported that nearly 50% of stress fractures in the lower extremity occur in the tibia and up to 20% in the fibula. Sports such as cross-country and track account for a large number of these stress fractures, but any sports requiring repetitive running and jumping can result in a stress fracture of the lower extremity.

Most tibia stress fractures occur in the posterior medial tibia. Anterior tibia stress fractures are considered to be problematic, often needing a prolonged period of nonoperative treatment or surgical management to allow them to heal. Fibula stress fractures tend to occur about 5 to 6 centimeters above the lateral malleolus in athletes, but they can occur at any point along the fibula.

Pathophysiology

Many risk factors have been implicated in the development of stress fractures of the tibia and fibula. Some proposed risk factors include running surfaces, footwear, mileage, weight loss, osteopenia/osteoporosis, running mechanics, foot type (pes cavus or pes planus foot types), and muscle fatigue. None have been shown to be a definitive risk factor, but they are believed to often occur in combination. Excessive contraction of the ankle plantarflexors is thought to play a role in fibula stress fractures.

Presenting Signs and Symptoms

Athletes will typically present with progressively worsening pain in the shins with running. Typically with medial tibial stress syndrome, or "shin splints," athletes may have reduction of their pain with running. With stress fractures, the pain tends to get progressively worse with longer periods of impact, as in running or jumping. Often, there is a focal area of pain rather than a large, diffuse area, as is commonly observed in shin splints. The athlete may limp with activity and often will have pain most of the time with just walking. There may have been attempts at taking rest for several days to weeks, only to have the pain recur quickly with resumption of activity. A recent increase in activity or mileage may have occurred.

Physical Exam Findings

Often on exam, the athlete will have a focal area of tenderness to palpation where the stress fracture is located. Pitting edema may be present in the area of the stress fracture. A limp may be present. It has been reported that placing a vibrating tuning fork over the tender area will cause a significant increase in pain, aiding in the diagnosis. Attempting a single leg hop on the affected side often is positive for pain, and many athletes will not want to attempt this as they may have already experienced significant pain with a similar maneuver. Evaluation for foot pronation or supination should be done, but

its usefulness may be limited as the athlete may be walking differently to avoid pain with walking.

Radiologic Findings

Initial evaluation should be done with plain-film X-rays. In the first few weeks of symptoms, it is not unusual to have normal X-rays. Many tibia stress fractures will not show up in radiographic images even after healing has begun. Fibula stress fractures will tend to give radiographic evidence of healing, evident by either a fracture line or callus formation, by 3 to 4 weeks after symptoms have started.

Early in the diagnostic process, it is often necessary to consider further imaging if the clinical suspicion is high for a stress fracture. Both bone scans and magnetic resonance imaging (MRI) scans are used, with MRI scans being slightly more sensitive and specific. MRI scans also have the advantage of being able to evaluate other adjacent structures besides the bone that may be causing pain, and there is no radiation involved. The MRI scan may also help distinguish between a stress reaction, where the bone has not progressed to failure of the cortical bone, and a true stress fracture.

Treatment

Essentially, all fibula stress fractures and the majority of tibia stress fractures are treated nonsurgically. Stress fractures of both the fibula and the tibia respond to rest from impact activity. Rest periods typically range from 4 to 6 weeks but may take up to 8 weeks. Athletes who are limping or having a difficult time with pain with general ambulation may need crutches, a pneumatic brace, or a walking boot for a few weeks to aid in the healing process and for pain relief. Avoidance of frequent use of anti-inflammatory medications is recommended due to the possibility of delayed healing that has been reported with the use of these medications for fractures.

Nonimpact cross-training, such as the use of an elliptical trainer, cycling, or swimming, should be recommended to maintain fitness. Once healing has occurred, gradual resumption of activity is recommended. Evaluation of footwear, running mechanics, and the potential need for over-the-counter or custom foot orthotics should be done to prevent recurrence.

Stress fractures of the anterior tibia frequently are treated surgically with an intramedullary nail. Nonoperative treatment may be undertaken, but it often takes 9 to 12 months for healing to occur.

Mark E. Halstead

See also Lower Leg Injuries; Sports Injuries, Overuse; Stress Fractures

Further Readings

Sherbondy P, Sebastianelli W. Stress fractures of the medial malleolus and distal fibula. *Clin Sports Med.* 2006;25(1):129–137.

Young A, McAllister D. Evaluation and treatment of tibial stress fractures. *Clin Sports Med.* 2006;25(1):117–128.

TIBIAL TUBERCLE AVULSION FRACTURE

Avulsion of the tibial tubercle occurs when the traction on the patellar tendon exceeds the strength of the tibial tubercle. The majority of tibial tubercle avulsions occur in adolescents during jumping sports, particularly due to an eccentric load to the patellar tendon during landing. Tibial tuberosity fractures have been reported almost exclusively in males.

Anatomy

The patellofemoral joint is the articulation of the femur (thighbone) and the patella (kneecap). The patella is a sesamoid (floating) bone within a large thick tendon. Above the patella, this tendon is termed the *quadriceps tendon*, and the continuation below the patella is termed the *patellar tendon*. As the quadriceps muscle contracts, it pulls on the quadriceps and patellar tendon, causing the knee to straighten.

The patellar tendon inserts onto the tibia (shinbone) on the tibial tubercle. In the growing adolescent, the physis (growth plate) of the tibia is located just under the knee joint. Above the physis, there are two centers of ossification, the larger tibial epiphysis and the smaller tibial tubercle apophysis, although in older adolescents, they may coalesce to form a continuous epiphysis.

Causes

This is usually an acute injury caused by either violent contraction of the quadriceps muscle against a fixed tibia (as in jumping) or flexion of the knee against a contracted quadriceps.

Symptoms

There will be swelling and tenderness over the front of the tibia, just below the kneecap. Fluid may be present in the knee, and a triangular fragment of bone may be felt. The injured knee may be held in mild flexion, and there will be difficultly extending it.

Diagnosis

A complete physical exam is done to look for swelling and tenderness. The degree of patella alta (high-riding kneecap) will be proportional to the severity of the injury. The patient will be unable to fully extend the knee.

X-rays of the knee are mandatory, with the lateral projection being the most important (see X-ray below). The physician must be aware that in children and adolescents (ages 9 to 17), the normal tibial tubercle may not be fully ossified.

Several different classification systems, most commonly the Watson-Jones, are used for tibial tubercle avulsion fractures. In general, the most important point of difference is whether the fracture is nondisplaced or displaced.

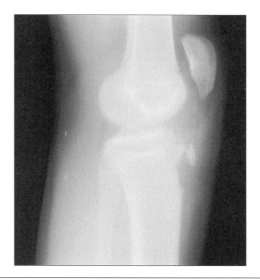

Lateral view of a tibial tubercle fracture

Source: Yi-Meng Yen, M.D.

(a)

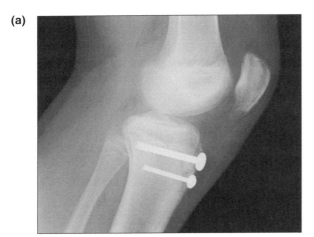

(b)

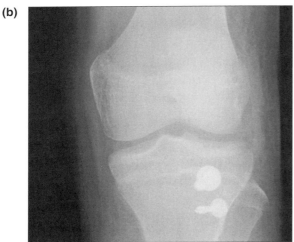

Tibial tubercle fracture after open reduction and internal fixation with two screws and washers; (a) lateral view and (b) anteroposterior view

Source: Yi-Meng Yen, M.D.

Treatment

Closed Reduction and Immobilization

In cases where there is minimal displacement of the tubercle, it is important to understand that the tibial tubercle is still being pulled by the force of the quadriceps into a displaced position. A closed reduction can be attempted and the knee casted. Even in a long leg cast, with the knee in full extension, there can still be tension on the tibial tubercle, so these fractures must be watched closely.

Surgery

Most specialists recommend open reduction and internal fixation of all displaced tibial tubercle fractures. This consists of making a vertical midline incision over the fracture site. The fracture is reduced (put back into place), and metal screws or pins are used to hold the fragment. The patellar tendon and other soft tissues may be sutured down as well to ensure that the screws or pins hold the fragment in place (see images a and b, left).

After Surgery

Depending on the quality of the fixation, patients are placed in either a brace that limits motion or a cast in extension. Crutches are used for touchdown weight bearing for a period of 5 to 6 weeks, at which time progressive full weight bearing can begin. Physical therapy is initiated to help the patient regain knee motion and strength. The patient is not allowed to resume impact activities until motion and strength are regained and the fracture has healed. This typically takes between 3 and 6 months.

Yi-Meng Yen

See also Avulsion Fractures; Tibia and Fibula Fractures; Young Athlete

Further Readings

Bolesta MJ, Fitch RD. Tibial tubercle avulsions. *J Pediatr Orthop.* 1986;6(2):186–192.

Christie MJ, Dvonch VM. Tibial tuberosity avulsion fracture in adolescents. *J Pediatr Orthop.* 1981;1(4):391–394.

Ogden JA, Tross RB, Murphy MJ. Fractures of the tibial tuberosity in adolescents. *J Bone Joint Surg Am.* 1980;62(2):205–215.

Skaggs DL. Extra-articular injuries of the knee. In: Beaty JH, Kasser JR, eds. *Rockwood and Wilkins' Fractures in Children.* Philadelphia, PA: JB Lippincott; 2006:937–984.

TITLE IX, EDUCATION AMENDMENTS OF 1972

Women's position within the world of sports has changed drastically over the past 40 years. This is in large part due to Title IX of the Education Amendments of 1972, legislation originally intended to provide women with improved access to higher education. Title IX states, "No person in the United States shall, on the basis of sex, be excluded from participation in, be denied the benefits of, or be subjected to discrimination under any education program or activity receiving Federal financial assistance."

Prior to this law, it was difficult to nearly impossible for a woman to pursue a career in any field other than nursing, education, social work, or library science. Females were also excluded from major sporting events. The first female to compete in an organized marathon was Kathrine Switzer, in 1967. She registered for the Boston Marathon as K. Switzer to hide her gender and avoid being denied participation. Title IX addressed this discrimination by including all federally funded programs within its purview, such as intramural sports, club sports, and varsity athletics. This new awareness of gender equity in sports led to the Amateur Sports Act of 1978. This act prohibits discrimination on the basis of gender, race, and physical disability in open, nonschool amateur sports. These would include Olympic, Pan American, world championship, and other international sporting events.

To further clarify the scope of this legislation, Title IX governs the overall equity of treatment and opportunity in athletics while giving schools the flexibility to choose sports based on the interests of the students, geographic influence, budget restraints, and gender ratio. In other words, it is a not a matter of women being allowed to participate in wrestling or that exactly the same amount of money is spent for a female as for a male basketball player. Instead, the focus is on the necessity for women to have equal opportunities with men on a collective, not on an individual, basis.

The impact of Title IX is far reaching. More females are participating in sports than ever before. In 1972, 1 in 27 high school girls played varsity sports. In 1988, this had improved to 1 in 3, whereas 1 in 2 boys participated in varsity high school sports. Women now view themselves as strong, competitive, and skilled athletes. In most circumstances, girls are encouraged by their parents at an early age to participate in sports. Parents have realized that the physical, psychological, and social well-being of their daughters is improved

through sports participation. Adolescents who participate in sports are less than half as likely to get pregnant as those with more sedentary habits. They often have greater confidence, self-esteem, and pride; indulge less in high–health risk behaviors such as smoking, drinking, and illicit drug use; are more likely to achieve academic success; graduate from college at a significantly higher rate; and suffer less from depression than those who do not participate in sports. These benefits may be due, in part, to the added benefits of sports, such as teamwork, goal setting, the pursuit of excellence in performance, and other achievement-oriented behaviors necessary for success in the workplace. Parents also realize that the quality of life for their children will likely depend on two incomes. This necessitates the training of daughters as well as sons, and sports participation is an excellent vehicle. Women's participation in sports is now deeply entrenched in core family values, with families enthusiastically supporting the sports participation of both their daughters and their sons.

The academic impact has also been demonstrated. In 1994, women received 38% of medical degrees, compared with 9% in 1972; earned 43% of law degrees, compared with 7% in 1972; and 44% of all doctoral degrees received by U.S. citizens, up from 25% in 1977. These statistics support the previously noted benefits of sports, including higher college graduation rates and greater academic success.

Not only are women participating in larger numbers in a greater number of sports, but advertisers have found themselves a whole new world of focus—the female consumer. Women are buying sporting goods not only for themselves but also for their spouses and children. In fact, women make 80% of the household retail buying decisions. In addition, they buy disproportionately to their participation. For example, female golfers constitute only 20% of all golfers but buy 50% of all golf products with the exception of clubs. The economic power of the active female has led advertisers to focus more attention on the female athlete and sporting goods companies to produce high-quality equipment designed specifically with the female athlete in mind.

With few exceptions, female athletes are making good role models for young girls. The image of the female athlete is positive: nonviolent, appreciative, and hardworking. This is in stark contrast to the image of the professional male athlete, who is often viewed as selfish and arrogant. Although the influx of money and the popularity of women's sports may lead to negative behavior among some women athletes, this has not yet been the case. The general public embraces the spirit and effort with which females approach sports.

As of 2008, female participation in sports is the highest in history, at 9,101 intercollegiate teams and 8.65 women's teams per school. The most popular sport is basketball, followed by volleyball and soccer. In the past decade, 2,755 new women's teams have been created. This growth has been attributed to many factors, including mothers who have benefited from the Title IX legislation encouraging their daughters' sports participation, law suits supportive of Title IX, societal acceptance of females as athletes, improved and increased media coverage, and advocacy groups such as the National Association for Girls and Women in Sports and the National Association of Collegiate Women Athletic Administrators.

Women's sports participation has never been more encouraged and accessible than it is today. Women athletes now enjoy the support of their families, peers, and physicians. Every time a woman takes her place on the playing field, gets in the blocks for a race, or takes the court, she does so with a host of women who came before her paving the way for her to have the opportunity to participate, to be accepted as a viable athlete, and to further perpetuate a culture of athleticism for women. The full impact of a generation of women who are now maturing and who are growing up with opportunities that their mothers and grandmothers never dreamed of having remains to be seen.

Michelle Wilson and Jeffrey A. Guy

See also Benefits of Exercise and Sports; Female Athlete; History of Sports Medicine; Mental Health Benefits of Sports and Exercise

Further Readings

Acosta RV, Carpenter LJ. *Women in Intercollegiate Sport: A Longitudinal Study: Thirty-One Year Update, 1977–2008*. Brooklyn, NY: Brooklyn College; 2008.

Birrell S, Cole CL, eds. *Women, Sport, and Culture*. Champaign, IL: Human Kinetics; 1994.

Guttmann A. *Women's Sports: A History*. New York, NY: Columbia University Press; 1991.

Lopiano DA. Modern history of women in sports. Twenty five years of Title IX. *Clin Sports Med*. 2000;19(2):163–173.

Verbrugge M. *Able-Bodied Womanhood*. New York, NY: Oxford University Press; 1998.

Women's Sports Foundation. *Wilson Report: Moms, Dads, Daughters and Sports*. East Meadow, NY: Women's Sports Foundation; 1989.

Toenail Fungus

In the United States, an estimated 10 million individuals suffer from *onychomycosis,* a fungal infection of the nails. Although the exact incidence is not known, studies suggest that between 2% and 26% of the general population worldwide are affected. Onychomycosis is commonly seen in conjunction with tinea pedis or may occur secondary to trauma to the nail. Although both fingernails and toenails can be infected, onychomycosis occurs approximately four times more frequently in toenails than in fingernails.

A large survey done in Europe in 1997 through 1998 on patients presenting to general practitioners' offices clearly indicated that sports-active individuals have a higher incidence of tinea pedis and onychomycosis than do nonathletes people.

All athletes, regardless of age or type of sport, are at risk of developing onychomycosis. Fungi are known to thrive in moist, warm environments—conditions found inside an athlete's shoe or in the contact of bare feet with infected surfaces such as shower stalls, pool decks, and locker room floors. Trauma to the skin or nails from friction, rubbing, or maceration provides the portal of entry for fungi.

Athletes are also susceptible to toenail problems because of the speed and intensity of play (e.g., in running), the frequent starting and stopping in a game (e.g., in tennis and racquetball), and the type or absence of shoes (e.g., in ballet, gymnastics, or swimming).

Clinical Variants of Onychomycosis

There are four main types or clinical variants of onychomycosis:

1. *Distal subungual onychomycosis:* This infection starts at the hyponychium, the tip of the undersurface of the nail, and migrates proximally through the underlying nail matrix. This is usually caused by *Trichophyton rubrum.* This subtype is the most common (see the first photo).

2. *White superficial onychomycosis:* This variant accounts for 10% of onychomycosis cases. It is most commonly caused by *Trichophyton mentagrophytes* and invades the superficial layers of the nail plate, forming white islands.

3. *Proximal subungual onychomycosis:* This type is the least common in healthy people and usually occurs in immunocompromised patients. It is most commonly caused by *Trichophyton rubrum,* which invades the nail via the proximal nail fold and migrates distally.

4. *Candidal onychomycosis:* This type is seen in patients with chronic mucocutaneous candidiasis. The nail plate thickens and turns a yellow/brown color. This type generally involves all the fingernails.

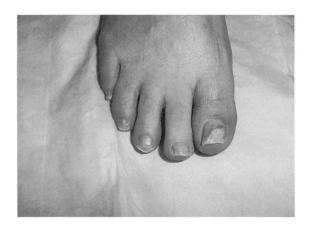

Patient with distal subungual onychomycosis, the most common type of onychomycosis

Source: Peggy R. Cyr, M.D.

Differential Diagnosis

Not all thick, dystrophic toenails are caused by fungi. Fifty percent of thick nails are infected by fungi. The practitioner should perform diagnostic testing to determine if fungi are present. Psoriasis involving the nail is most commonly confused with onychomycosis, and the two diseases may coexist. Pitting of the nail plate surface is seen in psoriasis but not in onychomycosis. Eczema, lichen planus, or habitual picking of the proximal nail fold may induce dystrophic changes in the nail plate. Leukonychia are white spots or bands that are present in the proximal nail plate and grow out with the nail; they may be confused with onychomycosis.

Treatment

There are many options available today for treatment of onychomycosis. The athlete's medical history, concomitant illnesses, and medications must be reviewed carefully. Presenting the patient with published data on the effectiveness of each treatment, as well as the possible side effects, will lead to a joint decision on how to proceed.

Topical Agents

Ciclopirox nail lacquer 8% (Penlac) is approved by the Food and Drug Administration (FDA) for use in mild to moderate onychomycosis caused by *Trichophyton rubrum* with no lunula involvement. The medication is applied once daily to the nail, 5 millimeters of the surrounding skin, the nail bed, and the undersurface of the nail. A new coating is placed over the old one each day, and the medication is completely removed with rubbing alcohol once a week. Treatment extends up to 48 weeks, with periodic debridement of the infected nails. More aggressive debridement may increase the effectiveness of the medication. Published cure rates in the United States are 29% to 36%. In non-U.S. studies, the cure rates were higher; from 46.7% to 85.7%. This method will require a motivated patient to complete the treatment course. There are little to no side effects other than possible redness or irritation of the skin surrounding the nail.

Nail Avulsion Combined With Topical Treatment

This method should only be used for painful, severely affected nails as the procedure is temporarily disabling and painful. Complete toenail removal with phenol/alcohol nail bed ablation is considered in older athletes who have totally dystrophic toenails that are not growing or growing very slowly. Systemic antifungals are doomed to failure in this scenario since improvement depends on the dystrophic nail growing out and being replaced by a new nail proximally. After the procedure, activity must be limited until the nail bed heals. Then, for 6 to 12 months, a bandage must be worn over the freshly healed skin to prevent blistering. After that time, the skin would have developed enough anchoring fibrils, enabling the athlete to engage in any kind of athletic activity without limitation. Debridement of the part of the affected nail that is not attached to the nail bed is encouraged for all patients.

Oral Agents

Griseofulvin (Gris-peg) and ketoconazole (Nizoral) have been available for many years but are no longer considered first-line treatment due to the need for a prolonged treatment course (10–18 months), the low success rates, and the high rates of relapse. Studies show that 90% of patients who were clinically cured after prolonged griseofulvin therapy relapsed 1 to 2 years later.

The newer triazole and allylamine antifungals have replaced griseofulvin and ketoconazole in the treatment of onychomycosis. These drugs, terbinafine (Lamisil), itraconazole (Sporanox), and fluconazole (Diflucan), all promptly penetrate the nail and nail bed, persist for months in the nail after discontinuation of treatment, and have good safety profiles. Each agent has potential drug interactions as well as different dosing options. The FDA approves the use of all these agents, except fluconazole, in treating onychomycosis.

Terbinafine (Lamisil) is the preferred treatment for onychomycosis. Dosing options are 250 milligrams (mg)/day for 12 weeks for toenails and 6 weeks for fingernails. Cure rates are 71% to 82%. There are fewer interactions with this medication than with the other oral antifungals. Another dosing option is 250 mg/day for 1 week every month for 11 or more months until a new nail has grown. In one study, the cure rate was 90%. Headache, rash, and gastrointestinal upset are possible but infrequent side effects. Rare but serious complications include cholestatic hepatitis, blood dyscrasias, and Stevens-Johnson syndrome. It is prudent to take liver function tests and check complete blood count before treatment starts and every 6 weeks during continuous-treatment protocols. If liver functions rise greater than two times above the normal, the medication should be stopped.

Itraconazole (Sporanox) in doses of 200 mg/day for 12 weeks for toenails and 6 weeks for fingernails or pulse therapy at 400 mg/day in the first week of each month can be prescribed. Two to three pulses are recommended for fingernails and three to four pulses for toenails. Liver enzyme monitoring is recommended for continuous therapy but is not considered to be needed for pulse therapy. Published cure rates are 35% to 80%. Because itraconazole is metabolized by hepatic cytochrome P450, significant drug interactions can occur with anti-arrhythmics, HMG CO-A (3-hydroxy-3-methylglutaryl-coenzyme A) reductase inhibitors, benzodiazepines, histamine blockers, and proton pump inhibitors. These interactions make this drug less desirable.

Fluconazole (Diflucan) in doses of 150 mg once weekly for 6 to 9 months can be used. This medication is the treatment of choice for onychomycosis caused by *Candida* but is also effective against other dermatophytes. Published outcomes show clinical improvement in 72% to 89% of the cases. Significant drug interactions can occur with benzodiazepines, cimetidine, HCTZ (hydrochlorothiazide), hypoglycemics, rifampin, theophylline, and coumadin.

Prevention

Most cases of onychomycosis can be prevented by early recognition and treatment of tinea pedis. Any athlete with a rash on his or her feet should have a potassium hydroxide examination of skin scrapings. The rash of tinea pedis may be maceration in the web spaces of the toes, scaling with or without erythema along the lateral aspect of the sole, or inflammatory vesicles along the instep. Dry moccasin scaling is another variation on the appearance of tinea pedis. Tinea pedis can be treated with topical antifungal cream (Spectazole) and antifungal powder (Zeasorb AF). There are numerous over-the-counter antifungal preparations, such as clotrimazole (Lotrimin) and tolnaftate (Tinactin). A simple approach is to place antifungal powder in all shoes in one's closet every Sunday so that compliance is enhanced as different shoes are worn throughout the week. Compliance is the big issue when it comes to long-term prevention strategies. Resistant or severe cases may require oral antifungal agents.

Athletes should use cotton socks for wicking away moisture and wear sandals in locker rooms, pool decks, and shower stalls. Properly fitting shoes are important to prevent microtrauma to the nails. Daily laundering of socks is recommended.

Ciclopirox 8% applied to the nail and nail fold two to three times per week may prevent recurrence after successful treatment of onychomycosis.

Return to Sports

There are no specific return-to-play NCAA (National Collegiate Athletic Association) guidelines for onychomycosis. Wearing sandals in locker rooms and showers is important, particularly until an athlete has been successfully treated.

The toenails may be the starting place for developing tinea on the other parts of the body. Tinea corporis gladiatorum has been described in wrestlers. Though the toenails of wrestlers are covered by shoes, examination of wrestlers with onychomycosis will reveal that many have exposed patches of tinea. Clearing the toenails eliminates the reservoir for fungus in these athletes, decreases the opportunity for development of tinea on exposed surfaces, and therefore decreases the possibility of its spread to other athletes.

Peggy R. Cyr

See also Dermatology in Sports; Fungal Skin Infections and Parasitic Infestations; Podiatric Sports Medicine

Further Readings

de Berker D. Clinical practice. Fungal nail disease. *N Engl J Med.* 2009;360(20):2108–2116.

Elewski BE, Leyden J, Rinaldi MG, Atillasoy E. Office practice-based confirmation of onychomycosis: a US nationwide prospective survey. *Arch Intern Med.* 2002;162(18):2133–2138.

Hinojosa JR, Hitchcock K, Rodriguez JE. Clinical inquiries. Which oral antifungal is best for toenail onychomycosis? *J Fam Pract.* 2007;56(7):581–582.

TORTICOLLIS, ACUTE

Acute torticollis, also known as *wryneck,* is a twisting of the neck causing the head to be tilted and rotated to one side. It is typically caused by spasms of the muscles on one side of the neck. Torticollis may be congenital (present at birth), but acute torticollis usually affects individuals between the ages of 30 and 60, with a greater incidence in females than in males. Athletes in any sport may develop torticollis for a variety of reasons. In contact sports, such as football or basketball, acute torticollis may develop from collisions to the head or torso, which strain the neck muscles. The effects of the collision may manifest immediately or even days later. In other sports, improper technique or overuse and repetitive motions, such as looking up during a tennis serve or shooting a rifle, place the neck in positions that may be prone to spasms.

Anatomy

The neck normally has seven vertebral bodies, which make up the cervical portion of the spine. A vertebral disk, which acts as a shock absorber for the neck and allows for smoother neck motion, separates each of the seven spinal segments. Attached to these segments are numerous ligaments, which provide stability, and muscles, which allow the neck to flex, extend, bend sideways, and rotate. The muscles that are primarily involved in acute torticollis, and can individually or collectively spasm, are the sternocleidomastoid, trapezius, occipitalis, splenius, and levator scapulae.

Causes

Acute torticollis involves irritation of the cervical nerves leading to abnormal neck contractions and is commonly, but not always, caused by some inciting incident, such as rapid head or neck movements or injury from whiplash or concussion. Often, individuals will develop acute torticollis from keeping their head and neck in awkward positions for prolonged periods of time (e.g., sleeping in a wrong position or on a new bed or pillow). If there is a history of forceful trauma to the neck, other etiologies to consider are fracture, dislocation/subluxation, slipped facets, or disk herniation. Medical causes that should not be overlooked and may have a similar presentation are bacterial or viral infections in the head or neck or underlying chronic inflammatory or neurologic diseases. Certain medications can also cause acute torticollis.

Symptoms

Acute torticollis typically presents 1 to 2 days following neck irritation, although symptoms may not develop for several weeks or months. It is usually painful in the neck muscles or down the spine, and the individual has difficulty turning the head to one side. The head may tilt in one direction as the chin tilts in the opposite direction. Involuntary head shaking may occur as a direct result of muscular spasm.

Diagnosis

Acute torticollis is diagnosed by a thorough medical history and physical examination. Special attention to recent or past neck injuries, acuity of onset, pain location and radiation, fevers, and medications can help in confirming the diagnosis. The presenting posture is the head bent sideways in one direction with the chin pointing in the opposite direction. Active range of motion of the neck is usually limited, and the examiner may be able to palpate spasm and elicit tenderness of the affected muscle. The physical examination should also include evaluation of the eyes, ears, nose, mouth, and pharynx. A complete neurologic examination, including the neck and upper extremity, should be performed, and if abnormalities are present, further workup is warranted.

X-rays of the cervical spine can be taken if there is a suspicion of fracture or subluxation. More advanced imaging studies, such as computed tomography (CT) or magnetic resonance imaging (MRI) scans, can be ordered if there is concern about infection (i.e., abscess) or deeper anatomic abnormalities (i.e., disk herniation). No specific laboratory studies are required for acute torticollis unless occult infection or chronic inflammatory conditions need to be ruled out. Electromyography (EMG) can be a useful tool to determine the degree of muscle or nerve involvement.

Treatment

Treatment for acute torticollis is primarily symptomatic. Frequently, the spasms will subside on their own after about a week. Noninvasive modalities include gentle passive stretching of the neck, massage, warm compresses, and a short course of wearing a soft cervical collar for comfort and to allow the muscles to relax. Medications that may provide some benefit include nonsteroidal anti-inflammatory drugs (NSAIDs) and benzodiazepines or other muscle relaxants. If symptoms are prolonged and continue for several weeks or months, botulinum toxin (Botox) injections can be administered, usually by a neurologist or other specialist. These injections help prevent involuntary muscle contractions.

Most of the time, acute torticollis improves with nonsurgical intervention. However, if the problem becomes chronic, selective denervation of the affected muscle (irreversibly severing the nerve supplying the contracted muscle) may be considered. Physical therapy involving manual stretching and strengthening and range-of-motion exercises are started after approximately 1 week.

Rupert Galvez and Jeffrey Guy

See also Neck and Upper Back Injuries; Neck Spasm; Sports Injuries, Overuse

Further Readings

Bland J. *Disorders of the Cervical Spine: Diagnosis and Medical Management.* Philadelphia, PA: WB Saunders; 1987.

Collins DR. *Differential Diagnosis in Primary Care.* Philadelphia, PA: Lippincott Williams & Wilkins; 2007.

Professional Guide to Diseases. 8th ed. Philadelphia, PA: Lippincott Williams & Wilkins; 2005.

Webb M. Acute torticollis. Identifying and treating the underlying cause. *Postgrad Med.* 1987;82(3):121–126.

TRANSSEXUAL ATHLETES

In all but a few sporting disciplines, Olympic competition follows the tradition of segregation of the sexes, which has been defended on the basis of the physiological differences that exist between adult males and females. Prior to puberty, there are no significant differences between the performance abilities of boys and girls. However, during puberty hormonal differences emerge that form the basis for the superior strength, power, and aerobic capacity that males possess, on average, compared with the average postpubertal female. Interestingly, however, as females have come to enjoy greater opportunities in sports, the performance gap between elite female and elite male athletes has become noticeably narrower. Nevertheless, it is still commonly accepted that it would be unfair to permit males to compete against females in the "gender-affected" sports (defined as those sports in which the physical strength, stamina, or physique of average persons of one sex would give them an advantage over average persons of the other sex).

In an effort to maintain the level playing field promised by sex segregation, for nearly three and a half decades, many sports governing bodies and the International Olympic Committee (IOC) pursued a program of "gender verification." The fear was that unscrupulous men might masquerade as women to compete against the "weaker sex," thereby unfairly gaining the laurels of victory. Although the stated goal of gender verification seemed reasonable—given the accepted system of sex segregation—in practice, such testing earned a rather inglorious reputation for inappropriateness and inaccuracy. After repeated public calls for its discontinuation, the IOC finally abandoned routine sex testing prior to the 2000 Sydney Games. Interestingly, since the present doping code demands inspection of the external genitalia at the time of urine collection, a mechanism remains in place for randomly assessing an athlete's phenotypic sex. Olympic medical regulations permit further medical intervention to determine an athlete's true sex should there be medical suspicion of improper participation.

In retrospect, gender verification failed in part because the methodology employed failed to accurately identify those genetic intersex states that confer a performance advantage. The phenotypic and genotypic combinations that are associated with the intersex states confound the commonly accepted definitions of what constitutes male and female and thus challenge the simple binary understanding of sex that society has accepted as normal. Similarly, transsexualism blurs the physiological borders between male and female in ways that challenge our accepted beliefs about sex. Indeed, the issue of how to integrate transsexual athletes into elite sports has proven to be quite contentious. The critical question is whether transsexual athletes (particularly postpubertal male-to-female [MTF] transsexual athletes) have an unfair performance advantage over other female athletes.

Transsexualism refers specifically to individuals who identify with (and wish to be accepted as a member of) the sex opposite to that assigned to them at birth. As such, it falls at one end of the transgender spectrum. Our current understanding suggests that transsexuals feel compelled to transition from their assigned birth sex to the opposite sex out of a prevailing sense that their true gender is at odds with their birth sex, a condition known as gender identity disorder. The resulting gender dysphoria is considered to be incurable, and the interventions to transform one's sex—which include exogenous administration of hormones and surgical sexual reassignment—are therefore merely palliative. Once transitioned from their assigned birth sex to their acquired sex, the transsexual's genotype and phenotype are disconnected, and it is only through ongoing manipulation of their hormonal milieu that transsexuals are able to maintain their acquired physiology.

Exogenous administration of sex hormones therefore represents the cornerstone of therapy for gender identity disorder and is the mechanism for effecting the desired physiologic cross-sex transition. Sexual reassignment surgery is available to those who wish to complete the phenotypic conversion. Studies of postpubertal MTF transsexuals have documented the effects of prolonged androgen suppression combined with estrogen supplementation, including significant decreases in total and regional muscle mass, muscle strength, and bone density and significant increases in total and regional fat mass. However, no peer-reviewed studies have been published describing the effects of long-term cross-sex hormone therapy on sports performance.

Consequently, it is unclear whether any significant physiologic performance advantage exists for the fully transitioned MTF transsexual athlete over an elite athlete who retains her female birth sex. Of course, those MTF transsexuals who transition after puberty will (at least partially) retain the acquired skeletal effects of testosterone exposure (e.g., height), which could prove advantageous in selected sports. However, given the wide-ranging physiological differences that exist between elite athletes, it seems likely that the abilities of the vast majority of transsexual athletes will fall within the existing spectrum of sex- and sport-specific athletic performance capacity. As a case in point, consider the pioneering MTF transsexual athlete Renée Richards. Although she achieved considerable success in tennis, her level of accomplishment did not outstrip prior levels of accomplishment attained by other athletes (who were presumably females at birth). Unfortunately, Richards was forced to overcome daunting obstacles (not the least of which was public scorn) in order to compete in her chosen sport.

The debate over whether transsexuals should be permitted to compete in sports as members of their acquired sex seemingly intensified when the IOC decided to critically examine the issue. After considerable deliberation, in 2004 the Committee voted to permit transsexual athletes who meet strict criteria to participate in the Olympics (see Table 1). The IOC's decision (the "Stockholm Consensus") led to an outcry of protest from those who feared that the existing competitive balance in elite women's sport would be upset by the influx of poorly feminized transsexuals. Despite these concerns, such a competitive imbalance has yet to materialize at the Olympic level, as no openly transsexual athletes competed in the Games of Athens, Torino, or Beijing. It is not known whether this reflects transsexual athletes' unwillingness to publicize their status or other factors (e.g., failure to qualify or simply the low number of elite transgender athletes).

It appears unlikely that the question of whether it is fair for postpubertal transsexual athletes to compete in sports against athletes who share their acquired sex will be resolved unless convincing new information is brought to bear on the matter. Of course, the difficulty in agreeing on what is fair lies in the fact that fairness is a subjective value. Even so, research should help inform the constituents whether consistent sport-specific performance advantages exist for the transsexual athlete, and education can help correct the misinformation and alleviate the prejudice that inevitably accompanies consideration of this issue. Meanwhile, in the United Kingdom, politicians have entered into the discussion. Shortly after the Stockholm Consensus was announced, Parliament revised its statutes concerning sex discrimination. The Gender Recognition Act (GRA) of 2004 provided transsexuals with the important legal right to be identified as belonging to their acquired gender. However, Section 19 of the GRA specifies that "in certain circumstances" transsexuals may be restricted

Table 1   Olympic Eligibility Criteria for Transsexual Athletes, Based on the Stockholm Consensus

Birth Sex	Acquired Sex	Timing of Intervention	Duration of Therapy	Sex Reassignment Surgery Required?	Legal Recognition
Male	Female	Prepubertal	Ongoing	Yes	Required
Female	Male	Prepubertal	Ongoing	Yes	Required
Male	Female	Postpubertal	2 years minimum	Yes	Required
Female	Male	Postpubertal	2 years minimum	Yes	Required

from competing in certain gender-affected sports to "ensure fair competition."

Apart from the ongoing debate, from a practical standpoint, the sports medicine practitioner who encounters a transsexual athlete should remember the unique aspects of transsexual physiology. Hormonal therapy is not without undesirable side effects, including (but not limited to) effects on cardiovascular health and hepatic function. Interestingly, however, one study of 293 female-to-male (FTM) transsexuals failed to demonstrate any significant increase in cardiovascular disease compared with the general population. The effect of hormonal manipulation on transsexual injury risk and recovery from injury remains largely unexplored. It is also critically important for all involved to remember that to be eligible to compete in the Olympic Games, the FTM athlete must obtain a Therapeutic Use Exemption (TUE) permitting exogenous administration of androgens. Failure to do so would constitute a doping violation. Of course, in light of the Stockholm Consensus, gender identity disorder is now an IOC-recognized diagnosis, and thus, FTM transsexuals should be eligible for a TUE providing they satisfy the strict IOC criteria governing transsexual participation.

Jonathan C. Reeser

See also History of Sports Medicine; Performance Enhancement, Doping, Therapeutic Use Exemptions; World Anti-Doping Agency

Further Readings

Cavanagh SL, Sykes H. Transsexual bodies at the Olympics: the International Olympic Committee's policy on transsexual athletes at the 2004 Athens Summer Games. *Body Soc.* 2006;12(3):75–102.

Gooren LJ. Olympic sports and transsexuals. *Asian J Androl.* 2008;10(3):427–432.

Liu PY, Death AK, Handelsman DJ. Androgens and cardiovascular disease. *Endocr Rev.* 2003;24(3): 313–340.

Mcardle D. Swallows and Amazons, or the sporting exception to the Gender Recognition Act. *Soc Leg Stud.* 2008;17(1):39–57.

Pilgrim J, Martin D, Binder W. Far from the finish line: transsexualism and athletic competition. *Fordham Intellectual Property Media Entertainment Law J.* 2003;13:495–550.

Teetzel S. On transgendered athletes, fairness, and doping: an international challenge. *Sport Soc.* 2006;9(2):227–251.

TRAVEL MEDICINE AND THE INTERNATIONAL ATHLETE

Travel medicine is the discipline devoted to the maintenance of the health of international travelers through health promotion and disease prevention. It is a multidisciplinary field, encompassing a wide variety of specialties and subspecialties, including infectious and tropical diseases, public health and preventive medicine, primary care, and geographic, occupational, military, and wilderness medicine. Recently, travel medicine has broadened to include migration medicine, immigrant health, and a focus on the impact of travel on receiving countries. Unlike many other health care specialties, depending on the country, travel medicine is often practiced by both nurses and physicians.

The worldwide focus and knowledge base of travel medicine distinguishes it from most other fields of medicine and nursing. Travel medicine practitioners must be aware of infectious disease risks and their magnitude, patterns of drug resistance, current outbreaks of illness, civil and military conflicts, and political barriers to travel at border crossings. In addition, they must have access to the most up-to-date information on travel-related vaccines and medications.

Today, the focus of travel medicine is on recreational tourists, business persons, overseas volunteers, missionaries, and the military. In addition, the current era of the increasing popularity of ecotourism and extreme travel has added a new dimension to the field. Professionals counsel increasing numbers of immune-compromised individuals, such as those with HIV (human immunodeficiency virus) infection, cancer, autoimmune disease, or organ transplants.

Health Advice to Travelers

Health risks are increasing for travelers to developing countries. These can easily be overcome, however, through the dissemination of accurate information. Public health organizations have excelled in gathering information on the extent of disease prevalence and on prevention and treatment. They have made such knowledge readily available to hospitals, physicians, and the travel industry. The news media can do much to disseminate information in ways that enhance the enjoyment of travel to the developing world, instead of frightening people away.

Travel advice is based on the recommendations of the Centers for Disease Control and Prevention (CDC) and the World Health Organization (WHO) and is supplemented by information provided by International SOS.

Before Traveling Out of a Country

Before traveling abroad, it is important to schedule an appointment with a health care provider at least 4 to 6 weeks in advance to discuss any needed vaccines or medications to prevent disease while traveling.

People with medical problems such as arrhythmias, clotting disorders, lung problems, or heart failure should discuss travel plans with their doctor even sooner. Even within small countries, diseases such as malaria might be a risk in one city but not in another, so it makes a difference to know exactly where a person will be going and what he or she will be doing. Also, the person must bring along a copy of previous immunizations. For the traveler's own safety, it is necessary, for all travel, that he or she is up-to-date on routine vaccinations. Most doctors also recommend hepatitis A and B vaccines for travelers. Based on travel plans, the doctor will then make recommendations about taking drugs to prevent malaria or vaccines to prevent yellow fever, typhoid, and other infectious diseases.

There are very few actual required vaccinations for travel, but this again depends on where the traveler will be going and when. The physician may refer the person to a travel medicine clinic if certain vaccinations are needed that are not readily available in regular clinics.

Those with underlying health problems should, with appropriate pretravel planning and behavioral modification during travel, be able to minimize the health risks associated with the travel. However, they must have realistic expectations concerning health maintenance and travel restrictions. Those

individuals at special risk have the option of making use of numerous resources that are now available to make travel an enjoyable and rewarding experience.

Travelers to developing countries, particularly those visiting friends and relatives, have the highest morbidity for infectious diseases, including typhoid, hepatitis A, malaria, tuberculosis, and HIV infection. This is associated with their lifestyle, behavior, culture, and beliefs. Improvements in travel medicine practice, including the development of new antimalarial drugs and novel vaccines, have been of little benefit to this group of travelers, as can be seen from the increasing trend of morbidity. Pretravel services are underused by this population, and there is little material adapted to the language and cultures of developing countries. A major shift in practice will be necessary to benefit these vulnerable travelers.

Preventing infection among business travelers is one of the key areas of the travel consultation. Prevention methods include timely vaccination, hygienic food and water, precautions against insects, and tuberculosis screening.

The business traveler, corporation, and medical practitioner have mutual responsibilities to ensure the health and safety of the traveler and consequently the success of the trip. The most effective way to manage this responsibility is through the use of medical practitioners with an expertise in both occupational and travel medicine. An effective travel consult should identify means for the prevention of disease and provide the appropriate anticipatory guidance to the individual who is travelling. In addition, the travel consultant should also address the potential health and safety liabilities to the company when clearing personnel for business-related travel. The corporate traveler and employer must have an effective plan for medical emergencies prior to the traveler's departure. On their return, long-term corporate travelers should have reentry physicals and health debriefings. Finally, to maximize preventive efforts, particularly in relation to future travel, business travelers should complete the vaccination series that were begun prior to travel.

Medical Support for Travelling Athletes

Professional and amateur sports require frequent travel. Athletes are confronted frequently with obstacles to optimal performance. The trainers, medical team, and staff face challenges in providing support while traveling and working.

Physical examinations should include screening, the review of past medical history and vaccinations, and physical and dental examination. This will help establish the team member's preparedness to face the challenges of international travel. This examination could identify medical problems such as travel anxiety, asthma, dental caries, gastrointestinal problems, allergies, diabetes mellitus, and coronary heart disease. All medical records of the athletes should be kept secure and accessible in the hand luggage during travel.

Large athletic events are frequently associated with outbreaks of infectious disease. All athletes and members of the team should have an up-to-date immunization status (i.e., measles, tetanus, diphtheria, polio, pertussis, rubella, and mumps). Medical team members and full-contact athletes (i.e., boxers, martial artists, and wrestlers) should have three doses of hepatitis B shots. Athletes traveling to developing countries should consider a hepatitis A vaccination. Athletes without any previous exposure to chickenpox should be vaccinated for varicella with two doses 4 to 8 weeks apart. Meningococcal and influenza vaccine should be considered. Vaccines against diseases such as rabies, typhoid, yellow fever, malaria, cholera, and Japanese encephalitis are recommended according to the guidelines of international agencies.

Education on preventing infectious disease during international competitions should be provided to athletes, coaches, and the staff accompanying the team. Recommended methods to prevent communicable disease during traveling are drinking bottled or purified water, hand washing with soap and water or using alcohol-based hand gel, washing or peeling fruits and vegetables before eating, eating fully cooked foods, and abstinence or use of condoms to avoid sexually transmitted infections.

The following measures should be taken to ensure preparedness for international travel. First, it should be assumed that nothing will be provided, regardless of the preparatory phase. Second, the teams should be self-sufficient. Third, communication with the host country is advisable beforehand (e.g., regarding electricity, water, telephones, the Internet, ice, examination tables, or towels). A travel health kit (first-aid items and antiseptic hand gel, antidiarrheal medication, thermometer) should be made available to athletes at all times. Medical health records of all athletes should be available. Weather forecasts should be reviewed before departure, and athletes traveling to high altitudes should have undergone acclimatization.

Problems arising during travel might relate to major time zone changes, modes of transportation, changes in climate and humidity, sun exposure, and differences in food, housing, language, and religion. Endemic infections such as hepatitis B, yellow fever, and typhoid may require clarification and appropriate immunization prior to travel. Immunization might require several months of preplanning to ensure adequate sero-conversion. Chemoprophylaxis for some diseases, such as malaria, should be initiated in advance.

Hygienic standards should be maintained during food preparation while traveling. At international competitions such as the Olympic Games, a diverse selection of food is available. This enables athletes and staff from around the world to have their normal diet.

Toxigenic *Escherichia coli* is a well-known agent responsible for "traveler's diarrhea." It can be communicated by contaminated water, so in case of any doubt about the safety of the water supply, the team should drink and brush their teeth only with bottled mineral water. Travel to a hot and humid environment warrants an adequate intake of fluid to prevent dehydration and hyperthermia. Sufficient consumption of fluids will change urine to a light color. This is a better indicator than thirst. Another monitoring method for dehydration is daily weight charting. Additional salt in the food or fluid is recommended.

It is important to plan air travel well to minimize the effects of traveling. Jet lag is due to the physiological changes that occur when the sleep-wake cycle is disrupted. Changes in hormone metabolism and body temperatures occur, which lead to feelings of confusion and exhaustion. Athletes should consider avoiding heavy training on arrival and instead participate in one or two light training sessions to ease their transition. It can take several days before these factors settle back into rhythm and maintain an appropriate balance. For every hour of time zone change, one day of accommodation may be required to overcome the effects of jet lag.

To minimize the effects of jet lag, athletes may try to adjust their sleep pattern over several days prior to departure to coincide with the time zone at the site of the competition. On the airplane flight, it helps to move around as much as possible, to avoid alcohol and coffee, and to ingest large amounts of fluid. It is recommended that athletes stay up on the day of arrival and try to adjust to the normal sleep pattern of the country in which they have arrived. Exercise after a long flight may prevent the malaise of jet lag. The use of high-protein meals and stimulating drugs such as caffeine, contained in beverages such as coffee and tea, may be temporarily useful for improving alertness at the time of arrival. Benzodiazepines could promote sleep during a long flight. Drowsiness and decrease of psychomotor performance are the side effects, which might decrease athletic performance. Therefore, these drugs should be reserved for traveling athletes with persistent insomnia, and their use should be supervised by a physician. Melatonin, a hormone that is secreted at night and plays a key role in circadian rhythms, is available as a drug. Conflicting evidence exists on the effects of melatonin on athletic performance and the amelioration of jet lag symptoms. Drowsiness and headaches might hinder sports performance if taken inappropriately. Athletes should use melatonin during flights if they are accustomed to the effects of this remedy. Long-distance travel should be interrupted for 1 to 2 days for a more gradual introduction to major time zone changes.

Motion sickness is another problem frequently encountered during traveling. Unstable air, mountainous roads, and heavy seas may trigger symptoms including nausea, vomiting, dizziness, headache, and malaise. Drugs such as dimenhydrinate, transdermal scopolamine, and meclizine when taken before travel may prevent symptoms of motion sickness.

Before setting off on the journey home, the same precautions for travel should be discussed with the team and athletes. Athletes with a medical problem or injury should be monitored closely, and preparations for their care at home should be made in advance. In case of a medical event, the team physician should prepare a health report on medical encounters, the type of injury or illness, treatments, and emergencies. The report may be presented to the local organizing committee and to the sports organizations back home. This approach will help explain the need for the medical services used and assist in preparations for future international athletic events.

Sercan Bulut and Hakan Yaman

See also Blood-Borne Infections; HIV and the Athlete; Infectious Diseases in Sports Medicine; Team Physician

Further Readings

Chicoine JF, Tessier D. International adoption. In: Keystone JS, Kozarsky PE, Freedman DO, Nothdurft HD, Connor BA, eds. *Travel Medicine*. Barcelona, Spain: Elsevier Science; 2004:275–281.

Cossar J.H. A review of travel-associated illness. In: Steffen R, Lobel HO, Haworth J, Bradley DJ, eds. Travel Medicine. Proceedings of the First Conference on International Travel Medicine, Zurich, Switzerland. Berlin, Germany: Springer; 1988:50–55.

Grimes P. Health advise to travelers. In: Steffen R, Lobel HO, Haworth J, Bradley DJ, eds. Travel Medicine. Proceedings of the First Conference on International Travel Medicine, Zurich, Switzerland. Berlin, Germany: Springer; 1988:501–504.

International Olympic Committee IOC Medical Commission. *Medical Support for Teams Travelling. Sport Medicine Manual* (A Publication of Olympic Solidarity, International Olympic Committee, Lausanne, Switzerland). Calgary, Alberta, Canada: Hurford Enterprises; 1990:453–457.

Kary JM, Lavallee M. Travel medicine and the international athlete. *Clin Sports Med.* 2007;26(3):489–503.

Keller P, Koch K. World tourism: facts and figures. In: Steffen R, Lobel HO, Haworth J, Bradley DJ, eds. Travel Medicine. Proceedings of the First Conference on International Travel Medicine, Zurich, Switzerland. Berlin, Germany: Springer; 1988:10–16.

Kozarsky EP, Keystone SJ. Introduction to travel medicine. In: Keystone JS, Kozarsky PE, Freedman DO, Nothdurft HD, Connor BA, eds. *Travel Medicine*. Barcelona, Spain: Elsevier; 2004:1–4.

Steffen R. Health risks for short-term travelers. In: Steffen R, Lobel HO, Haworth J, Bradley DJ, eds. Travel Medicine. Proceedings of the First Conference on International Travel Medicine, Zurich, Switzerland. Berlin, Germany: Springer; 1988:27–36.

TRIANGULAR FIBROCARTILAGE COMPLEX

The *triangular fibrocartilage complex* (TFCC) is a structure found in the wrist. The TFCC serves as the primary stabilizer of the distal wrist joint, as well as provides for cushioning from certain activities. It works in a similar fashion to the menisci found in the knee and is often called the "wrist meniscus." It can be injured either acutely during trauma or from repetitive overuse. There is some evidence that, over time, the TFCCs of all patients will begin to break down (usually beginning in the fourth decade of life) to a certain degree.

The TFCC is made up of several different structures. The primary components are the dorsal and palmar volar ligaments. These ligaments run from the radius to the ulna and provide for the structure of the TFCC. There is also a soft tissue disk that lies between these ligaments and provides extra support. Finally, a portion of the tendon sheath of the extensor carpi ulnaris (ECU) makes up a portion of the TFCC.

The TFCC can be injured either traumatically or through repetitive activity. Patients can suffer TFCC tears related to falls on their wrists and arms or from direct trauma to the ulnar side of the wrist. In particular, any trauma that results in the hand being forced downward against the ulna may result in a TFCC injury. TFCC injury from repetitive trauma and overuse is often seen in patients who perform activities that result in repetitive ulnar deviation of the wrist (e.g., lifting heavy weights, working with equipment such as hammers or drills). In addition, sports that result in repetitive compression of the wrist may result in TFCC tears; these sports include racquet sports, gymnastics, and diving. In addition, distal radius and ulnar fractures are often associated with TFCC tears.

The differential diagnosis of a TFCC tear includes, but is not limited to, fractures of the radius and/or ulna, tendinosis and tenosynovitis of the flexor or extensor tendons, displacement/snapping of the ECU tendon, injuries to other ligamentous or cartilaginous structures of the wrist (distal radioulnar joint [DRUJ], scapholunate, etc.), and arthroses of the wrist joint.

Diagnosis of a TFCC tear can be performed both clinically and radiographically. Typically, the patient will experience discomfort of varying degrees with palpation of the structure. Patients with small tears may experience little to no pain or limitations, while patients with larger and/or chronic tears may have constant debilitating pain both at rest and with use. The location of the tear will be important as well. Typically, the more peripheral a tear, the more likely it is to cause the patient discomfort; central tears of the TFCC can often be asymptomatic.

The outermost structure of the TFCC is easily palpated along the lateral wrist between the ulna and the lateral carpal bones (pisiform and hamate). Palpation of the structure can be accentuated with radial deviation of the hand. There may also be associated swelling around the structure, as well as "clicking" of the wrist, which may be heard or felt by the patient. Patients may also experience decreased grip strength and pain with resisted wrist dorsiflexion. The Apley Grind is the most commonly used diagnostic test. This test is usually performed with the physician gripping the hand of the patient and applying downward pressure, causing the hand to deviate toward the ulna. The hand can then have a twisting force applied to it, causing the TFCC to be compressed and exacerbating the pain.

Radiographic studies can also be of benefit in diagnosing TFCC injuries. Although the TFCC is a cartilaginous structure, X-rays can sometimes be helpful, for several reasons. With both trauma to the wrist and chronic pain, plain radiographs are often ordered to evaluate for bony injury. Evidence of an ulnar fracture of any form could alert the clinician to the possibility of a TFCC injury. More important, the shape of the ulna can help in making the diagnosis. In general, the lengths of the ulna and radius in the wrist are the same. However, in some patients, the ulna may be either longer or shorter than the radius; this is defined as positive or negative ulnar variance, respectively. Both positive and negative ulnar variance can be associated with a higher rate of TFCC injury.

To truly evaluate the TFCC, magnetic resonance imaging (MRI) is often required. This test allows visualization of the soft tissue of the wrist. This will often reveal swelling along the cartilage and sometimes a tear in the cartilage. The test can be made more accurate by the injection of contrast medium into the wrist. This procedure is called an *MR arthrogram*, and it can allow for better visualization of a TFCC tear, as the contrast material may actually track through the tear into other areas of the wrist where it was not injected. Computed tomographic (CT) arthrography may also be done, although it is typically not as accurate as MR arthrograms. Finally, the TFCC tear may be directly visualized through an arthroscopic procedure.

Treatment of TFCC tears can be both conservative and surgical. In general, nonoperative therapies are attempted first. Modalities such as protection from further injury, rest, and ice application are often helpful. Bracing is often used for mild and/or acute injuries as mild trauma to the TFCC may heal on its own. Bracing can be used with activities that cause pain and discomfort for the patient. At times, a cast can be used for a period of 2 to 4 weeks as well. This allows for immobilization as well as protection. This can be particularly helpful in cases of chronic TFCC injuries. Another option for treatment can be corticosteroid injection in or around the TFCC. This can be done for both diagnostic and therapeutic reasons. Also, both physical therapy and physiotherapy may be helpful. Finally, in cases that are resistant to conservative therapy, surgery can be an option. This surgery is usually accomplished arthroscopically and can be done for either acute or chronic tears. This intervention may result in either repair of the tear or excision of the fragments. Patients suffering from severe tears may be more likely to require surgical intervention. Also, if there are concomitant injuries to other structures of the wrist that require surgical intervention, then patients may undergo surgical correction of their TFCC injury at the same time.

Daniel S. Lewis

See also Triangular Fibrocartilage Injuries; Wrist Injuries; Young Athlete

Further Readings

Cohen S, Pannunzio M. Soft tissue injuries of the wrist in athletes. In: O'Connor FG, Sallis R, Wildner R, St Pierre P, eds. *Sports Medicine: Just the Facts.* New York, NY: McGraw-Hill; 2005:299–305.

Nagle D. Triangular fibrocartilage complex tears in the athlete. *Clin Sports Med.* 2001;20(1):155–166.

Verheyden J. Triangular fibrocartilage complex injuries. http://emedicine.medscape.com/article/1240789-overview. Updated June 23, 2009. Accessed June 14, 2010.

TRIANGULAR FIBROCARTILAGE INJURIES

The *triangular fibrocartilage complex* (TFCC) is a complex ligament-cartilage complex that sits between the distal ulna and the ulnar carpus. It serves as the main stabilizer of the distal radioulnar joint (DRUJ) and plays an important role in load bearing across the ulnar wrist. Tears of the TFCC are an important cause of both acute and chronic ulnar-sided wrist pain. This entry reviews the anatomy of the TFCC and discusses the classification, evaluation, and treatment of TFCC tears.

Anatomy/Function

The TFCC was first described by A. K. Palmer and F. W. Werner in 1981 and consists of an articular disk, a meniscus homologue, ulnocarpal ligament, dorsal and volar radioulnar ligament, and the extensor carpi ulnaris (ECU) sheath. It originates from the ulnar fossa of the distal radius and inserts into the base of the ulnar styloid. It is 2 millimeters (mm) thick on the radial side and 5 mm thick on the ulnar side. Distally, it inserts onto the lunate via the ulnolunate ligament (UL) and the triquetrum via the ulnotriquetral ligament (UT). The UL and UT ligaments are located volarly and are referred to as the disk carpal ligaments.

Blood supply is via the dorsal and palmar radiocarpal branches of the ulnar artery and the dorsal and palmar branches of the anterior interosseous artery. These vessels penetrate 10% to 40% of the periphery, leaving the central disk and radial portion avascular. As in the knee meniscus, peripheral tears are amenable to repair, whereas the central avascular portion does not heal.

As stated earlier, the primary function of the TFCC is as a stabilizer of the DRUJ. The volar portion of the TFCC prevents dorsal displacement of the ulna, and the dorsal portion prevents volar displacement of the ulna. Stability is achieved through selective tightening of the dorsal and volar TFCC during pronation and supination. The TFCC also increases the gliding surface for the radius and acts as a buttress to the proximal carpal row.

Another major function is to cushion axial loading through the ulnocarpal axis. The majority (80%) of axial load is carried by the radius; however, this can vary based on ulnar variance. Ulnar variance is a measure of the relative length of the ulna in relation to the radius. Studies have shown that a positive ulnar variance of 2.5 mm can increase load transmission by the TFCC to 42% while a negative ulnar variance of 2.5 mm can decrease load transmission to 4%. The increased load across the TFCC that occurs with positive ulnar variance accounts for its increased association with TFCC tears.

Examination/Evaluation

The most common symptom of a TFCC tear is ulnar-sided wrist pain with grinding or clicking during wrist range of motion. The mechanism of injury may be an acute fall onto an outstretched hand; a rotational injury with forced ulnar deviation, such as batting a baseball; or axial loading, such as in gymnastics. Chronic injuries result from overuse with repetitive rotation and loading of the ulnar wrist, also common in gymnasts. Isolated pain with pronation and supination may indicate injury to the articular disk, while constant pain with limited range of motion is associated with more peripheral tear.

Examination should include inspection for gross deformity, soft tissue swelling, erythema, and ecchymosis. Active and passive range of motion should include flexion, extension, pronation, supination, and radial and ulnar deviation. Patients are usually tender distal to the ulnar styloid in the soft depression just proximal to the pisiform. A painful click may be reproduced with repetitive pronation and supination of a clenched and ulnarly deviated wrist. Pain and/or clicking with the TFCC compression test may indicate a TFCC tear. This test involves wrist extension, ulnar deviation, and axial compression. DRUJ instability may be present, as evidenced by a positive "piano key sign," in which there is increased displacement of the distal ulna as the radius is held stable and the examiner forces or "shucks" the ulna in the volar and dorsal direction.

The ulna appears more prominent and ballottable, resembling a piano key.

Plain radiographs are a useful initial imaging modality for TFCC injuries because they may reveal a distal radius or ulnar styloid fracture and also allow for assessment of ulnar variance. The recommended views are zero-rotation PA (postero-anterior) and lateral. Triple-injection arthrography used to be the study of choice but has been shown to have poor correlation with arthroscopic findings and has fallen out of favor over the past 5 to 10 years. The utility of magnetic resonance imaging (MRI) is debatable, with sensitivity ranging from 17% to 100% in conflicting studies. A dedicated wrist coil can improve accuracy, but MRI is still not ideal for localizing tears. The gold standard is wrist arthroscopy, which can be used diagnostically and therapeutically.

Differential Diagnosis

Examination should also be centered on excluding other common causes of ulnar-sided wrist pain. Dorsal pain may be caused by tendinitis or subluxation of the ECU. Patients with ECU tendinitis will have pain with resisted wrist extension and ulnar deviation. Subluxation may be present with a palpable, painful snap when a flexed, ulnarly deviated wrist is supinated. Lunotriquetral (LT) instability should be evaluated for with ballottement and shuck tests of the LT joint. Volar pain may be caused by flexor carpi ulnaris (FCU) tendinitis or a fracture of the hook of the hamate or pisiform. FCU tendinitis will present with pain with resisted wrist flexion and ulnar deviation. Hook of the hamate fractures present with hypothenar pain and are often caused by direct trauma to the hypothenar region from grasping an object, such as the butt of a golf club.

Classification of TFCC Tears

In 1989, A. K. Palmer devised a classification system for TFCC tears, distinguishing acute tears from chronic tears and helping guide treatment strategies. Class I tears are acute, traumatic tears. They are further divided based on the location of the tear. Type IA tears are of the central, avascular portion of the articular disk. Type IB tears occur at the base of the ulnar styloid with or without a distal ulnar fracture. Type IC tears are of the ulnolunate or ulnotriquetral ligament at the carpal attachment. Type ID tears are radial sided with or without a sigmoid notch fracture.

Type II tears are chronic and degenerative in nature, describing a spectrum of damage by repetitive loading and positive ulnar variance called ulnocarpal abutment syndrome. Types IIA and IIB tears do not have frank perforation but thinning of the disk without and with chondromalacia of the lunate or ulna, respectively. Type IIC tears are frank perforations of the central disk with chondromalacia. Type IID tears are frank perforations of the disk with chondromalacia and a tear of the LT ligament. Type IIE tears describe end-stage disease with perforation, chondromalacia, LT tear, and ulnocarpal arthritis.

Treatment

The initial treatment for both acute and symptomatic chronic tears is a period of immobilization in a long arm cast for 4 to 6 weeks followed by physical therapy. A localized cortisone injection may provide some symptomatic relief as well. Acute, peripheral tears (Types IB and IC) that are not associated with positive ulnar variance do very well with nonoperative treatment. In contrast, acute avascular tears (Types IA and ID) and both acute and chronic tears associated with ulnar impaction do not heal well without surgical debridement and ulnar-shortening procedures. The emphasis should be on correcting positive ulnar variance as many studies have shown poor outcomes for simple TFCC debridement without ulnar shortening. Types IIA and IIB lesions may only require ulnar shortening without arthroscopic debridement as they do not have frank tears. Type IIC tears may be treated with a "wafer" procedure, in which a 2- to 4-mm section on the distal ulna is removed while keeping the styloid, TFCC, and ligaments attached. Type IID tears with LT instability require ulnar shortening along with LT ligament repair or possible LT fusion or pinning. Type IIE lesions require a salvage procedure.

The TFCC is a complex structure that stabilizes the DRUJ and supports axial load across the ulnar wrist. TFCC tears represent an important cause of ulnar-sided wrist pain. Injuries are often caused by acute falls on an outstretched hand or chronic overloading of the ulnar wrist. The most common symptom is pain with clicking during wrist motion, and examination will often reveal pain with a TFCC compression test. TFCC tears are associated with positive ulnar variance, which can be seen on plain radiographs. Tears are classified as acute and degenerative, and treatment for both types is a period of immobilization followed by therapy. Arthroscopy is indicated for unstable lesions and those refractory to nonoperative treatment. Ulnar shortening should be performed for those with ulnar impaction syndrome.

Rahul Kapur

See also Sports Injuries, Acute; Triangular Fibrocartilage Complex; Wrist Injuries

Further Readings

Ahn AK, Chang DC, Plate A-M. Triangular fibrocartilage complex tears. *Bull NYU Hosp Jt Dis.* 2006;64(3&4):114–118.

Triathlons, Injuries in

In the late 1970s, several endurance junkies started a contest to see who was tougher by swimming, biking, and running across the Hawaiian landscape. Over the decades that followed, the sport of triathlon has undergone a stunning rise in popularity. The individual medley of endurance sports (swim, bike, run) is now a well-accepted sport in the Olympics at the 1.5/40/10-kilometer distance and enjoys a wide and growing participation base across the world. Distances range from short, "sprint" races lasting less than 1 hour to longer-distance, "ironman" races that can take competitors up to 8 to 16 hours to complete. Some even extend this to ultradistances competed over several days. Races typically use road bicycles for the bike portion, but off-road races using mountain bicycles have been gaining in popularity as well. The medical and musculoskeletal issues that arise in the longitudinal care of triathletes are, for the most part, those that arise with training for each individual discipline. For those medical or other support personnel involved in race day coverage, however, a variety of other acute medical concerns may arise and need to be considered when planning for the medical coverage of such events.

Swimming

While competitive swimming involves training and racing using the four traditional strokes (butterfly stroke, backstroke, breaststroke, and freestyle) in an enclosed pool with clear, chlorinated water, a triathlon swim occurs in open water with variable conditions and with a multitude of other athletes. Mass start races are characterized by "pack" swimming, and this can occasionally lead to issues such as blunt trauma to the face/eyes and finger sprains from contact with other swimmers. Both hypothermia and hyperthermia have been seen during and after open-water swims. Triathletes will typically use wetsuits to combat the cooler water temperatures, and this will allow most athletes to tolerate long swims in temperatures as low as 10 °C (50 °F). Despite this, hypothermia can ensue both during the swim and after the swimmers exit the water, due to a phenomenon known as "after-drop." An athlete's core temperature can continue to drop after leaving the cold water as blood continues to perfuse the cooler extremities. This has led to injuries as athletes attempt to transition to the bike with impaired coordination and judgment as a result of hypothermia.

On the other end, the use of wetsuits in water greater than 25 °C (78 °F) can lead to elevations in core temperature and symptomatic hyperthermia (heat exhaustion, syncope, or heat stroke), and for this reason, wetsuit use is restricted above this temperature. Increases in core temperature and heat stress can be additive (from day to day and from event to event) and may progress during a race. Further elevations in core temperature accumulated during the bike and run segments could predispose an athlete to more symptomatic heat illness or exercise-associated collapse later. Heat exhaustion may present with confusion, weakness, cramping, or hypotension and may lead athletes to drop out of the race and present to the medical tent on their own. Heat stroke represents a progression of heat illness with system failure at the metabolic and organ levels. This is usually seen in the later stages of the run segment, with the

athlete's collapse or severe deterioration in the medical tent.

To those athletes accustomed to training in clear water with orderly passing, the chaos of group swims and the unpredictable water conditions (cold temperature, waves, currents) can lead to anxiety and panic attacks. This problem can be exacerbated when warmer water conditions preclude wetsuit use. Many of the weaker swimmers depend on the additional flotation provided by wetsuit use, and a last-minute prohibition of its use can cause significant anxiety. Severe panic attacks in open water raise concerns about near-drowning events or severe exacerbation of asthma in the triathletes, and these should be accounted for when planning race management. Other, less common medical concerns during open-water swims include bacterial infections from poor water quality (*Escherichia coli, Leptospirosis*), sudden death from cardiac embolism or fatal arrhythmias, and marine animal stings or attacks (e.g., jellyfish, coral, sharks).

Triathletes, however, still need to put in a significant amount of distance in the pool during training (albeit less than their competitive swimmer counterparts due to the bike and run training) and thus experience the same range of overuse injuries as swimmers do. The shoulder is, by far, the most commonly injured or painful area in swimmers. Shoulder stability is maintained by both the joint capsule and the rotator cuff and can be lost when either of the structures becomes weakened. The rotator cuff is a group of four muscles deep inside the shoulder that helps provide stability by holding the humeral head inside its socket. It also helps initiate the overhead motion of the arm up to shoulder level. To achieve full overhead motion, the scapula must also retract and tilt the shoulder socket upward. The muscles that accomplish this are the rhomboids, trapezius, and cervical paraspinals.

The tendons of the rotator cuff are prone to overuse and inflammation with the repetitive overhead motion of the swim stoke. When this happens, the tired or inflamed muscle-tendon unit becomes weaker. As this progresses, the cuff muscles no longer constrain the shoulder effectively, and the head of the humerus may elevate with arm motion, causing a painful impingement against the undersurface of the acromioclavicular (AC) joint. Load may also shift to the joint capsule and ligaments, as well as the labrum (the cartilage rim around the shoulder joint). Such an imbalance can lead to painful multidirectional instability or labral tears. The scapular muscles must increase their share of moving the shoulder when the cuff is weak, and this can eventually cause overuse and lead to neck and upper back pain. The importance of a strong rotator cuff as a shoulder stabilizer becomes even greater in those with a high level of flexibility (congenital or otherwise) as these athletes cannot depend on the stabilizing effect of the shoulder capsule and ligaments.

Swimmers also experience injuries to various other structures. The repetitive lumber spine extension and rotation forces during a swim stroke can lead to stress injuries to the posterior elements of the vertebra itself and, ultimately, to spondylosis or spondylolisthesis. Injuries to the knee, such as patellofemoral pain or chondromalacia, can also be seen. These are usually seen with greater use of breaststroke or eggbeater kick, but can also be seen in those athletes concurrently training for bicycling, such as triathletes.

Cycling

Cycling injuries range from acute trauma to chronic overuse injuries. Triathletes, like cyclists, put in a lot of miles on the bike during the training process, and the old adage that "it is not *if* you will crash but *when*" holds true for triathletes. The most common crash-related injury is "road rash," which is a traumatic abrasion or contusion caused by the body scraping against the pavement. Appropriately treated with good wound care, it heals and rarely causes a significant loss of training time. Fractures of the wrist (distal radius, scaphoid), clavicle and AC joint, and elbow (radial head) are relatively common, and fractures of the pelvis have also been reported. The speed of a crash can increase the severity of a fracture; however, it is the mechanism of impact with the ground that determines whether a fracture will occur. Off-road triathlons have the added risk of collision with a fixed obstacle or even penetrating trauma from tree roots. Head injuries such as concussion also can result when a rider strikes the ground, even if he or she is wearing a helmet. Helmets are mandatory during competition and should be used during training as well.

Nontraumatic injuries, however, dominate in terms of frequency of cycling injuries. Chronic neck pain is a frequent complaint and can result from the prolonged neck extension required for straight-ahead vision with normal positioning on standard handlebars. This can be exacerbated by the increased torso flexion/flat-back positioning required with aerodynamic time-trial bars. The pain can be due to muscle spasm and/or trigger points in the levator scapulae, trapezius, or cervical paraspinal muscles, as well as from cervical facet arthrosis or degenerative cervical disk disease. To some degree, this can be minimized with more upright positioning on the bike.

The use of the hands and wrist to support the upper body on the handlebars can lead to both ulnar nerve impingement in the Guyon canal laterally in the wrist as well as median nerve irritation in the carpal tunnel. Consistent use of padded cycling gloves helps reduce trauma to the ulnar nerve. Frequent hand position changes and avoidance of extremes of flexion or extension help combat median nerve irritation. Groin injuries are also quite common in cyclists. Chronic irritation of the perineal skin due to friction can lead to skin breakdown and subsequent abscess formation. This can be minimized with proper bike positioning, padded cycling shorts, and chamois cream to soften the pad. Compression of the pudendal nerve can also cause transient numbness in the genital area. Such compression is more common in triathletes who tend to ride on the nose of the bike saddle.

Knee problems are also quite common in cyclists and triathletes. The pedal stroke can put tremendous load on the patellofemoral articulation, and proper pedaling mechanics and bike positioning are imperative to avoid overloading the joint. Even with good form, an overly rapid progression of high-power/low-cadence pedaling too early in the season can overwhelm the quadriceps muscle's ability to maintain normal patellar tracking. Inflammation of the patellar joint surface (patellofemoral pain) or softening/erosion of patellar cartilage (patellar chondromalacia) can occur. Once established, patellofemoral pain can take months to resolve. Chronic quadriceps muscle tightness can add to the problem by increasing baseline compressive stress on the joint. Similar cartilage erosions can occur on the femoral side of the joint as well. Chronic stress and overuse can also cause a painful intrasubstance degenerative change (tendinosis) within the patellar or quadriceps tendon. The same degenerative changes and inflammation that occur in the tendons of the knee also can occur in the Achilles tendon of the ankle with overuse. The iliotibial (IT) band attachment on the outside of the knee is also frequently injured with repetitive knee bending and friction at its attachment site.

Running

Run training can cause similar problems with knee pain. Patellar and/or femoral chondromalacia, IT band syndrome, and patellar/quadriceps tendinosis are all common overuse injuries in runners with normal mechanics. Those with poor mechanics that result in knee valgus (knock-knees), however, can experience increased patellar maltracking and pain. Such mechanical issues include abnormal foot pronation and weak core and/or gluteal muscles. Rapid increases in mileage, a large amount of downhill running, and uneven running surfaces all can increase the likelihood of developing patellofemoral pain as well. Since triathletes tend to have stronger abdominal, gluteal, and quadriceps muscles from biking and swimming, they tend to have more issues with overuse patellofemoral pain, IT band syndrome, or plantar fasciitis in the foot. To some degree, the cross-training required in triathlon helps strengthen the muscles that protect triathletes from the abnormal mechanics seen in solo sport competitors.

A relatively common and insidious concern for triathletes, or for any other endurance athlete for that matter, is overtraining syndrome. At its worst, this can present as severe, chronic stress with pituitary suppression (decreased hormone levels, increased cortisol). The athlete feels tired, can't recover from training sessions, has elevated morning heart rates, can't reach maximum heart rate during exercise, and has symptoms of depression. There is a continuum of impairment in terms of clinical symptoms from minimal, with minor deficits in performance and mild depressive symptoms, to more significant, with mild immunosuppression (increased infections, etc.) and possible cardiac arrhythmias. Unless the symptoms are very severe, laboratory values are all within normal limits and the diagnosis is clinical. A more acute cardiac version has been seen in long-distance triathletes, who, following a race, have shown transient (6–8 weeks) depressions in cardiac function that fully reverse with rest. Chronic issues with muscle strains of the calf, quadriceps, or hamstring can also relate to insufficient recovery time or overtraining. The likelihood of suffering a more severe tear of a muscle or tendon with training or competition is increased when muscle or connective tissue is compromised and unable to withstand previously tolerated stresses.

A more concerning overuse injury, largely secondary to running, relates to stress fractures. Bone is a dynamic organ, and when impact stress overloads a bone's ability to adapt, a mechanical failure of the structure can occur. This may initially present as an inflammation of the periosteum (the membrane covering the bone). When this happens along the back edge of the tibia, where the soleus and posterior tibial muscles attach, it is called "shin splints." Left unchecked, this accumulation of mechanical stress above that which can be repaired may progress to bone marrow edema and eventually to cortical fracturing. This can occur in the tibia, fibula, metatarsal bones of the foot, tarsal bones of the ankle, pubic rami and symphysis of the pelvis, and femur. As part of the process of adaptation to training, bones become denser and better able to handle the mechanical stress. Thus at a certain level, quality rest/recovery can become just as important as quality training.

Conclusion

In general, triathletes experience the same overuse and traumatic injuries that their single-sport compatriots do. They simply have a larger exposure by training in all three disciplines. There are a few unique aspects associated with the open-water swimming and transitions, but the similarities outweigh the differences.

Andrew Hunt

See also Biking, Injuries in; Heat Illness; Stress Fractures; Swimming, Injuries in

Further Readings

Matheson GO, Carter D. Stress fractures & stress injuries in bone. In: Garrik R, ed. *Orthopedic Knowledge*

Update 3. Rosemont, IL: American Academy of Orthopedic Surgeons; 2004:273–283.

Moriarty J. Exercise in heat and heat injuries. In: Safran M, McKeag D, Van Camp S, eds. *Manual of Sports Medicine*. Philadelphia, PA: Lippincott Raven; 1998:95–105.

Van Gent RN, Siem D, Van Middelkoop M, Van Os AG, Bierma-Zeinstra SM, Koes BW. Incidence and determinants of lower extremity running injuries in long distance runners: a systematic review. *Br J Sports Med*. 2007;41(8):469–480.

Wanich T, Hodgkins C, Columbier JA, Muraski E, Kennedy JG. Cycling injuries of the lower extremity. *J Am Acad Orthop Surg*. 2007;15(12):748–756.

Weldon EJ, Richardson AB. Upper extremity overuse injuries in swimming. *Clin Sports Med*. 2001;20(3):423–428.

TRIGGER FINGER

Trigger finger is the most common atraumatic, painful complaint of the hand and the fourth leading reason a person is referred to a hand surgeon. Its incidence is 28 cases per 100,000 people per year, with a lifetime risk of 2.6%. Having diabetes increases this risk to 10%. Trigger finger initially starts as discomfort in the palm that worsens with movement of the digits and progresses to "locking" of the involved digit in flexion. Adults are affected more than children. Women are affected two to six times more than men. The dominant hand is the most commonly affected, and the digits that trigger in descending order of frequency are the thumb followed by the ring, middle, pinky, and index fingers. Peak age of incidence is 55 to 60 years, with a smaller peak under 8 years of age. The usual treatment involves a cortisone injection, which is curative up to 90% for all except individuals with diabetes mellitus and rheumatoid arthritis.

Anatomy

The flexor tendons connect the digits to the forearm muscles and are responsible for bending the digits. A membranous tendon sheath covers the outside of the tendon and is attached to the bones of the hand, starting at the metacarpal head (palm bone) and extending to the distal phalanx (last finger bone). Different areas of the tendon sheath are thickened and function as pulleys to direct the tendon in its path and to prevent bowstringing. Trigger finger occurs when there is a mismatch in size of the flexor tendon, most commonly caused by a nodule, and the pulley. The most common area for the tendon to get stuck at is the first annular (A1) pulley, located over the joint of the metacarpal (palm bone) and proximal phalanx (initial finger bone). Occasionally, triggering can occur at other pulley sites.

Causes

Trigger finger is often idiopathic. It does occur more commonly in people with metabolic problems such as diabetes mellitus and hypothyroidism and different rheumatologic conditions, including rheumatoid arthritis, psoriatic arthritis, amyloidosis, sarcoidosis, and pigmented villonodular synovitis. Interestingly, trigger finger is associated with duration of diabetes and not with sugar control in individuals with diabetes requiring insulin injection. Because repetitive finger movements due to one's occupation or sport can cause high tension across the A1 pulley, it is proposed to cause the development of fibrocartilaginous metaplasia of the pulley and tendon cells, thus creating the mismatch in size. Trigger finger commonly coexists with carpal tunnel syndrome, de Quervain tenosynovitis, and Dupuytren contracture. Sometimes, locking of the digit can occur if ligaments catch on the bony prominence of the metacarpal (palm bone) head, if there is swelling of the tendon at different locations, or if loose bodies are present in the metacarpal phalangeal joint. Rarely, a finger injury involving a laceration of the flexor tendon may present as a trigger finger from the cut portion of the tendon catching at the A1 pulley.

Symptoms

Initially, pain is only felt in the palm at the metacarpal phalangeal joint. The pain can also radiate along the palm or along the digit. Locking of the digit occurs during active flexion-extension activities, often reported to worsen on rising in the morning. The athlete may complain initially of painless clicking of the digit with flexion that progresses to painful catching. Long-standing cases of trigger finger may present as a stiff digit, which the person is unable to bend.

Diagnosis

Trigger finger is diagnosed clinically from a history of locking of the digit and observation of triggering in the physician's office. Sometimes, a nodule on the flexor tendon is felt at the metacarpal phalangeal joint. Snapping or crepitus may be felt along the flexor tendon at the A1 pulley while the finger is passively flexed and extended. Laboratory evaluation is only required if there is suspicion that the nodule is secondary to medical conditions such as diabetes mellitus, rheumatoid arthritis, hypothyroidism, or gout. Occasionally, a radiograph of the hand is performed to look for loose bodies in the metacarpal phalangeal joint and arthritic changes in the metacarpal head or accessory bones of the hand.

Treatment

If the triggering of a digit occurred with a specific activity, then avoidance of that activity will lead to resolution of the symptoms. Otherwise, the first-line treatment recommended involves an injection of steroid medication near the bump on the tendon. Oral or topical anti-inflammatory medications can be tried initially but are often unsuccessful. Splinting the involved digit with 15° of flexion at the metacarpal phalangeal joint can be tried, but this has a lower success rate in those with more severe disease, triggering of longer than 6 months' duration, and multiple trigger digits. Splinting needs to be done continuously for 6 weeks and has a success rate of up to 50%. Injection into the tendon sheath has a success rate of 90%, and if a second injection is required, it is half as beneficial as the first one. Steroid injection has a higher success rate in those with a palpable nodule, if the duration of symptoms is less than 6 months, and if the digit triggering is the thumb. Complications of steroid injection include dermal or subcutaneous fat atrophy, skin depigmentation, infection, and, very rarely, tendon rupture. If trigger finger persists despite the injection, surgical release can be curative and involves cutting the A1 pulley. This procedure is done under local anesthesia in the operating room as either an open or a percutaneous procedure. With the open technique, an incision is made over the A1 pulley site, and the pulley is divided under direct visualization. For the percutaneous technique, a 18-gauge needle is used to divide the pulley without direct visualization. Potential complications of either procedure include digital nerve injury, bowstringing of the tendon (especially if the A2 pulley is divided), infection, hematoma, and persistent pain. Other reasons for surgery to be considered include a digit that is stuck in flexion and cannot be reduced and trigger thumb in an infant. Occasionally, a reduction flexor tenoplasty is performed, which involves cutting out the bulbous swelling of the tendon so that the tendon is smooth and glides without hindrance through the pulley.

Bernadette Pendergraph

See also Carpal Tunnel Syndrome; Diabetes Mellitus; Finger Sprain

Further Readings

Akhtar S, Bradley MJ, Quinton DN, Bruke FD. Management and referral for trigger finger/thumb. *BMJ.* 2005;331(7507):30–33.
Kale S. Trigger finger. http://www.emedicine.com/Orthoped/topic570.htm. Published May 2008. Accessed July 11, 2008.
Ryzewicz M, Wolf JM. Trigger digits: principles, management, and complications. *J Hand Surg Am.* 2006;31(1):135–146.

TROCHANTERIC BURSITIS

Trochanteric bursitis is inflammation of the bursa that lies on the outside (lateral) aspect of the hip, known as the greater trochanter of the femur bone. Bursitis can result from both overuse (chronic) and trauma (acute). It is common in all types of athletic and nonathletic populations.

Anatomy

Bursae are small fluid-filled sacs that are usually found around joints or bony prominences. Their purpose is to create lubrication between two uneven surfaces and provide frictionless movement. In this case, the bursa lies between the femur's greater trochanter, which is the hard bony prominence on the outside of the hip, and a strong tendon known as the iliotibial (IT) band. The IT band runs from the top of the hip, down the side of the leg, to the knee. Its main function is to abduct the leg as if to kick one's leg out to the side. However, when moving the hip forward and backward, as when walking, running, swimming, and biking, the IT band tends to rub over the greater trochanter and may irritate the bursa. When the bursa becomes inflamed, it swells and becomes compressed between the bone and the tendon, thus creating pain.

Causes

Trochanteric bursitis is most often caused by overuse or direct trauma. Direct trauma such as a fall that causes the patient to land on the lateral hip region or a direct blow to the outer hip is more common in women and in the middle-aged or elderly population. However, direct trauma is frequently seen in contact and collision sports as well. These falls or blows will cause bleeding (hematoma) into the bursa, which then results in swelling. Usually, these hematomas are rapidly absorbed by the body, but not infrequently, they may result in scarring, adhesions, and calcifications, leading to a more chronic type of bursitis.

More commonly, chronic repetitive trauma is involved, which can occur from merely running or walking. Conditions that predispose patients to this type of trochanteric bursitis include postural abnormalities, which can be caused by scoliosis, degenerative spinal conditions, a wide pelvis (female runners), hip and knee arthritic conditions, leg length differences, flat feet, high-arched feet, overpronation of the feet, or even oversupination of the feet at heel strike. Improperly fitting shoes, worn-out shoes, running on uneven or hard (cement) surfaces, and sudden increases or changes in training are other causes of trochanteric bursitis. Another cause occurs in cycling when the seat is too high and the cyclist has to rock from side to side when pedaling, which results in repetitive sliding of the IT band over the bursa. At times, the bursitis develops spontaneously without any apparent cause.

Symptoms

Patients affected by trochanteric bursitis will complain of a deep ache or burning pain over the greater trochanter on the outside of the hip. It will usually be worse with activity and may be worse both after rising in the morning or after prolonged sitting. It may get better after the first few steps only to recur later after walking for a ½ hour or more. The pain may radiate down the side of the leg toward the knee or ankle or into the buttock. The pain is usually worse at night while trying to lie on the affected side.

Diagnosis

The diagnosis of trochanteric bursitis is usually clinical. A typical history can be confirmed on physical examination. There will be maximal point tenderness to palpation directly over the greater trochanter. Point tenderness just superior to the trochanter is usually more indicative of gluteus medius tendinitis, while point tenderness just posterior to the trochanter is more indicative of piriformis tendinitis. Pain will also be present during gait when the hip goes from flexion to extension. Pain may occur with passive hip adduction, abduction, or external rotation but not with internal rotation. Pain may also be present with active hip abduction. Rarely, a limp will be present.

An X-ray can be obtained to ensure that there are no bone spurs, calcifications, or arthritis that could be contributing to the problem. Occasionally, a magnetic resonance imaging (MRI) scan or a bone scan may be done if the diagnosis is unclear or if the problem does not resolve with treatment. These tests will help rule out tumor, occult fracture, or necrosis of the bone.

Treatment

The goals for treatment include reducing pain and inflammation, as well as preserving mobility and preventing recurrence. Treatment recommendations may initially include a combination of rest, heat and/or cold application, stretching and strengthening exercises, activity and shoe modification, pain medication such as acetaminophen or ibuprofen, and osteopathic manipulation along with correction of any anatomical or biomechanical asymmetry (orthotics/heel lifts). Cross-training incorporating low-impact activity such as biking, swimming, or using elliptical machines can minimize the pain and allow for continued exercise. Typically, resolution of symptoms occurs within 2 to 6 weeks of treatment. For persistent symptoms, more advanced treatments may be required, such as physical therapy, cortisone injections, or surgery.

While only a limited number of controlled studies have proven the usefulness of physical therapy for this condition, a specific and goal-directed program can often reduce symptoms. Physical therapy can be incorporated to teach the patient a home exercise program, emphasizing stretching specific tendons, including the IT band and tensor fascia lata, as well as stretching the external hip rotators, quadriceps, hamstrings, adductors, and hip flexors. Strengthening exercises should focus on the lower abdominals and the gluteal muscles. Other modalities used in physical therapy can also be employed, such as *phonophoresis*, which uses sound waves to allow for deep penetration of topical medications, and *iontophoresis*, which uses an electrical current to allow corticosteroids to penetrate the skin and minimize the inflammation to the bursa. Ultrasound therapy and soft tissue massage may also be helpful.

Cortisone injections are an important option within the comprehensive treatment plan. Randomized, controlled clinical trials have shown that corticosteroid and lidocaine injection for trochanteric bursitis is an effective therapy with a prolonged benefit. Trochanteric bursa injections are often performed without radiographic guidance, and a local anesthetic can first be used as a diagnostic injection. The needle is advanced to the greater trochanter (with contact on the bone being made to confirm depth and appropriate placement) and is then withdrawn slightly so that it is located within the bursa. The local anesthetic can then be injected directly into the bursa. If appropriate relief is achieved, this would be considered confirmation of trochanteric bursitis as the cause of the pain. This injection of local anesthetic can then be followed by the administration of steroids. An injection of 12 to 24 milligrams (mg) of betamethasone or 40 to 80 mg of methylprednisolone is commonly used. This injection may be repeated at 4 to 6 weeks if pain relief has been less than 50%. In most cases, in which the diagnosis of trochanteric bursitis seems straightforward from the clinical evaluation, a diagnostic injection with

local anesthetic is not necessary prior to the corticosteroid injection. Patients should be made aware of the risks of injection prior to the procedure.

Surgery is rarely indicated and is often reserved for severe cases that are recalcitrant to months of the conservative treatments discussed above. There are several surgical techniques that have been used in the past. One such technique involves excision of the bursa via incisions in the IT band over the greater trochanter. Another procedure is a trochanteric reduction osteotomy, which removes a portion of the trochanter. Arthroscopic bursectomy is the third option and allows for excision of the bursa using a scope. Finally, release and lengthening of the IT band is another surgical alternative. Surgical intervention carries the increased risk of anesthesia along with the direct surgical risks and should be considered only after appropriate nonoperative interventions have been exhausted.

Gregory Cibor and Sakina Kadakia

See also Gluteal Strain; Hip, Pelvis, and Groin Injuries; Iliotibial Band Syndrome

Further Readings

Browning KH. Hip and pelvis injuries in runners. *Phys Sportsmed*. 2001;29(1):23–34.

Cohen SP, Narvaez JC, Lebovits AH, Stojanovic MP. Corticosteroid injections for trochanteric bursitis: is fluoroscopy necessary? A pilot study. *Br J Anaesth*. 2005;94(1):100–106.

Craig RA, Jones DP, Oakley AP, Dunbar JD. Iliotibial band Z-lengthening for refractory trochanteric bursitis. *ANZ J Surg*. 2007;77(11):996–998.

Farr D, Selesnick H, Janecki C, Cordas D. Arthroscopic bursectomy with concomitant iliotibial band release for the treatment of recalcitrant trochanteric bursitis. *Arthroscopy*. 2007;23(8):905.e1–e5.

Leiberman JR. Trochanteric bursitis. In: Snider RK, ed. *Essentials of Musculoskeletal Care*. Rosemont, IL: American Academy of Orthopedic Surgeons; 1997:299–303.

Nuccion SL, Hunter DM, Finerman GAM. Hip and pelvis: adult. In: DeLee JC, Drez D, eds. *Orthopaedic Sports Medicine Principles and Practice*. Philadelphia, PA: Saunders; 2003:1446–1447.

Slawski DP, Howard RF. Surgical management of refractory trochanteric bursitis. *Am J Sports Med*. 1997;25(1):86–89.

Walker P, Kannangara S, Bruce WJ, Michael D, Van der Wall H. Lateral hip pain: does imaging predict response to localized injection? *Clin Orthop Relat Res.* 2007;457:144–149.

TRUNK INJURIES

Injury to the trunk during sports is common and generally includes muscle and bone injury, but it can also include more serious injury to the internal organs. Examples of muscle injuries include strains of large muscle groups, such as the rectus abdominus and perivertebrals. Bones such as the lumbar vertebrae can sustain chronic injury, as in spondylolysis, or acute injury, as with transverse process fracture in blunt trauma. However, the predominance of musculoskeletal injuries may lead the practitioner to overlook a more serious injury. Below are some important and sometimes life-threatening injuries to be considered in the athlete with injuries to the trunk.

Pneumothorax

A pneumothorax may occur spontaneously during a sporting event or acutely after blunt or penetrating trauma in sports activity. It occurs when air is introduced between the lung and the pleura, the membrane that surrounds the lungs. Depending on the mechanism with which the contact between these two surfaces was compromised, air can accumulate and compress the lung, resulting in chest pain and shortness of breath. This can lead to respiratory failure. If enough air accumulates, the pressure from this trapped air can compress the heart and limit its ability to fill and then pump blood, leading to cardiovascular collapse and death.

Spontaneous pneumothorax is caused by a ruptured bleb at the surface of the lung and leads to escape of air from the lung into the space between the lung and the pleura. It is most common in tall, thin males but can occur in any age-group or gender. It can occur at rest and also during vigorous exercise and can be mistaken for a musculoskeletal chest pain. The athlete generally will complain of moderate to severe pleuritic sharp pain on the left or the right, associated with varying degrees of shortness of breath. Generally, a spontaneous pneumothorax is small and stable, but it can progress to the life-threatening complications described above. The patient needs to be transported to a medical facility where imaging can be done and a thoracostomy performed to relieve the pressure. In the event that immediate transport is unavailable and the patient is experiencing cardiovascular collapse, an emergent decompression needle thoracostomy can be performed by qualified medical professionals.

Traumatic pneumothorax can be caused by blunt or penetrating forces. The force required to cause a pneumothorax from blunt trauma is generally significant and has associated injury, such as rib fractures. Rib fractures require only pain medication as treatment, but all suspected rib fractures require a plain radiograph to rule out the diagnosis of pneumothorax. For penetrating trauma, such as skate-induced chest wall laceration in ice hockey, a plain radiograph should be ordered to rule out the diagnosis of pneumothorax even when suspicion is low for it. Any lacerations or punctures to the chest wall should not be explored, as this can cause a pneumothorax in some cases. Complications and treatment are the same as described above.

Cardiac Contusion

High-speed blunt trauma to the chest can result in injury to the heart, the most dramatic effect of which is sudden death, or commotio cordis. Cardiac contusion in sports is rare but occurs when forces are transmitted from the ballistic (as in baseball) or opposing player (as in American football) to the chest of the athlete. The myocardium is bruised, which causes pain and can affect cardiac output and in rare cases can lead to failure. The diagnosis should be considered in any athlete who complains of chest pain after a high-speed impact. Evidence of significant injury, as with sternal fracture/injury or multiple anterior rib fractures, should increase suspicion of cardiac injury. Emergency evaluation includes a chest radiograph, electrocardiogram, and cardiac enzymes. If there is a high suspicion of cardiac contusion, an echocardiogram may be taken and/or the patient may be kept under observation.

Solid Abdominal Organ Lacerations and Contusions

Blunt trauma to the abdomen can occur in all contact sports, including football, men and women's hockey and soccer, and countless others from professional-level activities to recreational sports such as bodyboarding. Forces transmitted from an object, such as a helmet or a knee, to the abdomen can be absorbed by the liver, spleen, or kidney. In the event that these forces are sufficient to cause bleeding, these organs may become bruised and occasionally lacerate. Lacerations can cause bleeding within the organ and impair the functioning of the organ itself. This is often seen with a kidney laceration, which results in decreased long-term renal function. Occasionally, the bleeding is not contained within the solid organ, and blood accumulates in the abdomen. If the bleeding is brisk or the injury is not identified in time, this bleeding can result in severe blood loss and occasionally in death. If surgery is indicated, attempts should be made to stop the bleeding and preserve organ function. As both are not always possible, occasionally the damaged solid organ will need to be removed.

Solid organ injury should be considered under the right clinical circumstances. In cases where solid organ injury occurs, the history will include a mechanism that fits clinically. Examples of mechanisms of blunt solid organ injury include the impact of a football helmet on the abdomen or back, a high-speed hockey puck to the stomach, or a bodyboard lodged between the abdomen and the beach sand. The athlete will complain of abdominal or flank pain with or without nausea or light-headedness. The abdomen or flank is usually tender, and in cases of significant bleeding, the pulse rate may be high and blood pressure low. Any patient with possible solid organ injury should be transported immediately to a local emergency room.

Hollow Abdominal Organ Injury

Hollow organ injury, specifically large and small bowel trauma, is unusual after blunt trauma in athletics. Historically, the athlete will have a mechanism in which a forceful blunt trauma is sustained to the anterior abdomen. Mechanisms that can cause hollow organ injury include a fall from a bicycle with impact from the handlebars, a surfboard wedged between the sand and the surfer's abdomen, or a knock from a football helmet to the abdomen. In mild cases, the athlete may complain of minimal pain associated with nausea, as in the case of a minor small bowel contusion. In case of a ruptured viscus, the athlete will have severe pain and vomiting. On physical exam, the mild small bowel contusions may be normal save for some tenderness to deep palpation. This is in contrast to the patient with a ruptured viscus, who will have severe tenderness to light palpation, rebound tenderness, as well as other evidence of an acute abdomen. The vital signs may be unstable, with a low blood pressure and fast heart rate. An initial, upright chest X-ray is the fastest and most specific way of determining if there is air in the abdomen, which would indicate a perforated viscus. Computed tomography is the most sensitive study to find evidence of a ruptured viscus, and it will also show evidence of hollow viscus contusion and injury to the solid organs. A hollow viscus perforation is a surgical emergency, whereas a contusion can be monitored clinically.

Gian Corrado

See also Bruised Ribs; Chest and Chest Wall Injuries; Rib Fracture and Contusions

Further Readings

Kocher MS, Tucker R. Hip and pelvis injuries. In: Frontera W, ed. *Clinical Sports Medicine.* Philadelphia, PA: Elsevier; 2007:391–410.

Middlemas DA. Abdominal and pelvic injuries. In: Rehberg R, ed. *Sports Emergency Care: A Team Approach.* Danvers, MA: Slack; 2007:173–196.

Schwartz D. *Emergency Radiology.* New York, NY: McGraw-Hill; 2000.

Scuderi G. *Sports Medicine: Principles of Primary Care.* St Louis, MO: Mosby; 1997.

Tintinelli J. *Emergency Medicine.* New York, NY: McGraw-Hill; 1996.

TURF TOE

The term *turf toe* has become a commonly accepted name referring to a sprain involving the hallux (great toe) metatarsophalangeal (MTP) joint of the foot. The name was first coined in 1976 after it was found that the frequency of injuries to the MTP joint was much greater during competition on artificial playing surfaces. The injury is fairly common; it is seen most often in football, but it also occurs in other sports such as wrestling, basketball, and dance, among others. Because this particular joint plays a key role in running, sprinting, and cutting, an injury can result in significant functional disability. It is thought to be underreported and not always appreciated as the significant injury that it may be or can become if it is not appropriately managed.

Anatomy

The anatomy of the forefoot is intricate and quite complicated. The MTP joint of the hallux involves a metatarsal (long bone) with a rounded, cartilage-covered surface at the end, which joins with the concave base of the phalanx (toe bone). Stability of the MTP joint comes from medial (inside) and lateral (outside) collateral and metatarsosesamoid ligaments in addition to a strong plantar plate. There are also several different muscle tendons that run along either side and underneath the joint, attaching onto the phalanx. These structures together make up the intricate capsuloligamentous complex of the first MTP joint.

Motion in the joint consists primarily of plantarflexion (downward) and dorsiflexion (upward). Passive range of motion varies widely from 3° to 43° of plantarflexion and from 40° to 100° of dorsiflexion.

Causes

The two primary causes of turf toe are the advent of artificial playing surfaces and the coinciding introduction of flexible-soled turf shoes. Artificial playing surfaces were introduced in the 1960s, and with that came a dramatic increase in the number of turf toe injuries. This is due to the increased friction caused by the artificial surface and shoe interface. When artificial turf was introduced, players were typically wearing a grass cleat with a metal plate in the sole, which attached to the cleats and added stability to the forefoot. After playing on the artificial surface, players complained of traction problems, which led to the introduction of a flexible turf shoe. Both caused the incidence of turf toe injuries to increase dramatically.

As artificial turf ages, it stiffens. This has also been thought to contribute to the increasing incidence of turf toe injuries, although studies have not validated this hypothesis. Since natural playing surfaces are once again becoming the standard, it is expected that turf toe injuries will also decrease.

Mechanism of Injury

The most common mechanism of injury is hyperextension of the great toe. This often occurs with tackling in American football, where the forefoot is fixed on the playing surface with the heel raised in a dorsiflexed position. A force from the tackler is thus directed down the lower leg into the foot, causing an exaggerated dorsiflexion and subsequent hyperextension of the great toe. This hyperextension can lead to varying degrees of injury to the plantar plate, capsule, and collateral ligaments or the cartilage surface of the bone.

Although most turf toe injuries occur with hyperextension, other mechanisms have been described as well. Hyperflexion, or "sand toe" (termed so because of its high propensity in sand volleyball players), injury is sometimes considered a variation of turf toe, although it often has a different clinical course and, thus, may need to be considered separately.

Varus (bending inside) and valgus (bending outside) are two other described mechanisms. Valgus is most commonly seen in a football lineman who is pushing off from a stance. Varus is rarely seen but can occur when an outward force is applied to a fixed forefoot.

Diagnosis

The diagnosis is made by first eliciting how the injury occurred and, if available, watching a video replay of the incident. Patients may present with a single acute or multiple episodes of trauma. Classically, the MTP joint will exhibit tenderness, swelling, and pain with movement. At this point, if a turf toe diagnosis is suspected, X-rays with several different views should be obtained to assess for a capsular avulsion, sesamoid fracture or migration, impaction injury, or separation of a bipartite sesamoid. A magnetic resonance imaging (MRI) scan is usually ordered if there are abnormalities on X-ray. MRI is the best tool to assess soft tissue and cartilage damage, as well as further evaluate for bony abnormalities. This will aid in grading the injury, as well as formulating a treatment plan and making an overall prognosis.

Most injuries are graded on a scale of I to III, with III being the most severe. Grade I is a stretch injury to the capsuloligamentous complex, with minimal symptoms associated with it. Grade II is a partial tear to the capsuloligamentous complex, with pain with weight bearing, bruising, and restricted range of motion. Grade III is a complete tear of the capsuloligamentous complex, with an associated disruption of the plantar plate from the metatarsal neck, impaction of the phalanx into the metatarsal head, and sometimes movement of the sesamoids. There is severe pain, swelling, bruising, and motion restriction, along with inability to bear weight.

Treatment

The initial treatment of an acute turf toe injury should include the RICE protocol of *rest*, *ice*, *compression*, and *elevation*. Athletes with Grade I injuries often can return to play immediately, although often toe taping and/or using a stiff insole may be necessary or desired for protection. Grade II injuries will often require up to 2 weeks of rest. Patients with Grade III injuries should remain non–weight bearing for several days and have prolonged rest, usually for 4 to 6 weeks. The athlete should slowly progress from walking to running to cutting and, finally, sport-specific activities. Painfree range of motion of 50° to 60° of upward flexion has also been proposed as a criterion for returning to play. Operative treatment is reserved for the most severe turf toe injuries, including large capsular avulsions with an unstable joint and diastasis of a bipartite sesamoid, or after conservative therapy has failed.

Jeffrie C. Kindred

See also Foot Injuries; Hammertoe; Musculoskeletal Tests, Foot

Further Readings

Anderson JG, Bohay DR, Maskill JD. First ray injuries. *Foot Ankle Clin.* 2006;11(1):143–163.

Childs SG. The pathogenesis and biomechanics of turf toe. *Orthop Nurs.* 2006;25(4):276–280.

Coughlin M. Foot and ankle. In: DeLee JC, Drez D Jr, Miller MD, eds. *Orthopaedic Sports Medicine: Principles and Practice.* Philadelphia, PA: Saunders; 2003:2504–2510.

Kennedy R, Simons SM. Foot injuries. In: Frontera WR, Micheli LJ, Herring SA, Silver JK, eds. *Clinical Sports Medicine: Medical Management and Rehabilitation.* Philadelphia, PA: Saunders Elsevier; 2007:480–482.

Mullen JE, O'Malley MJ. Sprains—residual instability of subtalar, Lisfranc joints, and turf toe. *Clin Sports Med.* 2004;23(1):97–121.

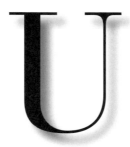

Ulnar Neuropathy

Ulnar neuropathy is inflammation or compression of the ulnar nerve, resulting in paresthesia (numbness, tingling, and pain) in the outer (ulnar) side of the arm and in the hand near the little finger. The ulnar nerve provides motor control to the muscles in the forearm and hand. It also provides the sensations of touch, temperature, and texture to the volar surface, or undersurface, of the forearm, the palm, and specifically the fourth and fifth digits of the hand circumferentially. Ulnar neuropathy that originates at the elbow is most common, although it can also be caused by injury to the nerve as it passes through the wrist.

Approximately 40% of Americans experience some form of ulnar neuropathy at least once during their lifetime. While the ulnar nerve is structurally identically in men and women, men tend to develop ulnar neuropathy more than do women. The reason may be that men generally have less fat overlying the elbow to protect the exposed nerve, or it may be due to differences in work- or sports-related stresses. The onset of ulnar neuropathy is often insidious. As a result, many of those who are affected are middle-aged or older adults. Demographic risk factors include a family history of diabetes, alcoholism, and HIV (human immunodeficiency virus) infection. Direct compression from pressure on the elbow can trigger ulnar neuropathy; therefore, people who have desk jobs and spend extended periods of time working on computers are at risk of developing the disorder. Ulnar neuropathy is variously known as *bicycler's neuropathy, cubital tunnel syndrome, Guyon canal syndrome,* and *tardy ulnar palsy*. Its occurrence is most notable in cyclists from prolonged compression on the nerve while gripping the bicycle handlebars; yet it is often seen in sports such as tennis, baseball, softball, and golf, where a significant amount of time is spent gripping sports equipment.

Anatomy

The anterior primary rami of the eighth cervical and first thoracic (C8 and T1) vertebrae contribute to form the medial cord of the brachial plexus. The medial cord leaves the axilla as the ulnar and median nerves. Though the ulnar nerve starts from the cervical nerve roots, its target motor and sensory innervations are located in the medial forearm and hand. The ulnar nerve travels along the posteromedial aspect of the arm, pierces the intermuscular septum, and courses beneath the medial head of the triceps. It enters the elbow at the ulnar groove between the medial epicondyle and olecranon. Then the nerve passes through the cubital tunnel into the forearm deep into the flexor carpi ulnaris. At the wrist, the ulnar nerve enters the hand distal to the ulnar styloid through the Guyon canal. The ulnar nerve is most susceptible to injury at these two tunnel sites. The muscles innervated by the ulnar nerve are the flexor carpi ulnaris, the flexor digitorum profundus, the palmaris brevis, the interossei muscles, the medial two lumbricals, the flexor

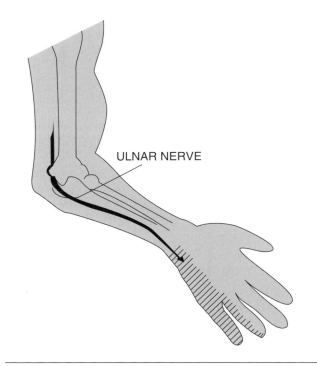

Figure 1   Course of Ulnar Nerve, Showing Sensory Innervation in the Forearm and Hand

pollicis brevis, the adductor pollicis, and the hypothenar muscle group. The ulnar nerve provides sensory innervation to the medial palmar and dorsal aspects of the forearm (including the elbow) and hand and supplies sensation to the small finger and medial one half of the ring finger (Figure 1).

History and Physical Exam

Ulnar nerve injuries can present initially as paresthesias anywhere along its sensory distribution. A typical complaint would be a feeling of "pins and needles" over the ring and small finger or medial forearm. Symptoms can include pain, weakness, and fine motor deficits. On examination, there may be clawing of the ring and small fingers or wasting of the intrinsic hand muscles.

Injuries at any point along the ulnar nerve can have distal manifestations in the hand and fingers. This makes it difficult to pinpoint the exact site where the ulnar nerve is injured. One exception is

lesions that occur at the Guyon canal. The dorsal cutaneous sensory branch of the ulnar nerve leaves the main ulnar nerve prior to the Guyon canal. Therefore, lesions at or distal to the Guyon canal would not present with dorsal sensory deficits. Identifying the correct location where ulnar nerve function is compromised affects rehabilitation and treatment recommendations. Other conditions in the differential diagnosis for ulnar neuropathy should be worked up if suspected, including C8-T1 radiculopathy, brachial plexopathy, thoracic outlet syndrome, peripheral polyneuropathy, and overuse syndromes.

There are certain provocative tests that may trigger ulnar nerve symptoms and help localize the lesion. These tests include the following:

- *Elbow flexion test:* Similar to the Phalen test for the median nerve and carpal tunnel syndrome, this maneuver can elicit symptoms due to cubital tunnel syndrome. The elbow is placed in full flexion with wrist extension for 3 minutes. A positive test is when numbness, tingling, and/or pain occur over the ulnar distribution.
- *Froment sign:* The patient is asked to hold a piece of paper between the thumb and the index finger. Patients with ulnar nerve injury will have difficulty holding onto the piece of paper and will compensate with the flexor pollicis longus muscle by flexing at the thumb's interphalangeal joint.
- *Tinel sign:* Percussion over the ulnar groove, medial epicondyle, cubital tunnel, or Guyon canal may reproduce symptoms. This is a very nonspecific test with variable results.
- *Wartenberg sign:* The small finger is in an abducted position at rest due to muscle weakness and asymmetric pull from unaffected muscles.

Imaging and Testing

Radiographs of the upper extremity are often obtained, but in the absence of associated musculoskeletal trauma, they rarely demonstrate abnormalities that aid in the diagnosis or treatment of ulnar neuropathy. The most frequent findings demonstrate degenerative changes, fractures, or bone spurs that can contribute to nerve impingement. Conversely, electrodiagnostic tests, such as nerve conduction studies and electromyography

(EMG), are extremely helpful to accurately localize the lesion and determine the severity of injury. Occasionally, there are multiple sites of injury to the ulnar nerve that can be distinguished on electrodiagnostic testing.

Specific Ulnar Nerve Injuries

Some specific ulnar nerve injuries are listed below.

- *Ligament of Struthers.* As the ulnar nerve passes through the intermuscular septum in the upper arm, it passes under a tough fascia layer called the arcade or ligament of Struthers. Here, the ulnar nerve can become entrapped. Conservative management tends to yield poor results; therefore, a surgical release of the ligament is often necessary.

- *Ulnar Groove.* The ulnar groove is a common site for ulnar nerve injury. Here, the nerve is at risk of being injured by direct trauma (fractures), traction injury such as valgus stress at the elbow from throwing (valgus overload syndrome), and recurrent subluxation of the nerve in and out of the groove. Compressive injury can occur at this site from leaning on the elbows or from the application of a tight cast, splint, or brace. Elbow flexion often reproduces or exacerbates the painful symptoms. Treatment options begin with conservative pain management and occupational therapy to maintain elbow range of motion and forearm strength. Biomechanical evaluation and loose protective padding or splinting around the elbow can help reduce the symptoms. Surgery (ulnar nerve release or ulnar nerve transposition) may be indicated if conservative treatment fails.

- *Cubital Tunnel Syndrome.* The ulnar nerve enters the forearm through the cubital tunnel under the medial epicondyle and olecranon. The borders of the cubital tunnel are the two heads of the flexor carpi ulnaris, the medial collateral ligament of the elbow, and the pronator aponeurosis. Ulnar nerve entrapment can occur anywhere along this tunnel. Injuries are typically due to repetitive motion. Treatment tends to be conservative and similar to the treatment, described above, for ulnar groove injuries. A surgical cubital tunnel release is reserved for those who fail conservative management.

- *Guyon Canal Compression.* The Guyon canal is formed by the pisiform bone, the hook of the hamate, the flexor carpi ulnaris, and the carpal ligament. The dorsal cutaneous sensory branch of the ulnar nerve leaves the main ulnar nerve proximal to the Guyon canal. Therefore, compressive lesions at or distal to the Guyon canal would not present with dorsal sensory paresthesias. Bicycle riding (*handlebar palsy*), push-ups, ganglion cysts, or lipomas can all cause ulnar nerve compression at the Guyon canal. Treatment includes activity modification (wrist padding or holding the handlebar from the side position instead of the top), stretching exercises, and nonsteroidal anti-inflammatory drugs (NSAIDs). Surgical interventions can be considered if symptoms fail to improve.

- *Hypothenar Hammer Syndrome.* Hypothenar hammer syndrome is caused by repetitive impact on the hand causing ulnar nerve injury at the Guyon canal. In addition to nerve injury, there can also be distal ischemia with arterial thickening, thrombosis, and possible aneurysm formation. In addition to the symptoms above, other complaints may include cold intolerance and pain over the palm of the hand. Treatment adjuncts to the above include vasolytic agents or vascular repair.

Conclusion

Ulnar nerve injuries are common. While the presenting symptoms are similar in most cases, it is essential to identify the exact anatomic location of compression or injury in order to properly treat this condition. Athletes who present with signs and symptoms of ulnar neuritis or ulnar neuropathy are often difficult to treat due to the frequent repetitive nature of the trauma induced from gripping sport-specific equipment. Modifications in grip technique as well as padding and other adjustments may help significantly alleviate the symptoms of this condition. When the etiology of the ulnar neuropathy is unclear, electrodiagnostic testing is helpful and should be performed. Referral to a sports or orthopedic specialist is indicated for refractory and frequently reoccurring cases.

Holly J. Benjamin and Brian Tho Hang

See also Elbow and Forearm Injuries; Handlebar Palsy; Musculoskeletal Tests, Hand and Wrist; Wrist Injuries

Further Readings

Kim RY, Wolfe VM, Rosenwasser MP. Entrapment neuropathies around the elbow. In: DeLee JC, Drez D Jr, Miller MD, eds. *DeLee and Drez's Orthopaedic Sports Medicine.* 3rd ed. Philadelphia, PA: Saunders;2010:Chapter 19.

Martin BD, Johansen JA, Edwards SG. Complications related to simple dislocations of the elbow. *Hand Clin.* 2008;24(1):9–25.

Pascuzzi RM. Peripheral neuropathy. *Med Clin North Am.* 2009;93(2):317–342.

Shapiro BE, Preston DC. Entrapment and compressive neuropathies. *Med Clin North Am.* 2009;93(2): 285–315.

Toth C. Peripheral nerve injuries attributable to sport and recreation. *Phys Med Rehabil Clin N Am.* 2009;20(1): 77–100.

ULTIMATE FRISBEE, INJURIES IN

Ultimate Frisbee (also known as *Ultimate,* in reference to a disc brand sometimes used in the sport) is a noncontact sport that is played in 42 countries by hundreds of thousands of men, women, and youth. In 2007, it was estimated that 824,000 people in the United States reported playing Ultimate at least 25 times a year. The Ultimate Player's Association (UPA) is the national governing body of the sport in the United States, while the World Flying Disc Federation (WFDF) provides international governance for the sport. Ultimate is played formally at the club, college, master's, and youth levels. In 2001, Ultimate debuted as a medal sport at the World Games in Japan.

Overview of the Sport

It is generally agreed that the sport was developed in 1968 on the east coast of the United States, and the first official rules for the game were codified in 1970. Despite having spread worldwide, the sport has had very little media coverage and is unfamiliar to many people. A brief overview follows.

The game is typically played by two teams of seven individuals on a regulation field that is 70 yards (yd; 64 meters [m]) by 40 yd (36.6 m) with end zones 25 yd (22.86 m) deep, approximating the dimensions of an American football field. Though any surface, indoors or outdoors, may be used, generally an Ultimate game is played outdoors on a grass field (variants of the traditional game include indoor and beach Ultimate). A plastic disc (the "Frisbee") whose regulation weight is 175 grams is used. Individuals try to advance the disc down the field, and scoring is achieved each time the offense completes a pass into the defense's end zone. Substitutions are allowed after scores or during injury time outs. A game is won when a specified number of points are accumulated (typically an odd number from 13 to 21), with two clear points on the opponents score, or after 80 minutes of play.

Physical contact between players, including picks and screens, is minimized in the game. The offense may advance the disc in any direction by completing a pass to a teammate. Players may not run with the disc after catching it. If a pass is not caught by a teammate, the defense immediately takes over possession and becomes the offense. Change of possession can also occur by the defense intercepting a pass or when an individual holds the disc for longer than 10 seconds. Ultimate is thus a transition game like basketball.

Several unique rules of Ultimate bear special mention. The game is self-refereed; that is, players are responsible for resolving any disputes at all levels of the game. Calls are typically made within the flow of play. There are clear rules for resolution of disputes, so self-refereeing does not lead to extended discussion or uncertainty about how to continue. The game, therefore, is interrupted much less frequently than many other team sports.

True to its origins in the countercultural 1960s, Ultimate is a sport that aims to be inclusive (teams are often of mixed gender) and in some important respects de-emphasizes competition. The sport places a high value on sportsmanship and fair play, codifying this in the rules as an overriding ethic known as the "Spirit of the Game." Ultimate players are often serious, motivated, and competitive athletes who nevertheless place a premium on the basic joy of play. According to Ultimate Players Association's *Official Rules of Ultimate* (11th edition), "such actions as taunting opposing players, dangerous aggression, belligerent intimidation, intentional infractions, or other 'win-at-all costs' behavior are contrary to the Spirit of the Game and must be avoided by all players" (sec. I. Introduction: B. Spirit of the Game, p. 2). Though this has not been studied, it may be expected then that there might be fewer injuries incurred consequent to fighting among players.

It can be difficult to find other sports with which to compare Ultimate. The sport combines the nonstop movement and athletic endurance of soccer with the aerial passing skills of football. Some commentators have even compared the game with rugby: Though widely dissimilar in their approach to contact, both games involve plenty of running and frequent, deliberate diving to the turf. Some rules of the game, such as self-refereeing and the codified sportsmanship ethic, are almost unique. Overall, Ultimate is a team sport fulfilling the expected requirements of a team sport such as soccer—for example, skill, fitness, sportsmanship, and organization.

Injuries

Like other sports defined as "noncontact," there is ample opportunity for Ultimate players to be involved in collisions, either with each other or with the ground. The nature of the game involves frequent cutting and sprinting, which can inevitably lead to muscle strains, ankle sprains, and knee injuries.

It is a common practice in Ultimate to dive full-length, propelling one's body horizontal to the ground, to catch a low disc. This maneuver is a signature moment in an Ultimate game, and is known as "laying out" or "going ho" (as in "going horizontal"). Laying out is a skill, like sliding in baseball, that can be taught properly: As the disc is caught, the whole body rolls in a twisting motion as it hits the ground, dissipating forces over a broad area from the ulnar aspect of the forearm to the torso and buttocks. Predictable consequences, including shoulder, arm, and rib injuries or severe friction injuries to the skin, can result if the layout is not executed correctly.

To perform at high levels, the player must be fit. As a transition game with little stoppage time, Ultimate places unresearched but predictable demands on the body. While on the field, players are almost continuously moving and are frequently sprinting. In terms of strenuousness, Ultimate would

likely then have similar physiological demands to soccer, another high-dynamic/low-static sport. It would be expected that players attempting Ultimate without the requisite levels of endurance, strength, speed, and flexibility would put themselves at higher risk of injury.

Unfortunately, there has been little research done on the injury patterns seen in Ultimate. A review of the relatively sparse literature found two surveys of injuries seen in the sport; the references can be found in the Further Readings at the end of this entry.

The first survey, published in 1991, assessed injuries that occurred in tournaments played in Europe from 1986 to 1990. The survey reported the following:

- Of all injuries, 66.6% affected the lower limbs; the most common injury involved a strain of the thigh muscle.
- Skin injuries, including friction burns, occurred at a higher rate than seen in other similar sports.
- "Minor" knee ailments such as patellar bursitis were more common than "major" injuries such as anterior cruciate ligament (ACL) tears.
- The pattern of knee injuries in general was quite different from that of many other sports and was found to be predominantly overuse injuries.

This study noted that three factors appeared to have the greatest influence on the sport's injury pattern: (1) the preparticipation fitness level of the player, (2) the organization of a tournament and squad size (more games and smaller squads allowing fewer substitutions, resulting in more frequent injury), and (3) the state of the field (hard, packed, and stony fields causing more skin and soft tissue injuries).

The study went on to recommend injury prevention practices, including clothing such as bike shorts and soft protectors on the elbows and knees to minimize the skin exposed to trauma. Though this has not been studied, such protective measures would be expected to minimize the number of lacerations, abrasions, and incidents of bursitis seen in the sport.

The second study, published in 2006, was based on a self-reported survey administered to athletes at an American tournament sponsored by the UPA in 2002. The survey asked players to report retrospectively injuries sustained in their careers; the study reported the following:

- Of the players surveyed, 71% had sought medical care.
- Eighty-eight percent had missed an Ultimate game or practice due to injury.
- Injuries included muscle strains (76%) and ankle (65%), knee (53%), shoulder (37%), head (30%), and rib (21%) injuries.
- A third of shoulder injuries occurred from a "layout" maneuver.
- A third of head injuries resulted in concussion.

The authors concluded, "The results of this survey demonstrate that Ultimate Frisbee injuries are common, that players are plagued with recurrent injuries, and that medical care is often sought."

Both studies noted that hand injuries were surprisingly infrequent. Given the fact that players must catch a typically fast-moving, hard plastic disc or as defenders be expected to block a throw at the point of release, hand injuries might be expected to be more common; however, in the British study, the rate of injury to the hand was only 5.7%, and in the American study, the rate was 8%.

Ultimate, like many other sports, can put participants at risk from environmental hazards, such as heat illnesses and lightning strikes. Other entries in this encyclopedia can be consulted to review the management of these conditions.

An unusual tradition in tournament Ultimate bears a final note: One of the regular prizes given out at some tournaments is for the "worst injury." Like "extreme sports" such as snowboarding or surfing or like a conventional and rugged sport such as rugby, there is a cultural emphasis in Ultimate on injuries as almost a badge of honor. Injuries preventing participation are not valued as they keep the participant from playing; but a laceration or severe abrasion that does not prevent play can be storied. Some have speculated that in such sports, injury rates may be higher as participants seek this unique "reward," playing intensely or beyond the limits of their endurance. It would be interesting to do more research on this phenomenon.

Overall, much more study specific to sports medicine is needed in this relatively new and growing sport. Increased injury surveillance can better elucidate injury patterns, and subsequent preventive measures might be put in place. Research into preparticipation conditioning levels might inform injury prevention practices. Investigations into environmental hazards or protective clothing might likewise reduce injury rates. Unique aspects of the sport—the "Worst Injury of the Tournament" award and "The Spirit of the Game"—could be studied and their effect on injury patterns and athletic health elucidated.

James Patrick Macdonald

See also Ankle Injuries; Foot Injuries; Knee Injuries; Overtraining

Further Readings

Marfleet P. Ultimate injuries: a survey. *Br J Sports Med.* 1991;25(4):235–240.
Reynolds KH, Halsmer SE. Injuries from ultimate Frisbee. *WMJ.* 2006;105(6):46–49.
Thornton A. Anyone can play this game: ultimate Frisbee, identity and difference. In: Wheaton B, ed. *Understanding Lifestyle Sports.* London, UK: Routledge; 2004:175–196.
Ultimate Players Association. *Official Rules of Ultimate.* 11th ed. http://www.boiseultimate.com/docs/11th_ed_Final_3_6_07.pdf. Accessed June 2, 2010.
Wikipedia. Ultimate (sport). http://en.wikipedia.org/wiki/Ultimate_%28sport%29. Accessed May 31, 2010.

Websites

Ultimate Players Association: http://www.upa.org
World Flying Disc Federation: http://www.wfdf.org

ULTRASOUND

Ultrasound technology has been used widely in the medical field for visualization and diagnosis of many conditions, including pregnancy, abdominal problems, and blood clots. More recently, the use of ultrasound in diagnosing and treating conditions in sports medicine has become more prevalent. Ultrasound imaging provides excellent visualization of tendons, ligaments, muscles, nerves, certain joints, and bones. It is exceptionally helpful in diagnosing tendon damage, ligament tears, and muscle strains. Sports medicine physicians frequently use ultrasound to make a particular diagnosis and guide their treatment recommendations.

Ultrasound Principles

An ultrasound machine uses a transducer that is connected to the monitor and computer of the machine (see photo, top of right column). The transducer is the device actually applied to the skin, using coupling gel, when images are being obtained. Electrical energy is transformed into sound waves by crystals in the transducer. This is called the piezoelectric effect and is fundamental to all ultrasound technology. Ultrasound is unique because it uses these sound waves to produce an image instead of using radiation, which is used for producing images for X-rays or computed tomography (CT). Ultrasound waves penetrate the skin and reflect back to the transducer after hitting certain tissues under the skin. This reflection of sound waves is converted into the images seen on the screen when performing a diagnostic ultrasound exam. Tissue that reflects the sound waves strongly appears bright white and is considered *hyperechoic.* (see image, bottom of right column). Tissue that poorly reflects sound waves appears dark and is considered *anechoic.* Tissue that falls somewhere in the middle of this spectrum is considered *hypoechoic.* Transducer frequency is an important concept for diagnostic ultrasound and is measured in megahertz (MHz). The higher the frequency of the transducer, the higher the resolution of the images obtained. However, higher-frequency transducers do not penetrate very deep, which limits the depth at which images can be obtained. Lower-frequency transducers penetrate deeper but do not provide as good image resolution as higher-frequency transducers.

Tendon Pathology

Athletes frequently encounter the pain of tendinitis when training and competing in their

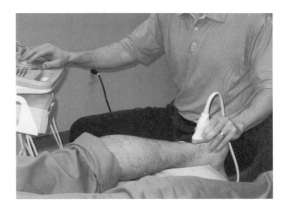

Ultrasound technique

Source: Photo courtesy of Joel M. Kary, M.D.

chosen sport. Tendinitis that does not heal well can become chronic, developing into tendinopathy. Tendinopathy occurs after the inflammatory response by the body has stopped but the tendon has not fully healed. Ultrasound demonstrates very well the changes associated with tendinopathy, such as partial tears, thickening, and cyst formation. Tendons normally appear as hyperechoic structures with fiber-like architecture and are imaged well with ultrasound due to their close proximity to the skin surface. A normal tendon will appear as smooth parallel lines of fibers without interruption or thickening, as demonstrated in the image of the Achilles tendon.

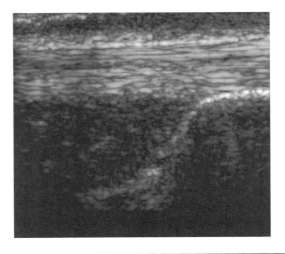

Normal Achilles tendon viewed with ultrasound. (Note that the image is necessarily of low resolution.)

Source: Photo courtesy of Joel M. Kary, M.D.

Tendinopathy, commonly found in patellar, quadriceps, and Achilles tendons, will appear thickened with areas of hypoechogenicity. Abnormal blood vessel formation sometimes occurs with tendinopathy, and this can be picked up using power Doppler settings. Power Doppler provides visualization of small blood vessels with slow flow rates, which is typical of abnormal blood vessels in tendinopathy. Ultrasound is superior to magnetic resonance imaging (MRI) when imaging tendons because it can provide high-resolution images of the individual fibers of the tendon. Tendon ruptures and tears also occur commonly in athletes. Once again, ultrasound images will clearly visualize the disruption of the tendon fibers and any blood filling the tear. In addition, the tendon can be viewed in motion while obtaining ultrasound images, providing a dynamic nature to the examination. This can be helpful in determining the size of the tendon tear and how many fibers are still intact. Rotator cuff tendon tears of the shoulder are common and are easily visualized using ultrasound.

Ligament Pathology

Ligaments appear as hyperechoic, tightly arranged, fibrillar structures providing a soft tissue connection between bones. Ligament sprains and tears occur in many sports, especially in those involving sprinting, sudden changes of direction, and jumping. Ultrasound provides excellent imaging of the superficial ligaments found in the elbow, ankle, and knee. Complete rupture of a ligament will appear as an interruption to the ligament fibers, usually with local fluid collection from the tear. Ultrasound provides an advantage, in comparison with other imaging modalities, when evaluating ligament tears. Because ultrasound allows for dynamic motion during evaluation, the ligament can be put under stress, and the amount of joint opening can be assessed. This is very helpful in determining the grade of a ligament tear and in prescribing appropriate treatment. Common ligament tears that can be diagnosed by ultrasound include the medial and lateral collateral ligaments of the knee, the ligaments of the ankle, and the ulnar collateral ligament of the elbow.

Muscle Pathology

Muscle tissue can be damaged during sports by a direct blow or sudden movements causing a tear. Muscle strains are exceedingly common in athletic participation and are readily visualized with ultrasound. Under visualization with ultrasound, muscle tissue appears as hypoechoic bundles separated by hyperechoic planes of tissue. Described another way, when viewed in long axis, muscle appears like veins in a leaf, and when viewed in cross section, it appears like a "starry night" pattern. A direct blow to a muscle can lead to accumulation of blood within the muscle tissue, known as a *hematoma*. This is seen as an anechoic or dark fluid collection within the muscle fibers and can be measured using ultrasound. Muscle tears are seen as discontinuity of the muscle fibers and can be accentuated by pressure from the transducer when doing an ultrasound examination.

Advantages of Ultrasound

The use of magnetic resonance imaging (MRI) or computed tomography (CT) in evaluating sports injuries can be quite expensive. In comparison, ultrasound is a less expensive imaging alternative providing superior images of many common sports injuries. Claustrophobia can be ruled out with patients undergoing ultrasound examination, which is done with the athlete seated or lying down on a comfortable exam table. Ultrasound examination can actually be performed as an extension of the physical exam, providing additional valuable information to the clinician. The body part being examined can be viewed in motion with ultrasound, observing the soft tissue and bony anatomy in "real time." This is particularly helpful in making the diagnosis of athletic injuries, the symptoms of which only occur when the tendon or muscle is in motion, such as a dislocating ankle tendon or a shoulder rotator cuff tendon getting compressed during the throwing motion. Another advantage of ultrasound is the ability to quickly perform comparisons of the injured body part with the uninjured side. As the technology has improved, ultrasound units have become more portable while still maintaining superior image quality. This portability is convenient in sports medicine as the unit can be used readily in the athletic training room or on the sideline. Ultrasound can be used to guide injections. The needle can be visualized during the entire injection, thereby ensuring accurate placement of the injection and avoiding damage to any nearby blood vessels or nerves.

Limitations of Ultrasound

The accurate use of ultrasound is operator dependent, and it requires extensive training and practice to become proficient. Errors can be made by not recognizing the difference between normal and abnormal anatomy. Athletes with a large body habitus provide a unique challenge as ultrasound waves have trouble penetrating deep enough to provide adequate images for diagnosis. Due to the inability of ultrasound waves to penetrate through bone, the visualization of deep joint structures and bone is best done using other imaging techniques such as X-ray, MRI, or CT.

Joel M. Kary

See also Achilles Tendinitis; Achilles Tendon Rupture; Joints, Magnetic Resonance Imaging of; Strains, Muscle; Tendinitis, Tendinosis

Further Readings

Bianchi S, Martinoli C. *Ultrasound of the Musculoskeletal System.* Berlin, Germany: Springer; 2007.

Jacobson JA. *Fundamentals of Musculoskeletal Ultrasound.* Philadelphia, PA: Saunders Elsevier; 2007.

Lento PH, Primack S. Advances and utility of diagnostic ultrasound in musculoskeletal medicine. *Curr Rev Musculoskelet Med.* 2008;1(1):24–31.

Nofsinger C, Konin JG. Diagnostic ultrasound in sports medicine: current concepts and advances. *Sports Med Arthrosc.* 2009;17(1):25–30.

URTICARIA AND PRURITUS

Urticaria, or "hives," represents a dermatologic allergic reaction, of which there are specific types. They are typically pruritic, white, or red nonpitting plaques.

Urticaria is caused by dilation of blood vessels and edema within the epidermis. Classic hives are typically 10 to 15 millimeters (mm) in diameter, will blanch with pressure, and typically result from an allergic trigger. For athletes, classic urticaria may result from exposure to medications such as aspirin or nonsteroidal anti-inflammatory drugs (NSAIDs), which may lead to mast cell degranulation. However, urticaria more commonly associated with exercise and sports are often smaller—2 to 4 mm typically. It is also known as *cholinergic urticaria.*

Cholinergic urticaria is part of a subgroup of urticaria known as *physical urticarias,* which are caused by physical stimulation. Physical urticarias represent 17% of all urticarias, and are most often seen in young adults. They include dermatographism, immediate-pressure and delayed-pressure urticaria, localized or generalized heat-induced urticaria, exercise-induced anaphylaxis, solar urticaria, X-ray–induced urticaria, and argon–laser induced urticaria. A person may have several types of physical urticarias, such as cholinergic urticaria along with solar urticaria. About 80% of all urticaria are idiopathic. About 10% to 20% of the population will suffer from urticaria at some point in their lifetime. If urticaria lasts for 6 weeks or more, it is defined as *chronic.* Chronic urticaria is most often idiopathic.

Cholinergic urticaria occurs when vasodilation of capillaries in the superficial dermis leads to increased transudate. It typically occurs when an antigen is bound by immunoglobulin (IgE) to release histamine from mast cells or basophils. As histamine levels increase, the level of pruritis also increases. Other factors, such as prostaglandins, leukotrienes, platelet-activating factor, and bradykinin and the complement system are also involved.

Cholinergic urticaria occur with any increase in core body temperature, which can occur with exercise. Aerobic activities and exercising in a hot environment are more likely to elicit urticaria. It is characterized by 2 to 4 mm wheals surrounded by large flares. It often starts within 2 to 3 minutes of exercise initiation, and starts on the thorax and neck and then spreads to the rest of the body. Tingling, itching, or a burning sensation on the skin may occur before the hives develop. The hives may coalesce, in which case they will resemble angioedema.

Wheezing and dyspnea may also develop in cholinergic urticaria. It may be difficult to identify cholinergic urticaria if the hives do coalesce. Those who are prone to cholinergic urticaria often also develop the same urticarial reaction with anxiety, a hot shower, sweating, or with any other elevation in body temperature. It is important to take a good history to determine if there are other triggers, such as with hot baths and showers, or with emotional stress and anxiety, or with ingestion of hot or spicy foods, to distinguish cholinergic urticaria from EIA (Exercise-induced anaphylaxis). Cholinergic urticaria is classically reproducible with exercise, stress, or hot showers, while EIA is not. There may be other signs of cholinergic stimulation, such as lacrimation, salivation, and diarrhea.

Cold urticaria is another type of urticaria that can be seen in athletes. It primarily occurs in cold-weather sports or in swimming. Wheals can be large or small, but they are generally confined to the area exposed to the cold. Diagnosis can be made with observation of hives on skin after 5 minutes of cold application and subsequent skin rewarming. The treatment consists of avoiding cold exposure and wearing protective warm equipment, as well as antihistamines.

The gold standard for diagnosis of cholinergic urticaria is passive warming, either in a warm bath or a sauna. An increase in the core body temperature of 0.7 °C to 1 °C is needed. In case there is a possibility that exercise-induced anaphylaxis is the true diagnosis, testing should be done under controlled conditions, with epinephrine, rescusitative equipment, and medical personnel at hand, and a IV set should be in place. Another test that is diagnostic is the methacholine test, where an intradermal injection of 0.01 milligram (mg) methacholine produces localized hives. However, the sensitivity is only about 30%. The passive heat challenge is the best test.

Treatment of cholinergic urticaria consists of avoidance of triggers primarily, such as bathing in hot water, and strenuous exercise in hot weather. Hydroxyzine, an H1 histamine antagonist, is an anticholinergic that has been shown to be most effective at reducing urticarial hives. Hydroxyzine, which is typically dosed at 100 to 200 mg over a 24-hour period, is most effective. In cases refractory to hydroxyzine, danazol anabolic steroid could be effective, but this treatment should be avoided at all costs, considering the side effects. Cyproheptadine may be used as adjunctive treatment if there is associated cold urticaria. Treatment of pulmonary symptoms with cromolyn sodium can be effective. For long-term treatment, an exercise program with gradual increases in duration and intensity may be effective in producing tolerance. Avoidance of obvious triggers, such as NSAIDs or aspirin before exercise is essential. Exercising with an EpiPen if there is any concern for EIA is important. However, care must be taken in athletes competing at NCAA (National Collegiate Athletic Association), Olympic, or professional levels to avoid certain medications that may be banned or restricted, such as anabolic steroids, albuterol, or decongestants.

Elizabeth Rothe and William W. Dexter

See also Allergic Contact Dermatitis; Allergies; Anaphylaxis, Exercise-Induced; Skin Disorders, Metabolic

Further Readings

Briner WW. Physical allergies and exercise: clinical implications for those engaged in sports activities. *Sports Med.* 1993;15(6):365–373.

Dice JP. Physical urticaria. *Immunol Allergy Clin North Am.* 2004;24(2):225–246.

Horan LF, Sheffer AL, Briner WW. Physical allergies. *Med Sci Sports Exerc.* 1992;24(8):845–848.

Hosey RG, Carek PJ, Goo A. Exercise-induced anaphylaxis and urticaria. *Am Fam Physician.* 2001;64(8):1367–1372.

Torchia D, Francalanci S, Bellandi S, Fabbri P. Multiple physical urticarias. *Postgrad Med J.* 2008;84(987):e1–e2.

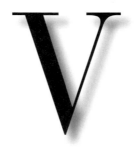

VEGETARIANISM AND EXERCISE

Vegetarian diets are common among athletes. A balanced vegetarian diet, meaning one guided by thoughtful and informed food choices, certainly may meet the needs of athletes and even be the foundation for some healthful lifelong habits. For young athletes, however, because growth is still occurring, the priority is to provide enough calories and nutrients for optimal growth and development while still supporting higher activity needs. This entry discusses the vegetarian diet as it relates to sports nutrition.

Individuals choose vegetarianism for a wide variety of reasons. Some of these include health benefits such as the prevention of certain chronic diseases, cultural beliefs, family practices, peer influences, and animal rights or environmental issues. Some athletes insist that a vegetarian diet may improve their performance. Others adopt a vegetarian diet to meet the increased carbohydrate demands of training or to assist in weight control. Of concern are those athletes who describe their dietary intake as "vegetarian" to hide restrictive dietary intake or to mask disordered eating behaviors.

Types of Vegetarian Diets

Many foods meet the criteria for a vegetarian diet. The term *vegetarian* is used to describe diets based exclusively on plant foods to those containing some animal foods. Table 1 outlines various vegetarian diets.

Vegetarian Diets and Performance

While there is no evidence that being a vegetarian gives any direct athletic advantage, healthy vegetarian athletes can perform as well as nonvegetarian athletes. A plant-based or vegetarian diet may be ideal for performance as it is generally high in complex carbohydrates. Only the caloric needs change, as plant-based diets are low in fats. Added fat, especially in the form of monounsaturated fats (olive oil, avocados, nuts, and peanuts), as well as essential fatty acids (fish and flax seed oils), may help provide additional calories to a vegetarian diet.

Vegetarianism does not greatly affect the fundamentals of optimal sports and performance nutrition. However, seeking advice from a dietitian may be beneficial in crafting an ideal performance nutrition plan.

Protein and Vegetarian Diets

Amino acids are the building blocks of protein. If a food contains the right combination of essential amino acids, it is called a *complete protein*. All animal-derived proteins and soy are complete. The remaining plant sources of protein contain many, but not all, of the essential amino acids and thus are considered *incomplete proteins*.

Previously, it had been suggested that vegetarians combine different plant foods at individual meals to ensure that all essential amino acids were provided at the same time. However, the American Dietetic Association has since stated that combining plant sources of protein meal by meal to meet

Table 1   Vegetarian Diets

Type of Vegetarian Diet	Diet Description
Fruitarian	Raw, dried, or cooked fruits, nuts, seeds, honey, and vegetable oils
Macrobiotic	Excludes all animal foods, dairy products, and eggs Uses only unprocessed, unrefined natural and organic cereals and grains Miso and seaweed are used as condiments
Vegan	Excludes all animal foods, dairy products, and eggs The vegan philosophy also excludes all animal products, including honey, gelatin, silk, wool, leather, and animal-derived food additives
Lacto-vegetarian	Excludes all animal foods and eggs Does include dairy products
Lacto-ovo-vegetarian	Excludes all animal foods Does include dairy products and eggs
Semivegetarian	Usually excludes red meat However, may include poultry, fish, eggs, and dairy products

the body's requirement for essential amino acids is unnecessary. Thus, as long as a variety of plant proteins are eaten throughout the day, adequate amino acids will be obtained.

A favorable eating regimen for vegetarian athletes is to ensure that protein-rich foods are included at each meal. Many athletes have limited time for meal preparation, particularly at lunch. Convenient and portable protein alternatives include ready-prepared beans (hummus, baked beans, and bean salad), nut and seed spreads (peanut butter and tahini), and ready-made luncheon meals made from soy or wheat gluten.

Along with including adequate protein, it is also crucial to obtain adequate calories so that protein is not used as an energy source. Athletes often have the misconception that the protein they consume is the only nutrient that is responsible for building more muscle. Actually, it is consuming enough calories that preserve protein for muscle repair and growth. Excess protein does not provide any advantage, and special protein supplements are generally not necessary. In summary, an athlete needs adequate protein, calories, and, most important, enough calories to spare, or make available, protein for growth and repair of tissues.

Meeting Vitamin and Mineral Needs

Athletes who are vegetarians have to include vegetarian alternatives in their diet that supplement certain vitamins and minerals that are commonly found in animal-based foods, such as vitamin D, riboflavin, vitamin B_{12}, iron, calcium, and zinc.

Vitamin D is important for bone health. Athletes need to ensure that they get adequate vitamin D from sun exposure and/or through fortified foods or supplements. Cow's milk, certain soy milks, and many breakfast cereals are fortified with vitamin D.

Riboflavin is low in vegetarian diets that do not include dairy products. It is an essential vitamin for the production of energy and thus important for athletes. Plant sources of riboflavin include fortified whole grains, soybeans, dark green leafy vegetables, avocados, nuts, and sea vegetables.

Vitamin B_{12} is needed for the production of normal red blood cells. Its deficiency may result in pernicious anemia and associated dementia. B_{12} is only found in animal products. The semivegetarian will obtain adequate B_{12} if fish and dairy products are consumed. The vegan will need to obtain B_{12}

through a supplement, nutritional yeast, fortified grains, or soymilk.

Calcium is essential for all athletes for optimal bone health. Vegetarians who do not include dairy products in their diet need to include calcium sources from plants or supplements. Athletes with low dietary calcium intake may have increased risk of bone fractures and stress fractures. Plant-based sources of calcium include kale, bok choy, turnip greens, and Chinese cabbage.

All athletes, especially female athletes, are at risk for iron deficiency. Iron plays a critical function in transporting oxygen throughout the body. There is also loss of iron due to heavy training. The absorption of iron from animal-derived foods is much higher than from plant sources. However, vitamin C significantly improves iron absorption from nonanimal sources. A diet rich in fruits and vegetables provides adequate vitamin C. Cooking in cast iron pots may also increase the iron content of certain foods. Iron-fortified breakfast cereals, spinach, beans, molasses, whole-grain products, textured vegetable protein, and some dried fruits (dried apricots, prunes, and raisins) are also good sources of iron.

In summary, with proper planning, athletes can choose a vegetarian diet that meets nutrient needs for athletic performance as well as for optimal health.

Jan Pauline Hangen

See also Dietitian/Sports Nutritionist; Eating Disorders; Female Athlete Triad; Nutrition and Hydration

Further Readings

Davis B, Melina V. *Becoming Vegan: The Complete Guide to Adopting a Healthy Plant-Based Diet.* Summertown, TN: Book Publishing Company; 2000.

Dorfman L. *The Vegetarian Sports Nutrition Guide: Peak Performance for Everyone From Beginners to Gold Medalists.* Hoboken, NJ: John Wiley; 1999.

Havala S. *Being Vegetarian for Dummies.* New York, NY: Hungry Minds; 2001.

Larson-Meyer DE. *Vegetarian Sports Nutrition.* Champaign, IL: Human Kinetics; 2006.

Wasserman D, Mangels R. *Simply Vegan: Quick Vegetarian Meals.* 4th ed. Baltimore, MD: Vegetarian Resource Group; 2006.

VOLKMANN CONTRACTURE

Volkmann contracture, also known as *Volkmann ischemic contracture,* is a permanent flexion contracture of the hand at the wrist, resulting in a clawlike deformity of the hand and fingers. It may affect a single finger or the flexor muscles of the entire forearm. It may result from injury to brachial artery and is usually associated with supracondylar fracture of humerus, sometimes consequent to a high-impact fall as in skateboarding or other sports. It can also result from an intense twist of the upper arm, falling on an outstretched hand, or severe contraction of muscles. Baseball pitchers and other athletes who participate in throwing sports such as javelin and discus are vulnerable to this condition.

Classification

Ischemia is defined as cell death due to lack of blood supply. The intensity of injury depends on the type of cell and its energy requirements.

Ischemic injuries are classified in various ways. One is according to the severity of involvement:

Grade I: Ischemia

Grade II: Ischemic contracture

Grade III: Ischemic contracture associated with nerve involvement

They may also be classified according to the structures involved:

Type I: Contracture involving forearm muscles with intrinsic muscles intact

Type II: Contracture involving forearm muscles associated with paralysis of intrinsic muscles

Type III: Contracture involving forearm muscles as well as intrinsic muscles

Type IV: Mixed type

Tsuge's classification comprises three types, according to the extent and the muscle groups involved.

Mild: It is characterized by flexion contracture of two or three fingers with minimal loss of sensation.

Moderate: The thumb gets stuck in the palm, and all fingers are flexed; the wrist may be flexed with associated loss of sensation.

Severe: All muscles in the forearm, including both the flexors and extensors of the wrist and fingers, are involved.

Anatomy

The brachial artery branches into the radial and ulnar arteries. The radial artery is superficially positioned, whereas the ulnar artery is deeply placed, passing deep into the pronator teres muscles. The ulnar artery gives rise to the common interosseous artery, which immediately divides into the anterior and posterior interosseous branches. The anterior interosseous artery provides blood supply to the flexors of the forearm and hand.

Causes

Ischemic contracture may be caused by the following:

- Fracture
- Compartmental syndrome
- Tight bandages
- Arterial embolus
- Arterial insufficiency
- Improper use of a tourniquet
- Improper use of a plaster cast

Volkmann contracture occurs when there is insufficient blood supply (ischemia) to the forearm and is the end result of an untreated or relatively inadequately decompressed compartment syndrome in which ischemic necrosis of muscles has developed. The key factor in all cases of ischemic contracture is reduction in compartment size or increase in the content of a closed, uncompromising osteofascial compartment, which is enough to cause occlusion of small vessels.

The blockade immediately results in ischemia of the nerve and muscle. If the pressure is not relieved in time, it may result in damage to muscle contracture and nerves.

Decrease in the compartment size can be attributed to the following causes:

- Constrictive casts and dressings
- Persistent localized external pressure

- Injuries due to heat
- Burn Escher
- Plastic surgery of facial defects

This can also be attributed to an increase in compartment content resulting from hemorrhage, bleeding diathesis, or anticoagulation.

Diagnosis

The hallmark symptom of Volkmann contracture is pain that does not improve with rest or nonsedative analgesics. It will continue to get worse as time passes, and if the pressure is allowed to persist, there will be decreased sensation and weakness.

Besides pain, symptoms include pallor, pulselessness, paresthesias (numbness), and paralysis. Aggravation of pain on passive stretch is the most reliable finding on physical examination. Other symptoms include decreased sensation, weakness, and induration of the forearm. Pulselessness and paralysis are late symptoms. The forearm may show swelling and is also shiny. There is a typical flexion contracture of the wrist along with clawing of the fingers.

An absolute diagnosis is made based on direct measurement of the compartment pressure. It is done by inserting a needle into the compartment that is attached to a pressure meter. When the pressure is above 45 millimeters of mercury (mmHg) or when it is within 30 mmHg of the diastolic pressure, a diagnosis of compartment syndrome is made. This is the general test to diagnose compartment syndrome.

Treatment

Early recognition and timely treatment of imminent Volkmann ischemia decrease the presentation and severity of late contracture and hand dysfunction. Ideal treatment requires a thorough examination of the extent of damage of the ischemia, followed by conservative therapy or operation.

Management presents considerable challenges. The success in achieving a potentially functional and aesthetically satisfactory result is greatest in the acute phase. A physician should be immediately consulted in case of an injury to the elbow or forearm and if swelling is also present.

Nonsurgical Treatment

If there is a forearm or elbow fracture, a proper initial splinting of the hand in functional position should be performed; the area must be kept still, and the arm should be raised above the level of the heart. This helps in preventing further injury and excessive swelling. When the extent of injury is determined, conservative treatment techniques such as rest and ice should be started to help decrease the swelling. Pain relief and anti-inflammatory medicines may be prescribed. Casts and surgery also may be indicated, depending on the injury. Bed rest or use of a protective device (a knee brace or wrist guard) is usually advised. Physiotherapy may also be of help in rehabilitation. Early mobilization, range-of-motion exercises, followed by stretching and strengthening exercises are part of rehabilitation.

Surgery

The best treatment is early surgical intervention to release the pressure in the forearm in order to prevent permanent injury to muscles and nerves. Reconstructive surgery to lengthen and sometimes transfer muscles may restore some hand function.

Muscle sliding is considered the most effective method. It results in the best preservation of resting length of muscle.

Other methods include the following:

- Tendon lengthening
- Neurolysis
- Scar excision
- Tendon lengthening
- Tendon transpositions
- Nerve grafting

Stage 1 Contracture

Muscle-sliding operation usually results in complete recovery. It consists of median nerve neurolysis and removal of necrotic debris. For isolated muscle injuries, tendon lengthening is recommended.

Stage 2 Contracture

Transposition of flexor tendons has an equal effect to muscle-sliding operation. It is an imperative procedure that helps in the prevention as well as control of imbalance deformity, its indication depending on the personal as well as professional profiles of the individual patient. A tendon transfer procedure alleviates the suffering from functional impairment and provides a far better alternative to permanent external splints. This is usually a secondary procedure for replacing function, which is done after evaluation of the functional motor loss.

Stage 3 Contracture

The primary treatment option is muscle-sliding operation. Some secondary procedures such as tendon transpositions and nerve grafts are often necessary.

Stage 4 Ischemic Contracture

Muscle-sliding operations may help in improving deficiency in extension; however, wrist arthrodesis is of great help. The aim of arthrodesis is to achieve a relatively painfree wrist by eliminating movement. In this procedure, the bones are fixed. This procedure is more beneficial for young, active patients or middle-aged patients but not for elderly patients. Extensor tendon transpositions may be of benefit.

Long-Term Prognosis

Prognosis is variable and depends on the severity of the disease and the stage at which intervention is made. If the pressure is released earlier by surgery, before the onset of any permanent damage, then the prognosis is excellent. High compartment pressure for a longer period of time can result in permanent nerve damage. Cubitus varus and loss of radial pulse are the other complications reported.

Mariam Shaheen and Maryam Tirmizi

See also Elbow and Forearm Injuries; Elbow and Forearm Injuries, Surgery for; Elbow Fracture; Forearm Fracture

Further Readings

Carson S, Woolridge DP, Colletti J, Kilgore K. Pediatric upper extremity injuries. *Pediatr Clin North Am.* 2006;53(1):41–67.

Gosset J. Ischemic and anoxic necrosis of the muscles of the forearm and hand (Volkmann's contracture) (author's transl) [in French]. *Ann Chir.* 1975;29(12):1059–1064.

Holden CE. Compartmental syndrome following trauma. *Clin Orthop.* 1975;(113):95–102.

Lanz U, Felderhoff J. Ischemic contractures of the forearm and hand. *Handchir Mikrochir Plast Chir.* 2000;32(1):6–25.

Mubarak SJ, Caroll NC. Volkmann's contracture in children: aetiology and prevention. *J Bone Joint Surg Br.* 1979;61(3):285–293.

Pedowitz RA, Toutounghi FM. Chronic exertional compartment syndrome of the forearm flexor muscles. *J Hand Surg Am.* 1988;13(5):694–696.

Shin AY, Chambers H, Wilkins KE, Bucknell A. Suction injuries in children leading to acute compartment syndrome of the interosseous muscles of the hand: case reports. *J Hand Surg Am.* 1996;21(4):675–678.

Tempka A, Schmidt U. Compartment syndrome of the hand. Diagnosis, therapy, results, late sequelae [in German]. *Unfallchirurg.* 1991;94(5):240–243.

Tsuge K. Management of established Volkmann's contracture. In: Green DP, Hotchkiss RN, Pederson WC, eds. *Green's Operative Hand Surgery.* 4th ed. New York, NY: Churchill Livingstone; 1999: 592–603.

Tsuge K. Treatment of established Volkmann's contracture. *J Bone Joint Surg Am.* 1975;57(7): 925–929.

VOLLEYBALL, INJURIES IN

Volleyball is the sport with the highest rate of jumping during practice and competition. Jumping seems to be the riskiest activity in volleyball because the majority of injuries are associated with jumping and landing. Defense is associated with a small number of injuries, while serving, passing, and setting are associated with even fewer injuries.

Epidemiologic studies of volleyball injuries have identified some of the risks of injury in the sport. The highest rate of injury in volleyball is associated with blocking, followed by spiking. These are also the two sport-specific activities that require a jump with every repetition.

Injury rates during competition have been evaluated. An injury is defined as "any condition causing the athlete to present to the medical staff during a tournament." In high-level play, a rate of injury between 1 per 25 hours and 1 per 50 hours is common. Injuries in American intercollegiate play have also been studied. "Any condition that resulted in missing a practice or match" is how an American intercollegiate group defines injury. Each practice or match was counted as one exposure. The rate of injury was about 4 per 1,000 athlete exposures in women's intercollegiate training and competition. This ranked volleyball second to softball for the lowest injury rate among 15 intercollegiate sports. Playing on a softer surface, such as sand, also seems to decrease the risk of injury.

Ankle Sprains

In volleyball, 15% to 60% of recorded injuries are ankle sprains. Ankle injuries are almost always associated with landing from blocking or spiking in the front court. The most common mechanism of injury occurs when the blocking player lands on an opposing spiker's foot that has come underneath the net and across the center line in the "conflict zone." The rules of volleyball allow a player's foot to cross this line beneath the net as long as some portion of the foot remains in contact with it. It often results in an inversion injury, where the ankle rolls outward. The ligaments on the outside, or lateral side, of the ankle are injured.

An ankle brace or orthosis is often recommended while actively rehabilitating, as it decreases the reinjury risk. Stirrup-style braces, particularly pneumatic-type orthoses such as the Aircast® brand, have been shown to decrease injury risk fourfold. The risk of reinjury is greatest during the first year after an initial injury, so it is recommended that braces be worn for a year after an ankle sprain. Braces have not been shown to decrease risk of injury in ankles that have not been previously sprained.

It may be possible to prevent a significant number of ankle sprains with a fairly simple prophylactic program. First, advise all players not to allow any part of their foot to touch the center line during practice. Second, identify "problem attackers." These are players who jump forward (doing a broad jump) when spiking the ball. These players should be coached to take longer last-approach steps and jump straight upward instead of out. A twofold decrease in ankle sprains may be anticipated. It should be easy to convince players that this is a good idea, because this technique actually results in a higher vertical jump.

Patellar Tendinitis (Tendinosis)

Patellar tendinosis (*jumper's knee*) is by far the most frequent overuse injury in volleyball. It is probably so common because of the high frequency of jumping inherent in the sport. Patellar tendinosis has been found to be more common in players who play more than four times weekly and are 20 to 25 years old. Players who have been in the sport for 2 to 5 years are also more likely to have symptoms. Plyometric training has *not* been associated with patellar tendinitis in these elite players. Most players with this condition have pain at the bottom part of the kneecap.

It may be possible to identify players who are at increased risk for patellar tendinosis. Those who can generate the greatest amount of power during jumping have been found to be at greater risk. These are also the players with the highest vertical jumps. Perhaps, they may not need as much jump training as their teammates. Deeper knee flexion at takeoff for jumping may also place players at greater risk. Coaching attention to proper jumping technique might help these players avoid injury.

Patellar tendinosis can usually be managed conservatively with ice, short-term anti-inflammatory medication, and alterations in training activity. Closed-chain eccentric strengthening of the quadriceps muscle can result in stronger fibers in the patellar tendon. An example of this sort of exercise would be leg presses where the athlete "works the negative." These exercises should be used to rehabilitate this condition.

Shoulder Tendinitis (Tendinosis)

The most common shoulder injuries in volleyball players are rotator cuff and biceps tendinosis as a result of overuse. They account for 8% to 20% of injuries in volleyball. Repetitively striking the ball overhead places a cumulative stress on the shoulder. Striking the ball at the highest point in the arm swing may place the shoulder at particular risk in this sport. These forces predispose the shoulder tendons to impingement with spiking and overhead serving. The tendons get impinged between the head of the humerus, or arm bone, and the acromion process, which sits above the shoulder.

A player who has shoulder pain and/or weakness should be evaluated by a physician, athletic trainer, or physical therapist. Sometimes, the entire shoulder girdle (including the shoulder blade) moves in an abnormal pattern. A rehabilitation program will often be prescribed. Abnormal shoulder blade movement should be addressed first. This usually involves shoulder retraction exercises. Then, rotator cuff exercises will help stabilize the ball in the socket.

Suprascapular Nerve Injury: A Volleyball-Specific Injury?

An unusual condition that may be present in up to one third of elite volleyball players is suprascapular nerve compression. Several factors may be involved with this problem, but the nerve is usually compressed by the bone of the shoulder blade near where it innervates the infraspinatus muscle. This is the muscle that externally rotates the shoulder. So players typically have isolated weakness of external rotation when a trainer evaluates their shoulder strength. Interestingly, the majority of the players with this condition do *not* have shoulder pain.

Players with this condition who have no pain probably do not require further evaluation or treatment. Findings of isolated external rotation weakness and infraspinatus atrophy should be noted on preparticipation physical exam for future reference, in case the player develops symptoms. In those with significant symptoms, such as shoulder pain, magnetic resonance imaging (MRI) may be helpful if surgery is being considered, because up to two thirds of affected individuals may have an abnormality called a ganglion cyst compressing the nerve.

Other Injuries

Volleyball players often suffer relatively minor hand or back injuries. These injuries are common yet rarely result in time missed from the sport. Sprain of the outside ligament of the thumb (metacarpal-phalangeal radial collateral ligament) is the most frequent hand injury seen in volleyball players. It often occurs with blocking and may require splinting or taping.

Low back injuries account for up to 14% of volleyball injuries. In teenage athletes, back pain should be evaluated by a physician, because back pain is unusual in this age-group and almost always occurs secondary to a condition that may respond to treatment. One such condition is spondylolysis, which is essentially a stress fracture of the low back. Athletes who have pain when they bend backward with their lower back (lumbar extension) should be evaluated by a sports medicine physician. This may occur in hitters, when they must repeatedly reach back behind their heads to contact the ball.

Severe knee injuries requiring surgery on the anterior cruciate ligament (ACL) are also rare, but these injuries seem to be more common in female players. A good way to evaluate female athletes who may be at risk for this injury is to observe players as they land after jumping off of a box. Those whose knees come together (into valgus) and touch on landing—"kissing knees"—should be considered for a program of exercises to prevent ACL injury.

William W. Briner, Jr.

See also Ankle Sprain; Musculoskeletal Tests, Shoulder; Patellar Tendinitis; Shoulder Injuries; Shoulder Injuries, Surgery for; Thumb Sprain

Further Readings

Ferretti A. *Volleyball Injuries: A Colour Atlas of Volleyball Traumatology.* Lausanne, Switzerland: FIVB Federacion Internationale de volleyball, Medical Commission; 1994.

Reeser JC, Bahr R. *Volleyball: Olympic Handbook of Sports Medicine and Science.* Oxford, UK: Blackwell Science; 2003.

Reeser JC, Verhagen E, Briner WW, Askeland TI, Bahr R. Strategies for the prevention of volleyball injuries. *Br J Sports Med.* 2006;40(7):594–599.

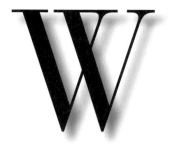

WARTS (VERRUCAE)

Warts, or *verrucae,* are common skin findings that are often considered benign. However, in the athletic population they have the potential to cause significant pain and, thereby, impair performance. Although warts are found in every age-group, children and young adults are the most commonly affected, and athletes are at particular risk.

Human papillomavirus (HPV) is a virus that infects the skin and mucous membranes. There are more than 150 different types of HPV that cause warts in various areas of the body. Recently, several types of HPV have received additional attention because of their association with cervical cancer. The HPV vaccine is aimed at minimizing the spread of subtypes 16 and 18. The vast majority of HPV infect the skin and cause cutaneous warts. These types of HPV have virtually no potential to cause cancer.

Transmission of HPV occurs when the virus comes into contact with areas of damaged, even minimally damaged, skin. Transmission can be skin to skin or skin to fomite, such as shower room floors. Participation in sports can cause trauma to the skin, particularly to the feet and hands. In addition, the shared use of shower facilities and weight training equipment introduces multiple potential sources of exposure to HPV.

It is difficult to know exactly when an HPV infection occurs, because there is a lag time between exposure to the virus and the appearance of the resultant warts. The viruses commonly have an incubation period of between 1 and 6 months. Once individuals are infected, they risk passing this infection to other areas of their own skin through activities that cause minor skin trauma, such as shaving or scratching. Most subtypes of HPV cause specific types of warts that have predilections for certain areas of the body.

Symptoms

Two types of warts that frequently affect athletes are common warts and plantar warts. Common warts make up approximately 70% of cutaneous warts. They can be found anywhere on the body, but these most frequently affect the backs of hands and fingers. In children, these warts often appear on the face and neck. These warts are often described as "irregularly surfaced domed lesions."

One study looked at the acquisition of new common hand warts in runners and members of the crew team at a university. Rowers experienced hand trauma through weight training and rowing. Runners, on the other hand, experienced hand trauma from weight lifting alone. The study noted a significant increase in new common hand warts in crew team members compared with track team members. The authors postulated that trauma to wet, macerated hands made crew team members more susceptible to HPV and the resultant common warts.

Plantar warts are found on the sole of the foot and often cluster in the areas that bear significant pressure. The ball of the foot and the heel are the two most commonly affected sites. Because of their location, plantar warts can become callused and appear to grow into the foot. These warts are often found in small groups and can produce significant pain during weight bearing. Athletes with plantar warts may feel the sensation of having a pebble in their shoe while running or walking. Several factors predispose athletes to plantar warts, including communal showers, excessive perspiration, and repetitive microtrauma to the foot.

It is important to note that plantar warts can cause symptoms similar to stress fractures; therefore, plantar warts must not be overlooked when investigating plantar foot pain. A case report describes a 24-year-old female tennis player who was forced to stop play in the middle of a tennis match. She had tenderness over the ball of her foot, and it was suspected that she had a stress fracture. Following 2 weeks of rest, she returned to competition, and again the pain returned. Notably, she had calluses over the painful area of her foot. These calluses were pared down, exposing multiple dark spots (the "seeds" commonly found in plantar warts). Her plantar warts were treated, and she subsequently returned to play.

This situation illustrates how debilitating plantar warts can be for an athlete and the need to include plantar warts in the differential diagnosis for foot pain. Part of the difficulty in diagnosing plantar warts is that they are often covered with a callus. Once the callus is removed, plantar warts have a characteristic appearance: multiple black speckles, which are actually small blood vessels. These small blood vessels are the hallmark of plantar warts and differentiate them from other skin findings.

Treatment

There are several options available for the treatment of both common and plantar warts. Treatment can be broken down into three categories: (1) observation, (2) mechanical destruction, and (3) stimulation of the patient's immune system. Given the fact that cutaneous warts are caused by viruses, the immune system can potentially eradicate the viruses and the resulting warts. Warts affect patients with intact and impaired immune systems alike. However, individuals with impaired immune systems may never be able to mount an immune response significant enough to fight HPV.

Most warts in a healthy patient will resolve spontaneously (without intervention) over months or years. One study demonstrated the spontaneous resolution of two thirds of warts over 2 years. However, this process may take longer and be less successful than interventional measures. The longer the warts remain, the greater the potential for spread to different areas of the skin and to other people. Furthermore, the spread of warts may result in larger or more numerous warts, which may be more difficult to eventually remove.

Although most warts will resolve without intervention, the option of observation is much less desirable for athletes whose performance is impaired due to warts. These individuals may be more appropriate candidates for mechanical destruction. Mechanical destruction can be accomplished through a variety of measures. The most common types of mechanical destruction include topical acids, freezing, and curetting. However, it is important to note that destructive measures, particularly curetting, have the potential to leave a scar. Such scars, especially in the case of plantar warts, can be painful and can potentially inhibit the athlete's ability to run or even bear weight on the affected foot. Therefore, athletes must be cautious with more aggressive means of wart destruction.

Topical acids are effective, safe if properly used, and available over the counter. Salicylic acid is a common preparation often used as a first-line interventional treatment for both common and plantar warts. However, instructions for application can be complex and, thus, decrease patient compliance with treatment. To maximize the efficacy of salicylic acid, a regimen that includes daily soaking, debridement with an emery board, topical application of the acid, and occlusion with duct tape should be followed. This stepwise treatment should be repeated every 24 hours. Several studies have demonstrated that topical acids are more effective and faster at eliminating warts than simple observation (no intervention).

Freezing, or cryotherapy, involves the use of liquid nitrogen or nitrous oxide to destroy warts. The wart is frozen using a cryogun until the entire wart and up to 2 millimeters (mm) of the surrounding tissue turn white. A second freeze after thawing makes this method more effective. Following the freeze, the affected area will blister and then gradually slough and heal over the next few weeks. The freeze destroys the wart but also stimulates the immune system that aids in the destruction of any remaining HPV. Although much less complex than topical therapy, this method has the potential to cause blistering and pain, particularly in the case of plantar warts. While in training, athletes must decide whether the functional impairment from their warts is severe enough to warrant the potential complications of freezing.

Occlusion with duct tape alone has been used by many practitioners and has been the subject of several studies. Although the exact mechanism of treatment with duct tape is not known, several theories have been proposed, including suffocation of warts, immune response stimulation, and mechanical debridement. In 2002, a study compared the efficacy of cryotherapy with that of duct tape occlusion. The results showed that duct tape occlusive therapy was significantly superior to cryotherapy in resolving common warts. However, two other studies have questioned the efficacy of duct tape occlusion as a successful therapeutic intervention. These studies demonstrated no significant differences in the resolution of warts when compared with placebo treatments such as corn pads or moleskin coverings. Though they showed a nonsignificant initial resolution of the wart, return of the wart was equally demonstrated. Questions still remain as to whether differences in the type of duct tape, silver versus transparent, could account for the divergent outcomes of these studies.

There are also various methods that have been used to stimulate the immune system to facilitate the destruction of HPV and the resulting warts. These methods are directed at enhancing the immune response both locally and systemically. Injection of *Candida* into the base of a wart is one way to generate a local immune response. The body's natural response to the fungus will supply the injected region with host cells that target the *Candida* as well as the viruses causing the wart. Similarly, topical agents such as imiquimod cream and diphenylcyclopropenone generate a local inflammatory response that enhances virus destruction. Interestingly, the H2 antagonist cimetidine (a medicine frequently used for the treatment of heartburn) has been used in an attempt to stimulate human immune cells to facilitate the regression of warts. Although early uncontrolled studies supported the efficacy of high-dose cimetidine, more rigorous double-blind controlled trials have contradicted these findings.

Conclusion

Warts are a common skin finding that have the potential to cause pain and impair performance in athletes. Although there are several methods for treating warts, preventive measures can help athletes avoid an HPV infection. Athletes who use communal showers should wear sandals and avoid direct contact with shower floors. Athletes may consider the use of drying agents to avoid moisture, which, by leading to maceration of the skin, increases the likelihood of infection with HPV. If athletes do develop warts, they should take into account the potential for side effects when selecting a treatment modality.

Thomas Trojian and Jeff Manning

See also Dermatology in Sports; Fungal Skin Infections and Parasitic Infestations; Skin Disorders Affecting Sports Participation

Further Readings

Esterowitz D, Greer K, Cooper P, Edlich R. Plantar warts in the athlete. *Am J Emerg Med.* 1995;13(4):441–443.

Habif T. *Skin Diseases: Diagnosis and Treatment.* New York, NY: Elsevier Mosby; 2005.

Levine N. Dermatologic aspects of sports medicine. *J Am Acad Dermatol.* 1980;3(4):415–424.

Micali G, Dall'Oglio F, Nasca M, Tedeschi A. Management of cutaneous warts: an evidence-based approach. *Am J Clin Dermatol.* 2004;5(5):311–317.

Roach M, Chretien J. Common hand warts in athletes: association with trauma to the hand. *J Am Coll Health.* 1995;44(3):125–126.

Stulberg D, Hutchinson A. Molluscum contagiosum and warts. *Am Fam Physician.* 2003;67(6):1233–1240.

WEIGHT GAIN FOR SPORTS

Many sports require an athlete to lose or maintain weight to optimize performance. Conversely, some sports and sports positions require weight gain for a greater competitive advantage. In some cases, the extra pounds can mean the difference between winning and losing. This entry describes how athletes may safely gain weight to achieve a competitive advantage.

Gaining weight is important for those who are underweight or who require greater strength. Gaining weight may also increase energy and endurance. Endurance is a person's ability to cope with intense and frequent exercise, such as distance running, swimming, or biking over long time periods or distances. Weight gain may also help an athlete to build muscle and increase strength. This strength may offer some athletes a protective advantage in sports such as football or hockey. The optimal time for gaining weight is during the off-season or at the beginning of the season.

Gaining weight may not be easy. In fact, often it is harder than losing weight, as athletes may use energy faster than they consume it. The question for the athlete is how to gain weight while still maintaining a healthful diet. In short, weight gain requires excess calorie intake. Each pound of weight gain requires 3,500 additional calories (cal; 1 cal = 4.2 joules). This is achievable by incorporating an extra 500 cal/day into the diet. If an athlete consumes an additional 500 cal/day for 1 week, then 1 pound (lb; 1 lb = 0.45 kilograms) of weight gain should be the outcome. Ideally, this should be combined with a resistance training program. The goal is not just to increase weight but also to increase lean muscle mass.

A combination of protein, carbohydrate, and fat is optimal for weight gain. The percentages of each of these macronutrients are approximately as follows: carbohydrate at 50% to 65%, protein at 15% to 20%, and fat at 25% to 30%. If these percentages are viewed as grams per day, the following is recommended: carbohydrate at 5 to 10 grams per kilogram per day (g kg^{-1} day^{-1}), protein at 1.0 to 1.7 g kg^{-1} day^{-1}, and fat at approximately 1 g kg^{-1} day^{-1}.

Maintaining a healthful diet of whole grains, fruits and vegetables, lean protein, and heart-healthful fats will help optimize performance. Weight gain, just like weight loss, takes time. The overall goal is to gain about 0.5 to 1 lb/week. Athletes trying to gain weight should consume three meals and two or three snacks each day. Skipping meals such as breakfast may make it more difficult to obtain the necessary calories needed to gain weight.

Weight Gain Methods

Many athletes think that additional calories should be obtained only from protein. Studies show that consuming excess protein (defined as more than 1.8 g kg^{-1} day^{-1}) may increase the oxidation of excess amino acids. Furthermore, excess protein may be converted to fat. Thus, a diet with too much protein has no advantage for muscle gain, when compared with a lower protein intake that is coupled with resistance training.

The speed at which weight gain occurs may depend on the athlete's genetic makeup, the calories consumed in excess of metabolic and training needs, the number of rest and recovery days per week, and the training program itself. Weight gain is achieved by ensuring that each meal and snack are made up of healthful, higher-calorie foods. Beverages are one easy way to increase calories. For example, instead of water, the athlete may add juice, milk, milk shakes, and instant breakfast drinks to meals or snacks. It is also important to snack regularly and carry healthful snacks each day to encourage snacking. Such snacks may include dried fruit, yogurt, cheese and crackers, nuts and peanuts, bran or fruit muffins, and multigrain bagels with cream cheese or nut butters.

Athletes may think that the need for extra calories gives them the right to eat whatever they want, but this may be detrimental to both performance and overall health. Substitutes may be found for many food items. For example, instead of using butter, canola or olive oil may be substituted. Mayonnaise may be replaced with avocado spread. Natural peanut butter may be spread on bagels, crackers, or bread instead of butter or cream cheese. Eating healthful foods in abundance is how an athlete gains weight safely and effectively. There is no need to add calories with fast food or junk food when calories are easily added by making favorable choices at meal and snack times.

Many athletes wonder whether protein supplements are helpful when trying to bulk up. These supplements are often marketed as ways to gain extra muscle quickly. However, the main reason why protein supplements help an athlete gain muscle is that they contain extra calories. Also, contrary to what some people believe, most athletes need only a small amount of extra protein to gain weight and muscle mass. The protein in the supplements is often too high. Caloric and protein needs may be met by eating a variety of healthy foods each day. If extra calories are needed, readily available weight gain drinks such as Ensure or Boost contain the extra calories and are marketed specifically for weight gain.

There are also unhealthful ways of gaining weight. A few of these are human growth hormone (HGH), anabolic steroids, and insulin. HGH use may increase the risk of diabetes, hypertension, joint pain, and possibly colon cancer. Anabolic steroids have been linked to many health problems, including breast growth and shrinking of testicles in men, voice deepening and growth of body hair in women, heart problems, liver disease, and aggressive behavior. Insulin is sometimes used in bodybuilding to increase the bulk of muscles. Insulin is a natural hormone secreted by the pancreas in response to high sugar levels. Its main use is to regulate sugar levels in the body. However, if one is not diabetic, taking insulin unnecessarily may cause the pancreas to stop producing insulin naturally, which might lead to diabetes.

Weight Gain Tips

Weight gain requires that an athlete eat consistently and not skip meals or snacks. Portions should be larger than normal, and calorically dense foods should be encouraged. Higher-calorie meals may also result from reading food labels to determine which foods have more calories than an equally palatable counterpart. For example, cranberry apple juice has more calories than does orange juice (170 vs. 110 cal/8 fluid ounces [oz; 1 oz = 29.57 milliliters]), granola has more calories than do Cheerios (700 vs. 100 cal/cup), and corn has more calories than do green beans (140 vs. 40 cal/cup).

In terms of individual food groups, the following guidelines may be helpful. Choose heavy breads such as honey bran, rye, and pumpernickel instead of lighter breads such as white bread. Choose cereals such as granola, instead of rice puffs or corn flakes. The caloric value of cereals may also be increased by adding nuts, raisins, and other dried fruits. When choosing fruits, bananas, pineapple, mangos, raisins, dates, and other dried fruits have more calories per serving than do watery fruits, such as watermelon, grapefruit, apples, and peaches. Starchy or sugary vegetables, such as corn, carrots, and peas, have more calories per serving than do less starchy vegetables, such as green beans, broccoli,

and summer squash. Lentils, lima beans, chili beans, and other beans are also high in calories. These foods are good choices, because they also provide both carbohydrates and protein. In terms of other protein foods such as meat, fish, and poultry, certain types and cuts are higher in calories. Dark meat of poultry, fatty fish such as salmon and trout, and some cuts of lean red meat are high in calories, including round or sirloin steak, ground round, fresh or boiled ham, or center-cut loin chops.

Jan Pauline Hangen

See also Dietitian/Sports Nutritionist; Lean Body Weight Assessment; Nutrition and Hydration; Obesity; Weight Loss for Sports

Further Readings

Applegate L. *Power Foods*. Emmaus, PA: Rodale Press; 1991.

Duyff RL. *Complete Food and Nutrition Guide*. Hoboken, NJ: John Wiley; 2006.

Gershoff S. *The Tufts Guide to Total Nutrition*. New York, NY: Harper & Row; 1990.

Manore M, Thompson J. *Sport Nutrition for Health and Performance*. Champaign, IL: Human Kinetics; 2000.

Rosenbloom C, ed. *Sports Nutrition: A Guide for the Professional Working With Active People*. Chicago, IL: American Dietetic Association; 2000.

Williams MH. *The Ergogenics Edge: Pushing the Limits of Sports Performance*. Champaign, IL: Human Kinetics; 1998.

WEIGHT LIFTING, INJURIES IN

Weight lifting is performed by itself as a competitive sport and by athletes in other sports as part of training programs to increase muscle strength, endurance, and power. The high amount of resistance and repetitive movements in weight lifting can cause both acute and chronic injuries to muscle, tendon, and bone. The body parts most commonly injured by weight lifting include the shoulders, knees, and lumbar spine. Although serious injuries can occur, most weight lifting injuries are relatively minor.

General guidelines should be followed to decrease the risk of injury from weight lifting. As in any other sport, athletes should perform a proper warm-up before weight lifting. This can

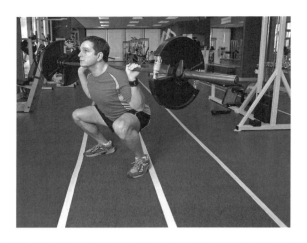

Personal trainer demonstrates proper technique for squat exercise with barbells.

Source: David H. Lewis/iStockphoto.

include stretching, cardiovascular exercises, or performing several repetitions of lifting light weights with controlled movements.

Proper technique is also critical to minimize the risk of injury. A spotter should be used when appropriate. Young athletes should always be under direct supervision when lifting weights.

To avoid injuries from overtraining, adequate time should be given for muscle recovery. Performance-enhancing substances should be avoided. Specific injuries and prevention techniques are discussed in the sections that follow.

Shoulder Injuries

The inherent instability of the glenohumeral joint combined with the high amount of weight used during exercises involving movements of the glenohumeral joint place soft tissues around the joint at risk of injury. Strains of the rotator cuff and deltoid muscles are common. Weight lifting exercises, such as front and lateral deltoid raises, and military presses that involve resisted overhead movements can place the athlete at risk for subacromial impingement.

In addition to the glenohumeral joint, the acromioclavicular joint is also stressed with repetitive overhead movements, dips, and bench press. Osteolysis of the distal clavicle joint is a relatively common condition in weight lifters.

Anterior shoulder structures, including the glenohumeral ligaments, are stressed during weight lifting exercises where the arm moves beyond the body in the coronal plane. This movement occurs when performing a bench press, behind-the-head latissimus pull-down, pec deck machine, and dumbbell chest fly through a full range of motion. A back squat is an example of a lower extremity exercise that can also stress the shoulder joint as it places the shoulder in excessive horizontal abduction and extension. Athletes with glenohumeral joint laxity are predisposed to injury with these exercises.

A rupture of the pectoralis major muscle is an example of a traumatic upper extremity injury that can occur while weight lifting. Although it is not a common injury, the injury classically occurs while performing a bench press. Rupture of the pectoralis major insertion requires surgical repair.

Shoulder Injury Prevention

Minor modifications to traditional weight lifting exercises can decrease the stresses on the shoulder joint that lead to the injuries discussed earlier. During the latissimus pull-down, the bar should always be lowered in front of, not behind, the head. A narrow grip during the latissimus pull-down and bench press will decrease stress on the anterior shoulder structures and acromioclavicular joint. Decreasing the range of motion with a bench press, cable fly, pec deck machine, and dumbbell chest fly so the arm stays anterior to the coronal plane of the body will also decrease stress on the anterior shoulder structures. When performing overhead movements, externally rotating the humerus will rotate the greater tuberosity and minimize the risk of subacromial impingement.

Maintaining proper muscle balance will also help decrease the risk of shoulder injury. Specifically, strengthening of the rotator cuff and scapulothoracic muscles is needed to avoid muscular imbalance, as most common weight lifting exercises strengthen the deltoid and anterior chest muscles.

Knee Injuries

Anterior knee pain is a common complaint of weight lifters. Anterior knee pain can be caused by strain or injury to any of several structures, including the patellar tendon and patellofemoral joint. Patellofemoral joint stresses are high during deep knee flexion in weight bearing, such as squatting, leg press, and lunges, especially when the exercise is performed beyond 90° of knee flexion. Knee extensions strengthen the quadriceps in a non–weight-bearing position. With this motion, the patellofemoral joint stresses increase as the knee extends beyond approximately 45°.

The menisci in the knee are also susceptible to injury during weight lifting. Acute and degenerative meniscal injuries can occur due to high loads on the tibiofemoral joint with the knee in a flexed position, such as during squats and lunges.

Knee Injury Prevention

Avoiding deep squats and lunges (limiting knee flexion to less than 90°) will minimize stress on the patellofemoral joint and meniscus. Non–weight-bearing knee extension exercises should be performed from 90° to 45° of knee flexion to minimize patellofemoral joint stress.

Lumbar Spine Injuries

Exercises that place excessive forces on the lumbar spine include squats and deadlifts. The most common injuries to the lumbar spine during weight lifting are muscle strains and stress injury or fracture to the pars intraarticularis (spondylolysis). Spondylolysis results from repeated hyperextension of the spine.

Athletes should maintain a neutral spine position whenever possible with all types of weight lifting exercises. Co-contraction of the multifidus with the deeper abdominal muscles (transverse abdominis, internal and external obliques) will stabilize the lumbar spine and avoid excessive forces from hyperflexion and hyperextension movements during weight lifting exercises. Excessive hyperextension during exercises such as military press, bench press, and squats should be avoided.

Special Considerations

Competitive Weight Lifting

Competitive weight lifting consists of power lifting and Olympic weight lifting. Competitive power lifts include deadlifts, squats, and bench press. Olympic weight lifts consist of the clean and jerk and the snatch. Athletes in these two competitive weight lifting sports want to reach as high a one-repetition maximum as possible and often lift weights three to five times their body weight. This requires the athlete to generate extremely large muscle forces and high joint torques.

Injuries to the lumbar spine and knees are the most common in Olympic weight lifting, whereas injuries to the lumbar spine and shoulder are the most common in power lifting. When performing a squat, power lifters position the bar lower on their back and lean their trunk more forward, resulting in less ankle dorsiflexion and a more posterior hip position, ultimately leading to less knee extension torque and less risk of knee injury. In contrast, when weight lifters perform the snatch, they are in a position of deep knee flexion, which increases stress on the knee joint. Although the low bar squat position used by power lifters results in less stress to the knee joint, it does increase stress on the anterior shoulder structures.

Youth and Weight Lifting

Weight lifting can be safe and beneficial for preadolescents and adolescents. An appropriately designed program will improve muscle strength and have general health benefits. It will not have any adverse effects on growth or lead to any medical risk in an otherwise healthy child. The increases in muscular strength seen in preadolescents are likely due to neural gains (changes in motor unit activation and recruitment) rather than due to muscle hypertrophy.

Free weights, elastic bands, exercise machines, and body weight are all various modes of resistance that can be used. Body weight resistance exercise is beneficial to emphasize proper technique and incorporate core strength. If exercise machines are used, they must be sized appropriately.

A weight training program for youth should emphasize proper technique, which requires appropriate supervision. A low to moderate resistance level should be used, with a higher number of repetitions (2–3 sets, 8–15 repetitions). The program can be performed two to three times per week.

Anna Thatcher and Jeffrey Vaughn

See also Core Strength; Resistance Training; Running a Strength Training and Conditioning Facility; Strength Training for the Female Athlete; Strength Training for the Young Athlete

Further Readings

American Academy of Pediatrics Council on Sports Medicine and Fitness; McCambridge TM, Stricker PR. Strength training by children and adolescents. *Pediatrics.* 2008;121(4):835–840.

Calhoon G, Fry AC. Injury rates and profiles of elite competitive weightlifters. *J Athl Train.* 1999;34(3):232–238.

Ellenbecker TS, Bleacher J. Modification of traditional exercises for shoulder rehabilitation and a return-to-lifting program. In: Ellenbecker TS, ed. *Shoulder Rehabilitation: Non-operative Treatment.* New York, NY: Thieme; 2006:107–123.

Fees M, Decker T, Snyder-Mackler L, Axe M. Upper extremity weight-training modifications for the injured athlete. *Am J Sports Med.* 1998;26(5):732–742.

Keogh J, Hume PA, Pearson S. Retrospective injury epidemiology of one hundred one competitive Oceania power lifters: the effects of age, body mass, competitive standard, and gender. *J Strength Cond Res.* 2006;20(3):672–681.

Malina RM. Weight training in youth—growth, maturation, and safety: an evidence-based review. *Clin J Sport Med.* 2006;16(6):478–487.

Raske A, Norlin R. Injury incidence and prevalence among elite weight and power lifters. *Am J Sports Med.* 2002;30(2):248–256.

Weight Loss for Sports

Weight loss is a reduction of the total body weight. This reduction is due to a mean loss of fluid, body fat, or adipose tissue and/or lean mass—namely, bone mineral deposits, muscle, tendon, and other connective tissue. Weight loss can be unintentional or intentional. Unintentional weight loss refers to the involuntary loss of weight secondary to genetics, some medical conditions, activities, or medications that decrease body mass. Intentional weight loss refers to the voluntary loss of total body mass in an effort to improve fitness, health, and/or appearance. Intentional weight loss in sports refers to the intentional loss of total body mass in an effort to improve fitness or athletic performance and/or to meet a sport-specific weight requirement. Weight loss occurs when an individual is in a state of negative energy balance. When the human body is spending more energy in work and heat than it is gaining from food or other nutritional supplements, it will use the stored reserves of fat or muscle. Although weight loss may involve loss of fat, muscle, or fluid, weight loss for the purposes of maintaining health should aim to lose fat while conserving muscle and fluid.

Weight Loss Techniques

The most often recommended weight loss techniques are adjustments to eating patterns and increased physical activity. Other methods of losing weight include the use of drugs and supplements that decrease appetite, block fat absorption, increase metabolism, or reduce stomach volume. Finally, surgery may be used in case of morbid obesity.

Dieting

One of the aspects of energy balance that affects body weight is energy intake. An examination of the weight loss literature shows that changes in energy intake play a significant role in reducing body weight. The currently available scientific evidence appears to indicate that the macronutrient content of the diet will affect body weight only when there is also a reduction in the total energy intake.

Athletes usually require a greater caloric intake than nonathletes. The actual energy intake (number of calories) depends on the athlete's body composition, weight, height, age, stage of growth, and level of fitness as well as the intensity, frequency, and duration of exercise activity. Athletes need to eat enough to cover the energy costs of daily living, growth, building and repairing muscle tissue, and participating in sports. Athletes need to be informed that weight is not an accurate indicator of body fat or lean muscle mass and that body composition measurements can be more helpful.

When athletes regularly restrict energy intake to less than 1,500 kilocalories per day (kcal/day; 1 kcal = 4,184 joules) for women and less than 1,800 kcal/day for men, they are at increased risk of poor nutritional intake. This level of energy intake is too low to meet the nutritional needs of the body and fuel the body for exercise, especially if physical activity is high.

Commercial programs recommend various combinations of macronutrient compositions for weight loss, including high-fat, high-protein, and high- and low-carbohydrate diets. Despite the popularity of many of these dietary approaches, the optimal macronutrient composition of the diet for weight loss has not been determined. Despite the different potential mechanisms for how changes in protein intake may affect weight loss, evidence from clinical trials supporting optimal protein and carbohydrate intake for long-term weight loss and weight maintenance is lacking.

Exercise

Scientific evidence suggests that the combination of dietary modification and exercise is the most effective behavioral approach for weight loss, and the maintenance of exercise may be one of the best predictors of long-term weight maintenance. Despite the importance of exercise, there is little evidence that suggests that exercise alone produces magnitudes of weight loss that are similar to what can be achieved with dietary modification. Also, when examining the effect of exercise on body weight, it has been suggested that there may be "responders" and "nonresponders" to the same exercise intervention. In general, daily guidelines for exercise are 60 to 90 minutes to prevent weight gain and over 90 minutes to maintain weight loss.

Behavior Modification for Weight Loss

Behavior modification for weight loss means lifestyle changes to develop a long-term healthy eating plan and exercise program. There is evidence that including behavioral principles within a weight loss program improves long-term outcomes. Maintaining contact with participants long term improves long-term weight loss outcome, and this is considered an important component of behavioral weight loss programs. Another important component of behavioral weight loss programs is self-monitoring of eating and exercise behaviors. There is consistent evidence that individuals who self-monitor these behaviors are more successful at weight loss than those individuals who are inconsistent with self-monitoring. The use of portion control diets may also improve weight loss outcomes by minimizing choice and providing specific guidance to adults that precipitates weight loss.

Pharmacological Treatment

All current guidelines consider pharmacotherapy to be an adjunct to lifestyle modification interventions and limit its use to patients with obesity or overweight patients with additional comorbidities (e.g., hypertension, dyslipidemia, or Type 2 diabetes).

Despite the interest in the potential use of pharmacotherapy for the management of body weight, there are few drugs approved for this use, and their safety and effectiveness have not been established for use beyond 2 years. Most available weight loss medications approved by the FDA are appetite-suppressant medications. These include sibutramine, phentermine, phendimetrazine, and diethylpropion. Appetite-suppressant medications promote weight loss by decreasing appetite or increasing the feeling of being full. These medications make the patients feel less hungry by increasing one or more brain chemicals that affect mood and appetite. Phentermine and sibutramine are the most commonly prescribed appetite suppressants in the United States. *Amphetamines are a type of appetite suppressant. However, amphetamines are not recommended for use in the treatment of obesity due to their strong potential for abuse and dependence.*

Another category of medication used for weight loss is orlistat. This medication reduces the body's ability to absorb dietary fat by about one third. It does this by blocking the enzyme lipase, which is responsible for breaking down dietary fat. When fat is not broken down, the body cannot absorb it, so it is eliminated, and fewer calories are taken in.

All weight loss agents should be used only under the direct supervision of a physician.

Pathologic Strategies and Health Concerns

Pathologic weight loss strategies include any weight loss behaviors or actions that are potentially harmful to the athlete. These strategies include restrained eating, chronic dieting, bingeing and purging, skipping meals, fasting, excessive exercise, dehydration, and laxative, diuretic, and emetic abuse.

Nutritional Deficiencies

To lose weight, athletes frequently restrict food intake by skipping meals, eliminating food groups, fasting, or eating only one to three foods a day. Severe energy restriction is especially a problem for female athletes, and this pattern can lead to the female athlete triad (amenorrhea, eating disorder, and osteoporosis). Female athletes typically need less energy than male athletes due to their smaller body size. In addition, even female athletes who are not dieting frequently have energy and nutrient intakes that are below the recommended levels.

Disordered Eating

For some athletes, chronic dieting to maintain a low body weight can be the first step toward developing a clinical eating disorder such as anorexia nervosa or bulimia nervosa. Persistent dietary restriction can lead to binge and purge eating. Bingeing includes consuming large quantities of food at one time, followed by purging through practices such as self-induced vomiting; the use of emetics, laxatives, or diuretics; and excessive exercise. Bingeing and purging are extremely dangerous practices that can lead to clinical eating disorders, tooth decay, poor performance, dehydration, and even death due to fluid and electrolyte imbalances.

Dehydration and Laxative Abuse

Dehydration is a practice commonly used for rapid weight loss in athletes needing to "make weight." One way of doing this is by exercising intensely in hot environments while wearing vapor-impermeable suits. Also, some athletes combine this activity with fluid restriction and the use of diuretics, emetics, and laxatives. This practice is extremely dangerous and has resulted in several documented deaths.

Charles A. Lascano and Mark Stovak

See also Dietitian/Sports Nutritionist; Lean Body Weight Assessment; Nutrition and Hydration; Obesity; Weight Gain for Sports

Further Readings

American Academy of Pediatrics Committee on Sports Medicine and Fitness. Promotion of healthy weight-control practices in young athletes. *Pediatrics.* 2005;116(6):1557–1564.

Bonci L. Nutrition. In: McKeag D, Moeller J, eds. *ACSM's Primary Care Sports Medicine.* Philadelphia, PA: Lippincott Williams & Wilkins; 2007:35–52.

Kruger J, Yore MM, Kohl HW 3rd. Physical activity levels and weight control status by body mass index, among adults—National Health and Nutrition Examination Survey 1999–2004. *Int J Behav Nutr Phys Act.* 2008;5:25.

Roth R. Diet and weight control. In: *Nutrition & Diet Therapy.* Clifton Park, NY: Thompson-Delmar Learning; 2007:273–288.

Stout A. Fueling and weight management strategies in sports nutrition. *J Am Diet Assoc.* 2007;107(9):1475–1476.

Williams PT. Asymmetric weight gain and loss from increasing and decreasing exercise. *Med Sci Sports Exerc.* 2008;40(2):296–302.

Wolinsky I, Driskell J. *Sports Nutrition: Energy Metabolism and Exercise.* Boca Raton, FL: CRC Press; 2008.

Websites

Food and Drug Administration: http://www.fda.gov
Weight-Control Information Network: http://win.niddk.nih.gov/publications

WINDSURFING, INJURIES IN

Windsurfing is a challenging and exhilarating aquatic sport that has gained worldwide appeal fairly quickly, including its introduction as an Olympic sport in 1984. There is something for everyone in this sport, whether you are a recreational amateur, Olympic competitor, or Professional Windsurfing Association champion. Exercise, excitement, thrill, and challenge are among the stimuli to participate, while trauma, injury, and overexposure to the elements represent the downside. Knowledge of the sport, proper equipment, and windsurfing skills help ensure that the positive aspects of windsurfing are enjoyed and the risks are avoided.

Windsurfing is an ingenious combination of Hawaiian-style wave surfing and the more accessible sport of wind sailing. The marriage of a one-person sailboard and a one-person sail by means of a universal (polyaxial) joint brought the intuitive burst to reality. Wave surfers are no longer limited to the few locations worldwide where the "perfect wave" might appear and impart massive kinetic power to propel a surfboard. Rather, one can now harness the more ubiquitous power of the wind to propel a sailor through the water and waves. The inception of the windsurfer was a "Eureka moment."

Basic Equipment

The sport of windsurfing requires a sailboard commonly referred to as a windsurfer and a rig consisting of sail, mast, and boom. The rig is attached to the sailboard by means of a universal joint that allows the rig to be tilted, pivoted, or flipped into various positions. The sailboard provides the flotation on which the sailor stands, sails, steers, and maneuvers through the water and waves. The rig supports the sail, which captures the wind power and allows the sailor to transfer it to the sailboard. Adjustments in the positions of the rig and sail provide the means by which to steer the board and finely balance the amount of wind power transferred to the board. A fin provides lateral resistance and lift to the board. Sail power and fin allow the windsurfer to hydroplane, making it the fastest sailing vessel on the water, capable of attaining speeds of over 50 miles (mi; 1 mi = 1.60 kilometers) per hour.

The booms may be aided by hand, or a harness may be worn to allow the sailor to hook into the straps attached to the booms. This permits the sailor to balance sail power against body weight, removing the burden from the arms and freeing the sailor to make fine adjustments to sail position. Foot straps are affixed to most sailboards, allowing the sailor to anchor his or her feet to the board and more efficiently transfer wind power to the board. Foot straps not only prevent the windsurfer from being thrown (catapulted) from the board but also provide a potential mechanism for injury to the lower extremities because they lock the feet in place and can thereby cause twisting injuries to the ankles and knees. Ancillary equipment includes gloves, booties, harness, wet suit, life jacket, and helmet.

The length and volume of windsurfers vary according to the ability of the sailor, the type of sailing intended, and the conditions of wind and water. Novice sailors and low wind conditions require larger boards for greater flotation and moderate-sized sails, which allow greater control. Slalom and freestyle sailing are accomplished on smaller boards, which are faster and more maneuverable but more difficult to sail. High wind days and wave sailing require that the smallest boards and sails be used. Sailors must carefully assess the wind velocity, water conditions, and local topography and their own sailing abilities prior to selecting the equipment used on any given day. Too small a board or rig on a low wind day may leave the sailor stalled or sunk (underpowered). Too large a board or rig on a high wind day may put the sailor in an uncontrollable situation, either blown off course or thrown about at the mercy of the wind and waves (overpowered).

What Can Go Wrong?

For the most part, windsurfing is a safe and enjoyable endeavor. Even an unsuccessful day of windsurfing is typically a "good day at the beach" with sun, water, waves, companionship, and recreation. Potential problems with equipment, weather conditions, or sailing ability may lead to injury. Medical studies estimate that the rate of injury to windsurfers is approximately 1.5 per year, with the majority of injuries being minor. These would include strains, sprains, contusions, or bruises, which rarely require medical attention. An ill-equipped novice sailor may develop hand blisters if improper gloves are worn or scrapes and scratches if no protective booties are worn. While

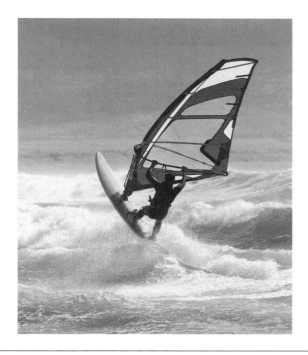

Windsurfer in Dingle Peninsula, County Kerry, in Ireland. Most of the injuries common to windsurfing are minor and include strains, sprains, contusions, or bruises.

Source: Ingmar Wesemann/iStockphoto.

learning to manipulate the sailboard and rig into correct positions, there is an intuitive inclination to force one's equipment into position rather than use simple physics and wind power to do the work. These undue efforts produce backaches, muscle strains, joint sprains, and contusions, which constitute the garden-variety problems that heal quickly. Beginners can avoid many of these struggles and injuries by taking lessons from certified instructors, consulting instruction manuals, or viewing the many excellent instructional videos that are available. *Windsurfing Magazine* and windsurf.com are good sources of information.

There are potentially serious, and frankly dangerous, situations that may lead to severe physical harm. Extreme overexposure to environmental elements can occur if a sailor is incapable of upwind sailing and consequently is blown downwind and away from the intended destination. Sailors have been stranded out at sea or even lost entirely. Equipment failure and major alterations in wind velocity or direction can produce similar results, blowing a sailor drastically off course. Prolonged exposure to the elements may lead to severe sunburn, dehydration, exhaustion, hypothermia, or drowning. These potential dangers underscore the importance of knowing your local conditions, the prevailing winds, the weather forecast, and equipment maintenance. Solo sailing is a hazard, and it is a windsurfing maxim to be with a "buddy sailor" and to know the whereabouts of rescue boats or vehicles. "Never leave your board" is another important maxim since it serves as your flotation device and may be kicked or paddled for long distances. Ancillary equipment such as a Coast Guard–approved life jacket, a wet suit, gloves, sunglasses, and booties help protect from exposure. Waterproof radios are expensive but may be crucial to the solo sailor who has ventured off course or become stranded. It is imperative to stay with your board, avoid solo sailing, and know the universal "sign of distress" to alert others to your plight. This involves sitting on your sailboard and raising both hands straight overhead and crisscrossing them back and forth.

Physical Injuries

Much of windsurfing's appeal is its overall safety. Being blown off course typically results in much paddling and walking rather than dramatic rescues. Similarly, most falls, collisions, or mishaps lead to splashy and refreshing immersions into the water, followed by uphauling or water starting to get back on course.

As a sailor progresses in his or her abilities, there is typically the urge to seek more challenge and greater speed and perform stylized turns, and wave jumping. Freestyle sailing involves phenomenal loops, rolls, and other aerial acrobatics. Higher speeds, crowded races, and advanced aerial maneuvers create the circumstances that may cause severe high-energy injuries. These injuries most frequently involve the lower extremities, affecting the knee, ankle, and foot. The lower extremity is placed at higher risk because of the foot straps that lock the foot onto the board. While the foot strap gives the sailor greater control over the board, the converse is unfortunately also true. Just as a ski bound to the foot of a skier can impart greater leverage and injury to the leg of a skier, the foot strap can impart greater leverage of the board and rig to the lower extremity of the sailor. If uncontrolled leverage due to a fall, aborted turn, or poor landing from a jump is transmitted to the vulnerable lower extremity, ligamentous tears may occur to the foot, ankle, or knee. Further leverage will cause complete rupture of ligaments or fracture of bone. Lower extremity injuries reported among windsurfers include midfoot sprains and complete disruption of the tarsal bones of the foot, known as Lisfranc fractures. The collateral ligaments of the ankle or knee may be disrupted, or the anterior cruciate ligament of the knee may be torn. Knee injuries of this severity are commonly associated with a "popping" sensation rapidly followed by pain, swelling, and difficulty bearing weight. Immediate emergency treatment involves *r*est, *i*ce, elastic *c*ompression, and *e*levation (RICE) followed by medical evaluation. Most sprains are partial tears and respond to rest, use of splints, and temporary use of a cane or crutches. Fractures, dislocations, or complete ligamentous disruption typically requires surgical treatment.

While most serious windsurfing injuries involve the lower extremity, other body parts are also at risk. The most common serious upper extremity injury is dislocation of the shoulder during high-velocity falls, catapults, or collision with other sailors. Chest wall contusions or rib fractures may result from collision with one's booms. Head, neck, and spinal injuries also have been reported and are typically associated with high-energy aerial acrobatics, collision with other sailors, or direct contact with the sea bottom. These catastrophic injuries may lead to concussions, skull fractures, vertebral fractures, spinal cord injuries, or death. Prevention, caution, and head protection are the keys to avoiding these catastrophic injuries. Windsurfers must follow sailing's "rules of the road," which determine who has the right of way on the water when conditions are crowded. Riders must know both their abilities and their limitations. Winds too strong, waves too high, and waters too crowded must signal caution. While helmets are not everyday requirements, they are an absolute must for high winds, crowded racing conditions, and freestyle sailing. Whenever in doubt, it is always prudent to decide on the side of caution.

Last, whether you are on home territory or on an exotic windsurfing vacation, it is important to do a little preparatory work researching your destination. Fortunately, most windsurfing destinations provide resources describing the local conditions, such as prevailing winds, water depths, rock or coral formations, and temperature extremes. Local flora and fauna may also provide potential hazards, such as sea urchins, needle fish, jellyfish, sharks, or marine bacteria, which may cause infection of scrapes or puncture wounds.

Peter P. Anas

See also Ankle Injuries; Bruised Ribs; Foot Injuries; Head Injuries; Rib Fracture and Contusions; Sunburn; Sunburn and Skin Cancers

Further Readings

United States Sailing Association. *Start Windsurfing Right!* 2nd ed. Portsmouth, RI: United States Sailing Association; 2001.

WOMEN'S HEALTH, EFFECTS OF EXERCISE ON

Cardiovascular disease (CVD) remains the leading cause of morbidity and premature mortality in women in the United States and most industrialized countries and, more recently, contributes to the significant disease burden in the developing nations. The prevalence of obesity and inactivity among Americans continues to rise. Exercise, for the physiologic reasons discussed below, has a beneficial effect in both preventing CVD among women and treating it once it occurs. Inactivity is also associated with multiple other cardiovascular risk factors, including obesity, diabetes, and hypertension. Furthermore, beyond its widely touted promotion of cardiovascular health among women, exercise has been shown to have multiple beneficial effects on other aspects of women's health. Among women, exercise has been shown to decrease the risk of colon and breast cancer, decrease the risk of osteoporosis, and boost cognitive and psychological well-being. In considering the myriad beneficial effects of exercise among women, it should be noted that these are independent of diet and weight loss.

Cardiovascular Adaptation to Exercise Training

Typical cardiovascular adaptations to regular aerobic physical training include lowered blood pressure and heart rate, mild increases in the dimensions of the heart cavity, augmentation of the amount of blood pumped by the heart, as well as increases in heart muscle mass. In addition to the structural changes that occur with training, changes in heart physiology also occur. These include an enhanced pumping and relaxation function of the right and left ventricles, the heart chambers that pump blood to the lungs and the aorta, as well as an increase in the amount of oxygen consumed by the body, known as the $\dot{V}O_2max$. $\dot{V}O_2max$ is widely considered to be the gold standard metric for cardiovascular fitness.

While the majority of cardiovascular adaptations to training are similar between men and women, unique cardiovascular adaptations to exercise in women have been described. While both men and women exhibit increases in their heart chamber sizes and muscle mass, the body surface–adjusted increases in mass are not as substantial in women as in men. In addition, females exhibit lower $\dot{V}O_2max$ compared with males, likely due to lower myocardial mass.

Additional physiologic differences between men and women may contribute to the improvement in $\dot{V}o_2$max observed with regular physical exercise. While the mechanism of increased $\dot{V}o_2$max in men appears largely due to increases in the volume of blood pumped by the heart, in women, the improvement appears to be related to the increased extraction of oxygen from muscle at the cellular level.

The Role of Exercise in the Reduction of Cardiovascular Risk Factors

Regular physical exercise is of great value in reducing established cardiovascular risk factors, including obesity, diabetes mellitus, and hypertension. In addition, there are a multitude of beneficial cardiovascular effects of regular physical exercise that result in physiologic, psychological, as well as biochemical improvements, all of which lead to a reduction in overall cardiovascular risk. These changes include reduction in the likelihood of obesity, improved blood pressure control in hypertensive individuals, reduction in serum cholesterol, decreased insulin resistance and other markers of inflammation, improved function and less stiffening of the large and small blood vessels, and reduction in the risk of pathologic blood clots. In contrast, physical inactivity and poor physical fitness are associated with a potentially harmful blood-clotting profile in middle-aged women with coronary heart disease.

Many women with multiple risk factors for heart disease are able to manage their risk factors through diet and exercise alone. For those women who require medical therapy to treat high cholesterol and high blood pressure, regular aerobic exercise provides an additional benefit.

Exercise in the Patient With Established CVD

CVD includes disease of the arteries of the heart, such as coronary artery disease (CAD), high blood pressure (hypertension; HTN), peripheral arterial disease (PAD), cerebrovascular disease, rhythm disturbances, diseases of the heart valves, and disorders of the small blood vessel not associated with actual blockages (small vessel disease). This entity of small vessel disease appears to be more common in women than men.

Exercise training is a significant component of rehabilitation of individuals who survive a heart attack (myocardial infarction; MI). Gradual, supervised regular physical exercise in survivors of MI not only introduces a healthy lifestyle habit to a potentially sedentary group but also enhances recovery from MI. Many of the benefits of exercise in this group include those described earlier but also include the psychological benefits afforded by regular physical activity. This is of particular value in this group due to the high prevalence of depression in survivors of MI and individuals who have undergone coronary artery bypass grafting. Female survivors of heart attack are much less likely than their male counterparts to participate in cardiac rehabilitation and currently miss out on the multiple beneficial aspects of this highly valuable but optional component of cardiovascular care.

The potential benefit of regular exercise in patients with PAD has also been demonstrated. A study examining the benefit of regular exercise in 118 patients with PAD demonstrated lower likelihood that the individuals who exercised would experience or die from a cardiovascular complication over the 5 years of follow-up.

Exercise can also lead to benefits among women with heart failure. Heart failure occurs when the heart can either not pump or not relax efficiently enough to deliver adequate blood supply to the body. Unfortunately, heart failure has reached epidemic proportions in the United States. Heart failure associated with abnormal heart relaxation (diastolic dysfunction) is common in women, particularly women over the age of 65. There is preliminary evidence available to suggest that regular physical activity not only treats the diastolic dysfunction but also treats the conditions that may be responsible for its presence in the first place, including obesity, high blood pressure, and diabetes. A recent large study examined regular aerobic exercise in men and women with reduced pumping function of the heart. This study found that regular aerobic physical activity leads to reductions in hospitalizations for heart failure and was not dangerous in this group of patients.

Exercise and Other Aspects of Women's Health

In addition to its beneficial effects on cardiovascular health, exercise has been shown to confer myriad other health benefits among women.

Exercise increases bone mineral density and, thus, prevents osteoporosis. Increased leisure-time activity, such as walking, has been shown to reduce the risk of hip fracture among postmenopausal women. It is worth noting that the beneficial effects of exercise may stem more from muscle strength, resistance, and balance training than from the intensity of the exercise itself. Furthermore, caution should be used in blanket recommendations to elderly women to exercise, as vigorous exercise among elderly patients may predispose them to the risk of falls and, thus, increase the risk of fracture.

In the realm of exercise and cancer, women who engage in regular physical activity have been shown to have a decreased risk of both colon and breast cancer. For women diagnosed with breast cancer, exercise has been shown to improve survival. As far as cancer risk is concerned, it is not entirely clear how much exercise confers risk reduction or at what stage of life. For breast cancer, it is postulated that exercise achieves this effect in women via reduction in adipose tissue and, thus, decreased overall estrogen production.

Finally, exercise has been shown to have numerous beneficial effects for women in terms of psychological well-being and cognitive function. Exercise has been shown to have utility in the treatment of major depressive disorder, with a dose-response effect, meaning that a certain level of exercise was necessary to achieve this response. Among women with premenstrual syndrome, exercise also seems to have a beneficial effect on both physiologic and psychological symptoms. Also for women with postpartum depression, a regular exercise program (three times per week) seems to mitigate depressive symptoms. Finally, among elderly women, a recent trial showed that a 6-month exercise intervention was associated with a modest improvement in cognitive function.

How Much and When?

Questions invariably arise when discussing the effects of exercise on women's health, namely, how much is exercise is enough and at what stage in life. These questions are difficult to assess because, as discussed earlier, exercise is associated with multiple different health benefits for women and each one may be associated with a different amount of exercise, at various stages of life. Thus,

these questions continue to be investigated. For now, basic recommendations by the Centers for Disease Control and Prevention as well as the American College of Sports Medicine exist, suggesting at least 30 minutes of moderate-intensity physical activity on most days of the week. Indeed, a recent study following both men and women between the ages 50 and 71 years over time found that adherence to these guidelines, namely, engaging in moderately intense physical activity greater than 3 hours/week, led to a risk reduction of 27% in death from any cause among women in this age-group. This reduced risk was independent of other cardiovascular risk factors and body mass index.

Though these recommendations for a minimal amount of exercise exist, this does not mean that more exercise is not additionally beneficial. Again, the type of exercise, its intensity, and the age of greatest benefit depend on what outcome is being assessed. A recent prospective analysis among elderly women suggests that women who had previously had a sedentary lifestyle and began exercising after 65 years of age had reduced mortality.

Specifically, those women who increased their physical activity levels to a calorie expenditure equivalent to 1 mile (1.60 kilometers) per day of walking from their initial routine, to a follow-up 6 years later, had a reduction in cardiovascular mortality, cancer, and all-cause mortality. This benefit was not seen among women who began exercising after 75 years of age. Women who were consistently active, both before and after the 6-year intervention, had a similar risk reduction to those who only began exercising when the study began. Interestingly, recent physical activity levels were a better predictor of longevity than past. Another study, looking at 40,000 women, showed not only that there is a direct association between physical activity and decreased mortality but that the greatest benefit was seen among women who go from a sedentary lifestyle to one involving moderate physical activity.

Conclusions and Future Directions

In sum, exercise confers multiple health benefits for women. In the realm of cardiovascular health, exercise both prevents disease and improves outcomes among women with existing CVD. Exercise also has a role in mitigating cardiovascular risk factors, including hypertension, diabetes, and obesity.

Outside cardiovascular health, exercise has been shown to reduce the risk of osteoporosis, cancer, depression, and cognitive decline. Active investigation continues into optimal exercise regimens for women to achieve these health benefits, though research to date suggests that a clear health benefit occurs for most women who begin exercising, even if they have been inactive in the past.

Malissa J. Wood and Lisa Rosenbaum

See also Benefits of Exercise and Sports; Exercise During Pregnancy and Postpartum; Female Athlete; Female Athlete Triad; Strength Training for the Female Athlete

Further Readings

Al-Khalili F, Janszky I, Andersson A, Svane B, Schenck-Gustafsson K. Physical activity and exercise performance predict long-term prognosis in middle-aged women surviving acute coronary syndrome. *J Intern Med.* 2007;261(2):178–187.

Ashton WD, Nanchahal K, Wood DA. Leisure-time physical activity and coronary risk factors in women. *J Cardiovasc Risk.* 2000;7(4):259–266.

Bensimhon DR, Leifer ES, Ellis SJ, et al; HF-ACTION Trial Investigators. Reproducibility of peak oxygen uptake and other cardiopulmonary exercise testing parameters in patients with heart failure (from the Heart Failure and A Controlled Trial Investigating Outcomes of Exercise Training). *Am J Cardiol.* 2008;102(6):712–717.

Feskanich D, Willett W, Colditz G. Walking and leisure-time activity and risk of hip fracture in postmenopausal women. *JAMA.* 2002;288(18): 2300–2306.

Holmes MD, Chen WY, Feskanich D, Kroenke CH, Colditz GA. Physical activity and survival after breast cancer diagnosis. *JAMA.* 2005;293(20):2479–2486.

Kushi LH, Fee RM, Folsom AR, Mink PJ, Anderson KE, Sellers TA. Physical activity and mortality in postmenopausal women. *JAMA.* 1997;277(16): 1287–1292.

Mai PL, Sullivan-Halley J, Ursin G, et al. Physical activity and colon cancer risk among women in the California Teachers Study. *Cancer Epidemiol Biomarkers Prev.* 2007;16(3):517–525.

McTiernan A, Kooperberg C, White E, et al. Recreational physical activity and the risk of breast cancer in postmenopausal women: the Women's Health Initiative Cohort Study. *JAMA.* 2003;290(10): 1331–1336.

Nagy E, Janszky I, Eriksson-Berg M, Al-Khalili F, Schenck-Gustafsson K. The effects of exercise capacity and sedentary lifestyle on haemostasis among middle-aged women with coronary heart disease. *Thromb Haemost.* 2008;100(5):899–904.

Raitakari OT, Porkka KV, Taimela S, Telama R, Rasanen L, Viikari JS. Effects of persistent physical activity and inactivity on coronary risk factors in children and young adults. The Cardiovascular Risk in Young Finns Study. *Am J Epidemiol.* 1994;140(3):195–205.

Scott JM, Esch BT, Haykowsky MJ, et al. Sex differences in left ventricular function and beta-receptor responsiveness following prolonged strenuous exercise. *J Appl Physiol.* 2007;102(2):681–687.

Stevenson ET, Davy KP, Seals DR. Hemostatic, metabolic, and androgenic risk factors for coronary heart disease in physically active and less active postmenopausal women. *Arterioscler Thromb Vasc Biol.* 1995;15(5):669–677.

Weuve J, Kang JH, Manson JE, Breteler MM, Ware JH, Grodstein F. Physical activity, including walking, and cognitive function in older women. *JAMA.* 2004;292(12):1454–1461.

WORLD ANTI-DOPING AGENCY

The World Anti-Doping Agency (WADA) is a private Swiss law foundation, founded in 1999, responsible for ensuring fair competition in sports around the world. Its mission is to promote, coordinate, and monitor the fight against doping in all its forms. The WADA Code provides the basic framework for the agency's work, that is, "to protect the athlete's fundamental right to participate in doping-free sport and thus promote health, fairness, and equality for athletes worldwide." The objectives of the agency are to preserve the integrity and value of sports and youth, actively promote the "level playing field" philosophy, and act independently, professionally, and without bias or influence.

WADA is composed and funded equally by the Olympic movement and governments of the world. It is situated in Lausanne, Switzerland, and has its headquarters in Montreal, Canada. In 1999, the International Olympic Committee (IOC) held the first World Doping Conference in Sport in Switzerland. It was attended by the sports movement and representatives of several governments in an effort to establish an organized and cohesive plan to control a growing, complex problem in the world of competitive sports. There were several important results of this conference, including the establishment of the World Anti-Doping Code (the Code), the International Convention Against Doping in Sport (the Convention), and the Copenhagen Declaration on Anti-Doping in Sport (the Declaration).

Because many governments cannot be legally bound by a nongovernmental document such as the WADA Code, the International Convention was drafted under the auspices of UNESCO (United Nations Educational, Scientific and Cultural Organization), the body responsible for education, science, and culture. The Convention was unanimously adopted at the 33rd UNESCO General Conference in 2005. Separately, the Copenhagen Declaration was finalized at the World Conference on Doping in Sport in 2005. This declaration is the political document that signals a government's intention to formally recognize and implement the Code. As of 2007, 192 countries have signed the Declaration, and 80 UNESCO member states have become part of the Convention. In addition, more than 570 sports organizations have adopted the Code.

WADA is made up of a Foundation Board, an Executive Committee, and several other committees. The Foundation Board and Executive Committee comprise equally members of the Olympic Movement and governments. Government representation is allocated according to the five Olympic regions: Africa, Asia, the Americas, Europe, and Oceania (Australia and New Zealand). The Foundation Board has 38 members and is the agency's supreme decision-making body. The board delegates the management and running of the agency, including the performance of activities and the administration of assets, to the Executive Committee. Other committees such as the Athletic Committee or the Health, Medical and Research Committee act as advisors and provide guidance for WADA programs.

WADA received $18.3 million from the Olympic Movement to fund its first 2 years. Since 2002, funding was sourced equally from the Olympic Movement and the governments of the world. The governments agreed to a regional formula, and within each region, governments agree internally to each of their individual shares.

WADA prioritizes its work to focus on seven areas emanating from the Code.

1. *Code adoption, implementation, and compliance:* The agency ensures that sports and government agencies accept the principles of the Code. It assists in organizing a systematic testing process and ensures adjudication of results.

2. *Science and medicine:* WADA promotes global research to stay current on doping substances and methods. In addition, it maintains the annual List of Prohibited Substances and Methods, accredits antidoping labs worldwide, and monitors "therapeutic use exemptions."

3. *Antidoping coordination:* The Anti-Doping Development Management System (ADAMS) is the web-based database management system in place to assist stakeholders in coordination and compliance.

4. *Antidoping development:* The agency facilitates coordination of activities in regions where there are limited antidoping activities, so that resources can be pooled.

5. *Education:* WADA coordinates effective strategies and education to assist stakeholders in their education programs.

6. *Athlete outreach:* Antidoping experts take every opportunity, including one-on-one interaction at sporting events, to answer questions and educate athletes and stakeholders about the dangers and consequences of doping.

7. *Out-of-competition testing:* The agency contracts with stakeholders to help fulfill their responsibility for "no-notice out-of-competition" testing.

The Prohibited Substances and Methods list, as well as many other resources for athletes and stakeholders, is available on the WADA website and is updated annually (www.WADA-ama.org). The general categories of banned substances include androgenic anabolic steroids and other anabolic agents, hormones (e.g., growth hormone, erythropoietin, and insulin), hormone antagonists and modulators, beta-2 agonists, diuretics, and masking agents. Gene doping is specifically prohibited as well, although at this time, there is no reliable testing for this. Blood doping and other methods to enhance oxygen transfer are prohibited.

There is a process, of course, to ensure that an athlete who needs a substance that could be considered a doping agent for medical reasons, such as insulin or albuterol, can use it in a medically responsible way to treat an illness or condition. A Therapeutic Use Exemption (TUE) application is submitted to the athlete's local sports federation for review by a panel of independent physicians, called a Therapeutic Use Exemption Committee (TUEC). Preapproval, with possible monitoring of medication levels, is determined by the local federation. WADA does not accept TUE applications, but it has the power to overturn an exemption that has been granted or overturn a denial if it is determined that international standards were not followed.

There are three basic criteria to determine if an athlete will be granted a TUE: (1) the athlete would experience significant health problems without taking the prohibited substance or method; (2) the therapeutic use of the substance would not produce significant enhancement of performance; and (3) there is no reasonable therapeutic alternative to the use of the otherwise prohibited substance or method.

The problem of doping is an extremely complex one, often with enormous financial, political, and cultural implications. WADA has created an intricate system with checks and balances, as well as international representation to work for and protect athletes and sporting events, large and small, around the world.

Michael O'Brien

Websites

International Olympic Committee: http://www.olympic.org
National Collegiate Athletic Association:
    http://www.ncaa.org
World Anti-Doping Agency: http://www.wada-ama.org

WRESTLING, INJURIES IN

Wrestling is a sport in which the clinician faces many unique challenges. A strong knowledge of infectious skin diseases and issues related to weight control is imperative for anyone concerned with this sport. Many common sports medicine injuries will be encountered in wrestling. One common injury definitely seen in wrestling is concussion.

Concussion

Concussion is defined as any impact to the head or to the trunk, chest, or neck that radiates force to the head. It is often believed that concussion needs to have loss of consciousness or amnesia associated with it, but this is not the case. Although common, these symptoms do not necessarily need to be present. Concussion is characterized by a spectrum of symptoms, including but not limited to headache, dizziness, nausea, vomiting, confusion, cognitive difficulties, and balance disturbances. These symptoms occur quickly after impact, are neurological in nature, and generally abate spontaneously over time. For an athlete experiencing symptoms, a complete physical examination, including a thorough neurological and mental status examination, should be performed. Diagnostically, a computed tomography (CT) scan or magnetic resonance imaging (MRI) scan is ordered by physicians to rule out further pathology, such as bleeding within the brain. Concussion is treated symptomatically. Only when an athlete is symptom-free, is not taking any medicines for symptom control, and has normal mentation can he or she be placed on a return-to-sport protocol. A symptomatic wrestler is never allowed to return to his sport.

Auricular Hematoma (Cauliflower Ear)

An auricular hematoma occurs from trauma to the cartilaginous portion of the ear. In this area, blood collects between the skin and cartilage. If not treated in a timely manner, the deformity to the ear can become permanent. Treatment is via aspiration of the blood before it clots and application of a pressure dressing or other device to avoid further bleeding and accumulation of blood.

Epistaxis (Nosebleed)

A nosebleed occurs most often when there is breaking of the small vessels at the front of the nose due to trauma. Quite often, wrestlers are prone to recurrent nosebleeds because of continued trauma to the nose. It is important to try to stop the bleeding as quickly as possible. This is done by tilting the head forward and pinching the nostrils until the blood stops. A cotton plug or dental gauze placed in the nose can continue to hold pressure so that a wrestler can finish the match. If the bleeding becomes recurrent, then cauterization of the nasal vessels can often lead to permanent relief of the symptoms.

Sprains and Strains

A sprain refers to an injury to a ligament where it is stretched or, in the worst case, completely torn. A strain refers to an injury to a tendon or muscle where it is "pulled" or partially torn. Sprains and strains can happen to any joint in the body and are common in wrestling due to the consistent contact between the wrestlers and the contact of the athletes with the mat surface. They are characterized by pain, swelling, redness, loss of motion, and loss of strength at a joint. During competition, sprains and strains can be treated by the PRICES protocol, which refers to *p*rotection of the joint, *r*est, *i*ce, *c*ompression, *e*levation, and *s*upport of the joint. Once a more severe injury is ruled out by either physical examination by a physician or further radiological studies, physical therapy, taping/bracing, and anti-inflammatory medications are used to try to treat these conditions. Unfortunately, many complete sprains, such as those of the anterior cruciate ligament, or tendon/muscle tears, such as that of the patella tendon, require surgical intervention to reestablish proper functioning of the affected joint.

Fractures

A fracture is a medical condition in which there is a break in the bone. It can happen to any bone in the body. In wrestlers, the bones that are frequently fractured are the nasal bones, the bones of the fingers or toes, and those of the wrist and ankle, though other bones may also undergo fracture. Fractures are identified by pain, swelling, bruising, and redness at a fracture site. Physicians are suspicious of a fracture if there is pain directly on a bone or if they can feel a break, or step-off, in the outer covering of the bone, or cortex, when they follow the smooth contour of a bone. There is also a loss of motion or strength if a joint is involved. In general, suspected fractures are splinted or braced at the site of competition, ice is applied, and the athlete is sent for confirmation of the fracture. X-rays, MRI, CT, or bone scan can confirm fracture in a wrestler. Fractures are treated by splinting or casting to allow bone alignment for healing. For those fractures whose alignment cannot be maintained by splinting or casting, surgery is necessary to insert hardware to keep the bone ends together in order to allow the fracture to heal.

Cervical Strain (Neck Strain) and Lumbar Strain (Back Strain)

This injury occurs when there is a strain or injury to the muscles of the neck/back, usually during a takedown or bridging. It is characterized by pain and sometimes spasm of the muscles that line the spinal column. As long as there is no injury to the spinal cord or column, this injury usually heals without much difficulty. Treatment is icing and anti-inflammatory medications to the neck/back as well as physical therapy to the neck/back muscles to stretch and strengthen them.

Dislocated Shoulder

This injury occurs when the humeral head, or top of the arm bone, becomes separated from the glenoid, or shoulder bone. There is often pain deep within the shoulder and possibly numbness down the arm on the same side. One can often see the top of the humerus, either in front or behind the glenoid. When this occurs, it is important to be sure that the athlete has normal neurovascular status and absence of obvious fracture before even considering reducing or putting the shoulder back in place. If there is no qualified person available, the arm should be splinted and the athlete sent to the hospital for reduction. An X-ray at the hospital can then aid in determining the position of the humerus, rule out fracture, and assist in the reduction. Once reduced, the shoulder is checked for further pathology with an MR arthrogram. If there is no further pathology, physical therapy should bring the shoulder back to normal function. If there is further pathology, often surgery is performed to repair the damaged soft tissue structures and prevent another episode of dislocation.

Acromioclavicular (AC) Separation (Separated Shoulder)

This occurs when a wrestler lands directly on his or her shoulder, usually during a takedown. This results in a sprain of the ligament between the acromium, or shoulder bone, and the clavicle, or collarbone. This is often demonstrated by the clavicle being elevated above the acromium. An X-ray can confirm this. This injury often responds well to physical therapy and usually does not require surgical intervention.

Brachial Plexopathy (Burner or Stinger)

This injury occurs when the neck is forcibly side bent as the shoulder on the same side of the body is depressed, causing a stretch of the brachial plexus, the site where the nerves that innervate the upper extremity on the affected side exit out the neck and through the shoulder area. This can happen when a wrestler is forcibly taken to the mat. The wrestler usually complains of burning pain from the base of the neck through the entirety of the affected extremity. The condition usually lasts seconds with an initial episode but takes longer to resolve after each successive episode. The pain usually resolves on its own in several seconds to several minutes depending on the number of past episodes a wrestler has endured. There is generally no work-up done by the physician unless the condition becomes chronic. In this case, X-rays are ordered to look for bony structural issues that may be causing the injury. These may be followed by MRI or CT scan to further evaluate both bony and soft tissue structures to determine if there is an anatomical reason for the injury and to determine whether the wrestler should be removed from the sport because of the danger of neurological damage from repetitive injury due to his or her anatomy. Initial stingers are usually returned to play once the symptoms have resolved. Those who have repetitive episodes will need further examination to make sure that anatomy is not contributing to the injury and usually undergo a cervical stretching and strengthening program to prevent further injury.

Ulnar Collateral Ligament Sprain of the Elbow

The elbow is essentially a hinge joint made from the coming together of the radius and ulna (the two smaller forearm bones and the larger humerus, or upper arm bone). Wrestlers typically suffer injury to the ulnar collateral ligament of the elbow, which is the ligament connecting the ulna and

humerus, when posting after a takedown or during an arm chop when the wrestler is beginning on the bottom position. Both these maneuvers can lead to stress on this ligament and a possible stretch, sprain, or tearing of the ligament. The physician can check the integrity of the ligament by putting force on it. If moves and "gaps" are more than on the opposite side, there is concern for a sprain or tear. An X-ray can determine if this is due to fracture. MRI can show the extent of damage to the ligament. A complete tear would require surgical repair in a wrestler. A sprain would require possibly bracing to let the ligament begin to heal, followed by physical therapy to regain normal elbow function.

Ulnar Collateral Ligament Tear of the Thumb (Gamekeeper's Thumb)

This injury occurs when the thumb is abducted or forced away from the rest of the hand. This movement may sprain or tear the ulnar collateral ligament that connects the proximal phalanx of the thumb to the first metacarpal. Wrestlers with this injury cannot oppose the thumb. An X-ray can rule out fracture at the joint. MRI can show damage to this ligament. Treatment involves casting or splinting of the thumb for sprains and surgery for complete tears.

Back Pain

Back pain in wrestling is usually due to a muscle strain or "pulled muscle" during competition. Some forms of back pain in wrestling are not due to muscle strain. One such cause is herniation of a vertebral disk. Disk herniation occurs when the soft jelly-like part of the disk escapes through a tear in the annulus fibrosis, which is the tougher covering of the disk. When radicular symptoms, pain or numbness occurring in either lower extremity or both, are present, the pain may be due to a herniated disk causing stenosis or pressure on the nerve that innervates that particular lower extremity. A less common cause of back pain sometimes found in wrestling is a spondylolysis, or stress fracture of the pars portion of the vertebra. This can occur due to the consistent flexion and extension of the back while wrestling. Physical examination, X-rays, MRI/CT scans, and bone scans can often elucidate which of these conditions is causing the back pain. Muscle strains, herniated disks (with and without stenosis), and annular tears are usually treated conservatively with rest, icing, physical therapy, and anti-inflammatory medications. Epidural injections, injection of cortisone at the area of disk herniation, or surgery, may be needed if pain cannot be treated conservatively. Return to sports is usually guided by pain tolerance in the wrestler unless neurological symptoms occur. Spondylolysis treatment is more controversial. Many physicians recommend physical therapy and return to sports when painfree. Others recommend bracing followed by physical therapy and then return to sports. There is no consensus on treatment for this condition.

Trunk Pain

Pain in the area of the trunk is common in wrestling. This is often caused by movements in which one wrestler grasps the other wrestler, trying to expose his or her back. Pain in the rib area can be due to rib fracture or due to a strain of the small muscles between the ribs, the intercostals. It can also be due to strain of any of the abdominal muscles. Symptoms of rib fracture or muscle strains in the trunk can include pain at the site of injury, pain with movement, or difficulty breathing. With pain, an immediate physical examination should be performed, including listening to the lungs, to be sure that a fractured rib has not pierced a lung, creating a pneumothorax. X-rays are diagnostic of rib fractures. Treatment for rib fractures as well as strains includes rest, icing, medications for relief and pain, and physical therapy. Return to wrestling after a rib fracture is allowed when the fracture has healed, to avoid pneumothorax. Pain is the guide for wrestlers with simple strains.

Groin Strain (Groin Pull)

A strain of the muscles of the groin can occur in an area where the external rotators or flexors of the hip are located. This injury is characterized by movement in these planes. These injuries are usually self-limiting but can take several weeks to heal. Treatment is usually with rest, icing, anti-inflammatory medicines, and rehabilitation.

Knee Meniscal Tear

The meniscus is the shock absorber found between the femur, or upper leg bone, and tibia, or lower leg bone. There is one on the inside of the knee, or medial, and one on the outside, or lateral. Meniscal tearing occurs during a plant-and-twist injury, such as getting a foot caught in the mat when the wrestler is attempting to escape his or her opponent. Wrestlers often report feeling or hearing a "pop" or "tear." This is often accompanied by swelling within the knee and pain at the knee joint line. Often, it is difficult to walk on the affected leg. Physicians can test the affected meniscus for tearing by performing the McMurray test. In this test, the physician attempts to catch a piece of the damaged meniscus between the femur and tibia by manipulating the knee. X-rays cannot reveal a meniscal tear. An MRI test usually can detect meniscal tears. Meniscal tears are treated usually by surgery to either repair the damaged meniscus, if good blood supply is present, or remove the damaged part of the meniscus in a procedure called a partial meniscectomy. Surgery is usually followed by physical therapy. Meniscal tearing that does not produce symptoms can also be treated by physical therapy with or without cortisone injection.

Patella Dislocation/Subluxation

The patella is also called the kneecap. It sits in the groove of the femur, or top leg bone, and aids in extension of the knee. It is stabilized at the top of the bone by the quadriceps tendon and on the bottom by the patellar tendon. With certain moves, the patella can reach the edge of the groove and almost slide over it, referred to as a subluxation. If the kneecap does in fact pass over the groove, it is referred to as a dislocation. The kneecap often moves laterally, or to the outside of the leg, with this movement. Patients often complain of hearing a "pop," have immediate pain and swelling at the knee, and may visualize the kneecap on the outside of the femoral groove. Often, the kneecap will go back into place as the wrestler moves secondary to the pain he or she has from the displacement of the kneecap. If it does not go back into place on its own, the kneecap is often stabilized with an immobilizer or a brace. The physician usually performs an Apprehension Test, where he or she places outside stress on the kneecap to see if the symptoms of kneecap subluxation/dislocation can be mimicked. X-rays are often taken to ensure that there is no fracture, and the physician will manipulate the kneecap back into place. This may be followed by an MRI test to be sure that there is no subtle fracture that was missed by the X-ray or that there is no tearing of important soft tissue structures holding the kneecap in place. Surgery may be necessary to repair these tissues. Physical therapy is then done to maximize function and strength, either after surgery or in the absence of soft tissue damage after a patella dislocation.

Prepatellar Bursitis

The patella has a fluid-filled sac, called a bursa, between it and the underlying soft tissue. This bursa is necessary to allow the soft tissue structures above the patella to pass over the bone without causing injury. In competition, wrestlers often land directly on their knees, causing a compressing force on the bursa as it is trapped between the bone and the mat surface. This can lead to an inflammation of the bursa or bursitis. The hallmark of a prepatellar bursitis is swelling just above the patella. The swelling feels like a fluid-filled sack and renders the knee painful when one tries to kneel on the affected knee. There are usually no tests used to diagnose this problem as its appearance itself is diagnostic. Often, the bursal fluid will recede on its own. If the fluid does not recede on its own, it can be aspirated by a physician. Once recovered, the wrestler can return to competition. If the bursa becomes infected, the condition is called a septic bursitis. Antibiotics are usually given to the athlete to treat the infection, and aspiration is delayed until the infection has cleared.

Ankle Sprain

An ankle sprain is caused when the foot either turns out (or everts) or turns in (or inverts) during activity as the body weight passes over it. The athlete at the time of the sprain sometimes hears a "pop" followed by immediate pain and swelling in the affected area of the ankle. Walking, or ambulation, is often difficult, and crutches must sometimes be used. Once an ankle sprain occurs, the ankle is usually immobilized and iced immediately.

The physician usually checks range of motion and strength to assess damage to the joint. Certain tests, such as the Anterior Drawer Test or Tilt Test, check the integrity of the ligaments after a sprain. X-rays are often ordered to rule out associated fractures. Weight-bearing X-rays may be performed to be sure that the bones of the ankle have retained their alignment or have held together the functioning unit of the ankle, called the *mortise*. MRI may be necessary to look at the soft tissue damage more intently or determine if there has been damage to the ligaments or soft tissue between the tibia and fibula that may necessitate early surgical intervention. Simple ankle sprains are generally treated with protection, rest, ice, compression, elevation, and support. Physical therapy is usually necessary to restore movement and function.

First Metatarsal Sprain (Turf Toe)

This condition refers to a sprain of the collateral ligaments—or ligaments that connect the two sides of a joint—that connect the first metatarsal, or last foot bone, to the proximal phalanx, or first toe bone. The condition gets its name commonly from football, where the first toe can be sprained when it gets caught in the artificial turf during play. The principle is the same in this case, as the toe gets caught in the mat and sprains the joint. The athlete commonly complains of loss of motion and/or strength, pain, swelling, and possibly redness at the site. After the physician checks motion and strength, X-rays may be obtained to be sure that there is no underlying fracture at the joint. If there is no fracture, treatment consists of applying ice to the joint, therapeutic taping, physical therapy, and sometimes shoe modification to make the sole of the wrestling shoe stiffer in order to keep the toe straight. Pain is usually the limiting factor for the athlete's return to play.

R. Robert Franks

See also Acromioclavicular (AC) Joint, Separation of; Ankle Sprain; Bursitis; Cervical Nerve Stretch Syndrome; Concussion; Ear Injuries; Fungal Skin Infections and Parasitic Infestations; Lower Back Injuries and Low Back Pain; Meniscus Injuries; Nose Injuries; Patellar Dislocation; Skin Infections, Bacterial; Skin Infections, Viral; Thumb Sprain; Wrestling, Injuries in

Further Readings

Agel J, Ransone J, Dick R, Oppliger R, Marshall SW. Descriptive epidemiology of collegiate men's wrestling injuries: National Collegiate Athletic Association Injury Surveillance System, 1988–1989 through 2003–2004. *J Athl Train.* 2007;42(2):303–310.

Hewett TE, Pasque C, Heyl R, Wroble R. Wrestling injuries. *Med Sport Sci.* 2005;48:152–178.

Jarret GJ, Orwin JF, Dick RW. Injuries in collegiate wrestling. *Am J Sports Med.* 1998;26(5):674–680.

Khalili-Borna D, Honsik K. Wrestling and sports medicine. *Curr Sports Med Rep.* 2005;4(3):144–149.

Pasque CB, Hewett TE. A prospective study of high school wrestling injuries. *Am J Sports Med.* 2000;28(4):509–515.

Wrist Dislocation

The wrist joint serves as a link between the hands and the upper body, and a great deal of force is transmitted through this joint. The specific arrangement of bones and the presence of ligaments provide flexibility to the joint. Although this flexibility helps in the movement of our hands and fingers, it also allows for dislocation.

Wrist dislocation means that the wrist bones have been knocked out of position or a bone has come out of place in the wrist joint. It is sometimes also referred to as carpal dislocation. Such an injury is common among athletes. It is usually experienced in sports with increased force vectors (height and speed), for example, adult inline skaters and football players. Other cases include falls from a height, as seen, for example, in gymnasts.

The most common cause of injury is high energy, but low-energy trauma has also been described as the cause of carpal dislocation in some reports.

Wrist dislocation is a serious injury and requires immediate emergency care. In a study by Larsen and Lauritsen, as many as 2.5% of all cases presented in various emergency departments of the United States are wrist injuries. Ten percent of all carpal injuries are subluxations and dislocations, perilunate dislocation being the most common type.

The initial evaluation and treatment of wrist injuries can be performed by emergency physicians and/or family practitioners. Early recognition of a dislocation and determination of proper treatment can prevent complications, including prolonged pain, discomfort, and surgery, and time lost from sports participation.

Anatomy

The wrist comprises 10 bones: 8 of these are the carpal bones, and the remaining 2 are (lower ends of) the forearm bones (see Figure 1).

The carpal bones are arranged in two rows and include the scaphoid, lunate, triquetrum, and pisiform in one row and the trapezium, trapezoid, capitate, and hamate in the other. The forearm bones are the radius and the ulna.

A complex set of ligaments holds the carpal bones together and assists in movement. These ligaments are named according to the bones they hold together. Dorsal ligaments are weaker than other ligaments; making this side of the joint more vulnerable to dislocations.

Types of Wrist Dislocation

Wrist dislocations can be divided into two types:

Perilunate dislocations: The lunate remains aligned with the radius, but the capitate dislocates. It is more common than lunate dislocation as the radial-lunate ligaments are stronger than the lunate-capitate ligaments. Seventy-five percent of the cases are associated with scaphoid fractures (known as trans-scaphoid perilunate dislocation).

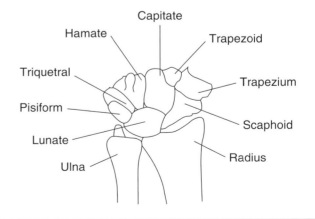

Figure I   Bones of the Wrist Joint

Lunate dislocations: In these, the lunate bone dislocates, and the other carpal bones remain in alignment. This type of dislocation is less common than perilunate dislocation.

Causes

Wrist dislocation can occur as a result of either of two causes:

1. *Repetitive activity:* Repeated stress on the carpal ligaments renders them more prone to injury, especially in athletes. In some cases, the overuse may be so great that the wrist bones slip.

2. *Trauma:* Sudden extreme pulling or stretching of the ligaments or a severe blow to the bones, commonly due to falling on an outstretched arm, can result in dislocation. This type of dislocation most commonly involves displacement of the lunate bone, but other bones of the wrist can also be involved.

Stages of Dislocation

Mayfield and coworkers have classified wrist dislocation into four stages:

Stage I: Scapho-lunate dislocation due to a tear in the ligaments holding these bones together

Stage II: Lunate-capitate subluxation that results from injury to the capito-lunate joint

Stage III: Lunate-triquetral dislocation resulting from injury to the ligament

Stage IV: Lunate dislocation resulting from injury to the dorsal radio-lunate ligament (the ligament that holds the lunate against the radius)

Clinical Evaluation

The evaluation of a wrist dislocation begins with a history and physical exam.

History

The typical history is one of a person who attempts to brace for a fall. The force of the body landing on the palm results in a dislocation. Sometimes athletes can dislocate their wrist on falling on an outstretched hand when they have mistimed a landing, as in gymnastics. Wrist dislocation is also seen in football, where defenders try to stop oncoming forces with resistance. Often the resistance is great enough to lead to a wrist dislocation.

Physical Examination

On physical examination, the following signs and symptoms are observed in a case of wrist dislocation:

- Extreme pain at the time of the injury that worsens with movement
- Loss of wrist and hand mobility or decrease in the range of motion
- Deformity or contortion of the wrist
- Tenderness around the wrist and hand area
- Swelling of the wrist
- Hand weakness (unilateral)
- Decrease in grip strength
- Numbness and paralysis of the hand in case of severe injury (due to pressure, pinching, or cutting of blood vessels or nerves)

Sometimes neither the patient nor the physician is able to appreciate the severity of the trauma, and the dislocation may present itself after a delay. Therefore, during the evaluation of a patient with wrist injury, dislocation should always be suspected.

Diagnostic Tests

Sometimes tests are required to make the diagnosis of a wrist dislocation. Tests that can be done include the following:

X-rays of the wrist: Radiographs of both hands are taken for comparison, and bone alignment is checked along various planes/axes.

Bone scan: A radioactive tracer is injected into the blood and gets attached to all the bones of the body. A computer scan generates a picture of the skeleton by reading the radiation levels. Any abnormalities are easily observed.

Magnetic resonance image (MRI) of wrist: An MRI scan provides good resolution of soft tissue as well as bone.

Wrist arthroscopy: This is a surgical procedure used to diagnose and treat problems inside a joint. Small incisions are made around a joint, and a pencil-sized instrument called an arthroscope is inserted. The arthroscope contains a miniature lens and camera, which project the three-dimensional images of the joint onto a screen.

Arthrography: It is useful in detecting tears of the ligaments.

Treatment

Nonsurgical Approach

All types of injuries need to be assessed by a physician. If there is no evidence of fracture and the injury is not very severe, the wrist bones may align themselves properly and heal with time. There may be a need for repositioning the bones to reduce the dislocation. If there is an associated wrist fracture, surgery is performed to restore the joint to its normal position.

Surgical Approach

Surgical reconstruction or replacement of the joint is required in acute or recurring dislocations. It is performed under anesthesia. The surgeon opens the hand and wrist area and aligns the bones properly. In case of major damage, other devices such as surgical screws may also be used.

Associated Measures

Along with treatment, the following measures should be incorporated to enhance successful healing:

- Elevation of the wrist
- Rest and immobilization, perhaps with a sling for 2 to 8 weeks
- Ice, which helps in reducing acute pain and swelling
- Compression of the wrist (cold compresses may be used)
- Elastic (ACE) wrap
- Cast or splint for a wrist dislocation
- Physical therapy for a wrist dislocation, including exercises designed to build up the muscles of the hand and wrist, helpful in restoring full functional strength and motion in the hand and wrist
- Occcupational therapy for a wrist fracture

Symptomatic Treatment

The following medications may be included in this treatment:

Nonsteroidal anti-inflammatory drugs (NSAIDs): These lower the elevated body temperature and relieve pain without impairing consciousness and have anti-inflammatory effects.

Narcotic pain medication: These are strong pain relievers and cause loss of feeling.

Prevention

Use of gloves, wrist guards, or tapes, if the sport permits, can provide some protection to the wrist. Implementation of proper technique and maintenance of good strength and good flexibility can prevent wrist injuries. In case of an injured wrist, the patient should return to play only after achieving full recovery.

Return to Sports

The dislocated joint and the injured ligaments require a minimum of 6 weeks for complete healing. On returning to work, the patient may support the wrist with a tape or a brace initially if he or she is required to perform lifts or bear weight on the involved wrist.

Sometimes, undergoing special exercise programs, physical therapy, or occupational therapy to restore full strength may be necessary. A physician should be consulted in all cases before resuming routine physical activities.

Ammara Iftikhar and Mariam Shaheen

See also Wrist Fractures; Wrist Injuries; Wrist Sprain; Wrist Tendinopathy

Further Readings

Alt V, Sicre G. Dorsal transscaphoid-transtriquetral perilunate dislocation in pseudarthrosis of the scaphoid. *Clin Orthop Relat Res.* 2004;(426): 135–137.

Elstrom JA, Perry CR, Virkus WW, Pankovich A. Fractures and dislocations of the wrist. In: *Handbook of Fractures*. New York, NY: McGraw-Hill Professional; 2005:182–189.

Martinage A, Balaguer T, Chignon-Sicard B, Monteil MC, Dreant N, Lebreton E. Perilunate dislocations and fracture-dislocations of the wrist, a review of 14 cases [in French]. *Chir Main*. 2008;27(1):31–39.

Mayfield JK, Johnson RP, Kilcoyne RK. Carpal dislocations: pathomechanics and progressive perilunar instability. *J Hand Surg Am*. 1980;5(3): 226–241.

Walker B. Sports injuries of the wrists and forearm. In: *The Anatomy of Sports Injuries*. San Francisco, CA: North Atlantic Books; 2007:95.

WRIST FRACTURE

In sports, the wrist is one of the most vulnerable parts of the body. Wrist fractures are among the most common sports-related injuries. Surveys have shown that women, beginners, and younger athletes are more prone to wrist injuries, and it is recommended that they wear wrist guards that help protect the wrist from injury.

Wrist fracture is the most common fracture in patients under 65 years of age and accounts for about one sixth of all factures seen in hospital emergency departments. It is defined as a break in one or more of the bones in the wrist, but when clinicians are describing wrist fracture, they are usually referring to a fracture of the distal end of the radius (one of the two bones in the forearm, the other being the ulna). The other bones of the wrist joint may also be broken, but the term *wrist fracture* usually implies a fracture of the end of the long bone of the forearm.

Fractures of the wrist most commonly occur as the result of a person extending his or her hand to break a fall, due to which a large amount of force is applied to the wrist, causing the fracture (usually seen in sports where a fall on a hard surface is likely, such as skating, basketball, and hockey); or they may be due to a large force being directly applied to the wrist (e.g., a direct blow during contact sports or a blow from a stick, as in hockey or lacrosse). Injuries related to sports, car accidents, and falls from a height are important contributing causes of wrist fracture. In older individuals, osteoporosis may play a significant role by making the bones brittle and more susceptible to fractures, even with minor trauma.

Anatomy

The wrist is made up of two long bones in the forearm (ulna and radius) and eight short bones (carpal bones). The radius is located on the thumb side of the forearm, while the ulna is located on the side of the little finger. The carpal bones are situated in two rows (four in each) at the wrist joint and have synovial joints between them, but movement at these joints is restricted. The ulna and radius are joined at the proximal radio-ulnar joint near the elbow and the distal radio-ulnar joint at the wrist.

The wrist joint is a complex synovial joint between the distal end of the radius and the end of the ulna with the proximal row of carpal bones (the distal row of carpal bones make the carpo-metacarpal joints with the metacarpal bones of the hand). The joint between the radius and ulna is fixed due to the articular disk covering the end of the ulna. The surfaces of carpal bones form a convex contour that articulates with the concave surface of this articular disk and radius. At each joint, the end of the bones is covered by a cartilage, which allows for smooth movements. The bones are held together by ligaments. The joint cavities are filled with synovial fluid, which reduces friction. This arrangement allows for movement at the wrist around two axes, side to side, and the bending and straightening of the wrist. Rotation of the wrist is brought about by combinations of these movements.

In addition, there are a number of nerves and blood vessels traversing this region that may be damaged due to injury to the wrist.

Classification of Wrist Fractures

Generally, the different patterns of fracture of the wrist are the Colles fracture, the Smith fracture, the Barton fracture, and the Chauffer fractures. The classification of fractures is based on the pattern of injury involved, the behavior and outcome of that pattern, and the need to distinguish between conditions requiring different treatment strategies. Furthermore, the fracture may be extraarticular or intraarticular (extending into the joint cavity or not), it may be a closed injury or a compound fracture, and comminution (the amount of crumbling at the fracture site) may be extensive or minimal.

In assessing the stability and determining treatment, many features of the fracture must be considered, such as radial shortening, radial angulation, comminution, articular incongruity, accompanying soft tissue injuries, and associated ulnar fractures.

In addition, other bones of the wrist may also be broken in wrist fractures, the most common being the scaphoid (carpal bone articulating with the radius) (Figure 1a) and the "hook" of the hamate (Figure 1b).

Symptoms and Evaluation

Wrist injuries inflicted in vehicle accidents or sports or in any other way can result in wrist fractures. The first symptom experienced by the person is pain that occurs immediately after the injury and does not subside. The intensity of pain varies with different kinds of fractures and from person to person. Other symptoms may be swelling and tenderness around the wrist, bruising around the wrist, limited range of motion of the thumb and wrist, and visible deformity of the wrist. These symptoms can also be due to other conditions, so it should not be assumed that there is a fracture. A doctor should be consulted.

Diagnosis can be made by observing the deformity of the distal radius, but it should be confirmed by an X-ray. Computed tomography (CT) scans and magnetic resonance imaging (MRI) can also be helpful in confirming the diagnosis if fractures are not seen on X-ray immediately after the injury.

Treatment

The treatment differs widely depending on the nature and severity of the injury. The treatment plan consists of the following:

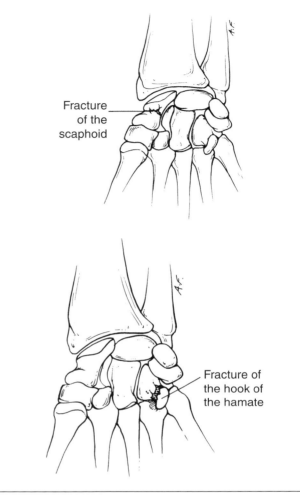

Figure 1   Wrist Fractures

Note: (a) Fracture of the scaphoid and (b) fracture of the hook of the hamate.

- It involves approximating the pieces of the fractured bone together, which may require anesthesia and also may require surgery.
- The pieces of bone should be kept in position while the bone heals and the ends join.

After the reduction of the fracture, different modalities may be employed to hold the bone in place (stabilization):
- A cast may be used with or without surgery.
- Internal fixation may be done with a metal plate and screws.

- Percutaneous pin fixation may be done.
- External fixation may be done.
- A combination of these modalities may also be used.

The typical treatment is immobilization with a plaster of paris cast for 5 to 6 weeks to allow union of the bones. The use of other modalities depends on the nature and extent of the injury, and appropriate treatment for each case is determined by the surgeon. For athletes requiring the use of their wrist, such as in tennis, motocross, or cycling, recovering from a fracture without stiffness is important. This is done by performing surgery only when necessary to realign the bones and treating postsurgery without a cast to allow early motion of the wrist and fingers. Due to the functional importance of the hand, the period of immobilization is kept to a minimum to avoid dysfunction of the hand and wrist. The more motion these patients have, the easier it is to resume their sport.

Follow-Up and Recovery

It is common practice to repeat X-rays at about 1 week during the follow-up period. Follow-up is also needed to determine when the cast may be removed, when the fracture has healed and the rehabilitation is complete. Removal of the cast is followed by rehabilitation for 1 month or more, a short period of which may involve the use of a wrist brace for comfort.

Return to sports should be decided by the patient's physician. Braces should be used to stabilize the wrist during sports or even normal activities. In most cases, athletes can return soon after the immobilization with some protection for the wrist or after adequate postoperative healing, as recommended by the doctor. When the pain subsides, the athlete should work on strengthening the wrist and improving its function, as directed by the doctor. This is usually achieved by performing stretching exercises such as

- wrist range of motion,
- wrist stretch,
- wrist extension stretch,
- wrist flexion stretch, and
- forearm pronation and supination.

These are followed by strengthening exercises such as

- wrist flexion,
- wrist extension, and
- grip strengthening.

It is important during fracture healing that the flexibility of the fingers and hand be maintained. The patient may start hand and wrist exercises as soon as the wrist is stable, to recover the flexibility, strength, and function of the wrist. It is recommended to stay off sports for 6 weeks at least, but the time for recovery varies according to the severity of injury, on any associated injury, and on factors related to the individual. Full recovery may take 6 to 12 weeks, when the patient may resume normal activities, but it is not unusual for maximal recovery from a wrist fracture to take several months. Some patients may, however, have residual stiffness or pain, and even arthritis may develop. On occasion, reconstructive surgery or additional treatment may be required.

Prevention

Certain risk factors increase the chance of developing wrist fractures:

- Advancing age
- Postmenopause
- Poor nutrition
- Osteoporosis
- Decreased muscle mass
- Contact sports such as soccer or rugby
- Skating, bike sports, skateboarding
- Vehicle accidents

Risk of injury may be avoided by following these simple guidelines:

- Putting oneself at risk for trauma should be avoided.
- The diet should include adequate calcium and vitamin D.
- Proper safety equipment should be used in sports training and contests.
- Fair play and a healthy competitive spirit should be practiced.

- Rules must be enforced to minimize risk of injury to players.
- The athletes should be provided proper coaching and training by qualified specialists.

Prompt medical attention should be easily available to the athlete at all times, especially in cases of emergency.

Aun Raza Shah, Muhammad Zeshan Ali, Mohammad Bilal, and Sanniya Khan Ghauri

See also Musculoskeletal Tests, Hand and Wrist; Taping; Wrist Injuries; Wrist Sprain

Further Readings

Abbaszadegan H, von Sivers K, Jonsson U. Late displacement of Colles' fractures. *Int Orthop.* 1988;12(3):197–199.

Azzopardi T, Ehrendorfer S, Coulton T, Abela M. Unstable extra-articular fractures of the distal radius: a prospective, randomised study of immobilisation in a cast versus supplementary percutaneous pinning. *Br J Bone Joint Surg Br.* 2005;87(6):837–840.

Fernandez D, Jupiter J. *Fractures of the Distal Radius.* 2nd ed. New York, NY: Springer; 2002.

Goldfarb CA, Yin Y, Gilula LA, Fisher AJ, Boyer MI. Wrist fractures: what the clinician wants to know. *Radiology.* 2001;219(1):11–28.

WRIST INJURIES

The wrist is frequently injured in sports. Sprains are the most common wrist injury, accounting for 20% to 50% of injuries, followed by contusions (15%–30%) and fractures (5%–35%). Distal radius fractures are the most common fracture seen in emergency departments; scaphoid fractures are the most common carpal fracture. Acute injuries of the wrist occur in sports such as football, hockey, and snowboarding, most often from falls. Falls resulting in wrist injuries can also be seen in recreational activities such as rollerblading and biking. Overuse wrist injuries occur in sports such as golf, gymnastics, and racquet sports. It is important to recognize wrist injuries and ensure appropriate treatment to avoid impairments that may affect not only sports participation but also activities of daily living.

Wrist injuries are more common in children and adolescents than in adults participating in sports. Wrist and hand injuries account for between 3% and 20% of all athletic injuries in the younger population. Possible reasons to explain this increased frequency of wrist injuries in young athletes include increased sports participation by younger athletes; the increased popularity of "extreme" sports; the use of age- or size-inappropriate equipment; increased risk of injury of the immature musculoskeletal system in children, particularly with excessive frequency or intensity of certain sport-specific activities; and poor sport-specific techniques, poor supervision, and inadequate coaching.

Anatomy

The joints of the wrist include the radiocarpal joints and the distal radioulnar joint. The radius articulates mainly with the scaphoid. The ulna articulates primarily with the lunate. Movement at the radiocarpal joints includes flexion-extension and radioulnar deviation. Movement at the distal radioulnar joint includes pronation-supination.

The carpal bones in the wrist consist of a proximal row, including the lunate, triquetrum, and pisiform, and a distal row, including the trapezium, trapezoid, capitate, and hamate. The proximal and distal rows of carpals are bridged by the scaphoid bone. The ossification centers of the carpal bones appear on X-rays in a predictable pattern. The capitate appears first at less than 1 year of age, followed by the hamate, triquetrum, lunate, scaphoid, trapezius, trapezoid, and pisiform. All ossification centers are apparent on X-rays by 10 years of age. The distal radial epiphysis appears by 1 year of age, whereas the distal ulnar epiphysis becomes visible by 6 to 7 years of age. These physes close by 16 to 18 years of age, when skeletal growth has been completed. Knowledge of the appearance of these ossification centers and epiphyses can help avoid confusion between normal structures and possible fractures and bony injuries in children and adolescents.

Wrist stability is imparted by several extrinsic and intrinsic ligaments. The carpal bones are stabilized by the intercarpal ligaments and allow for transmission of forces across the wrist. There are many extrinsic tendons that traverse the wrist, including the wrist flexors (flexor carpi radialis, palmaris longus, flexor carpi ulnaris) and wrist extensors (brachioradialis, extensor carpi radialis longus, extensor carpi radialis brevis, extensor carpi ulnaris).

Evaluation of Injuries

Details of Injury

The mechanism of injury, including the position of the wrist, the direction and magnitude of the involved force, and subsequent symptoms of weakness, pain, or instability, can help determine the cause of wrist pain. Acute injuries are usually the result of a *fall on an outstretched hand* (FOOSH). Striking a solid object with a piece of equipment, such as a bat, golf club, or tennis racquet striking the ground, can result in a fracture of the hook of the hamate. Rotational stress to the distal radioulnar joint, as well as forced ulnar deviation and rotation, may result in a tear to the triangular fibrocartilage complex (TFCC). More severe wrist injuries may prevent an athlete from returning to activity immediately following injury.

The exact location of pain helps narrow the differential diagnosis. Wrist injuries may result in mechanical symptoms such as clicking, snapping, or swelling. Previous injuries to the upper extremities may predispose an athlete to wrist injuries. Other important details such as hand dominance, type of sport, position played, level of performance, and occupation may affect management of the injury.

Physical Findings

Wrist injuries may cause obvious deformity, swelling, or bruising of the wrist. The athlete may hold the wrist in various positions to avoid pain. The range of motion of the injured wrist may be decreased flexion-extension, supination-pronation (hand down/hand up), and radial-ulnar deviation. Normal range is 20° of radial deviation and 60° of ulnar deviation. Comparing the range of motion of the injured wrist with that of the uninjured side can emphasize any decreased movement of the injured wrist. Decreases in wrist movement can also be seen when the hands are placed in the "prayer position" and "reverse prayer position." The prayer position evaluates wrist extension. The patient apposes the palms with the elbows flexed and the wrists extended. Normal range of motion is 70° of wrist extension. The reverse prayer position evaluates wrist flexion. The patient apposes the dorsal aspects of the hands with the elbows and wrists flexed. Normal range of motion is 80° of wrist flexion.

Bony injuries of the wrist may result in tenderness to palpation or deformity. Bony prominences that may be tender to palpation include the distal forearm, the radial snuffbox, the base of the metacarpals, the lunate, the head of the ulna, the radioulnar joint, the pisiform, and the hook of the hamate.

Special tests of the wrist that may point to a specific injury include the Watson test and TFCC integrity. The Watson test evaluates scapholunate stability. The examiner places a thumb on the scaphoid tuberosity with the patient's wrist in ulnar deviation. The wrist is then deviated radially while the examiner applies pressure on the scaphoid. A positive test for scapholunate dissociation occurs if the patient feels pain dorsally over the scapholunate ligament or the examiner feels the scaphoid move dorsally. Assessment of TFCC integrity involves placing the athlete's wrist in dorsiflexion and ulnar deviation and then rotating the wrist. A positive test for a tear of the TFCC occurs when overpressure causes pain and occasional clicking at the ulnar aspect of the wrist.

Wrist injuries may result in nerve damage or injury to the blood vessels in the wrist as well.

Investigations

In the setting of a traumatic wrist injury, routine X-rays can show possible fractures. X-rays should include posterior-anterior (PA), lateral, and PA with radial and ulnar deviation views. If a ligament injury is suspected, a PA view with a clenched fist can indicate possible injury. The normal PA view should demonstrate a smooth line joining the proximal ends of the proximal row of carpal bones and the "C" shape of the midcarpal joint (the Gilula arcs). On the normal lateral view of the wrist, the proximal pole of the lunate fits into the concavity of the distal radius, and the convex head of the capitate fits into the distal concavity of the lunate. These bones should be aligned with each other and the base of the third metacarpal.

Specialized X-ray views can be ordered for specific suspected injuries. If a scaphoid fracture is of concern, scaphoid views should be obtained. A carpal tunnel view with the wrist dorsiflexed allows the hook of the hamate and ridge of the trapezium to be inspected.

Other modalities that are helpful to diagnose wrist pain, such as ganglions or occult fractures, include ultrasound, radionuclide bone scan, computed tomography (CT) scan, and magnetic resonance imaging (MRI). Ultrasonography is helpful to assess soft tissue abnormalities such as tendon injury, ganglions, synovial cysts, or thickening. Bone scans are helpful to rule out subtle fractures. CT scans can also evaluate fractures that may not be apparent on plain films. MRI can evaluate soft tissue injuries, such as a tear of the scapholunate ligament, more effectively than CT. Arthroscopy is an increasingly used procedure for diagnosis and therapy. It is an excellent tool for detecting scapholunate tears and is the investigation of choice for patients with ulnar-sided wrist pain that persists following an acute injury (see Table 1).

Prevention of Injury

Many wrist injuries in sport can be prevented. The use of protective wrist guards has been shown to reduce wrist fractures in sports such as snowboarding and inline skating. Studies have shown that the incidence of wrist fractures was reduced by half in participants who wore wrist guards while snowboarding. Similar studies on inline skating found that athletes who did not wear wrist guards were more than 10 times more likely to injure their wrist than those who did wear wrist guards.

In younger athletes, it is important to use age- and size-appropriate equipment to reduce injury. For instance, studies on youth soccer have shown that distal radius fractures are more common in younger children using an adult-sized ball than in those who use a junior-size ball.

Return to Sports

Return-to-play recommendations vary somewhat according to the specific injury, the treatment modality, and the sport-specific demands of the individual athlete. In general, full unprotected return to play is not allowed until the athlete has regained full active and passive range of motion and almost full strength of the affected wrist. Bony or ligamentous injuries usually require 3 to 6 weeks to heal. Athletes should not participate in sports unless the injury is appropriately immobilized in a cast or splint. Wrist injuries do have the potential for delayed or failed healing despite appropriate initial

Table I Types of Wrist Injuries

Acute	Chronic
Distal radius fracture	Ganglion cyst
Scaphoid fracture	Intersection syndrome
Wrist ligament sprain/tear	Kienböck disease
Hook of hamate fracture	de Quervain tenosynovitis
Triangular fibrocartilage complex (TFCC) tear	Dorsal pole of lunate and distal radius impingement (gymnasts)
Distal radioulnar joint instability	
Scapholunate dissociation	Tendinopathy (flexor carpi ulnaris, extensor carpi ulnaris)
Carpal bone dislocation	Posterior interosseous nerve entrapment
Carpal tunnel syndrome	Inflammatory arthropathy
	Degenerative joint disease
	Nonunion of scaphoid fracture

treatment, requiring subsequent surgical intervention. Therefore, early referral to an orthopedic or hand surgeon is recommended for follow-up. Another consideration in determining when an athlete is ready to return to sports is the safety of the injured athlete as well as the other participants. If an athlete is considering returning to sports wearing a protective device, permission should be obtained from trainers, coaches, and officials.

Laura Purcell

See also Colles Fracture; Musculoskeletal Tests, Hand and Wrist; Wrist Dislocation; Wrist Fracture; Wrist Sprain; Wrist Tendinopathy

Further Readings

Bae DS. Injuries to the wrist, hand and fingers. In: Micheli LJ, Purcell LK, eds. *The Adolescent Athlete.* New York, NY: Springer; 2007:223–263.

Forman TA, Forman SK, Rose NE. A clinical approach to diagnosing wrist pain. *Am Fam Physician.* 2005;72(9):1753–1758.

Garnham A, Ashe M, Gropper P. Wrist, hand and finger injuries. In: Brukner P, Khan K, eds. *Clinical Sport Medicine.* 3rd edition. Sydney, Australia: McGraw-Hill Professional; 2007:308–339.

Kocher MS, Waters PM, Micheli LJ. Upper extremity injuries in the pediatric athlete. *Sports Med.* 2000;30(2):117–135.

Rettig AC. Athletic injuries of the wrist and hand. Part I: traumatic injuries of the wrist. *Am J Sports Med.* 2003;31(6):1038–1048.

Rettig AC. Athletic injuries of the wrist and hand. Part II: overuse injuries of the wrist and traumatic injuries to the hand. *Am J Sports Med.* 2004;32(1):262–273.

WRIST SPRAIN

A *sprain* is an injury to a ligament. Ligaments are a type of tissue that connects bones to bones and provides stability to joints. One may think of ligaments as analogous to ropes. *Sprain* comes from the French word *espraindre,* which means "to wring." A wrist sprain is an injury to the ligaments of the wrist. Often, sprains occur from falls or sports-related injuries that involve forcibly bending the wrist backward (hyperextension) or excessive pressure through the long axis of the joint (axial loading), with subsequent damage to the ligaments of the wrist joint.

Anatomy

The wrist comprises many different types of structures, including eight small bones (called carpal bones), multiple ligaments, cartilage—a firm covering of the bones (e.g., the tip of your nose), and specific junctions with the bones of the hand (metacarpals) and forearm (radius, ulna). The joint where the radius and ulna are connected near the hand is called the distal radial ulnar joint (DRUJ). This joint is particularly susceptible to injury during falls.

Several structures in the wrist deserve particular mention, including the triangular fibrocartilage complex (TFCC). The TFCC is a special type of tissue (a mix between fibrous tissue and cartilage) that absorbs stress during axial loading of the wrist and limits lateral movement of the carpal bones. Throwing a "jab" or "punch" in boxing, for example, would be axially loading the wrist joint. This special cartilage (TFCC) also stabilizes the DRUJ.

There are two types of ligaments in the wrist—extrinsic, which connect the radius and ulna to the carpal bones, and intrinsic, which connect the carpal bones to each other.

Extrinsic ligaments have two components, *volar*—the palmar or underside of the wrist and hand, and *dorsal*—the backside (knuckle side) of the wrist and hand.

The volar radiocarpal ligaments are stronger and thicker than the dorsal and so provide the majority of motion stability in the wrist. The most important ligament of this group is the radioscaphocapitate, which attaches the radius (forearm bone) to the scaphoid and capitate (carpal bones). Intrinsic ligaments are also called interosseous ligaments. They originate on the carpal bones and are within the capsule of the wrist.

The most common ligament indicated in wrist sprains is the scapholunate, which is an intrinsic ligament between the scaphoid and lunate bones. It comprises dorsal collagen bundles that provide a structure that lends to its superior stability. Another important interosseous ligament is the lunotriquetral, connecting the lunate and triquetrium carpal bones.

Classification of Injuries

Sprains are classified based on severity, ranging from mild to moderate to severe injury. Typically, Grade I sprains represent the least amount of injury—a stretching of the ligament fibers—and result in minimal or no loss of function at that joint. Grade II sprains usually equate to a partial tearing of the ligament. This may be observed by increased swelling and pain of the joint along with moderate dysfunction. The most serious of wrist sprains would be a complete tear of the ligament, a Grade III sprain. This results in an unstable joint and requires immobilization (splinting) and often referral to a specialist.

Injury Setting and Symptoms

Wrist sprains occur in many settings and due to a variety of reasons, including direct injury, chronic repetitive trauma and loading activities, or falls and sports-related injuries. Sprains are more common in adults than in children due to the different anatomy of the developing bones in children. In younger populations, similar injuries more often produce fractures of the immature bone rather than damage to the ligaments. Commonly, skiing, skating, snowboarding, and inline skating are sports associated with wrist sprains, but they can occur in any contact or noncontact sports under certain conditions. At times, specific wrist injuries are classified as *falls* on an *outstretched hand* (FOOSH), such as fractures of the scaphoid bone or disruption of the scapholunate ligament.

Patients with wrist sprains may report feeling a tear or hearing a pop during the event. Areas of the wrist or hand may swell, demonstrate bruising, or be painful to touch. Patients have difficulty and pain with movement of the wrist. Wrist and hand anatomy is intricate, and diagnosing an injury may present a difficult task, so an evaluation should include a detailed history, a careful physical exam, and often radiographs. The exam should consist of general inspection, a neurovascular evaluation, palpation of bony prominences and ligaments, and assessment of joint range of motion and stability.

Treatment

Sprains usually heal completely within 4 to 6 weeks. Conservative treatment involves splinting in a neutral position with either a brace or a compressive elastic wrap, rest from painful activity, application of ice packs, and taking nonsteroidal anti-inflammatory drugs (NSAIDs) to reduce swelling and for pain relief. After a period of immobilization and before returning to full activity, patients should exercise to improve wrist range of motion and strength. This may include work with a resistance band or weights for wrist extension, flexion, and ulnar and radial deviation (ulnar deviation: side movement in the direction of the little finger; radial deviation: side movement in the direction of the thumb).

Grade III sprains or complete tears of ligaments may require surgical correction and repair. These injuries represent unstable joints, and the wrist must be immobilized at the discovery of injury to prevent additional or more serious injury.

While most wrist sprains heal with conservative therapy and without other intervention, some important conditions must not be missed due to varying treatments and risk of adverse events. These include injury to the TFCC, carpal bone dislocation (displacement), DRUJ, or any fracture of the carpal bones or forearm bones (radius or ulna).

Tanika M. Pinn

See also Wrist Fracture; Wrist Injuries; Wrist Tendinopathy

Further Readings

Bencardino JT, Rosenberg ZS. Sports-related injuries of the wrist: an approach to MRI interpretation. *Clin Sports Med.* 2006;25(3):409–432.

Giunta YP, Rocker JA, Adam HM. Sprains. *Pediatr Rev.* 2008;29:176–178.

Griffin LY, ed. *Essentials of Musculoskeletal Medicine.* 3rd ed. Rosemont, IL: American Academy of Orthopaedic Surgeons; 2007.

Parmelee-Peters K, Eathorne SW. The wrist: common injuries and management. *Prim Care.* 2005;32(1):35–70.

WRIST TENDINOPATHY

Overuse wrist tendon injury, or *tendinopathy*, occurs regularly in athletes participating in sports with repetitive wrist and hand movement. Unlike more proximal tendinopathies (e.g., rotator cuff), which are typically degenerative and noninflammatory, symptoms from wrist tendinopathy frequently involve inflammation of the outer tendon sheath, known as paratenonitis. The most common wrist tendinopathies in athletes involve the dorsal/extensor aspect of the wrist, such as de Quervain disease, intersection syndrome, and extensor carpi ulnaris (ECU) paratenonitis.

Risk factors for athletic wrist tendinopathy include muscle weakness or imbalance, overuse from training load, improper technique or equipment, and inadequate rest. The accurate diagnosis of wrist tendinopathy requires skilled history taking and physical examination, and advanced imaging is infrequently necessary. Treatment of inflammatory tendinopathy of the wrist includes rest, noninvasive anti-inflammatory modalities (e.g., ice, anti-inflammatory medications), risk factor modification, and occasional local corticosteroid injection. With an accurate diagnosis and a treatment plan customized for the athlete, the sport, and the severity of the condition, most athletes with wrist tendinopathy return to their sport quickly and very rarely have long-term limitation.

Anatomy

Tendons consist of longitudinally oriented, closely grouped collagen bundles with an outer covering called the paratenon. In areas such as the wrist, where tendons bend at acute angles over bone, the paratenon is thicker and lined with synovium and is called a tendon sheath. The synovium of the tendon sheath both provides mechanical resistance to shearing forces and produces synovial fluid, lubricating the tendon to decrease frictional injury.

Wrist tendons are divided into extensor tendons, which run over the dorsal aspect of the wrist, and flexor tendons, which run over the volar/palmar aspect of the wrist. The side of the wrist closest to the radius (and thumb) is referred to as the radial aspect of the wrist, and that closest to the ulna (and fifth finger) is referred to as the ulnar aspect of the wrist. The relative anatomic course of each of these wrist and finger tendons is represented in Figure 1 (extensors) and Figure 2 (flexors). The dorsal/extensor wrist is divided into six compartments, numbered from the radial to ulnar aspects, the first two of which are frequently involved in athletic wrist tendinopathies. The first dorsal compartment consists of the abductor pollicis longus (APL) and extensor pollicis brevis (EPB) tendons. The second dorsal compartment includes both extensor carpi radialis brevis (ECRB) and extensor carpi radialis longus (ECRL) tendons.

Pathology

Tendinopathy is a broad term that includes tendinitis, tendinosis, and paratenonitis. *Tendinitis*

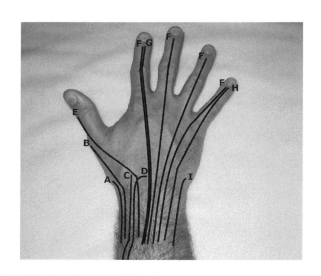

Tendons of the dorsal aspect of the wrist: (a) abductor pollicis longus, (b) extensor pollicis brevis, (c) extensor carpi radialis longus, (d) extensor carpi radialis brevis, (e) extensor pollicis longus, (f) extensor digitorum, (g) extensor indicis, (h) extensor digiti minimi, and (i) extensor carpi ulnaris

Source: Photo courtesy of Jeffrey D. Smithers, M.D.

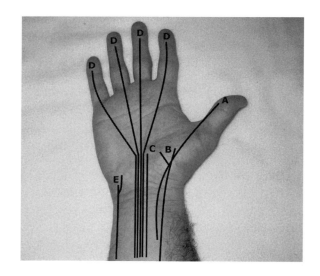

Tendons of the volar aspect of the wrist: (a) flexor pollicis longus, (b) flexor carpi radialis, (c) palmaris longus, (d) flexor digitorum (superficialis and profundus), and (e) flexor carpi ulnaris

Source: Photo courtesy of Jeffrey D. Smithers, M.D.

refers to inflammation of the tendon substance and rarely occurs without the presence of underlying degenerative tendon change, or *tendinosis*. *Paratenonitis*, or alternatively *tenosynovitis*, involves inflammation of the paratenon/tendon sheath, can occur alone or in combination with tendinosis, and constitutes the majority of wrist tendinopathy. However, elite and older athletes also often have some component of underlying tendinosis contributing to their symptoms.

De Quervain disease and intersection syndrome are the two most common athletic wrist tendinopathies. De Quervain disease is a paratenonitis of the tendons in the first dorsal compartment. Intersection syndrome, while not a classic paratenonitis, represents inflammation of the crossover area where the musculotendinous junctions of the first dorsal compartment meet with the tendons of the second dorsal wrist compartments. Less common wrist tendinopathies in sports include the separate syndromes of ECU and FCU (flexor carpi ulnaris) paratenonitis along with the infrequent flexor carpi radialis (FCR) paratenonitis and carpal tunnel syndrome from paratenonitis of the digital flexor tendons.

Causes

Wrist tendinopathy in athletes results from chronic microtrauma due to tendon overuse. While athlete ageing and tendon underuse can contribute to degenerative tendon changes, most wrist tendinopathies are caused by a combination of numerous factors, the most important being excessive repetition of wrist and hand motion. Such motion is required in many sports, including racquet sports (tennis, squash), golf, baseball, volleyball, gymnastics, rowing, and rock climbing. Other factors contributing to wrist tendinopathy include muscle imbalance or weakness, improper technique (e.g., excessive wrist radial deviation on the tennis forehand), improper equipment (e.g., size of the bat or racquet handle), and inadequate recovery time.

Causative sports for specific wrist tendinopathies are those that involve motions isolating the involved tendons. For example, de Quervain disease affects two tendons exerting their action on the thumb and is common in sports that require strong or repetitive thumb motion, such as racquet (tennis) and other hand grip sports (rowing and golf). Intersection syndrome involves tendons that

act on both the thumb and the radial aspect of the wrist, is caused by repetitive wrist extension in radial deviation, and is encountered in many of the previously mentioned sports, along with weight lifting and downhill skiing. ECU paratenonitis and tendinosis occur from excessive wrist extension in ulnar deviation and are seen especially in racquet sports, golf, and rowing. FCU paratenonitis is also common among golf and racquet sport athletes.

Clinical Evaluation

History

Suspicion for wrist tendinopathy in an athlete generally stems from pain over the involved tendon(s). Pain from paratenonitis is typically constant and proportional to activity level and can be seen in athletes of all ages. Patients with paratenonitis usually report a recent increase in the duration or intensity of their sports activity and often note accompanying swelling, stiffness, and wrist "squeaking." Alternatively, athletes with tendinosis will complain of more intermittent pain and will usually have a remote history of overuse. Patients with tendinosis will also typically complain of pain that starts during the warm-up phase, decreases during activity, and increases during the cooldown and recovery phases. Finally, patients with tendinosis will describe a course of pain that begins as sharp and intense and becomes more dull and achy over time. Because paratenonitis can be seen in combination with tendinosis, symptoms from both processes can co-occur.

Accompanying symptoms such as paresthesia, weakness, radiation of pain, blunt trauma, fever, and overlying skin changes should be ruled out in the athlete with tendon pain. The presence of these symptoms should prompt consideration of more extensive differential diagnosis and work-up. Of note, rheumatologic conditions such as rheumatoid arthritis affect the synovium, causing both arthritis and paratenonitis, and should be suspected in an athlete with recurrent or diffuse paratenonitis.

Physical Examination

A thorough examination of the affected forearm, wrist, and hand along with comparison with the nonaffected side is necessary in evaluating athletes with suspected wrist tendinopathy. They will have pain to tendon palpation, especially under tension with manual muscle testing. As with most inflammatory conditions, patients with wrist paratenonitis will have associated palpable swelling and increased temperature over the affected area of the tendon. Patients with wrist paratenonitis can also have crepitus and occasional catching with passive movement of the involved joint, as in passively flexing and extending the wrist in ulnar deviation to evaluate ECU paratenonitis. Finally, the athlete will often have pain with the tendon in full stretch, such as the Finkelstein maneuver, in which the patient is asked to make a clenched fist about the adducted thumb and the examiner subsequently places the patient's wrist in ulnar deviation. Pain over the radial styloid (distal radius) with this maneuver is highly specific for de Quervain disease.

Imaging

Clinical assessment with history and physical examination is usually sufficient for accurate diagnosis and classification of wrist tendinopathy. Plain radiographs in tendinopathy are routinely negative, and advanced imaging is rarely required. However, in cases recalcitrant to initial therapy or where more significant tendon disruption is suspected, magnetic resonance imaging (MRI) and ultrasound can serve as helpful adjuncts. On the MRI scan, paratenonitis demonstrates increased (fluid) signal in the tendon sheath on T2 and STIR (short inversion time inversion recovery) sequences, whereas tendinosis shows less uniform increased intratendinous signal on the same sequences. Ultrasound examination of paratenonitis demonstrates anechoic signal (representing fluid) in the surrounding tendon sheath, and in tendinosis, it shows hypoechoic intratendinous regions.

Treatment

The mainstay of wrist tendinopathy treatment is conservative therapy relying on relative rest, ice, analgesics (e.g., oral or topical nonsteroidal medications), physical therapy, and short courses of wrist bracing or splinting, to include thumb spica immobilization in cases of de Quervain disease. In paratenonitis, use of topical (e.g., iontophoresis) or systemic corticosteroid treatment can be beneficial,

and local injections of topical anesthetic and corticosteroid into the tendon sheath by skilled hands are often effective in confirming the diagnosis and treating the condition. In cases with underlying tendinosis, anti-inflammatory treatments do not treat the underlying degenerative pathology and cannot prevent recurrence. The most widely accepted treatment modality for tendinosis is eccentric muscle strengthening of the affected muscle-tendon unit. In all tendinopathies, adjustment of the underlying modifiable risk factors, such as errors in technique, training schedule, or equipment, must always be addressed for adequate treatment and prevention of recurrence. In rare cases where the athlete's wrist tendinopathy does not respond to conservative treatment, surgical release of the tendon sheath or debridement of the degenerative tendon may be indicated.

Conclusion

Wrist tendinopathy from tendon overuse commonly affects athletes participating in tennis, golf, and other sports requiring repetitive wrist and hand motion. Inflammation of the tendon sheath surrounding the tendon, or paratenonitis, is the most common underlying pathology in these cases and often responds to conservative therapy with relative rest, analgesics, and anti-inflammatory modalities without long-term sequelae.

Jeffrey D. Smithers

See also Colles Fracture; Musculoskeletal Tests, Hand and Wrist; Wrist Dislocation; Wrist Fracture; Wrist Sprain

Further Readings

DeLee JC, Drez D Jr, Miller MD. *DeLee and Drez's Orthopaedic Sports Medicine*. 3rd ed. Philadelphia, PA: Elsevier; 2009:1321–1335.

Honing EW. Wrist injuries. Part 2: spotting and treating troublemakers. *Phys Sportsmed*. 1998;26(10):63–70.

Moore JS. De Quervain's tenosynovitis: stenosing tenosynovitis of the first dorsal compartment. *J Occup Environ Med*. 1997;39(10):990–1002.

Rettic AC. Athletic injuries of the wrist and hand. Part II: overuse injuries of the wrist and traumatic injuries to the hand. *Am J Sports Med*. 2004;32(1):262–264.

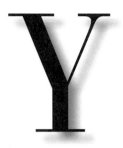

YOUNG ATHLETE

Youth participation in sports has increased dramatically in recent years. Children are becoming involved at younger and younger ages and are training with increasing intensity. Understanding their unique needs with respect to injury patterns, changing body habits, and psychological development is key to dealing with the child athlete. A sensible approach to training that takes into consideration skill level and motivation, as well as physical and emotional development, will help prevent injuries and promote enjoyment of the sport. For the child who becomes involved in competition, acquisition of skills and fitness must be balanced with avoidance of overtraining. It is important to have some knowledge of the types of injuries our young athletes sustain and an understanding of the prevention and rehabilitation of these injuries. Finally, the most influential people in the child athlete's life, coaches and parents, need to help the child keep winning in perspective.

Uniqueness of the Child Athlete

Growth and development are the most important features that distinguish young athletes from adults. The changing mechanical properties of growing bones and tissues give rise to maturation-related injuries. Bone growth occurs first, followed by a secondary lengthening of muscle–tendon units and ligaments. Many experts feel that during a growth spurt, there is a relative decrease in flexibility before the soft tissues catch up with bone growth. This decrease in flexibility places the child at risk for injuries such as Osgood-Schlatter apophysitis or patellofemoral pain. The imbalances in muscle strength and flexibility that occur during these periods of growth are risk factors for both sudden (acute) injuries and overuse injuries. Growing bones themselves are weakened because bone matrix formation and mineralization do not occur at the same rate. As a result, children's bones are less dense than those of adults.

The types of bony injuries sustained by children are quite different from adult injuries. For example, a similar mechanism of injury may produce a displaced or comminuted fracture in an adult bone, but it may only cause bending (plastic deformation) of the softer bone of the child athlete. The inherently weak growth plate (physis) is involved in 30% of all fractures of the long bones of children. During different stages of development, the relative strength of the physes changes, with the time of the greatest vulnerability to injury being the onset of the adolescent growth spurt. At such times, if stressed, the musculoskeletal system will break down at the growth plates before the adjacent ligaments tear. In prepubescence and again in late pubescence after growth has slowed, the physes may actually be stronger than the adjacent ligaments; therefore, true sprains are more likely to occur than injuries to the physes.

The main concern with growth plate injuries is the potential for altered growth. This also depends on the child's stage of development. For example, repetitive microtrauma to the wrists in gymnasts during early puberty may result in a temporary decrease in growth of the growth plate at the lower portion of the forearm (the distal radial physis). Normal growth is restored once the trauma stops. The same injury to a midpubertal gymnast may result in permanent loss of growth.

Other areas of growth tissue occur at the tendon insertions of large muscle groups. These sites are known as apophyses and are subject to injuries unique to the growing athlete. A common site of apophyseal injury is the insertion of the patellar tendon into the top of the shin (tibial tubercle). Repetitive stress at this site can cause either apophysitis or avulsion fracture. Apophyseal injuries will be discussed later in this entry. It is important to remember that the tissues of the young athlete are in transition, which has a great bearing on the types of injuries sustained.

The child athlete differs from the adult in other ways as well. The response of the cardiovascular system and the body's control of temperature (thermoregulation) to exercise in children is different from that in adults. Thermoregulation will be discussed in greater detail later. Regarding cardiovascular differences, children generally use more oxygen for a given activity and rely on anaerobic metabolism less than adults do during exercise. They tend to have higher heart rates and pump less blood from the heart with each beat (lower cardiac stroke volume) as well. This can affect how well the child tolerates physical activity. In addition, reaction time decreases as the child matures.

With increasing strength and endurance, particularly in the latter half of childhood, speed of movements and general skills increase. Thus, the innate tools that the child athlete has at his or her disposal vary with physical maturation. This should be kept in mind when setting goals for the child in sports.

Thermoregulation: Exercise in the Heat

Approximately 80% of energy released during exercise is in the form of heat. If the mechanisms for heat loss are not functioning properly, the athlete may experience a 1 °C increase in body temperature per 5 minutes of activity. If this is allowed to continue, it would be potentially fatal within 20 minutes. Mild dehydration, as little as 1.2%, may make it even more difficult to control body temperature.

Once water deficits are greater than 3%, there is a significant risk of heat illness. Heat-related illnesses include a spectrum of conditions ranging from heat cramps, which are painful, sustained muscle contractions, to life-threatening heat stroke.

Uniqueness of Children

The thermoregulatory mechanisms in children are slightly different from those in adults. Compared with adults, children produce more heat per kilogram (kg) while walking and running. They begin to sweat at a higher core temperature and sweat less per square meter. They have a lower cardiac output at a given metabolic level and less blood flow to the skin for removal of heat by convection. Their larger body surface area per kilogram results in increased heat exchange between the environment and the skin, causing greater heat stress. Their thermoregulatory impairment from dehydration is also greater.

Children are slower than adults to acclimatize to heat. Acclimatization involves physiologic changes that increase tolerance to exercise in the heat. This adaptation is influenced by age, duration of exposure to heat, rate of body heat production, severity of environmental stress, and the preexisting level of conditioning of the athlete. These differences in thermoregulation place the child athlete at increased risk of heat illness, especially in extreme heat.

Prevention of Heat Illness

Prevention of heat illness addresses environmental conditions, hydration, clothing, conditioning, and acclimatization. Activity should be modified in the face of high ambient temperature or humidity. For temperatures less than 19 °C (67 °F), the players most susceptible to heat stress should be under close observation. Unlimited supplies of drinking water should be available on the field, and athletes should be encouraged to take fluids when ambient temperatures are between 19 and 25 °C (67 and 77 °F). Water breaks should be scheduled every 20 to 25 minutes. For temperatures above 25 °C (77 °F), practice sessions should be reduced and, if possible, scheduled for early morning or late afternoon. Susceptible players, such as those with a history of heat illness, should be withheld from participation. At any temperature, if relative humidity is greater than 95%, activity should be modified as per the requirements for temperatures >25 °C.

Athletes may lose 2% to 3% body weight before thirst develops, at which point performance is already impaired. To ensure adequate hydration, adolescent athletes should be encouraged to drink 235 milliliters (ml; 8 ounces [oz]) of water 10 to 15 minutes prior to workout and 235 to 350 ml (8–12 oz) at 20- to 30-minute intervals throughout the practice. Younger, smaller athletes will need slightly less than this amount (approximately 150 ml of cold tap water every 30 minutes for a 40-kg child). After workout, drinking to quench thirst will replenish only one third to one half of fluid losses; therefore, athletes should weigh themselves before and after workout (without clothes) and should drink 1 liter/kg lost (2 cups/pound). Plain water is adequate for most activities of young athletes.

Appropriate clothing for training in the heat is lightweight, single layer, and absorbent. As much skin as possible should be exposed to air, and sweat-saturated articles of clothing should be changed. If helmets are worn, they should be removed between drills, because a significant proportion of heat loss occurs via the head. Sauna suits for weight reduction should never be permitted.

Athletes should start the season as physically fit as possible. A preseason conditioning program will give the child a good baseline fitness level, which will not only decrease the risk of heat illness but also help prevent other problems such as overuse injuries. An attempt should be made to acclimatize the athlete before beginning a strenuous program or before travel to a warm climate.

Common Injuries Associated With the Child Athlete

Several injuries occur more frequently, or in some cases uniquely, in the skeletally immature athlete. These injuries can be divided into either acute or overuse types. Acute bone injuries encountered exclusively in the child athlete include *growth plate* (physeal) *injuries* and *apophyseal avulsion fractures,* which occur when large tendons pull off (avulse) fragments of bone and growth cartilage at the sites where tendons and bones join. Other fractures seen in children (torus, greenstick, plastic deformation) occur because of a lesser degree of mineralization and thinner cortices than in adult bones. There are also several overuse injuries that are seen primarily in young athletes. The most common of these are discussed in this section.

Acute Injuries

Growth Plate Injuries

At certain times during development, growth plates are weaker than the surrounding soft tissues; therefore, when a joint is placed under abnormal stress, such as a sudden, forceful inversion of the ankle, the result is a fracture through the growth plate. This is accompanied by swelling and tenderness on the outer aspect of the ankle. There may be some tenderness over the ligaments, but if there is bony tenderness over the lateral ankle, it is likely to be a growth plate injury. This relative weakness of the physes is maximum at the onset of the growth spurt. Immediate management includes ice, elevation, and compression. Immobilization and crutches may be necessary for pain control. Early institution of physical therapy will restore function and help prevent reinjury. It is possible for young athletes to sprain ligaments rather than injure physes, particularly adolescents nearing physical maturity and prepubescent athletes.

Avulsion Fractures

Children with open physes also have apophyses at the insertion of large tendons into bone. Like growth plates, these cartilage structures are subject to injury, particularly during rapid growth. The most common acute injury to the apophysis is an *avulsion fracture.* Avulsion fractures are typically seen in 14- to 17-year-old males. These occur frequently around the pelvis, into which several large muscles insert. These athletes will complain of severe pain at the affected site and inability to continue activities. Pain will worsen with contraction of the muscle responsible for the avulsion injury. Athletes should apply ice and use crutches during the acute phase. Relative rest with early institution of physical therapy will hasten the recovery. Full range of motion and normal strength should be regained prior to return to sports participation.

Overuse Injuries

Overuse injuries result from repetitive micro-trauma to bones and soft tissue. Growth is a risk factor for overuse injury in the young athlete. Growth cartilage is inherently weak when compared with the adjacent bone and is unable to withstand excessive repetitive stress. Many experts feel that flexibility decreases with growth, as muscles and tendons are stretched by the growing bones. Muscle tightness is a well-known risk factor for overuse injury among athletes of all ages. Training error is another recognized risk factor for overuse injury. Examples of training errors include sudden increases in training intensity or duration. These errors are encountered frequently in the context of summer sport camps, where children may increase their participation in a given physical activity from a few hours per week to a few hours or more each day.

Little League Elbow

Little League elbow refers to a number of different conditions that cause pain about the elbow. The forces generated during throwing result in valgus stress to the elbow, with compression on the outer aspect and tension on the inner aspect of the joint. Specific diagnoses can include medial epicondyle apophysitis, overgrowth of the radial head, osteochondritis dissecans of the radial head, and premature closure of the radial growth plate at the elbow. If there is swelling and decreased range of motion in the joint, there may be a problem with the cartilage and bone of the joint or there may be a loose body in the elbow. The child should be referred to a physician for evaluation, and further pitching should be avoided until an assessment has been done. Management includes avoidance of aggravating activities and initiation of physical therapy for range of motion followed by strength exercises. Once pain has resolved, range of motion is full, and careful evaluation of the throwing technique to correct errors that may have contributed to the injury is done, *gradual* return to play is possible. If the number of throws per week is limited to not more than 300, it may help prevent some of these injuries.

Osgood-Schlatter Apophysitis

Osgood-Schlatter apophysitis is a painful response to repetitive stress at the patellar tendon/tibial tubercle junction. Injury of the apophysis results in pain with jumping and running and tenderness to touch. Swelling may be seen over the tibial tubercle on the upper portion of the lower leg. This condition is most often observed in young athletes who have patellar maltracking or who have recently undergone a growth spurt. In the latter situation, muscles about the knee become very tight, placing added stress on the extensor mechanism. A similar stress injury (Sinding-Larsen-Johansson syndrome) occurs at the lower pole of the patella. The presentation of Sinding-Larsen-Johansson syndrome is similar to that of Osgood-Schlatter, except that the point of maximal tenderness is the lower portion of the patella. Reassurance is the first part of treatment for Osgood-Schlatter apophysitis. Athletes and their parents need to know that this condition will resolve when growth is complete. In the meantime, attempts must be made to decrease pain and secondary inflammation and to prevent recurrence. The child should be advised to stop any jumping or running activities until the pain and swelling have subsided. Application of ice three or four times per day while the symptoms are severe may be enough to reduce the pain. Nonsteroidal anti-inflammatory drugs, or NSAIDs, are of limited use other than as analgesics, unless there is significant secondary soft tissue swelling present. A home exercise program must begin immediately to work on hamstring and quadriceps stretching. When the pain has decreased, strengthening of these muscles can begin. The athlete is permitted to return to full activity only when jumping and running are pain free. A strap brace may be placed over the patellar tendon to reduce the pull of the quadriceps on the tibial tubercle. A knee pad to protect the tibial tubercle from direct trauma may reduce incidence of flare-ups. This condition can recur and occasionally can lead to avulsion fractures of the tibial tubercle.

Osteochondritis Dissecans

Osteochondritis dissecans (OCD) is an injury that affects a localized area of cartilage on the joint surface (articular cartilage) of bone, along with a small portion of underlying (subchondral) bone. Although the exact cause of this condition is not entirely clear, there appears to be some localized insufficiency of the blood supply to the bone, likely exacerbated by repetitive trauma or compressive forces. As the bone loses its blood supply, the overlying articular cartilage and subchondral bone may become unstable. In more severe cases, the bone and cartilage fragment becomes a loose body in the joint. OCD in the knee usually occurs on the inner aspect of the lower end of the thighbone (femur). This condition is also seen in the outer aspect of the elbow in Little League elbow and in the ankle (talus). A child with OCD of the knee may present with intermittent joint swelling, pain, and limited range of motion. Management depends on the severity of the OCD and the maturity of the child. In a growing child with intact cartilage overlying the bony defect, full range of motion, and no locking, nonsurgical treatment may be adequate. The child is restricted from impact activities such as jumping and running, and early physical therapy is initiated to maintain or regain range of motion. Other treatments may include limitation on weight bearing or use of bracing. Resistive weight training should be withheld for 6 to 12 weeks until bone healing occurs. It may be as long as 6 to 12 months before the athlete can resume full activities. Arthroscopic surgery may be necessary in the presence of mechanical symptoms such as locking, if magnetic resonance imaging (MRI) suggests an unstable fragment, or if more conservative treatment does not result in healing after 3 to 6 months.

Sever Apophysitis

Sever apophysitis is an injury to the calcaneal apophysis that results in tenderness at the insertion site of the Achilles tendon in the heel. Children will usually present with posterior heel pain after activity. The condition occurs in both feet in two thirds of cases and typically occurs between 7 and 14 years of age. On examination, the most tender point is the back of the heel at the Achilles tendon insertion. There may be pain with passive stretching of the calf muscles or with active plantarflexion of the ankle (downward). Squeezing the heel (squeeze test) is usually painful. To unload the painful heel, weight bearing and gait may be altered. This may result in pain and tenderness of the Achilles tendon or under the arch of the foot, clinically suggestive of Achilles tendinosis or plantar fasciitis. Treatment includes heel cups to decrease stress on the apophysis, cessation of all painful activities, and institution of physical therapy. The therapy is aimed at reducing secondary inflammation through application of ice, as well as increasing the flexibility and strength of the calf muscles. When the pain has subsided, the athlete can increase physical activity as long as the pain does not recur.

Spondylolysis

Spondylolysis is a stress fracture of the pars interarticularis, which is one of the posterior elements of the spine. This injury is most commonly encountered in sports that require repetitive extension of the spine, such as gymnastics, figure skating, and ballet. Football and hockey players may also develop this injury from the repetitive stress of sled training or body checking, respectively. The athlete will complain of low back pain with extension movements of the spine. The athlete may note tightness of the hamstrings on the affected side. On examination, there is often some degree of muscle spasm alongside the defect in the lower back. Provocative tests such as extension of the spine (arching backward) will reproduce the symptoms. There will be a relative tightness of the hamstrings on the affected side. When dealing with gymnasts and dancers, it is important to remember that they are usually extremely flexible; therefore, left and right asymmetry should be noted.

Plain X-rays may show the fracture, but a special bone scan, SPECT (single-photon emission computed tomography), will be able to definitively diagnose the lesion. Treatment involves cessation of the offending activities. A rigid, custom polypropylene brace is often used to limit extension. The brace is worn for 23 hours a day, with 1 hour out for physical therapy and showering. Once the athlete is painfree in the brace, return to modified activity is allowed. Duration of bracing is generally 6 months to allow for bony healing. Many athletes are able to return to their sport while wearing the brace.

"It Is Not Whether You Win or Lose . . . "

It has been shown that children have a much greater likelihood of dropping out of sports where the greatest emphasis is on winning. It is easy for the child athlete to begin to equate winning with success and losing with failure. Fear of failure places an enormous amount of stress on the child athlete. If a child feels that his or her "success" depends on a win, then every competitive situation becomes even more stressful and every loss adversely affects self-worth. Winning is an important goal in competitive sports, but it needs to be kept in a healthy perspective. While striving to win, the sense of success should come from putting out maximal effort. Young athletes should feel that even though they make mistakes or lose games, as long as they are trying their best, their parents and coaches will approve. This will greatly enhance the child's enjoyment of the sport, making continued participation much more likely.

Prevention Techniques

When discussing prevention in sports, one must differentiate between physical and psychological injury. The physical injuries discussed in this entry include overuse and acute trauma, as well as heat illness. Prevention of overuse injuries involves addressing risk factors before they become problematic. Preparticipation physical examinations can identify muscle imbalances and other physical factors that may predispose the athlete to injury. Preseason conditioning can reduce the risk of injury to muscles and tendons. Athletes should be educated regarding specific preventative techniques such as stretching muscles when warm and aggressively working on flexibility during growth spurts. To allow tissues to adapt to increasing work loads, training should not increase more than 10% per week. Prevention of acute injuries involves ensuring adequacy of equipment (e.g., football helmets) and striving to ensure that young athletes are matched up based on size and maturation rather than age. Rules that are meant to minimize serious trauma (e.g., no spear tackling in football) should be adhered to. Prevention of heat illness was covered earlier in this entry.

Prevention of psychological injuries is an important part of dealing with young athletes. Psychological stress occurs when athletes perceive that the demands placed on them exceed their skills. If failure is perceived as catastrophic, the stress on the athlete increases significantly. If personal value becomes dependent on success, this also adds to stress. As a result, if stress levels become too high for the athlete to cope with, he or she may withdraw from sports. If training continues, the child may develop physical symptoms such as headache or abdominal pain as a direct result of the stress or as a mechanism to avoid participation. Such situations can be avoided by addressing the causes of stress. De-emphasizing winning can significantly reduce stress. Coaches play a key role in reducing stress among athletes by enhancing enjoyment of the sport. They can provide immediate reinforcement for good plays and good efforts. Correcting errors should be done in a positive way by explaining how correct techniques will be beneficial. Coaches should not emphasize the errors that the young athlete has made. Mistakes should never be met with disapproval or yelling.

Parent-induced stress can be difficult to address. This occurs in situations where the child becomes an extension of the parents, who want their little athlete to either follow in their footsteps ("star" athlete parents) or succeed where they have fallen short. The following guidelines for parents may be helpful in these situations.

1. Parents should remain seated in the spectator area during the contest.

2. Parents should not yell instructions or criticism to their children.

3. Parents should make no derogatory comments to players, parents of the opposing team, officials, or league administrators.

4. Parents should not interfere with their children's coach. They must be willing to relinquish the responsibility for their child to the coach for the duration of the contest.

Conclusion

Because of the many benefits, both physical and mental, of sports participation children need to be encouraged to become involved. Ideally, the sport should choose the child, which means that the suitability of the child for a particular sport is considered before he or she begins. For example, a child with pes cavus (high-arched feet) may be better suited to swimming than running; however, in most cases, the child is already involved in his or her sport when problems arise. It is the role of the coach, parent, and physician to monitor the effects of the activity on the child. Intervention before problems arise can be accomplished by addressing risk factors early. When injuries occur, adequate rehabilitation will help prevent recurrence. The concept of "winning at all costs" should not be ingrained in the child athlete; rather, enjoyment of the sport should be the primary goal. It is important to remember that the elite young gymnast is not only an athlete but a child as well.

Merrilee Zetaruk

See also Apophysitis; Cardiovascular and Respiratory Anatomy and Physiology: Responses to Exercise; Juvenile Osteochondritis Dissecans of the Knee; Osgood-Schlatter Disease; Overtraining; Spondylolysis and Spondylolisthesis; Temperature and Humidity, Effects on Exercise

Further Readings

American Academy of Pediatrics Committee on Sports Medicine and Fitness. Climatic heat stress and the exercising child and adolescent. *Pediatrics.* 2000;106(1, pt 1):158–159.

Brenner JS; American Academy of Pediatrics Council on Sports Medicine and Fitness. Overuse injuries, overtraining, and burnout in child and adolescent athletes. *Pediatrics.* 2007;119(6):1242–1245.

Bruce EJ, Hamby T, Jones DG. Sports-related osteochondral injuries: clinical presentation, diagnosis, and treatment. *Prim Care.* 2005;32(1):253–276.

Emery KH. Imaging of sports injuries of the upper extremity in children. *Clin Sports Med.* 2006;25(3):543–568.

Frick S, Jones ET. Skeletal growth and development as related to trauma. In: Green NE, Swiontkowski MF, eds. *Skeletal Trauma in Children.* Vol. 3. 4th ed. Philadelphia, PA: Saunders; 2009:1–18.

LaBella CR. Common acute sports-related lower extremity injuries in children and adolescents. *Clin Pediatr Emerg Med.* 2007;8:31–42.

Mountjoy M, Armstrong N, Bizzini L, et al. IOC consensus statement: training the elite child athlete. *Br J Sports Med.* 2008;42(3):163–164.

Patel DR, Baker RJ. Musculoskeletal injuries in sports. *Prim Care.* 2006;33(2):545–579.

Purcell L. Sport readiness in children and youth. *Paediatr Child Health.* 2005;10:343–344.

Soprano JV, Fuchs SM. Common overuse injuries in the pediatric and adolescent athlete. *Clin Pediatr Emerg Med.* 2007;8:7–14.

Tofler IR, Butterbaugh GJ. Developmental overview of child and youth sports for the twenty-first century. *Clin Sports Med.* 2005;24(4):783–804.

Zetaruk MN. The young gymnast. *Clin Sports Med.* 2000;19:757–780.

Zetaruk MN. Lumbar spine injuries. In: Micheli LJ, Purcell L, eds. *The Adolescent Athlete: A Practical Approach.* New York, NY: Springer; 2007:109–140.

YOUTH FITNESS

Fitness is a state of well-being that allows the body to function efficiently and effectively during school, work, leisure, and sports activities. In general, there are two main categories of fitness. *Health-related fitness* is said to include cardio-respiratory endurance, muscular strength, muscular endurance, flexibility, and body composition, whereas *skill-related fitness* components include agility, coordination, reaction time, balance, speed, and power. Both are associated with numerous physiological and psychological benefits during childhood and adolescence. In addition, positive behaviors that are acquired during the school-age years are likely to be carried over into adulthood. Thus, youth who enjoy fitness activities and learn how to live a physically active life are more likely to become active, healthy adults.

Current Health and Fitness Status

Although youth tend to be more active than adults, nowadays fewer children and adolescents walk or ride their bicycles to school, and sedentary pursuits such as television viewing and "surfing" the Internet have decreased youngsters' need to move. A majority of children do not participate in any organized physical activity during nonschool hours, and physical education and recess periods are unfortunately viewed as expendable in some school districts. It is becoming more apparent that the lack of daily physical activity along with the greater accessibility to energy-dense foods is contributing to the increasing prevalence of obesity among school-age youth.

These trends have significant implications for the present and future health of children and adolescents, given the increased prevalence of cardiovascular disease risk factors and obesity-related comorbidities such as Type 2 diabetes, heart disease, and cancer. If current trends continue, the health-related consequences of physical inactivity and childhood obesity will likely pose an unprecedented burden on youth, their families, and our health care system. As a result, the promotion of safe, effective, and enjoyable fitness activities for children and adolescents with different needs, goals, and abilities has become a major public health issue.

General Youth Fitness Guidelines

Children and adolescents should be encouraged to be physically active as part of play, recreation, sports, and school activities. Researchers and health care providers recommend that school-age youth participate daily in 60 minutes or more of moderate to vigorous physical activity that is developmentally appropriate, that is enjoyable, and that involves a variety of activities. This recommendation provides a reasonable standard that even sedentary boys and girls can achieve with a modest commitment to physical activity and support from their parents and schools. Youth can increase the amount of time they have for physical activity by reducing sedentary leisure pursuits such as television viewing, computer use, telephone conversations, and video games. Sedentary youth should gradually increase the amount of physical activity by about 10% per week until they reach the 60-minute goal.

Since youth will rarely perform prolonged periods of physical activity without rest or recovery, youth should be encouraged to accumulate their physical activity requirement throughout the day rather than perform a continuous bout of physical activity at a predetermined intensity. While continuous moderate-to-vigorous physical activity is not physiologically harmful, it is not the most appropriate method of exercise for youth, who tend to enjoy nonsustained activities or games. Watching children on a playground supports the premise that youth tend to have short bursts of physical activity followed by brief rest periods to recover and recharge. Participation in age-appropriate fitness activities is more likely to become a lifelong habit if youth experience success, gain confidence in their physical abilities, establish a base of general fitness, and become aware of the health benefits of physical activity.

Health- and Skill-Related Fitness Activities

Unlike most adult fitness programs that isolate fitness components, youth fitness programs should provide participants with the opportunity to improve both health- and skill-related components of fitness. While the components of health-related fitness relate specifically to health enhancement and disease prevention, skill-related components are necessary to perform daily activities as well as recreational pursuits and sports skills.

Health-Related Fitness Activities

While most youth can accumulate 60 minutes of daily physical activity, health-related activities including aerobic games, strength training, and flexibility exercises must be punctuated with brief rest periods. Stop-and-go games or circuit training activities that alternate higher-effort and lower-effort segments have proven to be effective. While the standard means of assessing aerobic exercise intensity in adults is heart rate monitoring, this type of assessment is problematic for healthy children, who have great difficulty finding and counting their pulse rate during exercise. Moreover, there is little need for healthy children to monitor their heart rate response because adult target heart rate formulas are inappropriate for youth under 16 years of age. Generally, simple observations may be sufficient for determining physical exertion during youth fitness activities.

Despite traditional concerns associated with youth strength training, research clearly demonstrates that strength training can be a safe, effective, and worthwhile activity for children and adolescents provided that age-appropriate training guidelines are followed. Although there is no scientific evidence to suggest that the risks and concerns associated with youth strength training are greater than those of other sports and recreational activities in which children and adolescents regularly participate, youth strength training programs must be competently supervised, properly instructed, and appropriately designed. In general, if a child is ready for participation in some type of sport activity (generally at age 7 or 8), then he or she may be ready to strength train. Different types of equipment, including free weights (e.g., barbells and dumbbells), child-size weight machines, elastic bands, medicine balls, and body weight exercises, have proven to be safe and effective for children and adolescents.

While flexibility is a well-recognized component of health-related fitness, long-held beliefs regarding the traditional practice of warm-up static stretching have been questioned. Research findings suggest that static stretching immediately before exercise has no significant effect on injury prevention and can have a negative influence on strength and power performance in children and adolescents. Children and adolescents should perform low- to moderate-intensity dynamic activities (e.g., walk, jog, hop, skip, and jump) during the warm-up period and static stretching exercises during the cooldown period. Because gains in flexibility are specific to the flexibility exercises performed at each joint, youth should perform a variety of static stretches for the upper body, lower body, and midsection. The cooldown may actually be the ideal time to perform static stretching exercises because the muscles are already warmed up and participants need to recover from the exercise session with less intense activities.

Skill-Related Fitness Activities

Most youth programs focus primarily on enhancing the health-related components of fitness and underemphasize the importance of developing skill-related fitness abilities that are characteristic of how children move and play. Games, activities, and exercises that involve skipping, hopping, twisting, kicking, and throwing can help youngsters develop the necessary prerequisite movement skills prior to facing the demands of more demanding fitness programs and sports training sessions. With competent instruction and quality practice time, children and adolescents can learn the skills needed for successful and enjoyable participation in recreational activities and organized sports.

Leadership and Instruction

The challenges associated with promoting youth fitness should be met with enthusiastic leadership, creative programming, and effective age-specific teaching strategies. A major objective of youth fitness programming is for physical activity to become a habitual part of children's lives and, if possible, persist into adulthood. With this objective in mind, parents, teachers, and youth coaches must strive to increase participants' self-confidence in their physical abilities. To achieve this objective, clear instructions should be provided so that participants can experience success and develop a sense of mastery of a specific skill. Thus, the focus of youth fitness programs should be on positive experiences instead of stressful competition in which most children fail.

Professionals should understand the uniqueness of childhood and adolescence and should genuinely appreciate the fact that youth are active in different ways and for different reasons compared with adults. Professionals who choose to work with children and adolescents need to relate to youth in a positive manner and understand how they think. Participation in a youth fitness program is a personal choice. Thus, it is unlikely that children will continue in a program if they do not understand the games or are unable to perform the exercises. Along with the primary objective of engaging youth in fun physical activities, professionals who work with children and adolescents are also responsible for class management, quality instruction, transition periods, and skill development. Needless to say, the development of successful youth fitness programs requires preparation, coordination, and understanding of the physical and psychosocial uniqueness of childhood and adolescence.

Avery Faigenbaum

See also Pediatric Obesity, Sports, and Exercise

Further Readings

Faigenbaum A. *Youth Fitness*. San Diego, CA: American Council on Exercise; 2001.

Institute of Medicine. *Preventing Childhood Obesity. Health in the Balance*. Washington, DC: National Academies Press; 2005.

Rowland T. Promoting physical activity for children's health. *Sports Med.* 2007;37(11):929–936.

Strong W, Malina R, Blimkie C, et al. Evidence based physical activity for school-age youth. *J Pediatr.* 2005;146(6):732–737.

Glossary

acclimation The process of adjusting physiologically or psychologically to different environmental conditions, such as altitude or temperature

acetabular labrum A ring of fibrous cartilage that runs along the socket of the hip joint

acetabulum The socket of the hipbone in which the head of the femur rests, forming a ball-and-socket joint

achondroplasia The most common form of dwarfism, a genetic disorder that affects the development and maturation of bone from cartilage

acromioclavicular (AC) joint The joint located at the top of the shoulder between the acromion and the clavicle

actinic conjunctivitis An eye disease characterized by inflammation of the conjunctiva due to prolonged exposure to ultraviolet light

acute fracture Break of bone or cartilage in which the fracture line is sharp and the surrounding bone appears normal

acute injury An injury that occurs with a rapid onset after a single event

adhesion Fibrous band of scar tissue that forms between tissues not normally bound together, often resulting from injury

agonist A contracting muscle that is resisted by an antagonist muscle

air embolism Any obstruction of the circulatory system caused by the entry of air bubbles into the bloodstream, often through ruptured alveoli

all-around development The emphasis on the development of the three primary attributes of athleticism, flexibility, and musculoskeletal and cardiovascular capacities

allograft The surgical transplant of tissues or organs between different individuals of the same species

ALPSA (anterior labral periosteal sleeve avulsion) A lesion at the distal end of the shoulder associated with shoulder dislocation

alternative medicine Healing practices that fall outside the realm of conventional medical practice, such as homeopathy, acupuncture, naturopathy, or herbalism

alveoli Tiny air sacs within the lungs that facilitate the exchange of carbon dioxide and oxygen; the terminal points of the airways within the lungs

amenorrhea The absence or abnormal cessation of a menstrual period in a premenopausal female when menstruation should be present

anabolic-androgenic steroid A synthetic drug that is used to stimulate muscle and bone growth by mimicking the male hormone testosterone

anaerobic threshold   The point during exercise when the body begins to work the muscles without the use of oxygen; the limit at which aerobic exercise can be maintained

aneurysm   An abnormal blood-filled swelling of an artery or vein from weakness of the blood vessel wall

ankle inversion test   A range-of-motion test performed on the ankle; positive tests reveal a potential tear of the calcaneofibular ligament of the ankle

annular ligament   A strong band of fiber that surrounds the wrist or ankle joint

anomalous coronary arteries   Congenital variation in the origin, pathway, termination, number, or structure of the coronary arteries; most anomalies are clinically silent and do not affect quality of life

anorexia athletica   A condition in which people engage in excessive exercise to lose weight, typically associated with anorexia nervosa

anorexia nervosa   A condition in which people intentionally starve themselves for fear of gaining weight, usually characterized by extremely low body weight and body image distortion

antagonist   The counterpart of the contracting, or agonist, muscle responsible for the lengthening or stretching of the agonist

anterior apprehension test   A clinical test for assessing the instability of a shoulder, in which apprehension with abduction and external rotation of the joint suggests anterior instability

anterior drawer test   A measure of the stability and integrity of the anterior cruciate ligament of the knee

aortic stenosis   A cardiovascular disease characterized by the abnormal narrowing of the aortic valve between the left ventricle and the aorta

Apley grind test   A commonly applied diagnostic test in which the physician grips the hand of the patient and applies downward pressure, causing the hand to deviate toward the ulna

Apley scratch test   A clinical test used to assess the range of motion of the shoulders by asking the patient to scratch his or her back

Apley test   A clinical test used to assess knee or shoulder injuries

apophysis   A natural swelling or outgrowth, or protuberance, on any part of a bone

apophysitis   An inflammation of an apophysis

apprehension test   A clinical test used to assess the location and severity of injuries, which is performed by manipulating a patient's joints and gauging his or her pain response

arachnoid mater   The weblike protective covering of the brain and spinal cord; the middle of the three layers of meninges

arrhythmogenic right ventricular dysplasia   A genetic disorder of the heart that is characterized by abnormal, arrhythmic ventricular contractions

arteriovenous malformation   A congenital disorder characterized by an abnormal connection of veins and arteries, often resulting in internal bleeding and headaches

arthrofibrosis   A condition most often associated with the knee, characterized by the growth of scar tissue resulting in limited joint mobility

arthroscopic portal   Small incision through which arthroscopic surgery is performed

arthroscopy   A minimally invasive surgery that allows the physician to examine the interior of a joint and diagnose and treat common knee, shoulder, and other joint problems

articular (hyaline) cartilage   A tough, fibrous connective tissue that forms on the surface of bones within joints and aids in joint mobility

aseptic necrosis   A condition in which the lack of blood supply to the bone may cause bone tissue death

ataxia   The lack of motor coordination or the inability to coordinate skeletal muscle contractions

athlete's heart syndrome   A medical condition in which the heart enlarges in response to the physiologic stresses of strenuous physical training; typically benign but difficult to distinguish from more serious cardiovascular illnesses

athlete's nodules   A general term for relatively hard, discrete, roughly spherical, abnormal cutaneous masses occurring in individuals who engage in sports

athletic pseudonephritis   The occurrence of protein and white and red blood cells in the urine in response to strenuous physical activity, often mimicking the problems associated with kidney disease but clearing up completely after 3 days of rest

atlantoaxial instability   Increased flexibility of the ligaments between the atlas and the axis, the two bones at the top of the spinal column, with neurologic symptoms occurring when the spinal cord is affected

atlas (vertebra)   The uppermost cervical vertebra of the spine

atopy   An allergic reaction that becomes apparent almost immediately in response to a stimulus; genetically determined hypersensitivity to an allergen

ATP (adenosine triphosphate)   A complex chemical compound derived from adenosine that is formed by the energy released from food and is used to perform cellular metabolic functions; energy molecule of a cell

auditory exostosis   Benign bony growth located in the external auditory canal; frequently present in athletes who engage in water sports

autograft   Tissue that is taken from one site and grafted onto another in the body of the same individual

avascular necrosis   Death of the cells in a bone or joint due to depletion of blood supply

avulsion   A painful separation of a muscle from its attachment to a bone

avulsion fracture   Bone fracture that occurs when a tendon pulls off a piece of bone from a larger bone mass, usually as a result of a violent or forceful muscle contraction

axial compression test   A test performed by pressing on the top of the patient's head with his or her neck in a neutral position; test is positive if the pain is aggravated

axial pain (syndrome)   Pain referring to the central part of the body; back pain distinguished from the limbs

axis   The second uppermost cervical vertebra, which provides a pivot for turning the head

axon   A long extension of a neuron responsible for conducting a signal away from the cell body

balance   The capacity to remain in a controlled position without falling or losing coordination

Bankart lesion   A tear of the anterior glenoid labrum that is caused by violent movement of the arm

Basilar skull fracture   Fracture that occurs at the base of the skull or the portion underneath the brain

belly press test   A clinical test used to assess the function of one of the four muscles of the rotator cuff located within the shoulder, the subscapularis; performed with the patient in a standing position with his or her hand on the stomach, pushing as hard as possible

Bennett fracture   A bone fracture of the first metacarpal between the thumb and wrist

bipartite   Consists of two parts or divisions

Blount disease   A growth disorder of the tibia in which the lower leg angles inward; characterized by a bow-shaped lower leg

bony Bankart lesion   A fracture of the front lower portion of the glenoid; *see* Bankart lesion

bony edema   A swelling of a bone that occurs following an injury

boutonniere deformity   A deformity of the finger in which the joint nearest to the knuckle is bent inward due to misalignment of the tendons

bowlegs   Legs that bend outward instead of angling inward; the opposite of knock-knees

boxer's fracture   A fracture in the fourth or fifth metacarpal, which comprises the knuckles

brachial plexus   An arrangement of nerves that conducts signals from the spine to the shoulder and allows for movement of the arm

bronchitis   A respiratory disorder characterized by inflammation of the mucus membranes lining the bronchial tubes

bronchoconstriction   Constriction of the bronchioles (airways in the lungs) due to the tightening of surrounding smooth muscle; can cause coughing, wheezing, and shortness of breath

bulge   Swelling or outward protrusion

bulimia nervosa   An eating disorder characterized by episodes of binge eating followed by behaviors designed to prevent weight gain, such as purging, fasting, or excessive exercise

bursa (*pl.,* bursae)   A small, fluid-filled sac that provides a cushion between bones and tendons and/or muscles around a joint. Aids in reducing friction between bones and allows free movement

bursitis   Painful inflammation of a bursa caused by pressure, repetitive stress from overuse, or infection

cam impingement   An abnormal shape of the proximal femoral epiphysis that causes the femoral head to fit awkwardly within the socket, resulting in mild to severe pain

capsulorrhaphy arthropathy   A disease afflicting the shoulder characterized by deterioration of the joint surface due to previous repairs of recurrent dislocations

cardiovascular drift   A phenomenon that describes an increase in heart rate with prolonged exercise (greater than 10 minutes) despite the exercise continuing at the same intensity

catharsis   In psychiatry, the process of release of repressed memories, ideas, or emotional tension

cauda equina syndrome   A serious neurological condition characterized by a dull pain and numbness in the buttocks, genitals, and/or thigh with uncontrolled bladder and bowel function due to compression of the spinal nerves

central nervous system   The part of the nervous system consisting of the brain and spinal cord; responsible for integrating environmental signals

cerebral edema   An excess accumulation of fluid in the intracellular and extracellular spaces of the brain; a serious condition requiring emergency treatment

cerebrospinal fluid   The fluid surrounding the brain and spinal cord that protects the spinal cord and provides nutrients

cervical spine   The part of the vertebral column comprising the first seven vertebrae inferior to the skull

chair sign   A clinical test to check for elbow stability and integrity, in which the patient is seated with elbows flexed at 90°, with forearms supinated and arms abducted, and then tries to rise from the chair pushing down only with the arms

chiropractic   An alternative or complementary medical system that focuses on maintaining correct alignment of the musculoskeletal system; spinal manipulation is the most common treatment method, and many people visit chiropractors for treatment of low back pain

chondrolysis   Disappearance of the cartilage on the joint surface of the femur (articular cartilage) as a result of disintegration or dissolution

chondromalacia   A degeneration or softening of the articular cartilage

chondromalacia patella   A softening of the cartilage on the articular surface of the patella that causes pain, particularly during flexion

chondroplasty   The smoothing of torn cartilage on the joint surface

chronic exertional compartment syndrome   An exercise-induced neuromuscular condition that causes swelling and pain in the arms and legs

closed fracture   A fracture that does not pierce the skin

coarctation of the aorta   A congenital disorder characterized by narrowing of the aorta, thereby decreasing blood flow to the body

coccyx   The end of the spinal column; the base of the spine where the vertebrae are fused

co-contraction   A type of contraction when both agonist and antagonist muscles fire at the same time

Colles fracture   A fracture to the distal end of the radius bone located in the forearm

comminuted fracture   A fracture involving extensive fragmentation of bone

commotio cordis   Sudden heart failure due to a severe blow to the chest; most common in extreme contact sports

compartment   A group of related muscles found in the same area of the body

compartment syndrome   An acute medical issue characterized by the overuse of the same muscle or muscle group and decreased blood flow in a confined anatomical space

complementary medicine   A diverse set of systems of holistic medicine based on philosophies other than those used in conventional Western medicine; often called *preventive medicine*

compound fracture   The former term for a broken bone that has gone through the skin; now called *open fracture*

concentric movement   The part of the movement where the agonist muscle contracts, for example, the lifting motion of an exercise

concussion   An injury to the brain caused by a violent blow or rapid shaking; a mild concussion may involve no loss of consciousness; severe concussion may cause prolonged unconsciousness. An athlete who has had a concussion should return to play only with a physician's approval

conditioning   Development of physical fitness through adaptation of the body and its various systems to a program of exercise

conduction   The act of transmitting heat, sound, or nervous impulses from one area of the body to another

condyle   A rounded epiphysis of a bone usually encased in the articular cartilage

contralateral   Of or relating to the opposite side

contusion   A blunt force injury that does not break the skin but causes underlying tissue damage, with bleeding under the skin (bruising)

convection   The transfer of heat via gas or liquid

coordination   The ability to conduct more than one set of muscle movements in unison

coracoid   The bony prominence of the scapula

costochondritis   An inflammation at the point where the ribs fuse with the sternum

crepitus   A grinding noise or sensation within a joint or the lungs

cruciate   Cross-shaped

crutch palsy   Compressive injury to the nerve complex (the brachial plexus) located in the underarm

cyanosis   A medical condition characterized by a bluish discoloration of the skin or mucous membranes; a symptom that indicates a dangerously low level of oxygen in the discolored area

de Quervain disease   *See* de Quervain tenosynovitis

de Quervain tenosynovitis   A painful inflammation of the tunnel that surrounds the two tendons that control the movement of the thumb

debridement   Surgical removal of dead, damaged, or infected tissue and foreign matter from a wound or burn

deep vein thrombophlebitis   The formation of a blood clot within a vein, typically located in the leg; causes the extremity to become swollen, painful, red, and/or warm

dehydration   An excessive deficiency of body water

dens   A superior projection of the vertebral body that goes up into the anterior ring of the atlas

depressed skull fracture   A skull fracture in which fragmented bones press into brain tissue and cause neurological trauma

dermatophyte   A parasitic fungus that infects the skin

dermis   The deep vascular layer of the skin located beneath the epidermis

diabetes mellitus   A condition characterized by hyperglycemia, resulting from the inability to appropriately control blood sugar and regulate insulin levels

diaphragm   A muscular partition between the thoracic and abdominal cavities that regulates breathing

diaphragmatic breathing   The act of breathing deep within the lungs by focusing on lowering the diaphragm rather than expanding the chest

diaphysis   The main shaft of a long bone

diastatic skull fracture   Fracture that occurs along the growth plates or sutures of the skull

disability   A physical or mental impairment that prevents a person from performing one or more major life activities

disk herniation A condition of the vertebral column in which a tear in the outer, fibrous ring (nucleus pulposus) of an intervertebral disk allows the soft, central portion (anulus fibrosus) to bulge out, commonly known as a *slipped disk*

disk-osteophyte complex A medical condition where the soft tissue of the intervertebral disk extrudes beyond its normal parameters

displaced Pertaining to the removal from the normal position, location, or place

distraction test An orthopedic test performed on the knee; positive tests indicate a ligamentous injury of the knee

diuretic Any substance that increases the amount of urine production by the kidneys and reduces the amount of water in the blood, thereby decreasing the blood volume

dorsal Pertaining to the back surface of a body part, such as the backside (knuckle side) of the wrist and hand

dorsiflexion Backward flexion or bending toward the dorsal side; flexing the ankle and pointing the toes upward

drawer test An orthopedic test that is used to detect torn cruciate ligaments in the knee

dura *See* dura mater

dura mater The outermost layer of the meninges, the membranes surrounding the brain and spinal cord

dysesthesia A condition characterized by an unpleasant, abnormal sensation such as burning, caused by lesions of the nervous system

eccentric contraction A condition that occurs when the force generated by the muscle cannot overcome the resistance placed on the muscle; also, a lengthening contraction of the muscle

eccentric movement A movement in which the agonist muscle elongates

ecchymosis The escape of blood within subcutaneous tissue that results in discoloration or bruising

echocardiogram A sonar imaging scan used to study the structure and motions of the heart

edema A swelling of tissue due to the accumulation of excess fluid

effusion The discharge or outpouring of a fluid into a body cavity

electrocardiogram A medical record that is used to measure the electrical rhythms of the heart

endogenous Produced, occurring, or caused by factors within the body of an object or organism

endotenon A thin retinacular structure investing each tendon fiber

endurance The ability to withstand stress and hardship or sustain an activity over time; a measure of stamina

epicondyle A protrusion of a bone above the condyle that provides the surface area to which ligaments and tendons can attach

epidermis The outermost layer of the skin surface of vertebrates, which is on top of the dermis

epidural space The space between the dura mater and the lining of the spinal canal

epiphysis The rounded end of a long bone

epitenon A component that surrounds the tendon and contains the vascular, lymphatic, and nerve supply and is in turn surrounded superficially by the paratenon

erythema An abnormal red discoloration of the skin due to the dilation of cutaneous blood vessels

euhydration   A normal state of body water content

evaporative heat loss   The loss of body heat due to the evaporation of sweat from the body

excision   Surgical removal of a portion or all of an organ or other structure

exercise-associated hyponatremia   Dangerously low levels of sodium within the blood due to excessive exercise

exercise-induced hematuria   The presence of blood within the urine due to excessive exercise

exogenous   Produced, occurring, or caused by factors outside the body of an object or organism

extra-axial hemorrhage   Blood loss within the intracranial space; increases pressure, causing headaches

extreme-risk injury   Injury needing immediate medical attention

extrusion   A bulge or protuberance, pushing out

facet joints   Small joints located between adjacent vertebrae

fascia   A continuous sheet of connective tissue that separates and bonds together muscles and other organs

fasciotomy   A surgical procedure in which fascia is removed from the body to relieve tension and pressure

female athlete triad   A medical condition seen in some female athletes, characterized by disordered eating, amenorrhea, and osteoporosis

FEV$_1$ (forced expiratory volume in 1 second)   The volume of air an athlete can expel in the first second of a forced expiration; the most important parameter examined in determining airway obstruction

first-degree strain   A minor strain characterized by only a few muscle fiber tears

flail chest   A severe medical condition characterized by fragmentation of the ribs due to stress

flexibility   The ability of a muscle or extremity to relax and yield to stretch forces

focal fibrocartilage dysplasia   An uncommon, normally harmless bone lesion that causes deformity of the long bones in youth

fontanelle   The gaps located between the bones of the cranium in an infant or fetus

foramen (*pl.*, foramina)   Any opening or orifice within the body

Freiberg disease   An osteochondrosis affecting the metatarsals (long bones of the foot)

Freiberg sign   The reproduction of pain caused by passive internal rotation of the hip with the leg in an extended position

fulcrum test   By placing the left hand under the glenohumeral joint to act as a fulcrum, the apprehension test becomes a fulcrum test

functional limitation   Any health problem that prevents an individual from completing a task

ganglion cyst   A small, abnormal, fluid-filled sac (usually less than 2 centimeters) that develops near a joint capsule or tendon sheath

gastrocnemius soleus (calf muscle) strain   A strain or tear, with the sensation of a pop being felt, due to the simultaneous stretching and active contraction of the muscle

genu valgum   A medical condition characterized by an inward curvature of the legs so that the knees touch when a person is standing straight; commonly known as *knock-knees*

genu varum   A medical condition characterized by an outward curvature of the legs; commonly called *bowlegs*

GLAD lesion (glenolabral articular disruption)   Lesion characterized by a labral tear associated with an injury to the glenoid articular cartilage

glenohumeral joint   The shoulder joint that functions as a ball-and-socket joint; composed of the glenoid socket and the humeral head

glenohumeral ligaments   Three bands of connective tissue that strengthen the glenohumeral joint

glenoid   Any shallow depression of a bone resembling a pit or socket

glenoid labrum   A rim of articular cartilage that surrounds the margin of the glenoid cavity in the shoulder blade

glial cell   Nonneuronal cell that provides nutrients and removes waste from other neural cells

glycogenolysis   The process by which glycogen is broken down in the liver into individual molecules of glucose

gout   A form of arthritis caused by a buildup of uric acid in the joints

gradual progressive throwing   A shoulder rehabilitation technique in which throwing motions help stabilize the shoulder

gray matter   A large component of the central nervous system comprising glial cells, neuronal cell bodies, dendrites, axons, and capillaries

grind test   A clinical test used to determine the integrity and problems associated with the meniscus of the knee

Hawkins-Kennedy test   A test that attempts to cause external compression of the rotator cuff and consequently re-create the patient's pain

hemarthrosis   Bleeding into joint spaces

hematocrit   The volume percentage of red blood cells in a blood sample

hematoma   Swelling formed by excess accumulation of blood

hematopoiesis   The production of blood cells

hemorrhage   A copious discharge of blood from the blood vessels

hemothorax   Accumulation of blood located within the pleural cavity, or the area surrounding the lungs

hepatitis   Inflammation of the liver caused by certain viruses or other factors such as alcohol abuse or medications

hepatomegaly   Abnormal enlargement of the liver

heterotopic bone formation/ossification   The formation of bone in abnormal locations, such as in soft tissue or muscle

Hill-Sachs lesion   A depression in the head of the humeral epiphysis due to a forceful impact against the glenoid rim

hip dysplasia   An abnormal formation and deterioration of the hip socket that is characterized by excessive pain and arthritis

hip impingement   A condition that is characterized by excessive friction within the ball-and-socket hip joint

hip quadrant test   A clinical test that indicates arthritis, avascular necrosis, and/or an osteochondral defect within the hip

Homans sign   A sign of deep vein thrombosis; is positive when pain is located within the calf muscles

hop test   A clinical test used to measure the horizontal and vertical power of the legs by performing three consecutive jumps

hydrogenation   A form of chemical reduction, a chemical reaction between molecular hydrogen (H_2) and another compound or element, usually in the presence of a catalyst; commonly employed to reduce or saturate organic compounds

hyperpronation   The extreme inward rotation of the foot during gait

hyperalgesia   An increased response to pain caused by damage to the peripheral nerves

hyperesthesia   A state of abnormal increase in sensitivity to sensory stimuli

hyperlipidemia   An excess quantity of lipids in the blood

hypertrophic cardiomyopathy   A condition where the heart muscle becomes abnormally enlarged, limiting the amount of blood that can enter the heart and thereby reducing pumping ability

hyphema   A collection of blood in the anterior chamber of the eye often caused by trauma; causes blurry vision, pain, and tearing

hypodermis   The lowermost subcutaneous level of the three skin layers

hypohydration   *See* dehydration

hypothalamus   The part of the brain responsible for the control of endocrine glands and the autonomic nervous system

hypoxia   Decreased availability of oxygen to body tissues

iatrogenic   Describing inadvertent harmful consequences or complications resulting from medical treatment

idiopathic   A disease of an unknown origin

iliotibial band   A band of fascia that spans from the iliac crest of the pelvis region to the knee joint; can become inflamed due to excessive running

impingement   Striking or excessive pressure on a tissue, often from encroachment by adjacent structures

infective endocarditis   An inflammation of the membrane that lines the cavities of the heart and forms part of the heart valves, generally caused by an infection

influenza   An acute, highly contagious viral disease; also referred to as the *flu*

inguinal hernia   A protrusion of the intestines through the inguinal canal where the flesh of the abdomen meets the thigh

injury, catastrophic   An extremely serious injury that may result in disability and loss of bodily functions, with full recovery doubtful

injury, nonfatal   A broad range of types of injury from acute to catastrophic with no life-threatening issues

injury, serious   An injury in which mortality is probable

integrative medicine   A combination of alternative and conventional medicine to provide a more comprehensive healing plan for the patient

intersection syndrome   Inflammation of the crossover area where the musculotendinous junctions of the first dorsal compartment meet with the tendons of the second dorsal wrist compartments

interval training   An exercise strategy in which an athlete raises his or her exercise intensity above the anaerobic threshold for a short period of time and then dips back below the threshold and keeps exercising

intervertebral disk   A fibrocartilaginous disk that provides cushion and support between two adjacent vertebrae

intervertebral foramen   An opening between vertebrae that transmits nerves from the spine throughout the body

intraarticular dilation   An expansion within the joint

intra-axial hemorrhage   A hemorrhage that takes place within the central part of the body

iontophoresis   Therapy that uses small electric currents to deliver medicine into tissues of the body

ipsilateral   Positioned on or affecting the same side

irrigation   Cleansing injured tissue by rinsing with sterile saline, with or without antibiotics in the solution

ischemic necrosis   A condition in which the lack of blood supply to the bone may cause bone tissue death

isometric contraction   A contraction that generates muscle force but in which no joint movement occurs, such as holding a squat for 10 seconds

isotonic contraction   A contraction that occurs when the muscle contracts and joint movement occurs

jerk test   A clinical test used to determine the integrity of the knee joint (possible torn meniscus), also called Hughston's jerk test, to distinguish from the simple knee-jerk test of neurological reflex by tapping the patellar tendon.

Jobe's empty can test   A clinical test used to determine the integrity of the supraspinatus tendon

joint aspiration   The removal of fluid from within a joint

joint effusion   The escape of intraarticular fluid

joint integrity   A measure of the stability and durability of a joint

joint of Luschka   Small synovial joints between adjacent lower-cervical vertebral bodies—a frequent site of arthritis formation

Jones fracture   A fracture of the fifth metatarsal of the foot

knock-knees   A condition in which the legs curve inward at the knees; *see* genu valgum

kyphosis   An abnormal backward curve in the spinal column

labrum   A thickened portion of connective tissue that surrounds the sockets of the shoulder and hip joints

Lachman test   A test that is used for examining the integrity of the anterior cruciate ligament of the knee

lactate threshold   The point at which lactic acid buildup in the muscles begins to impair performance

lamina (*pl.*, laminae)   A broad plate which extends from the pedicle to the median line of the vertebra, two laminae fusing to complete the roof of the vertebral arch

laminectomy   Surgical removal of any part of the lamina

lateral epicondylitis   A painful inflammation of the tendon that wraps around the elbow; also called *tennis elbow*

lateral pivot-shift test   A clinical test used to evaluate the anterolateral structures of the knee

lift-off test   A clinical test used to check the stability of the shoulder

ligaments   Fibrous connective tissues responsible for connecting bones, cartilage, and other structures

linear fracture   A fracture that runs parallel to the axis of the bone

load and shift test   An orthopedic test used to check for the stability and integrity of the shoulder

loose body   A free-floating piece of bone or cartilage that has broken away and is moving around a joint

lordosis   An inward forward curve of the lower spine

lucid interval   A temporary improvement in a patient's condition following a traumatic brain injury, after which the patient's condition deteriorates

Ludloff sign   A test checking the ability to flex the thigh while sitting down; is positive if patients fail to perform the test, and negative if performed effectively

lumbar   The portion of the spinal column between the thorax and the pelvis, commonly called the lower back

luteal phase   The second half of the menstrual cycle lasting from ovulation to menstruation

malleolar bursitis   Swelling and pain over the ankle bone caused by irritation of the bursa, a fluid-filled sac that aids in reducing friction between moving bones

McMurray test   A test used to determine whether a meniscal tear is present in the knee by bending the lower leg, straightening it out, and rotating it; is positive if pain is found around the area of the meniscus

medial and lateral patellar glide test   A test used to determine the stability of the lateral retinaculum in the knee and the medial aspect of the knee

medial epicondylitis   An overuse injury, commonly known as *golfer's elbow,* that causes pain in the inside of the elbow

medial tibial stress syndrome   An overuse injury, commonly known as *shin splints,* causing irritation in the shinbone, which is located in the front of the lower leg

mediastinum   The central cavity surrounded by the lungs, containing the heart, proximal aorta, and vena cava and lined by a protective tissue, the pericardium

meninges   Protective coverings of the brain and spinal cord, consisting of three layers from outermost to innermost—namely, the dura mater, arachnoid, and pia mater

meniscal cartilage   The cushioning tissue of the knee between the femur and the tibia

meniscus   A structure consisting of both the lateral and the medial cartilage of the knee, acting as a pad between the joints of the femur and the tibia and providing a smooth surface for the joints to glide on

menorrhagia   Excessive menstruation that lasts for more than 7 days

metabolic ketoacidosis   A condition that usually affects patients with diabetes when the body has very low levels of insulin and starts to break down body fat, leading to the formation of a high concentration of ketone bodies, and thus causing the blood to become too acidic

metaphysics   The study of reality in relation to such questions that may not be answered scientifically; also, the study of subjects relating to mind and matter

metatarsalgia   An overuse injury that causes pain in the middle region of the forefoot

microfracture   A surgical technique in which tiny holes are made in the exposed bone in an area of the joint where the full thickness of the cartilage has been completely damaged

microtrauma   The term given to microscopic injuries such as microtears in muscles, tendons, and tissues

milk test   An orthopedic measure to test elbow instability

Monteggia fracture   A break in the ulna bone of the forearm, along with dislocation of the radial head

Morton neuroma   Irritation, pain, and swelling of the nerve located between the third and fourth toes of the foot

moving valgus stress test   A test used to determine whether the medial collateral ligament (MCL) of the elbow is torn

MR (magnetic resonance) arthrogram   A test used to examine the joints in the body, such as the knee or shoulder, in which a contrast-enhancing dye is injected to facilitate viewing by magnetic resonance imaging

muscle hypertrophy   The increased cross-sectional size of the muscle fibers

muscle strength   The ability of the muscle to create force against physical objects

muscular endurance   The ability of a muscle to perform and maintain repeated muscle contractions over long periods of time

myocarditis   An inflammation of the heart muscle (myocardium)

myocardium   Cardiac muscles that make up the bulk of the heart wall

myofascial release   The adding of pressure with the thumb over the muscle spasm to decrease the contraction

myositis ossificans   The formation of bone within muscle tissue; occurs after the tissues surrounding the muscles are damaged in a traumatic injury

Neer test   A test that attempts to cause external compression of the rotator cuff and consequently recreate the patient's pain

nerve impingement   (or "pinching" of the nerve) Refers to pain in or impaired function of a nerve that is under pressure

nerve root   A part of a collection of nerve fibers that branch off from the spinal cord. Dorsal roots are composed of sensory fibers that bring information into the spinal cord. Ventral roots are composed of motor neurons that carry commands from the spinal cord to the muscles and internal organs

nerve tracts   A collection of nerve fibers located in the central nervous system (CNS)

neurons   Nerve cells; the conducting cells of the nervous system that receive and transmit information through chemical and electrical signals

Noble compression test   A test used to check for iliotibial band syndrome

nondisplaced   A type of fracture in which the bone maintains its normal alignment after breaking

nonpurging-type bulimia nervosa An eating disorder involving excessive eating along with attempts to compensate afterward through diet pills, fasting, or excessive exercise

nonunion A fractured bone that failed to heal properly

nuchal ridge A thick crest located on the back of the neck and base of the skull (occipital bone)

nucleus pulposus A gelatinous substance found in the center of intervertebral disks of the spinal column; aids in shock absorption

Ober test A test used to evaluate the shortening of the iliotibial tract muscle

O'Brien test A test used to evaluate acromioclavicular joint injury in the shoulder

OCD *See* osteochondritis dissecans

occipitocervical injuries An injury of the cervical spine in which the cranium dislocates from the neck, a severe injury that can be fatal if not treated immediately

odontoid process A toothlike structure found in the second vertebra of the neck

open fracture A fracture in which the bone penetrates through the skin, also called a compound fracture

orthorexia nervosa An eating disorder characterized by an excessive concern with eating healthy foods (not officially recognized as a medical diagnosis)

orthosis A support device used to brace or correct the function of specific limbs—for example, arch supports that are used to correct foot function

os acromiale Pain in the shoulder due to the failed fusion of the bone at the front of the shoulder roof known as the acromion

os odontoideum A separation of the top of the dens from the C2 vertebral body

ossicle The smallest bones in the body, of which three are located in the middle ear

osteoarthritis A form of arthritis; a degenerative disease that affects joints and also leads to the gradual breakdown of cartilage and the formation of "bone spurs" on joints

osteoblasts Cells in the body that are responsible for bone formation

osteochondral injury An injury that affects the articular cartilage and the bone underneath

osteochondritis Inflammation of bone and cartilage

osteochondritis dissecans (OCD) An injury in which fragments of cartilage and bone are separated from the end of the bone and are loose in the joint space

osteochondrosis The necrosis or breakdown of growth centers in the pediatric or skeletally immature patient followed by regeneration or healing

osteoclast A body cell that not only breaks down bone tissue but also absorbs it back into the body

osteolysis The active resorption of bone matrix by osteoclasts as part of an ongoing disease process

osteonecrosis A condition in which the lack of blood supply to the bone may cause bone tissue death

osteopenia A condition in which the level of bone mineral density is below normal levels, but not as severe as in osteoporosis

osteophyte An abnormal growth of bone in damaged joint areas, more commonly known as a *bone spur;* commonly seen in osteoarthritis due to the nature of degenerative joints

osteoporosis   A disease that causes bones to lose density, strength, and tissue over a period of time, leaving bones fragile and more susceptible to injuries such as fractures

osteotomy   A surgical procedure that involves cutting the bone to promote proper alignment and healing in the affected joint area; can be used for arthritis treatment and to fix bones that may have grown incorrectly

otalgia   Ear pain, of which there are two types: (1) pain originating from the outside of the ear, or *referred otalgia*, and (2) pain that originates from within the ear, or *primary otalgia*

otorrhea   A discharge of fluid from the ear canal

Ottawa ankle rules   A set of guidelines established to help physicians determine whether X-rays are needed to diagnose possible fractures in the foot or ankle

Ottawa knee rules   A set of guidelines established to help physicians determine whether X-rays are needed to diagnose knee injuries

outer annulus   The outermost layer of fibrocartilage in an intervertebral disk, tears or ruptures of which may permit extrusion of the nucleus pulposus into the surrounding tissue

overreaching   A condition in which an athlete trains excessively, causing stress, fatigue, and sometimes poor athletic performance

Pace sign   A test used to determine whether a patient has piriformis syndrome, a compression of the sciatic nerve by the piriformis muscle of the thigh

paraplegia   Partial or complete paralysis of the lower extremities caused by a spinal cord defect or traumatic injury

paratenon   The external covering of the entire tendon

paratenonitis   Inflammation of the paratenon, the outermost layer of the tendon

paresthesias   The occurrence of abnormal nerve sensations such as tingling, burning, itching, and "pins and needles," sometimes caused by nerve damage

parietal pleura   A specialized skinlike surface that lines the thoracic cavity

patellar tendinosis   Inflammation or long-term damage to the tendon that connects the bottom of the kneecap to the top of the shinbone

patellar tendon   The attachment of the quadriceps muscle to the tibia

patellar tilt test   A test used to assess the tightness of the lateral side of the knee and also pain around the kneecap (patella)

Pavlik harness   A soft brace used for babies less than 6 months old with thighbone fractures

periodization   The process of splitting up time into blocks; in sports medicine, the splitting up of a training regimen into phases

periosteum   A membrane/tissue covering all bones

peripheral nervous system   Composed of the nerves outside the brain and spinal cord, which also connect the central nervous system to the sensory organs, limbs, and muscles

pertussis   A contagious bacterial disease that causes violent coughing, commonly known as whooping cough

pes planus   A condition in which the arch of the foot collapses and touches the ground, commonly called *flat feet*

petechiae   Round red spots that are visible on the skin due to bleeding under the skin

phalanges (*sing.,* phalanx)   The bones of the fingers and toes

pharmacokinetics   The study of what happens to a drug after it is taken into the body, that is, how it is metabolized

phonophoresis   A technique using ultrasound to help the body absorb therapeutic drugs through the skin

physiatrist   A physician who specializes in physical and rehabilitation medicine

physis   The growth plates at the ends of long bones

pia mater   The innermost layer of the meninges, the membranes surrounding the brain and spinal cord

pincer impingement   A form of hip abnormality in which the front edge of the hip socket sticks out too far

piriformis sign   A test used to determine whether the pain originating in the gluteus maximus causing referred pain down the leg is due to piriformis syndrome

pivot-shift test   A test used to determine the stability of the anterior cruciate ligament (ACL) in the knee

plantar fascia   A series of connective tissues that start from the heel and support the arch in the foot

plantarflexion   Bending of the foot in a downward direction

pleura   A membrane that surrounds the lungs and also covers the diaphragm and lines the inner chest wall, forming a potential space for lung expansion

pleural cavity   The body cavity that surrounds the lungs

plica syndrome   An inflammation of the plica (*see* plicae) found in the knee

plicae   Bands of synovial tissue located in the lining of a joint

plication   A surgical procedure used to tighten tissues by folding them into tucks and suturing them

pneumomediastinum   A pathological condition consequent to trauma to the chest in which air leaks from the injured lungs into the middle of the chest (mediastinum)

pneumonia   An inflammation of the lungs caused by infection

pneumothorax   A serious condition that occurs following the collapse of a lung, in which air collects in the pleural space surrounding the lungs and makes breathing difficult

popliteal   Refers to the structures in the back of the knee, such as veins, nerves, arteries, and so on

positive J sign   A test that shows the patella tracking laterally as the knee changes from flexion to extension

posterior drawer test   A test to evaluate the posterior cruciate ligament (PCL) in the knee, especially for tears and ruptures

posterior Lachman test   A test used to diagnose a torn anterior cruciate ligament (ACL)

posterior sag test   A test used to determine instability in the posterior cruciate ligament

posture   The position in which the body is held upright against gravity while standing or sitting down

power   A force that is exerted over a period of time

progressive muscle relaxation   A set of skills whereby the athlete is trained to control the tension of his or her muscles by alternatively consciously flexing them, holding the tension, and then slowly releasing them

progressive overload   The increased stress placed on the body during exercise

prolotherapy   A form of therapy that involves injection of a substance into the body to strengthen weakened tissues and also alleviate pain

proprioception   The ability to sense the position and movement of muscles

protrusion   An extension beyond the usual limits

pseudocyst   An abnormal sac that resembles a true a cyst but lacks membranous lining

pterygium   An abnormal growth that begins on the white of the eye and invades the cornea, the clear tissue covering the iris and the pupil, which may result from overexposure to sunlight and can be surgically removed. May also refer to a winglike triangular membrane abnormally occurring in the neck, eyes, knees, elbows, ankles, or digits

pudendal nerve compression syndrome   Pain in the pelvic area due to compression activities such as cycling

pudendal nerve entrapment syndrome   Chronic pain in the pelvic area due to stretching, inflammation, or compression of the pudendal nerve

pulmonary contusion   Bruising of the lungs that causes pain and difficulty in breathing

pulmonary edema   Excess fluid buildup in the lungs; can be caused by circulatory problems such as congestive heart failure

pulse oximetry   A method in which the oxygen saturation of the hemoglobin is monitored

purging-type bulimia nervosa   A type of disorder in which the bulimia patient uses vomiting, laxatives, diuretics, or enemas to rid the body of consumed calories

purpura   Bleeding under the skin characterized by purple or red discoloration spots

push-up sign   A test for posterolateral instability in the elbow

pyrogen   A substance that causes a rise in body temperature and subsequent fever; released by certain bacterial infections

quadriceps tendon   The tendon above the patella (kneecap)

radiation heat loss   The loss of heat from the body, most significant between sunset and sunrise, due to infrared emission

radicular pain   Muscle weakness, tingling, numbing, and pain due to the compression of a spinal nerve root

radicular symptom   Pain manifested in the legs or arms due to a compressed spinal nerve root

radiculopathy   The inflammation of spinal nerve roots

reduction   The technique of returning a fractured bone to its proper alignment

release test   A test in which a force that decreases the patient's pain is removed, causing the pain to return

relocation test   A test used to determine whether anterior instability is present within the shoulder

Renee creak test   A test used to diagnose pain and tightness in the iliotibial band; is positive if pain is present when standing on the affected leg with knee flexion at 30°

retromalleolar groove   A concavity located in the fibula, which when abnormally shaped can lead to tearing of the peroneus brevis (PB) tendon

reversibility   Reduction or complete loss of fitness as the result of not training

rheumatoid arthritis   An autoimmune disorder that causes chronic inflammation in the joints and can also affect other organs in the body

rhinitis   An inflammation of the mucous membrane inside the nose, commonly known as a stuffy nose, that is associated with the common cold and allergies

rhinorrhea   Fluid nasal discharge; "runny nose." Following head injury, may indicate leakage of cerebrospinal fluid, a serious condition requiring prompt medical attention

ribs, false   Five ribs, located inferiorly to the true ribs, called "false" because not directly connected to the sternum

ribs, floating   The lowest two sets of ribs attached to the vertebrae in the lower back

ribs, true   The uppermost seven pairs of ribs, attached to the sternum

rickets   A disorder that leads to the weakening and softening of bones in children; caused by lack of vitamin D and, in some cases, lack of adequate calcium intake

righting reflexes   A neuromuscular response that enables the body to regain its normal position when it has been displaced

rotator cuff   A structure composed of four muscles that stabilize the shoulder joint and allow shoulder movement, namely the supraspinatus, infraspinatus, teres minor, and subscapularis

sacrum   The triangular bone located in the base of the spine, composed of five fused sacral vertebrae forming the rear of the pelvis

sarcopenia   The degenerative loss of muscle mass and strength due to aging

second-degree strain   An injury in which the muscle is overstretched, causing inflammation and pain; involves most of the muscle fibers tearing and difficulty performing certain movements

second impact syndrome   A condition involving a second concussion before the first has properly healed; a serious, often fatal injury in which the brain rapidly swells up, causing an increase in the intracranial pressure

secretory phase   The second half of the menstrual cycle

septal hematoma   Bleeding within the nasal septum

sequestration   An abnormal separation of a part from a whole, such as a portion of a bone by a pathological process or a portion of the circulating blood into the surrounding soft tissue from a broken blood vessel

Sever disease   Pain in the heel due to the inflammation of the growth plate (calcaneus) located in the back of the foot

shear injury   An axonal injury to the brain due to accelerated rotational forces

shoulder capsule   A structure that provides extra stability to the shoulder joint

SLAP lesion (superior labrum anterior-posterior)   An injury to the glenoid labrum, located in the shoulder

slipped disk   A condition of the vertebral column in which a tear in the outer, fibrous ring (nucleus pulposus) of an intervertebral disk allows the soft, central portion (anulus fibrosus) to bulge out. *See* disk herniation

slump test   A physical examination to evaluate the sciatic nerve in cases of pain in the spinal and lower extremities

Smith fracture   An injury to the distal radius (forearm bone)

spasm   An involuntary contraction of a muscle

specificity   A measure of a test's ability to rule out a disease

Speed test   A test to evaluate whether pain is present in the bicipital groove of the shoulder

spica   A body casting to treat fractures

spinal stenosis   A narrowing of the space enclosed by the spinal column, causing pressure on the spinal cord

spirometry   A test used to measure the breathing capacity of the lungs

spondylolisthesis   Forward displacement of a vertebra over a lower segment due to a congenital defect or fracture in the pars interarticularis

spondylolysis   The breaking down of a vertebra, usually leading to small stress fractures from an overuse injury

spondylolytic   A term used to describe a patient with a degenerative disorder of the pars interarticularis, a structure found in the vertebrae

spondylosis   A degenerative disorder that affects the intervertebral disks in the spine, often referred to as spinal osteoarthritis

sports concussion   A head injury caused by either mild or severe impact during sports activity that causes the brain to shake violently within the cranium

sports hernia   A condition that occurs when muscles and tendon in the lower abdomen become weakened, usually causing chronic groin pain in athletes; not a true hernia

Spurling test   A test for pain in the neck originating from the spinal nerve roots

Stener lesion   A condition that occurs when the ulnar collateral ligament (UCL) tears and the surrounding tissue of the overlying thumb tendon gets lodged between the torn UCL fibers

stenosis   A condition in which the blood vessels and tubular organs become narrowed and constricted

strain   The stretching or partial tearing of the muscle, resulting in inflammation and pain

strength   The ability of a muscle to generate and resist physical force

stress fracture   A small crack in a bone, usually caused by overuse

stress fracture test   A bone scan used to evaluate the injured area on the bone

stretch reflex   A muscle contraction in response to stretching within the muscle; also known as a myotatic reflex

stroke volume   The amount of blood that is pumped out of a ventricle in the heart during a contraction

structural tolerance   The ability to withstand weeks or months of high-volume training without the incidence of injury, illness, or fatigue that may lead to overtraining

Stryker notch view   An X-ray view used to evaluate for Hills-Sachs lesion after a dislocation

subacromial impingement   Pain in the shoulder caused by friction between the rotator cuff and acromion

subarachnoid space   The meningeal space located between the arachnoid and the pia mater

subchondral bone   A bone layer that underlies the articular cartilage

subcutaneous emphysema   A pathological condition that occurs when air is trapped beneath the tissues in the skin of the chest, neck, and face

subdural space   The space between the dura mater, the outermost meningeal layer, and the underlying arachnoid mater, caused by an injury or a pathologic process such as a subdural hematoma

subluxation   A condition that occurs when the patella, commonly called the kneecap, becomes partially dislodged from its normal position

subtalar neutral position   The normal position of the foot when one walks

sulcus sign   A test to evaluate the presence of inferior instability within the glenohumeral joint

superior retinaculum   The ligament binding the extensor tendons closest to the ankle joint

surfer's ear   A condition that occurs when the ear canal becomes blocked due to abnormal bone growths, called exostoses, caused by prolonged exposure to cold water and wind

surfer's myelopathy   A nontraumatic spinal cord injury in which blood flow to the spine is interrupted when the back is hyperextended, sometimes causing partial or complete paraplegia

swan-neck deformity   A hand deformity in which the distal joint of the finger is pointed inward and the proximal joint outward

synchondrosis   A cartilaginous joint that joins bone to bone, such as the sternocostal joints where the first ribs join the sternum

syncope   A temporary loss of consciousness, commonly known as fainting

synostosis   A condition in which two separate bones fuse together as one

synovial cyst   A cyst that is filled with synovial or joint fluid to produce its characteristic bulge

synovial fluid   The lubricant that serves to reduce friction of the articular cartilage within the joint capsule

synovial tendon sheath   A membrane consisting of an outer fibrotic sheath and an inner synovial sheath, which may be found in areas subject to increased mechanical stress where efficient lubrication is required

synovitis   An inflammation of the synovium, the tissue that lines the joints

synovium   A soft tissue that lines the joints and produces synovial fluid

syringomyelia   A disorder characterized by the formation of a cyst in the spinal cord

tachycardia   A heart rate faster than normal

tarsal coalition   A condition in which two bones in the back of the foot (tarsal bones) are fused

tendinitis   The inflammation of the tendon; rarely occurs without the presence of underlying degenerative tendon change

tendinopathy   Tendon injuries such as tiny tears, pain, and inflammation

tendinosis   A noninflammatory repetitive injury to the tendon resulting in microtears that do not heal properly

tendon A band of fibrous connective tissues that connect a muscle to a bone

tenodesis stabilization Procedures that are indicated for patients with lateral ankle instability with failed anatomic repair; consists of a suture of the end of a tendon to a bone

tenosynovitis An inflammation of a tendon and its sheath

tenotomy A surgical procedure that involves cutting or releasing a tendon

tension pneumothorax A condition that forms a one-way valve, allowing air to enter the pleural space but not to escape; the buildup of air within the pleural space producing pressure on the lungs, thus making breathing difficult

tetraplegia A traumatic spinal injury that causes complete paralysis of all limbs

therapeutic exercise A therapy with goals such as improving musculoskeletal function, recovering from injuries, and providing relaxation

thermoregulation Control of body temperature

third-degree strain The most severe type of strain, which occurs when a muscle has been completely ruptured due to an injury

Thomas test A test used to evaluate whether a patient can extend the hips

Thompson test A test used to evaluate for an Achilles tendon rupture

thoracic kyphosis An abnormal forward curvature of the upper back region

thoracic spine The middle region of the spine, consisting of 12 vertebrae

tibia vara A growth disorder of the upper shinbone, causing a bowlegged appearance

tinea capitis A contagious infection of the scalp caused by a fungus, commonly called ringworm

tinea corporis A contagious fungal infection affecting the skin, commonly known as ringworm

tinea cruris A fungal infection affecting the groin area, commonly called jock itch

tinea pedis A fungal infection of the foot, commonly known as athlete's foot

Tinel test One of two tests used to diagnose the presence of carpal tunnel syndrome

tophi The buildup of uric acid in joints, bones, and cartilage

torticollis A pathological condition involving uncontrolled spasms of the neck muscles so that the neck remains in a twisted position with the head tilted and turned to one side

toss The act of disengaging a member of a cheerleading team from either a pyramid or a base arrangement

traction apophysitis An inflammation of an unfused apophysis caused by excessive pull of an attached tendon

training load The product of all three fundamental components of training: frequency, duration, and intensity

trans fat An unsaturated fat that is made into a solid by adding hydrogenated oils during manufacturing

Trendelenburg test A test to evaluate hip function, specifically of the gluteus medius muscle, in which the patient is asked to stand on one leg

triangular fibrocartilage complex A structure found in the wrist that is made up of several different structures, the primary components are being the dorsal and palmar volar ligaments

trochanter   Two bony projections located near the end of the thighbone

trochlear groove   The concave surface in the knee joint where the patella makes contact with the femur

tuberosity   A protuberance on a bone, especially where a muscle or ligament is attached

turf toe   Pain at the base of the great toe caused by jamming the foot

uncinate process   Any hooklike process, such as that keeping a vertebra from sliding backward off the vertebra below it

uric acid   A heterocyclic compound of carbon, nitrogen, oxygen, and hydrogen with the formula $C_5H_4N_4O_3$; a chemical created when the body breaks down substances called purines

valgus   Bowlegged position

valgus stress test   A test to evaluate the medial collateral ligament (MCL) in the knee

varus   Knock-kneed position

varus stress test   A test to evaluate the lateral collateral ligament (LCL) in the knee

vertebra (*pl.*, vertebrae)   Any of the separate segments comprising the vertebral column; there are normally 33 of them, differing in size and structure according to location

vertebral foramen   The opening in the center of the vertebra through which the spinal cord passes

vesicle   A small sac containing fluid

visceral pleura   A membrane covering the lungs and lining the inner wall of the chest

V̇o₂max   Refers to the peak oxygen uptake and the body's ability to use it during exercises that increase in intensity over time

volar   Refers to the the palmar surface, or underside of the wrist and hand

volar plate   A thick ligament found in the fingers preventing hyperextension injuries

West Point view   A specially positioned X-ray view used to detect a Bankart lesion of the shoulder

white matter   The portion of the brain containing myelinated nerve fibers; also part of the central nervous system

"winging"   Lifting off of the medial border of the scapular shoulder

xerosis   A condition in which the skin is abnormally dry

Yergason test   A test that is conducted by having the patient flex the elbow and rotate the hand from a palm-down position to a palm-up position while the examiner resists the motion

Zanca view   An X-ray view used to evaluate the acromioclavicular (AC) joint in the shoulder

Appendix A

Taping and Bracing Techniques

The step-by-step procedures in this appendix describe the basic taping and bracing techniques used today in sports medicine. The following table lists the various supplies typically used in these procedures.

Table 1   Taping Supplies and Equipment

Type	Properties	Size	Brands	Uses
Adhesive spray	Typically aerosol spray that makes the skin more adhesive	Cans come in various sizes of 4 to 12 oz	Tuff Skin	First step before applying any tape or elastic wrap. Always ask about potential allergy before applying
Elastic wraps	Made of cotton with elastic properties	Can vary in size from 2 to 6 in. and length of 5 to 11 yd	Ace Wrap	Can be used for initial injury for compression or used for spicas and wraps to provide support
Adhesive stretch tape	Stretchy tape with adhesive properties to stick to skin or other products such as padding	Can vary from 1 to 4 in. and 2.5 to 5 yd	Powerfast Lightplast	Can be used for compression or to secure padding
Nonadhesive stretch tape	Stretchy tape that sticks to itself	Can vary from 1 to 4 in. and 2.5 to 5 yd	Powerflex Activ-Flex Cohesive stretch tape	Can be used for compression or used as the basis of some tape jobs when prewrap is not needed
Prewrap	Made of foam and provides an under layer before the tape is applied	2¾ in. × 30 yd	Mueller Cramer	Placed under most taping procedures to decrease chafing and blisters
White zinc tape	Nonelastic tape with adhesive properties to stick to skin or other products	Can vary from ½ to 4 in. and 2.5 to 5 yd	Coach Zonas Jaybird Cramer	Used as the primary tape in most procedures due to its nonelastic properties

Note: 1 inch (in.) = 2.54 centimeters; 1 yard (yd) = 0.91 meters; 1 ounce (oz) = 28.35 grams.

This appendix includes discussions of 19 of the most common taping procedures, organized by body region:

1. great toe taping
2. arch taping
3. closed basket weave
4. Achilles taping
5. medial tibial stress syndrome taping
6. McConnell taping
7. knee hyperextension taping

8. medial collateral ligament taping
9. patellar tendinitis strap
10. thigh compression wrap
11. hip spica for adductor strain
12. rib compression wrap
13. shoulder spica for acromioclavicular taping

14. elbow hyperextension tape
15. ulnar collateral ligament taping
16. lateral epicondylitis strap
17. wrist hyperflexion taping
18. buddy taping
19. thumb spica

Great Toe Taping

Great toe taping is applied after injury to the first metatarsophalangeal (MTP) joint of the great toe after a hyperextension or hyperflexion injury and is associated commonly with "turf sports," such as football, soccer, and field hockey. The goal of taping is to limit excessive and/or painful extension or flexion of the MTP joint.

Procedure

Materials. Adhesive spray, 1½-inch (in.; 1 in. = 2.54 centimeters [cm]) white tape, 1-in. white tape.

Positioning and Preparation. The patient is made to lie in the supine position with the knee in extension, foot in relaxed position, and great toe in neutral position. Apply adhesive spray to the foot and great toe where the tape will be applied.

Application

1. Apply an anchor around the midfoot with the 1½-in. white tape. Apply the second anchor with the 1-in. tape around the great toe distally.

1.

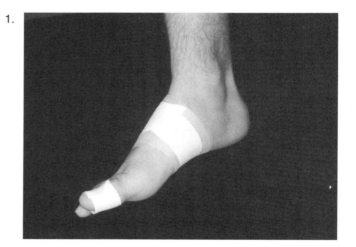

2.

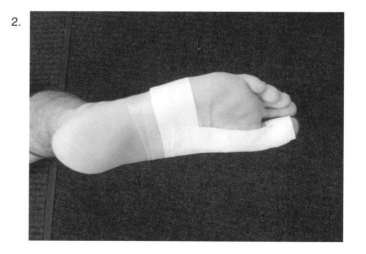

2. Apply a fan strip with the 1-in. white tape from the second anchor on the distal great toe. Position the great toe into slight flexion within the painfree range. Secure the first fan strip to the initial anchor. Repeat two to three times with additional fan strips to secure the great toes in painfree position.

3. To secure the fan strips, place the 1½-in. white tape over the initial anchor and the 1-in. white tape over the second anchor.

Final Assessment. Check for circulation and ensure that the application has limited the painful motion and is functional for the athlete.

Additional Notes

4. To limit painful flexion, reverse the fan strips, applying ventrally while placing the great toe in slight extension.

5. To gain additional support for cases of multidirectional instability and/or pain, apply toe spica consisting of two 1-in. white tape strips crossing over the medial MTP joint of the great toe prior to the final anchors. Secure with anchors as described above.

3.

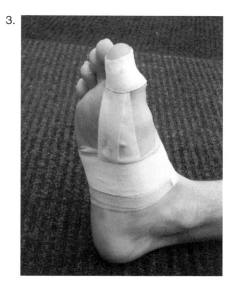

4.

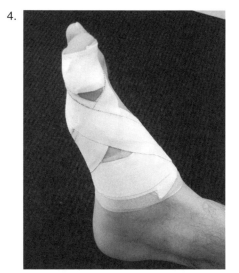

5.

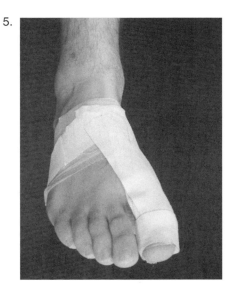

Custom/Prefabricated Items. Great toe extension may also be limited by prefabricated steel inserts or a precut plantar fascia strip.

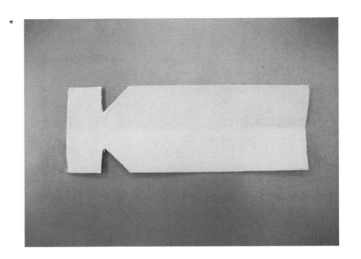

Arch Taping

Arch taping is applied to those individuals who require additional support to their arch in an effort to prevent excessive pronation. With this goal, excessive motion may be limited during gait, and pain in the lower extremity structures irritated by this motion may resolve.

Procedure

Materials. Adhesive spray, 1½-in. white tape, 1-in. white tape.

Positioning and Preparation. The patient is made to lie in the supine position with the knee in extension and the foot in relaxed position. Lightly spray the arch with the adhesive spray, and let it dry.

Application

1. Gently apply a half-anchor of the 1½-in. white tape around the metatarsal heads, pulling from the lateral to the medial direction.

2. Apply the 1-in. white tape in an X pattern with three "Xs" running from the first metatarsal head around the heel and returning to the fifth

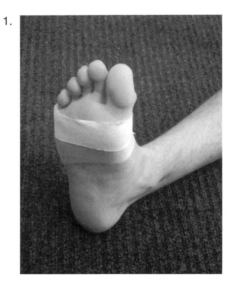

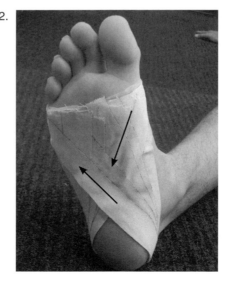

metatarsal head and three "Xs" running from the fifth metatarsal head around the heel and returning to the first metatarsal head. Overlap each "X" while filling in the arch space. Use a minimum of six "Xs" to fill in the entire arch space.

3. Apply the 1½-in. white tape half-anchors, pulling lateral to medial to cover the arch. Anchors should start proximal and continue distally. Be sure to cover all the loose ends.

4. Complete by securing with two full 1½-in. white tape anchors around the metatarsal heads.

Final Assessment. Check for circulation, and ensure that the application has limited the painful motion and is functional for the athlete.

*Custom/Prefabricated Items. Supporting the arch can also be achieved by purchasing off-the-shelf orthotics or custom shoe inserts.

3.

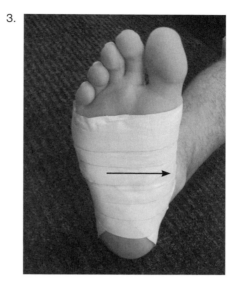

4.

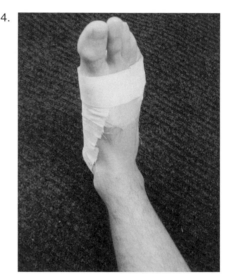

*

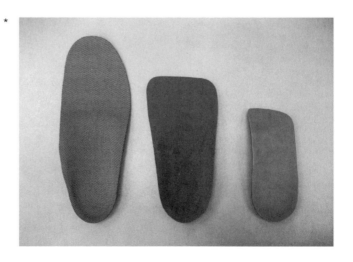

Closed Basket Weave

The closed basket weave is used after an inversion ankle sprain and is one of the most commonly seen tape procedures in sports medicine. It can be used both as a prevention measure and to limit inversion after injury.

Procedure

Materials. Heel and lace pads, adhesive spray, 1½-in. white tape, prewrap.

Positioning and Preparation. The patient is made to lie in the supine position with the knee in extension and ankle in a dorsiflexed position. Lightly spray the ankle with the adhesive spray, and let it dry.

Application

1. Apply at least one heel and lace pad at the front of the ankle and the other at the back where the Achilles tendon inserts into the calcaneus. Secure the pads with the prewrap, and cover the area where the tape will be applied.

2. Apply one anchor of the 1½-in. white tape 6 in. above the malleoli, adhering the prewrap to the skin. The second anchor should be placed around the midfoot while avoiding direct compression of the base of the fifth metatarsal.

3. Apply a stirrup running from the medial to lateral direction, from the medial proximal anchor to the lateral side, extending just above the anchors on both sides; this should cover the posterior one third of the malleoli. Apply the first

1.

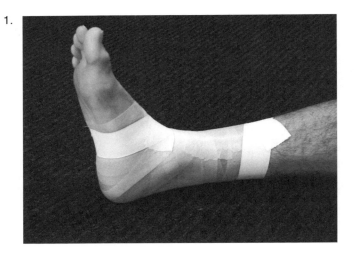

2.

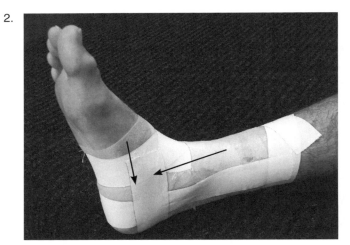

3.

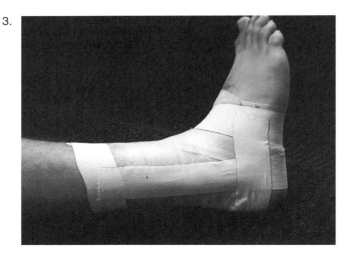

horseshoe starting directly on the metatarsal anchor along the first metatarsal, traveling behind the heel, and ending along the fifth metatarsal. Apply horseshoes always from the medial to lateral direction unless your goal is to limit eversion, in which case the pull would be in the opposite direction.

4. Apply each additional stirrup in the same fashion while overlapping by half the width of the tape. The second stirrup should cover the middle one third of the malleoli, with the third stirrup covering the anterior one third. Apply horseshoe strips in the same manner, with each strip slightly shorter than the previous, leaving a staircase appearance. Apply the stirrups and the horseshoes in an alternating fashion.

5. Follow the third horseshoe up the leg until you have completely enclosed the ankle and have ended just past your initial anchor. These strips should continue to be applied by overlapping half the width of the tape. Apply additional arch support until the bottom is enclosed.

6. Start applying the tape on the lateral malleolus, and pull around the arch of the foot to begin a figure-eight pattern.

4.

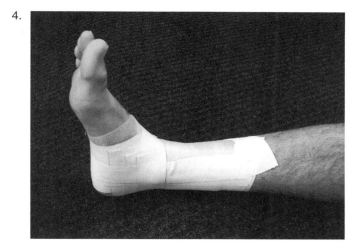

5.

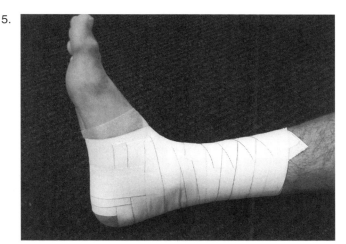

6.

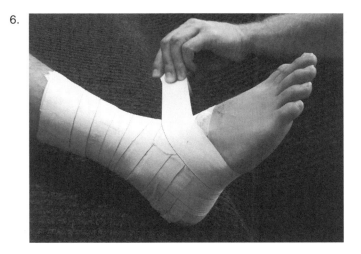

7. Continue the figure-eight pattern by completing a full turn around the ankle so that the roll of tape ends on the medial side, moving downward toward the medial malleolus.

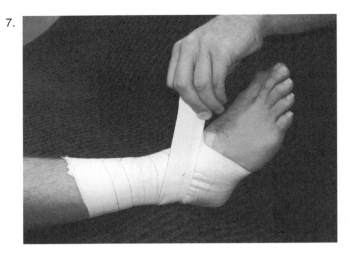

8. From this position, direct the roll of tape to the outside of the heel, and apply a heel lock, ending with the roll of tape moving in a caudal position.

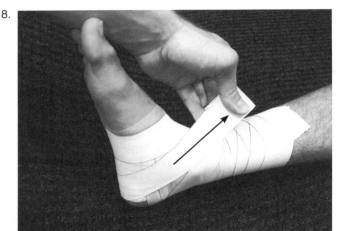

9. Continue by pulling the tape up and around the ankle with a complete turn.

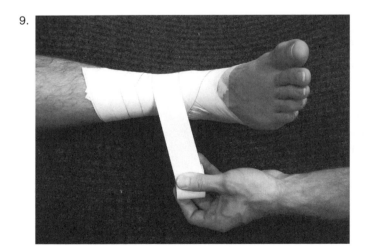

10. Once around the ankle, continue along the lateral ankle, moving toward the medial side of the heel, and apply another heel lock.

11. Once around the ankle, the tape may finish anywhere. Additional figure-eight and heel locks may be added depending on the severity of the injury or the size of the athlete.

Final Assessment. Check for circulation, and ensure that the application has limited either the painful motion or the inversion and is functional for the athlete.

Custom/Prefabricated Items. A number of ankle braces can be purchased with the benefits of self-application and increased cost-effectiveness.

10.

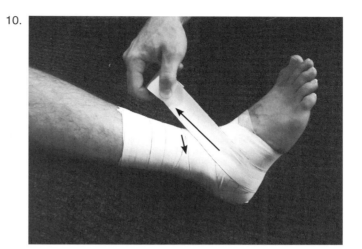

11.

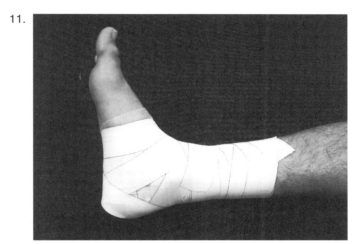

*

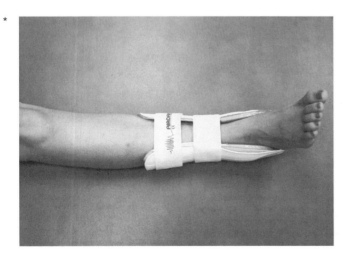

*

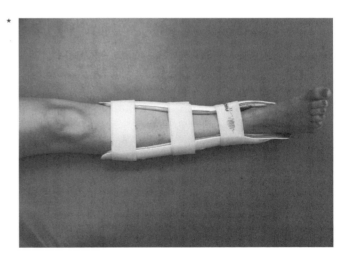

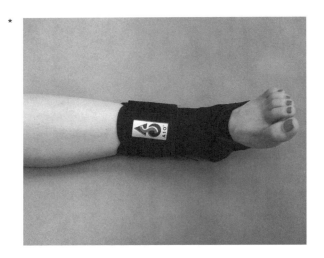

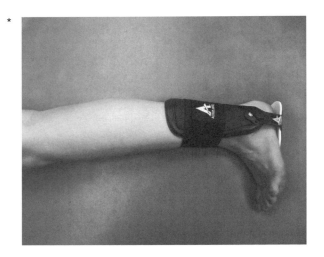

Achilles Taping

Achilles taping is applied to those individuals who suffer from pain with plantarflexion and where additional support and help with this motion are required. The goal of this tape job is to assist in the motion of plantarflexion and alleviate pain and discomfort.

Procedure

Materials. Prewrap, adhesive spray, 1½-in. white tape, 3-in. heavy-duty tape.

Positioning and Preparation. The patient is made to lie in the prone position with the knee in extension and the foot in relaxed position, slightly plantarflexed. Lightly spray the foot and ankle with the adhesive spray.

Application

1. Apply the prewrap around the foot, ankle, and lower leg. Apply an anchor of the 1½-in. white tape around the metatarsal heads and the other anchor 6 in. above the malleoli. Starting dorsally on initial anchor, apply the 3-in. heavy-duty stretch tape running to the anchor on the lower leg while the foot maintains a relaxed position. The first strip should run in a straight fashion.

1.

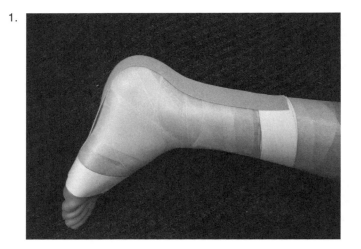

2.

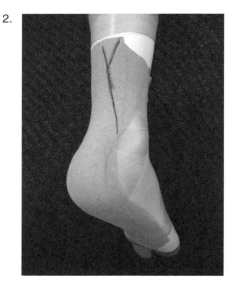

2. Apply two additional 3-in. heavy-duty stretch tape strips with each crossing over the painful site to form an X pattern.

3. Cover the anchors with the 1½-in. white tape, ensuring that there are no loose ends.

Final Assessment. Check for circulation, and ensure that the application has limited the painful motion and is functional for the athlete.

3.

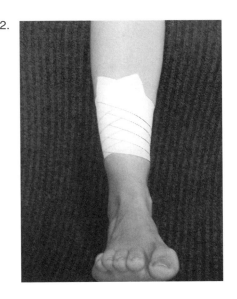

Medial Tibial Stress Syndrome Taping

Medial tibial stress syndrome (MTSS) or shin splint taping is applied to those individuals who suffer from pain in their lower leg during activity. Also known as an *open spiral*, the goal of this taping is to compress the musculature of the anterior lower leg to alleviate pain.

Procedure

Materials. Adhesive spray, 1½-in. white tape.

Positioning and Preparation. The patient is made to lie in the supine position with the knee in extension and foot in relaxed position. Lightly spray the lower leg with the adhesive spray, and let it dry.

Application

1. Apply a strip of the 1½-in. white tape starting laterally, or opposite to the painful side and 2 in. below. Wrap the tape around lower leg while squeezing the Achilles tendon, and end the strip just past the starting point. Always pull the tape so that the painful area moves toward the tibia.

2. Continue to apply additional strips in the same fashion. Be sure to overlap

1.

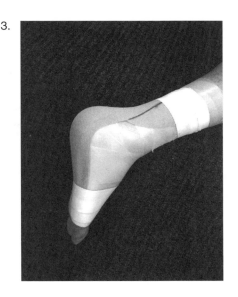

2.

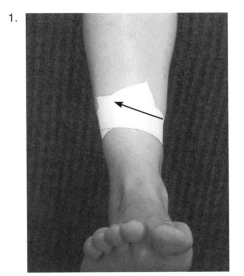

half of the previous strip. Each strip is applied tightly. Continue strips application until you are 2 in. above the painful site. Each individual strip should overlap and enclose the previous strip. Complete by applying a full anchor on both proximal and distal ends.

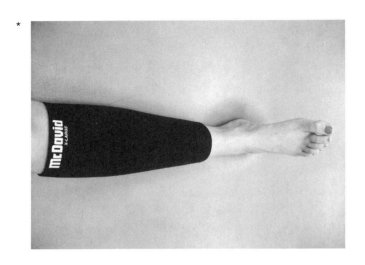

Final Assessment. Check for circulation, and ensure that the application causes limited pain and is functional for the patient.

*Custom/Prefabricated Items. A number of commercial compression sleeves are available that re-create the same effect.

McConnell Taping

McConnell taping is applied typically to treat patellofemoral stress syndrome (PFSS), which typically occurs with abnormal tracking of the patella. The goal of taping the patella is to restore proper tracking mechanics of the patella and to decrease or relieve painful knee biomechanics.

Procedure

Materials. Adhesive spray, 2-in. coverall, 1½-in. leukotape, scissors.

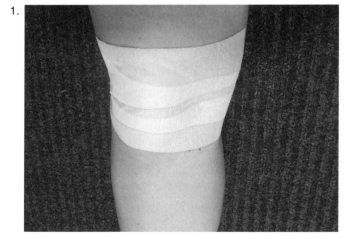

Positioning and Preparation. Check the skin for wounds and irritation. Remove excessive hair with a razor. The patient should be made to lie in the supine position on a table with the knee fully extended; the quadriceps should be fully relaxed to allow patella mobility. Apply adhesive spray to the knee where the tape will be applied, and allow it to dry.

Application

1. Cut strips of coverall long enough to cover the patella and the medial knee. Then apply these strips as a base covering the patella and medial knee.

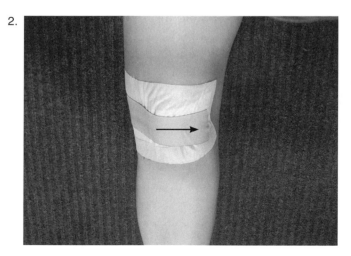

2. To limit lateral tracking, apply a strip of leukotape laterally on the patella, then pulling medially and placing the other end over the medial knee. Cut off the excess tape.

3. Apply two or three more strips as described above, covering the patella.

Final Assessment. Check the range of motion (ROM) of the knee and the comfort of the tape. Ensure that the application has limited the painful motion and is functional for the patient.

Additional Notes

4. To ensure that the tape will remain on and not fall off prematurely during activity, you may wrap it with nonadhesive stretch tape.

5. To limit tilting in other directions, pull the leukotape in the opposite direction of the motion that you are trying to limit.

Custom/Prefabricated Items. Abnormal patella tracking can also be altered by using a commercial brace with a patella buttress.

3.

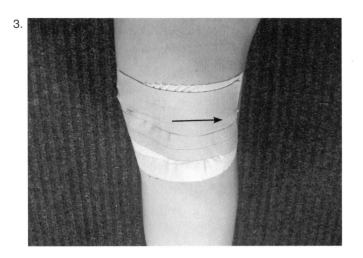

4.

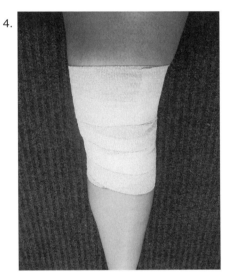

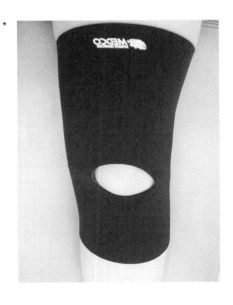

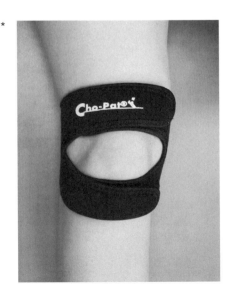

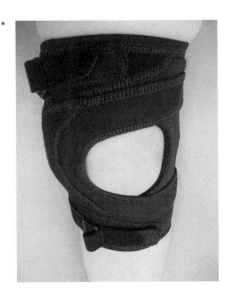

Knee Hyperextension Taping

Knee hyperextension taping is applied when a knee hyperextension injury has occurred. The goal of this tape job is to limit painful knee extension.

Procedure

Materials. Adhesive spray, prewrap, 2-in. heavy-duty elastic tape, 3-in. adhesive elastic tape, scissors.

Positioning and Preparation. Check the skin for wounds and irritation. The patient should be standing with the affected knee flexed 25° to 35° or within a painfree ROM. The patient should have a good portion of his or her weight over the affected leg and with the quadriceps contracted so that the wrap is not too tight. Apply adhesive spray to the lower leg and thigh where the tape will be applied.

Application

1. Apply the prewrap over the entire area that will be taped, starting at the midthigh and continuing distally to the midgastrocnemius. (*Note:* The longer the level of the tape job, the more effective it will be in preventing painful ROM.) Apply two anchors with the 3-in. adhesive elastic tape over the prewrap, one on the midthigh and the other on the midgastroc.

2. Apply strips of the 2-in. heavy-duty elastic tape in an X pattern behind the knee. The first strip should be applied laterally on the thigh anchor, crossing the posterior knee and ending at the medial anchor on the gastrocnemius. Cut off the excess heavy-duty elastic tape.

3. The second strip is applied medially on the thigh anchor, crossing the posterior knee and ending on the

1.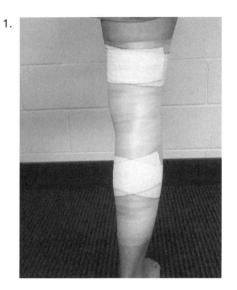

2.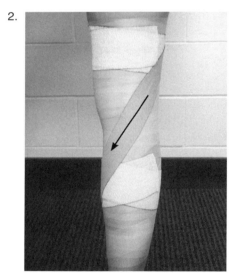

3.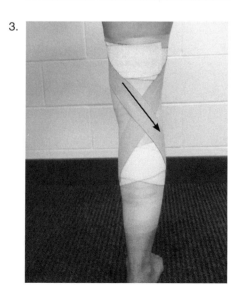

lateral anchor on the gastroc. Cut off the excess heavy-duty elastic tape.

4. Apply two more strips as described above, creating an X pattern behind the knee.

5. Cover the distal anchors up to the tibial tuberosity with the 3-in. adhesive stretch tape. Cover the proximal anchors distally with the 3-in. adhesive stretch tape, ending 3 in. above the superior patella. *Note:* To ensure normal tracking of the patella, do not cover the patella with the tape.

Final Assessment. Check the ROM of the knee and the comfort of the tape. Ensure that the application has limited the painful motion of the knee and is functional for the athlete.

4.

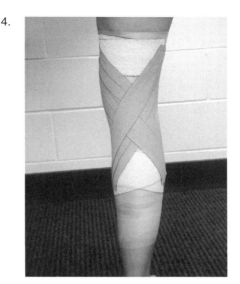

5a.

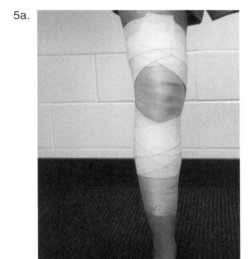

5b.

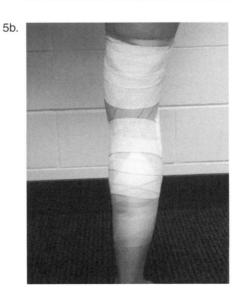

Custom/Prefabricated Items. Off-the-shelf braces with an ROM lock can limit the painful ROM—such as a knee immobilizer.

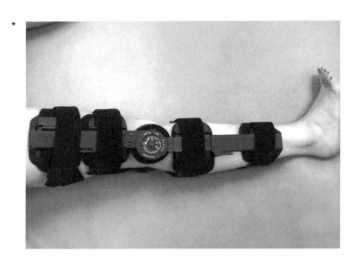

Medial Collateral Ligament Taping

Collateral ligament taping is applied when either the medial collateral ligament (MCL) or the lateral collateral ligament (LCL) is sprained. The goal of this tape job is to protect the ligament from further injury.

Procedure

Materials. Adhesive spray, prewrap, 1½-in. white tape, 3-in. adhesive elastic tape.

Positioning and Preparation. Check the skin for wounds and irritation. The patient should be standing with the affected knee slightly flexed and within a painfree ROM. The patient should have a good portion of his or her weight over the affected leg and with the quads contracted so that the wrap is not too tight. Apply adhesive spray to the knee and thigh where the tape will be applied.

Application

1. Apply the prewrap over the entire area that will be taped; starting at the upper thigh and continuing down to the midgastrocnemius. Apply two anchors with the 3-in. adhesive elastic tape on the upper thigh and midgastroc.

2. Apply strips of the 1½-in. white tape in an X pattern over the MCL.

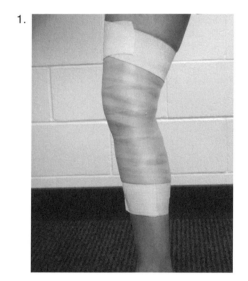

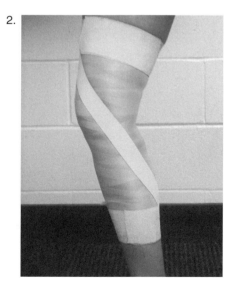

The first strip will be applied on the anterior thigh anchor, crossing the medial joint line and ending at the posterior anchor on the gastrocnemius.

3. The second strip will be applied on the posterior thigh anchor, crossing the medial joint line and ending on the anterior anchor on the gastroc.

4. Apply two or three more strips as described above, creating an X pattern over the medial joint line.

5. Cover the distal anchors up to the tibial tuberosity with the 3-in. adhesive stretch tape. Cover the proximal anchors distally with the 3-in. adhesive stretch tape ending 3 in. above the superior patella. *Note:* Do not cover the patella with the tape, to ensure normal tracking of the patella.

3.
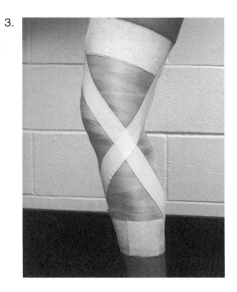

4.
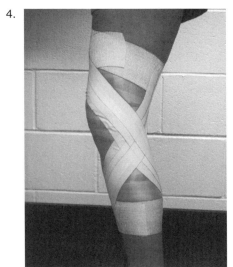

5.
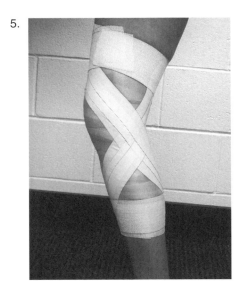

*Final Assessment. Check the ROM of the knee and the comfort of the tape. Ensure that the application is functional for the patient and gives support to the MCL.

Additional Notes

To tape for an LCL sprain, follow the previous steps, with the X pattern applied over the LCL.

*Custom/Prefabricated Items. Off-the-shelf braces with a medial stabilizer can be applied.

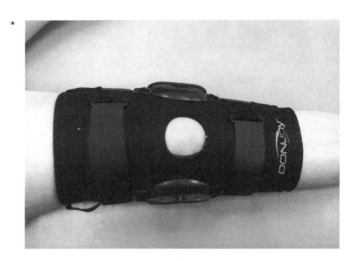

Patellar Tendinitis Strap

A patellar tendinitis strap is applied for a patient suffering from patella tendinitis (jumper's knee) or Osgood-Schlatter disease. The goal of this tape job is to decrease pain by applying pressure to the tendon and decreasing the stress of the tendon on the tibial tuberosity, where it inserts.

Procedure

Materials. Prewrap, 1½-in. white tape.

Positioning and Preparation. Check the skin for wounds and irritation. The patient should be standing with the affected knee slightly flexed and within a painfree ROM.

Application

1. Apply the prewrap, encircling the knee over the patella six to eight times with equal tension.

2. Apply three strips of the 1½-in. white tape anteriorly in the center of the prewrap.

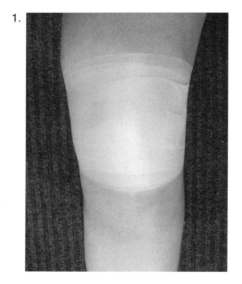

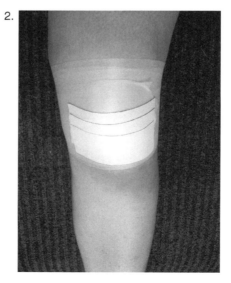

3. Roll the prewrap and tape from the proximal to distal direction to create a strap. Place the strap over the patellar tendon.

Final Assessment. Check the ROM of the knee and the comfort of the tape. Ensure that the application has adequate pressure on the patellar tendon and is functional for the patient.

*Custom/Prefabricated Items. Jumper's knee straps can be purchased over the counter to re-create this tape job.

3a.

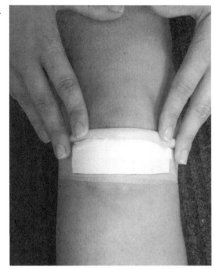

3b.

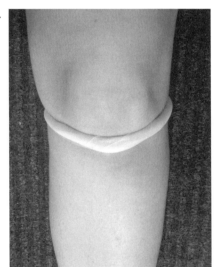

*

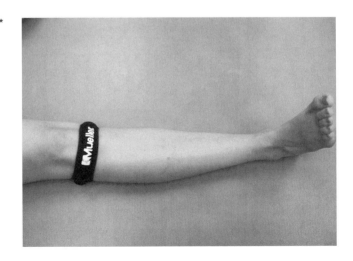

Thigh Compression Wrap

A thigh compression wrap may be applied after an injury such as a contusion or muscle strain to either the hamstring or the quadriceps muscle group. The goal of this wrap is to compress the muscle group and the origin of pain while providing support.

Procedure

Materials. Adhesive spray, 6-in. single elastic bandage, 1½-in. white tape. *Note:* Depending on the size of the patient, you may have to use a larger elastic wrap, 6 in. × 5 yards (yd), 6 in. × 11 yd, or 4 in. × 11 yd (1 in. = 2.54 cm; 1 yd = 0.91 meters [m]).

Positioning and Preparation. The patient should be standing with the involved knee flexed between 20° and 30° while keeping the majority of the patient's weight on the involved side. Apply spray on the area to be wrapped, and allow it to dry.

Application

1. Begin distal to the site of pain, and apply the compression wrap around the area to be treated in a herringbone fashion with the "Xs" central over the site of pain.

2. Continue proximally overlapping the compression wrap by half the width of the wrap.

3. Secure the wrap with the 1½-in. white tape by placing an "X" over the painful area, and anchor at the top and bottom.

Final Assessment. Check for circulation, and ensure that the application has limited the painful motion and is functional for the athlete.

1.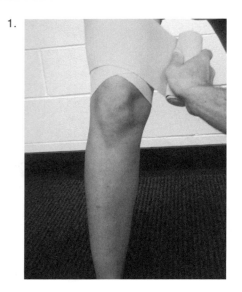

2.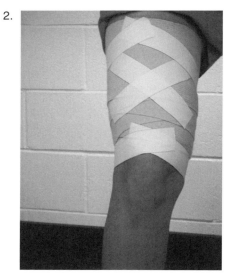

3.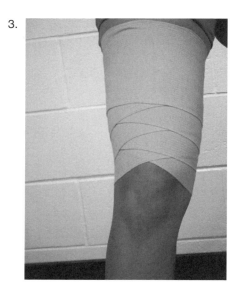

Custom/Prefabricated Items. Commercial compression sleeves, both with and without additional padding, are available.

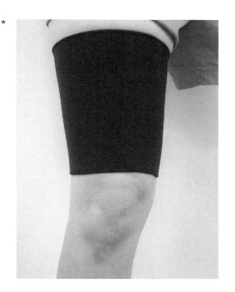

Hip Spica for Adductor Strain

A hip spica may be used for a number of conditions, including support of the adductor and hip flexor groups in addition to securing padding after an injury to the hip bone, or "hip pointer." The goal of this supportive wrap is to compress the muscle group and origin of pain while providing support and aiding in the natural motion of the muscle group.

Procedure

Materials. Adhesive spray, 4-in. double-elastic bandage, 1½-in. white tape. *Note:* Depending on the size of the patient, you may have to use a larger elastic wrap, such as 6 in. × 11 yd.

Positioning and Preparation. The patient should be standing with the involved leg placed in an internally rotated position. Ask the athlete to assume a slightly forward-lunge position that flexes the knee and causes the hip to adduct. Gently spray the thigh area that will be

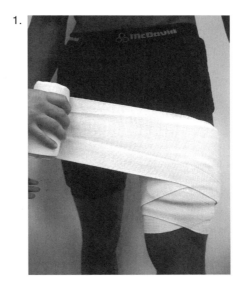

wrapped, which acts as the anchor for this tape procedure. *Note:* For maximum support, have the athlete wear spandex or tight shorts so that the wrap can be as close to the body part as possible.

Application

1. Secure the wrap to the leg by anchoring the wrap around the thigh while pulling laterally to medially.

2. Continue wrapping up and around the trunk, crossing deep in the groin over the adductor muscle group.

3. Finish the wrap on the thigh, and secure with the 1½-in. white tape by tracing the pattern once around the thigh and trunk. Add more tape strips as needed.

4. To secure the wrap further, you can trace the pattern of the wrap with the 3-in. adhesive elastic tape.

Additional Notes

To provide supportive taping for the hip flexor, begin in a similar fashion to the hip adductor wrap but with the patient in a slightly forward-lunge position with a slight forward bend at the trunk. Pull the wrap from medial to lateral, and place an "X" over the site of pain or the hip flexor group.

Custom/Prefabricated Items. Commercial compression garments can be purchased that offer focal and general compression.

2.
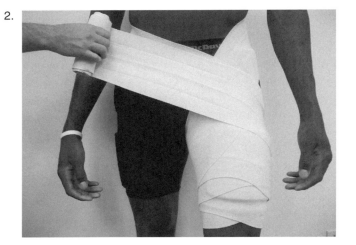

3.
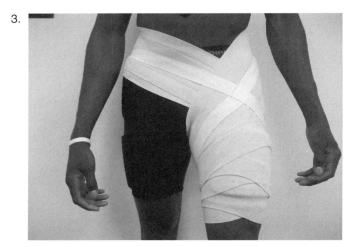

4.
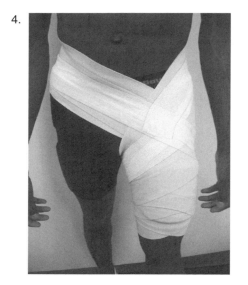

Rib Compression Wrap

A rib compression wrap is used to relieve the pain of a rib fracture or intercostal strain, secure a protective pad over an injured site, or control swelling. The goal of the wrap is to provide support to the injured area and decrease pain.

Procedure

Materials. Adhesive spray, 4-in. × 5-yd elastic wrap, 1½-in. white tape. *Note:* Depending on the size of the patient, you may have to use a larger elastic wrap, 6 in. × 5 yd, 6 in. × 11 yd, or 4 in. × 11 yd.

Positioning and Preparation. Check the skin for wounds and irritation. The patient should be standing with the arms abducted. Apply adhesive spray to the torso where the elastic bandage will be applied.

Application

The procedure described below is for a rib fracture. The injured area is marked "+."

1. Start the wrap superiorly to the injured site, encircling the torso and overlapping about 2 in. each time around.

2. Work your way caudally, covering the injured site and ending over the wrap superiorly to the injured area.

3. Apply two to three strips of the 1½-in. white tape at the end of the wrap to secure it.

1.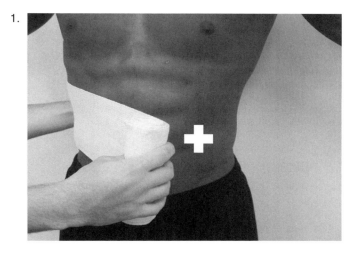

2.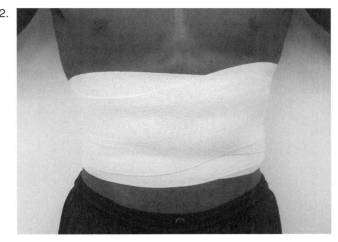

3.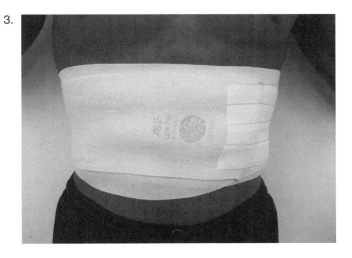

4. To secure the wrap, you may encircle the wrap and tape with the 3-in. adhesive elastic tape.

Final Assessment. Check the ROM of the torso and the comfort of the athlete during respiration. Ensure that the application provides support to the injured site and is functional for the athlete.

*Custom/Prefabricated Items. Rib belts can be purchased off the shelf to obtain similar results.

4.

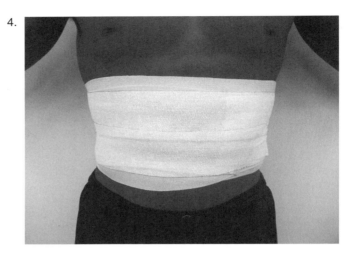

*

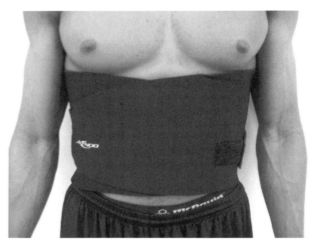

Shoulder Spica for Acromioclavicular Taping

The acromioclavicular (AC) wrap may be applied after an injury to the AC joint from direct contact, such as tackling in football or forced horizontal adduction. The goal of this wrap is to provide protection and general compression to the AC joint and shoulder in general.

Procedure

Materials. Adhesive spray, compression wrap (various widths and lengths), 1½-in. white tape.

Positioning and Preparation. The patient should be placed in a standing or seated position with the involved arm at the side and the hand on the hip.

1.

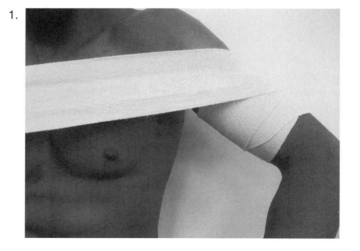

Spray the humerus with the adhesive spray, as this will act as the anchor for this tape procedure.

Application

1. Begin wrapping the midhumerus in a clockwise fashion (lateral to medial), and continue in a spiral fashion while overlapping by half the width of the wrap, moving distal to proximal for at least two times around the humerus.

2. Pull medially across the chest and under the opposite axilla, and continue around the torso. Apply the greatest amount of tension over the shoulder and the least amount of tension as you wrap around the torso. Encircle the humerus again.

3. Repeat the pattern at least twice or as needed depending on the size of the patient and the support needed. End the wrap on the arm. Secure the wrap with the 1½-in. tape by tracing the pattern on the humerus.

Final Assessment. Check for circulation, and ensure that the application has limited the painful motion and is functional for the athlete.

Additional Notes

In association with many AC joint injuries, an "AC pad" is often applied directly over the AC joint to provide padding to the injured joint below. Apply the AC pad if needed prior to securing the AC wrap.

Custom/Prefabricated Items. Other commercial items that are commonly used to support the shoulder either after injury or during actual play include the Sully Stabilizing Brace.

2.

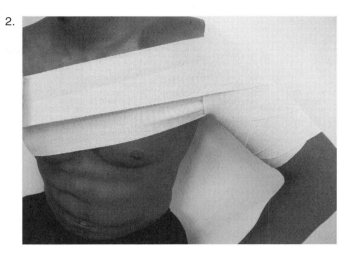

3.

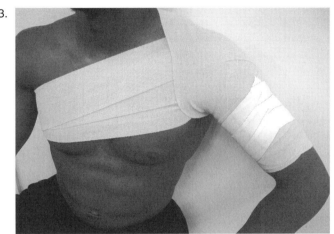

*

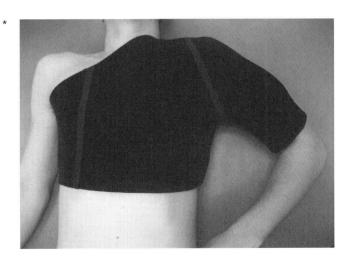

Elbow Hyperextension Tape

Elbow hyperextension taping is very similar to the knee hyperextension taping technique. This is applied when an elbow hyperextension injury has occurred, with the goal of limiting painful extension.

Procedure

Materials. Adhesive spray, prewrap, 2-in. heavy-duty adhesive elastic tape, 3-in. adhesive elastic tape, scissors.

Positioning and Preparation. Check the skin for wounds and irritation. The patient should have the affected elbow in slight flexion within a painfree range and supinated. Apply adhesive spray to the forearm and humerus where the tape will be applied.

Application

1. Apply the prewrap over the entire area that will be taped; starting at the midhumerus and continuing distally to the midforearm. (*Note:* The longer the level of the tape job, the more effective it will be in preventing painful ROM.) Apply two anchors with the 3-in. adhesive elastic tape, one on the midhumerus and the other at the midforearm.

2. Apply a strip of the 2-in. heavy-duty adhesive elastic tape over the anterior elbow. The first strip will begin on the anterior anchor of the humerus and follow the midline of the humerus distally to the forearm, where it ends at the second anchor at the midforearm. Cut off the excess heavy-duty elastic tape.

3. The next two strips will create an X pattern over the anterior elbow. The second strip will be applied laterally on the distal humeral anchor, crossing the anterior elbow and ending at the medial anchor on the forearm (ulna). The third strip will be applied medially on the

1.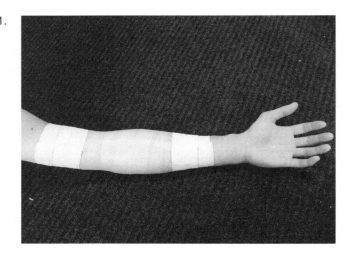

2.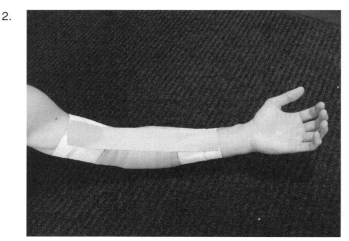

3.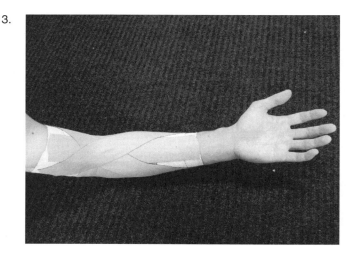

distal humeral anchor, crossing the anterior elbow and ending at the lateral anchor on the forearm (radius). Cut off the excess heavy-duty elastic tape.

4. Cover the tape job with the 3-in. adhesive elastic tape. *Note:* Do not cover the olecranon process with the tape, to ensure ease of movement.

Final Assessment. Check the ROM of the elbow to make sure that it is within the painfree ROM and functional for the patient. Check the distal capillary refill and the comfort of the tape for the patient.

*Custom/Prefabricated Items. Off-the-shelf braces with an ROM lock can limit the painful motion of the elbow.

4.

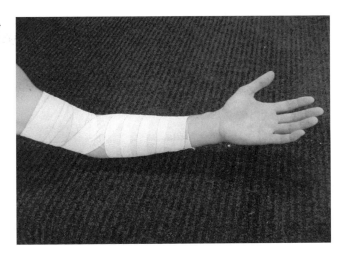

*

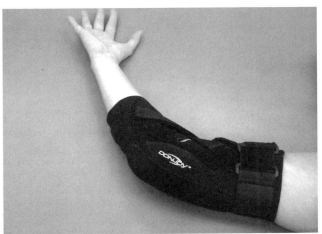

Ulnar Collateral Ligament Taping

This taping procedure is similar to the collateral ligament taping of the knee. Collateral ligament taping is applied when either the ulnar collateral ligament (UCL) or the radial collateral ligament (RCL) is sprained. The goal of this tape job is to protect the ligament from further injury.

Procedure

Materials. Adhesive spray, prewrap, 1½-in. white tape, 3-in. adhesive elastic tape.

Positioning and Preparation. Check the skin for wounds and irritation. The patient should be standing with the

1.

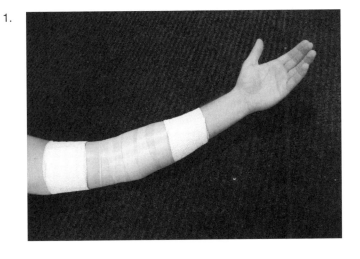

affected elbow slightly flexed within a painfree ROM and supinated. Apply adhesive spray to the forearm and humerus where the tape will be applied.

Application

1. Apply the prewrap over the entire area that will be taped, starting at the midhumerus and continuing distally to the midforearm. Apply two anchors with the 3-in. adhesive elastic tape over the prewrap, one on the midhumerus and the other on the midforearm.

2.
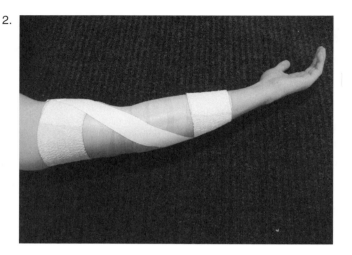

2. Apply strips of the 1½-in. white tape in an X pattern over the UCL. The first strip will be applied on the anterior humeral anchor, crossing the medial joint line and ending at the posterior anchor on the forearm.

3.
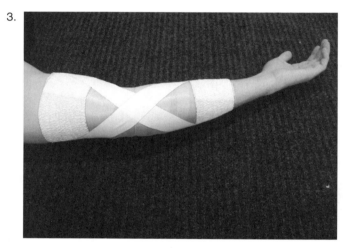

3. The second strip will be applied on the posterior humeral anchor, crossing the medial joint line and ending on the anterior anchor on the forearm.

4. Apply two or three more strips as described above, creating an X pattern over the UCL.

5. Cover the tape job with the 3-in. adhesive elastic tape. *Note:* Do not cover the olecranon process with the tape, to ensure ease of movement.

Final Assessment. Check the distal capillary refill and the comfort and function of the tape for the patient.

Additional Notes

To tape for an RCL sprain, follow the previous steps but with the X pattern applied over the RCL.

*Custom/Prefabricated Items. There are various off-the-shelf braces that can be purchased that will re-create the function of the tape procedure for the UCL.

4.

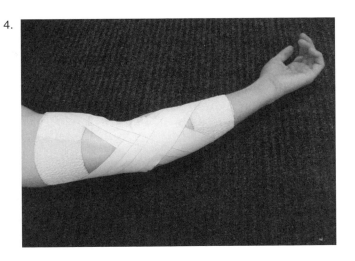

5.

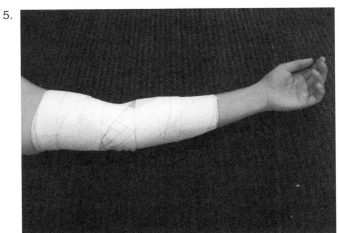

*

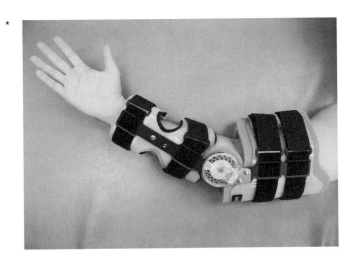

Lateral Epicondylitis Strap

A lateral epicondylitis strap is used for a patient suffering from lateral epicondylitis (tennis elbow). The goal of this tape job is to decrease pain by applying pressure to the common extensor bundle to decrease the stress of the extensor muscles on the bony attachment.

Procedure

Materials. Prewrap, 2-in. adhesive elastic tape, 1½-in. white tape.

Positioning and Preparation. Check the skin for wounds and irritation. The patient's arm should be in a relaxed supinated position.

Application

1. Apply the prewrap around the elbow two to three times distal to the lateral epicondyle, approximately ½ in.

2. Apply six strips of the 1½-in. white tape in the center of the prewrap distal to the lateral epicondyle.

3. Cover the prewrap and the 1½-in. white tape strips with the 2-in. adhesive elastic tape.

1.

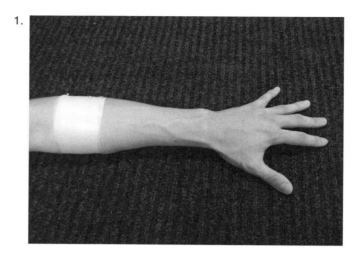

2.

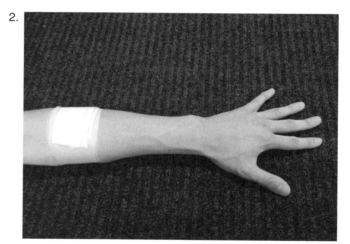

3.

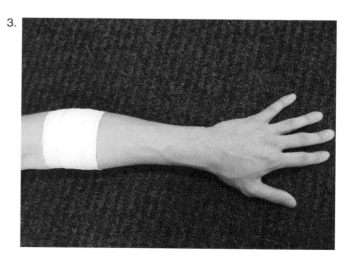

Final Assessment. Check the distal capillary refill and the comfort and function of the tape for the patient.

*Custom/Prefabricated Items. Prefabricated lateral epicondylitis straps can be purchased over the counter.

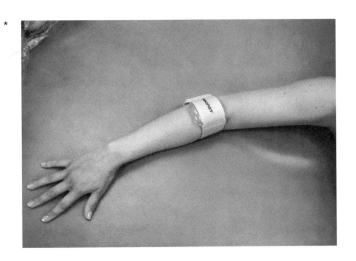

Wrist Hyperflexion Taping

Taping to the wrist is applied after an injury to any of the carpal bones or the wrist in general or to limit painful motion. The goal of this tape job is to provide stability and limit painful motions about the wrist to allow it to be used in athletic participation.

Procedure

Materials. Adhesive spray, 1½-in. white tape, prewrap.

Positioning and Preparation. Place the patient's wrist in a neutral position with the fingers abducted. Spray the area to be wrapped, and apply the prewrap as needed.

Application

1. Begin by applying two anchors on the midforearm and one around the hand just proximal to the metacarpophalangeal (MCP) joints. Be sure to keep the MP joints uncovered while slightly folding the tape before it crosses the thumb crease.

2. Apply parallel strips starting at the anchor on the hand and running to the anchor on the forearm. Complete

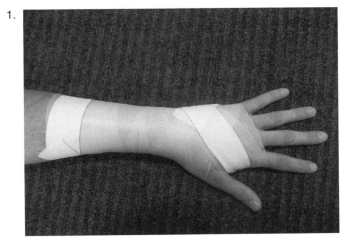

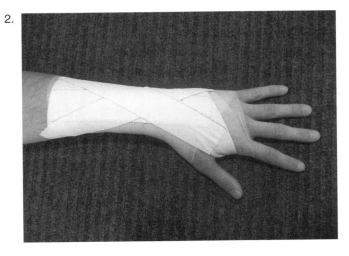

by applying at least two "Xs" in a similar fashion, crossing over the carpals. Apply parallel strips and "Xs" to the opposite side. If needed, add additional strips to the side in which you intend to limit the most motion (the dorsal side to prevent flexion and ventral side to prevent extension).

3. Close the entire forearm with the anchors.

4. Apply two figure-eight patterns starting on the dorsal side at the ulnar styloid process. Pull the tape between the thumb and the index finger, making sure that you place a small fold in the tape as it crosses through.

3.

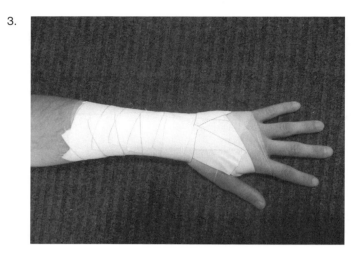

4a.

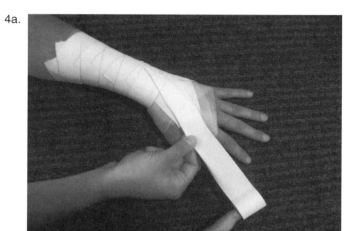

4b.

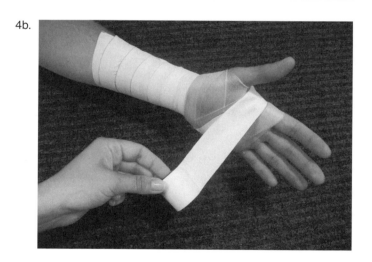

5. Continue to pull the tape across the palm to the dorsal side of the hand.

6. Continue to pull around the wrist, and end on dorsal side of the wrist. Repeat as necessary.

Final Assessment. Check for circulation and ensure that the application has limited the painful motion and is functional for the athlete.

*Custom/Prefabricated Items. Various prefabricated splints are available, such as the wrist splint. The velcro allows effortless application by the patient.

5.

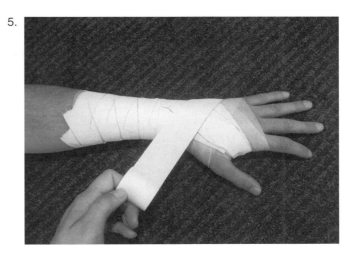

6.

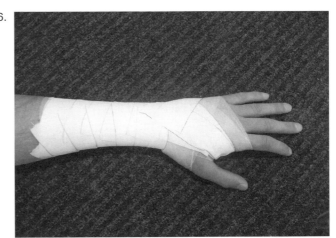

*

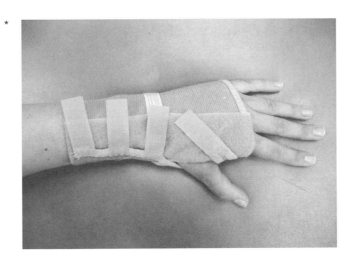

Buddy Taping

Buddy taping is the easiest and most common taping procedure for a patient to apply. It is typically used when an interphalangeal (IP) joint has been sprained. The goal of this tape job is to use one digit as a support for the injured digit to protect the sprained IP joint from further injury.

Procedure

Materials. Adhesive spray, 1-in. white tape.

Positioning and Preparation. Check the skin for wounds and irritation. The patient's hand should be relaxed and placed in a painfree position. Apply adhesive spray to the digits where the tape will be applied.

Application

The following taping procedure is for a sprained proximal IP of the fourth digit. For any other digits, simply repeat the steps as indicated.

Additional Notes

This is typically a procedure for a sprain in the second to fifth digits; this procedure is not used for the first digit. For a sprained first digit, see the section Thumb Spica.

1. Place the third digit next to the fourth digit in a comfortable, painfree ROM.

2. Apply a strip of the 1-in. white tape to encircle the proximal phalanges of the third and the fourth digits.

3. Apply a second strip of the 1-in. white tape to encircle the middle

1.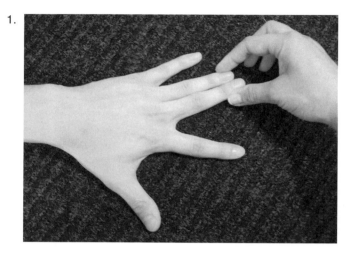

2.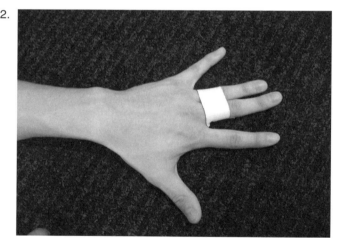

3.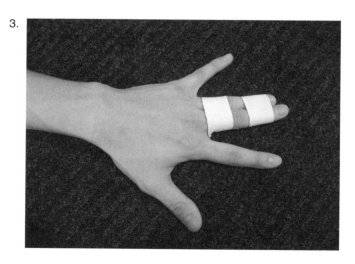

phalanges of the third and the fourth digits.

Final Assessment. Check the distal capillary refill of the third and fourth digits. Ensure that the tape is giving support to the fourth digit and is functional for the patient.

*Custom/Prefabricated Items. Various prefabricated splints are available, such as the aluminum finger splints and the Stax plastic finger splints.

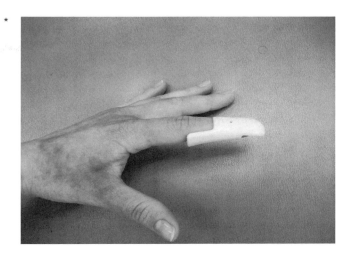

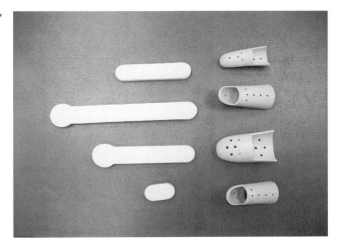

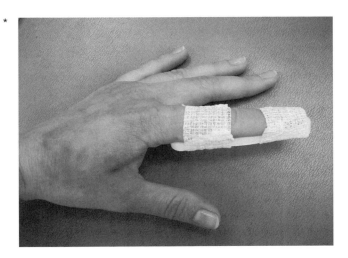

Thumb Spica

The thumb spica is used when the MCP joint of the first digit has been sprained. The goal is to limit multidirectional instability and prevent painful motion.

Procedure

Materials. Adhesive spray, prewrap, 1-in. white tape, 1½-in. white tape.

Positioning and Preparation. Check the skin for wounds and irritation. The patient should be relaxed, with his or her thumb slightly abducted and extended into a painfree position. Apply the adhesive spray to the first digit and the distal wrist where the tape will be applied.

Application

The following procedure is for a hyperflexion injury to the MCP of the first digit. To prevent hyperextension of the joint, follow the steps below, but place the X pattern on the volar aspect of the thumb.

1. Cover the thumb, the proximal hand, and the distal wrist with the prewrap.

2. Place two anchors with the 1½-in. white tape encircling the wrist.

3. Begin a strip of tape on the dorsal aspect of the anchors on the distal wrist. Continue this strip distally, crossing the lateral joint line of the MCP joint of the first digit.

1.
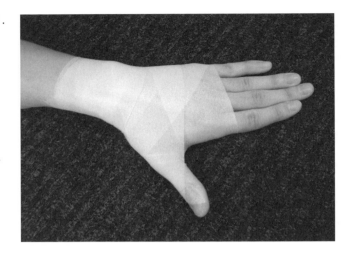

2.
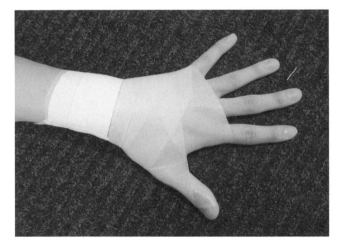

3.
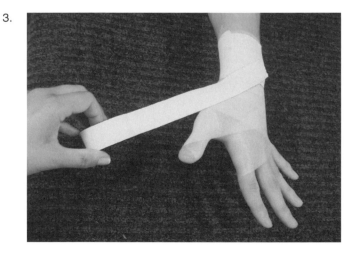

4. Continue the tape around the joint, crossing over the posterior aspect of the MCP joint of the first digit and ending on the volar aspect of the anchor on the wrist. You should have created an X pattern on the dorsal aspect of the MCP joint of the first digit.

5. Apply one or two more strips as indicated above, moving more distally on the first digit. *Note:* Do not cross the IP joint of the first digit.

6. Cover the anchors on the wrist with the 1½-in. white tape.

Final Assessment. Check the distal capillary refill of the first digit. Ensure that the tape prevents painful hyperflexion and is functional for the patient.

Additional Notes

Use caution when removing the tape from the first digit, so as to prevent damage to the distal phalanx; removing the tape with scissors is recommended.

4a.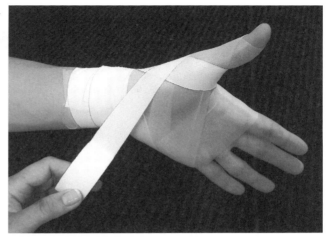

4b.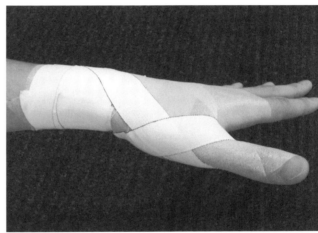

5.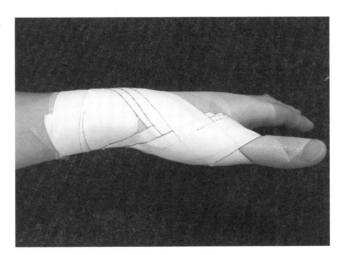

Custom/Prefabricated Items. Prefabricated thumb braces can be purchased to obtain similar results.

6.

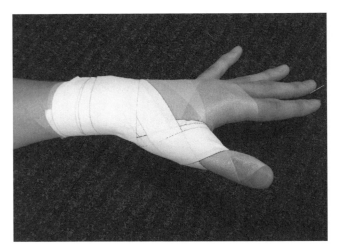

*

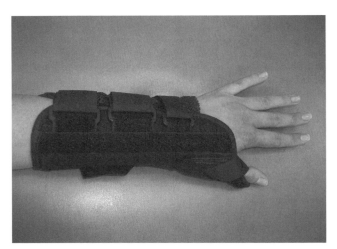

Conclusion

Just as all medical procedures have evolved, so too has the advancement of both taping and bracing applications. Although taping after the initial injury is rare, taping and bracing for support and protection during athletic participation and activities of daily living is a well-established practice that continues to undergo refinement based on sound knowledge and the practical experience of trained practitioners.

Arthur Horne and Cheryl Blauth

Further Readings

Beam JW. *Orthopedic Taping, Wrapping, Bracing and Padding*. Philadelphia, PA: FA Davis; 2006.

Firer P. Effectiveness of taping for the prevention of ankle ligament sprains. *Br J Sports Med*. 1990;24(1):47–50.

Herrington L. The effect of corrective taping of the patella on patella position as defined by MRI. *Res Sports Med*. 2006;14(3):215–223.

Perrin DH. *Athletic Taping and Bracing*. Champaign, IL: Human Kinetics; 1995.

Ubell M, Boylan J, Ashton-Miller J, Wojtys E. The effect of ankle braces on the prevention of dynamic forced ankle inversion. *Am J Sports Med*. 2003;31(6):935–940.

Appendix B

Organizations

American Alliance for Health, Physical Education, Recreation and Dance (AAHPERD)

> **Website:** http://www.aahperd.org
> **Publications:** *Research Quarterly, Health Education*; *Journal of Physical Education, Recreation and Dance*

An alliance of associations providing support to professionals involved in physical education, recreation, fitness, sports and coaching, dance, and health education and promotion.

American Association for Physical Activity and Recreation (AAPAR)

> **Website:** http://www.aahperd.org/aapar

An association linking professionals in education with community-based programs, promoting creative and active lifestyles through physical activity and recreation across the life span.

American Council on Exercise (ACE)

> **Website:** http://www.acefitness.org

A nonprofit organization that protects against ineffective fitness products, while also providing ongoing public education, outreach, and research, and sets certification and continuing education standards for fitness professionals.

American School Health Association (ASHA)

> **Website:** http://www.ashaweb.org

An association that organizes and advocates for effective school health policies that contribute to optimal health and academic outcomes for all school-age children.

American Sport Education Program (ASEP)

> **Website:** http://www.asep.com

An organization providing an educational program for coaches based on sports sciences such as sport physiology, sport psychology, and sport biomechanics.

American Swimming Coaches Association

> **Website:** http://www.swimmingcoach.org
> **Publication:** *Journal of Swimming Research*

A swimming association dedicated to enhancing coaching and building a stronger swimming community.

Canadian Fitness Professionals (CAN-FIT-PRO)

> **Website:** http://www.canfitpro.com

An organization providing education and certification for fitness professionals throughout Canada.

Cooper Institute for Aerobics Research

> **Website:** http://www.cooperaerobics.com

A nonprofit, founded in 1970, that has established an international reputation for research and education in preventive medicine.

Exercise Safety Association (ESA)

Website: http://www.exercisesafety.com

A national organization for fitness professionals providing certification and membership as well as fitness instructor training.

International Fitness Professionals Association (IFPA)

Website: http://www.ifpa-fitness.com

An association affiliated with Doctors Fitness Centers (DFC) and the Fitness Institute of Technology (FIT), providing fitness professionals the education and certification necessary to treat more than 65 different diseases, disabilities, and dysfunctions.

Joint Commission on Sports Medicine and Medical Science

Website: http://www.jcsportsmedicine.org

A voluntary forum that meets annually to discuss current issues in the profession as well as those that concern the future of sports medicine.

National Alliance for Youth Sports (NAYS)

Website: http://www.nays.org

An organization whose aim is to make the sports experience safe, fun, and healthy for youth by ensuring that the adults involved have proper training and information.

National Association for Health & Fitness (NAHF)

Website: http://www.physicalfitness.org

A nonprofit organization that promotes physical fitness, sports, and healthy lifestyles by fostering and supporting governors' and state councils and coalitions that promote and encourage regular physical activity.

National Association of Speed and Explosion (NASE)

Website: http://www.naseinc.com
Publication: *Sportspeed*

An educational organization and certification agency that includes coaches, strength and conditioning coaches, personal trainers, educators, and physicians focusing on the improvement of speed in short sprints to enhance athletic performance.

National Athletic Trainers' Association, Inc. (NATA)

Website: http://www.nata.org
Publication: *Athletic Training Journal*

A professional membership association for certified athletic trainers geared toward enhancing and advancing the athletic training profession.

National Council of Youth Sports (NCYS)

Website: http://www.ncys.org

An organization that represents more than 185 organizations (44,000,000 youth in organized sports) in the youth sports industry and promotes physical activity in youth via organized sports.

National High School Coaches Association (NHSCA)

Website: http://www.nhsca.com
Publication: *Coaches Quarterly Magazine*

A national nonprofit association that centers on the influence and professionalism of coaches and provides insurance coverage and educational programs for its participants.

National Institute for Fitness and Sport (NIFS)

Website: http://www.nifs.org

An Indiana-based nonprofit organization that conducts research for enhancing health and athletic performance and provides physical fitness programs and health and fitness education for individuals and corporations.

National Operating Committee on Standards for Athletic Equipment (NOCSAE)

Website: http://www.nocsae.org
Publication: *NOCSAE Manual*

A committee that develops performance standards for the protective equipment used in a variety of sports and commissions scientific research on the mechanisms of athletic injuries.

National Strength and Conditioning Association (NSCA)

> **Website:** http://www.nsca-lift.org
> **Publications:** *National Strength and Conditioning Association Journal, Journal of Applied Sport Science Research*

An association that promotes and disseminates research on strength and conditioning to improve athletic performance and fitness.

National Youth Sports Safety Foundation (NYSSF)

> **Website:** http://www.nyssf.org

A national nonprofit organization working to minimize the number and severity of sports-sustained youth injuries.

President's Council on Physical Fitness and Sports (PCPFS)

> **Website:** http://www.fitness.gov
> **Publication:** *PCPFS Newsletter*

A volunteer committee working with the U.S. Department of Health and Human Services to engage, educate, and empower Americans of all ages to adopt a healthy lifestyle that includes regular physical activity and good nutrition.

Sport in Society, National University Consortium for Sport in Society

> **Website:** http://www.sportinsociety.org
> **Publication:** *Journal of Sport and Social Issues*

An organization based at Northeastern University that promotes the use of sports to help prevent interpersonal violence, improve the health of impoverished youth, and foster social diversity.

U.S. Consumer Product Safety Commission (USCPSC)

> **Website:** http://www.cpsc.gov

The U.S. federal agency charged with protecting consumers and families from products that may pose a hazard or threat.

Sports

Amateur Athletic Union of the United States (AAU)

> **Website:** http://www.aausports.org
> **Publication:** *InfoAAU*

A national nonprofit, volunteer, multisport organization dedicated to the promotion and development of amateur sports and physical fitness programs.

American Junior Golf Association (AJGA)

> **Website:** http://www.ajga.org
> **Publication:** *AJGA Tour Talk Newsletter*

A nonprofit organization dedicated to the growth and development of competitive junior golfers striving to earn college golf scholarships.

Canada Games Council

> **Website:** http://www.canadagames.ca

The governing body for the Canada Games: a private, nonprofit organization that promotes ongoing partnerships with organizations at the municipal, provincial, and national levels and provides support in organizational planning, ceremonies, marketing, and sponsorship.

Canadian Association for the Advancement of Women and Sport and Physical Activity (CAAWS)

> **Website:** http://www.caaws.ca/e

An association supporting and promoting women in sport while providing leadership and education.

Canadian Blind Sports Association (CBSA)

Website: http://www.canadianblindsports.ca

The national governing body for goalball, advocating for the blind and visually impaired within the sports system.

Canadian Centre for Ethics in Sports (CCES)

Website: http://www.cces.ca

A nonprofit organization devoted to promoting ethical conduct in sport and responsible for the implementation and management of Canada's Anti-Doping Program.

Canadian Colleges Athletic Association (CCAA)

Website: http://www.ccaa.ca

The national governing body for college sports in Canada.

Canadian Deaf Sports Association (ASSC-CDSA)

Website: http://www.assc-cdsa.com

An organization that supports deaf athletes who meet the requirements for participating in international competitions, especially the Pan American Games for the Deaf, the Deaflympics, and the World Deaf Championships.

Canadian Interuniversity Sport (CIS)

Website: http://www.cis-sic.ca

The national governing body of university sports in Canada, comprising 52 member universities.

Canadian Wheelchair Sports Association (CWSA)

Website: http://www.cwsa.ca/en/site

A national sports organization, founded in 1967, representing wheelchair athletes.

Coaches of Canada

Website: http://www.coachesofcanada.com

The national organization that represents, promotes, and regulates the profession of athletic coaching in Canada.

International Amateur Swimming Federation (IASF)

Website: http://www.fina.org

The world governing body for swimming, diving, water polo, synchronized swimming, and open-water swimming, promoting the development of swimming worldwide.

National Association for Girls and Women in Sports

Website: http://www.aahperd.org
Publication: *The Women in Sport and Physical Activity Journal*

An association within the American Alliance for Health, Physical Education, Recreation and Dance that advocates for girls and women in sports.

National Association for Sport and Physical Education (NASPE)

Website: http://www.aahperd.org/naspe
Publication: *Journal of Physical Education and Recreation*

An association within the American Alliance for Health, Physical Education, Recreation and Dance dedicated to enhancing knowledge and increasing support for quality physical education programs.

National Collegiate Athletic Association (NCAA)

Website: http://www.ncaa.org

The national governing body for intercollegiate athletics in the United States.

National Dance Association (NDA)

Website: http://www.aahperd.org/nda
Publication: *Journal of Physical Education, Recreation, & Dance*

An association that strives to promote quality dance by providing leadership, disseminating research, and collaborating with external partnerships.

National Federation of Interscholastic Coaches Association (NFICA)

An association that aims to improve the athletic participation experience while establishing consistent standards and rules for competition.

National Intramural-Recreational Sports Association (NIRSA)

Website: http://www.nirsa.org
Publications: *NIRSA Journal, NIRSA Newsletter*

A research and educational resource for collegiate recreational sports that promotes superior recreational programs, facilities, and services for diverse populations.

Special Olympics

Website: http://www.specialolympics.org

An international organization that holds a competition every 2 years as well as yearlong training for people who have intellectual disabilities.

Special Olympics Canada

Website: http://www.specialolympics.ca

A national nonprofit organization that provides sports training and competition opportunities for athletes with intellectual disabilities.

United States Olympic Committee

Website: http://www.teamusa.org

A committee responsible for training, entering, and underwriting the full expenses for the U.S. teams in the Olympic, Paralympic, Pan-American, and Parapan-American Games, as well as overseeing the process by which U.S. cities seek to be selected as a host to these games.

United States Soccer

Website: http://www.ussoccer.com

The governing body for soccer in the United States, promoting the development of soccer at all recreational and competitive levels.

United States Sports Academy

Website: http://www.ussa.edu

An independent, nonprofit, accredited sports university providing programs in instruction, research, and service to prepare those pursuing careers in the profession of sports.

US Figure Skating (USFS)

Website: http://www.usfsa.org

The national governing body for figure skating and a member of the International Skating Union (ISU) and the U.S. Olympic Committee (USOC), comprising member clubs, collegiate clubs, school-affiliated clubs, and individual members.

USA Athletic Congress (USAAC)

Website: http://www.usaac.org
Publication: *American Athletics Annual*

An association that promotes good sportsmanship by recognizing athletes who have excelled within their respective sports, working in conjunction with international federations and national governing bodies to improve sports participation around the world.

USA Gymnastics

Website: http://www.usa-gymnastics.org

The national organization for gymnastics, encouraging participation and excellence and setting the rules and policies that govern gymnastics in the United States.

USA Swimming

Website: http://www.usaswimming.org

The national governing body for swimming in the United States.

USA Volleyball

Website: http://www.usavolleyball.org

The national governing body for volleyball in the United States.

Women's Sports Foundations (WSF)

Website: http://www.womenssportsfoundations.org
Publications: *Women's Sports and Fitness, Headway*

A foundation that advocates for equal opportunity for women in sports, focusing on the psychological, physical, and social benefits of sports participation.

Sports Medicine

Academy for Sports Dentistry (ASD)

Website:
http://www.academyforsportsdentistry.org
Publication: *Sports Dentistry Newsletter*

A forum for medical professionals, coaches, and trainers to exchange ideas pertinent to sports dentistry, as well as for the collection and dissemination of research regarding the prevention and occurrence of dental injuries among athletes.

American Academy of Orthopaedic Surgeons (AAOS)

Website: http://www.aaos.org
Publications: *AAOS Report, The Bulletin*

An association of musculoskeletal specialists that provides education and practice management services for orthopedic surgeons and allied health professionals, advocates for enhanced patient care, and disseminates orthopedic knowledge to the public.

American Academy of Pediatrics (AAP) Committee on Sports Medicine & Fitness (COSMF)

Website: http://www.aap.org/sections/sportsmedicine

A division of the American Academy of Pediatrics, providing educational programs, policy statements, collaborative partnerships, media outreach, advocacy work, and research awards to promote safe physical activity and the highest level of treatment in pediatrics.

American Academy of Physical Medicine and Rehabilitation (AAPMR)

Special Interest Group on Sports Medicine

Website: http://www.aapmr.org
Publications: *Archives of Physical Medicine and Rehabilitation, Journal of Physical Medicine*

An academy representing patients with, or at risk for, temporary or permanent disabilities and helping physicians acquire the continuing education, practice knowledge, leadership skills, and research findings needed to provide quality patient care.

American Academy of Podiatric Sports Medicine (AAPSM)

Website: http://www.aapsm.org

An academy that helps further the understanding, prevention, and management of lower extremity injuries in sports through professional education, scientific research, public awareness, and membership support.

American College of Sports Medicine (ACSM)

Website: http://www.acsm.org
Publications: *Medicine and Science in Sports and Exercise, Sports Medicine Bulletin, Exercise and Sport Sciences Reviews*

An association that promotes healthy lifestyles through the diagnosis, treatment, and prevention of sports-related injuries as well as the advancement of exercise science and the dissemination of research.

American Medical Society for Sports Medicine (AMSSM)

Website: http://www.amssm.org

A forum for primary care sports medicine physicians to promote professional relationships and advance the discipline of sports medicine through education, research, advocacy, and quality patient care.

American Optometric Association (AOA) Sports Vision Section (SVS)

Website: http://www.aoa.org/x4787.xml
Publication: *SVS News and Views*

An association that is specific to optometric sports vision, striving to advance care through education, injury prevention, and enhancement of visual performance.

American Orthopaedic Society for Sports Medicine (AOSSM)

Website: http://www.sportsmed.org
Publication: *American Journal of Sports Medicine*

A national organization of orthopedic surgeons committed to sports medicine education, research, communication, and fellowship.

American Osteopathic Academy of Sports Medicine (AOASM)

Website: http://www.aoasm.org
Publication: *Clinical Journal of Sports Medicine*

An educational forum for primary care physicians and health care professionals to attend to the quality of health care, promoting fitness and exercise guidelines and providing a collegial environment to expand the knowledge of sports medicine.

American Physical Therapy Association (APTA)

Website: http://www.apta.org
Publication: *Physical Therapy*

A national organization committed to the advancement of physical therapy practice and research, promoting the prevention, diagnosis, and treatment of movement dysfunctions and the improvement of the physical health and functional abilities of all members of the public.

British Association of Sport and Exercise Medicine (BASEM)

Website: http://www.basem.co.uk

The oldest sport and exercise medicine association in the United Kingdom (founded in 1953) and the official UK representative to both the European Federation of Sports Medicine Associations (EFSMA) and the International Federation of Sports Medicine (FIMS), dedicated

to the promotion of good health through physical activity and the provision of sports medicine expertise to optimize athletic performance at all levels.

Canadian Academy of Sports Medicine (CASM-ACMS)

Website: http://www.casm-acms.org

An organization of physicians dedicated to the practice of medicine as applied to all aspects of physical activity, including health promotion and disease prevention.

Canadian Athletic Therapists Association (CATA)

Website: http://www.athletictherapy.org/en/index.aspx

A nonprofit organization dedicated to promoting injury prevention, emergency services, and rehabilitative techniques for active individuals.

Canadian Physiotherapy Association (CPA)

Website: http://www.thesehands.ca

An association of physiotherapists, physiotherapy support workers, physiotherapy students, and affiliate members dedicated to advancing the field of physiotherapy and improving the health of all individuals.

Canadian Society for Exercise Physiology (CSEP)

Website: http://www.csep.ca
Publication: *Canadian Journal of Applied Physiology*

An organization of professionals involved in the scientific study of exercise physiology, exercise biochemistry, fitness, and health.

Gatorade Sports Science Institute (GSSI)

Website: http://www.gssiweb.com

A research and educational facility that studies with scientists around the world the effects of exercise, the environment, and nutrition on the human body.

International Federation of Sports Medicine (FIMS)

Website: http://www.fims.org

An international organization dedicated to the study of sports medicine as well as the dissemination of findings to help athletes maximize their potential.

International Society of Arthroscopy, Knee Surgery, and Orthopedic Sports Medicine (ISAKOS)

Website: http://www.isakos.com

An international society that provides a forum for surgeons to advance the exchange and dissemination of information on education, research, and patient care in arthroscopy, knee surgery, and orthopedic sports medicine.

National Collegiate Athletic Association (NCAA) Committee on Competitive Safeguards and Medical Aspects of Sports

Website: http://www.ncaa.org
Publications: *The Sports Medicine Handbook, Injury Surveillance Annual Report*

A committee whose mission is to provide expertise and leadership to the NCAA to help it promote a healthy and safe environment for student-athletes through research, education, collaboration, and policy development.

Society for Adolescent Medicine (SAHM)

Website: http://www.adolescenthealth.org
Publication: *Journal of Adolescent Health Care*

A multidisciplinary organization of health professionals with the common goal of understanding the health needs and concerns of adolescents and enhancing public awareness through education, research, clinical services, and advocacy activities.

Sport Physiotherapy Canada

Website: http://www.sportphysio.ca

An organization, founded in 1972, dedicated to providing therapy, rehabilitation, and counseling to athletes before, during, and after injury.

Index

Entry titles and their page numbers are in **bold**.

fats, **1**:368
herbals, **1**:370, **2**:577
immune system and, **2**:702
for mental satisfaction, **3**:993
minerals, **1**:369–370, **3**:992–993,
   3:993
proteins, **1**:368, **3**:991, **3**:1162,
   4:1538–1539
vitamins, **1**:369, **3**:992–993,
   4:1528–1529
wound healing and, **1**:5
*See also names of specific supplements
   and vitamins*
Dieting, **4**:1542–1543. *See also* **Nutrition
   and hydration; Weight loss for
   sports**
Dietitian/Sports nutritionist, **1**:236,
   1:370–371, **1**:371
Diffuse axonal injury, 1:372–374,
   2:635 (table)
anatomy of, **1**:372
epidemiology of, **1**:372
imaging of, **1**:373, **2**:634
prevention of, **1**:374
primary injury in, **1**:372
secondary injury in, **1**:372–373
in sports, **1**:373–374
See also **Concussion;
   Head Injuries**
Diffusing capacity of the lung for carbon
   monoxide (DLCO) test, **1**:109
Digestive system. *See* **Gastrointestinal
   problems**
Digit, locking of. *See* **Trigger finger**
Digital cascade, **3**:907, **3**:907 (image)
Dill, D. B., **2**:668
Dinghy racing, **4**:1253–1254
DIP joint. *See* Distal interphalangeal
   (DIP) joint
Direct current electrical stimulation,
   2:422, **2**:425
Direct inguinal hernia, **2**:603
Direct pars repair, **1**:134
Dirkin compression test,
   3:910–911, **3**:910 (image). *See also*
   Compression tests
Disability
   in ABCDE approach, **2**:427, **2**:509,
      2:511, **2**:515–517
   defined, **3**:1090, **4**:1586
See also **Physically and mentally
   challenged athletes**
Disabled individuals
   diversity of, in sports, **1**:377,
      1:380–381
See also **Physically and mentally
   challenged athletes**
Discoid meniscus, 1:374–376
anatomy of, **1**:374
causes of, **1**:374
diagnosis of, **1**:375
imaging of, **1**:375

physical examination and history for,
   1:375
return to activity, **1**:376
surgery for, **1**:375–376
symptoms of, **1**:375
treatment of, **1**:375
See also **Knee injuries; Meniscus
   injuries**
Discus (track-and-field event), **4**:1529
Disease prevention. *See* **Exercise and
   disease prevention**
Disease-modifying antirheumatic drugs,
   1:99
Diseases. *See names of specific diseases*
Disk herniation. *See* Herniated disk
Diskectomy, **4**:1264
Disk-osteophyte complex,
   1:256, **4**:1587
Disks, intervertebral. *See* Intervertebral
   disk
Dislocations
   cervical, **1**:258–259
   dental, **1**:353–354
   elbow, **2**:413–415, **3**:1115–1117
   fieldside treatment of, **2**:519
   finger, **2**:519, **2**:523–526, **2**:533
   hip, **2**:653–656
   patella, **2**:781–782, **3**:1032–1035
   PIP joint, **3**:1164–1167
   shoulder. *See* **Shoulder dislocation**
   wrist, **4**:1557–1560
See also **Acromioclavicular (AC) joint,
   separation of; Sternoclavicular
   (SC) joint, separation of;
   Subluxation**
Disordered eating. *See* **Eating disorders**
Displaced, defined, **4**:1587
Displaced fracture, **2**:559, **2**:560, **4**:1477,
   4:1478. *See also* **Fractures;** *and
   names of specific fractures*
Displaced ribs, **3**:1222. *See also* **Rib tip
   syndrome**
Distal biceps tendon musculoskeletal
   test, **3**:895
Distal biceps test, **3**:895
Distal groove, in the nail unit, **2**:712
Distal interphalangeal (DIP) joint,
   2:528
anatomy of, **1**:45
in hand and finger injuries, **2**:624,
   2:625 (table), **2**:626
in jersey finger, **2**:554, **2**:629, **2**:729,
   2:730
in mallet finger, **2**:629, **3**:835
in musculoskeletal tests, **3**:909
PIP joint dislocation and, **3**:1165
Distal radioulnar joint (DRUJ), **2**:557
   in triangular fibrocartilage complex,
      4:1501, **4**:1502, **4**:1504
   in wrist injuries, **4**:1563, **4**:1566
See also Falls on the outstretched hand
   (FOOSH); Radius; Ulna

Distal radius growth plate, **2**:610
Distal subungual onychomycosis,
   4:1491, **4**:1491 (image)
Distance healing, **1**:307
Distance running, injuries in. *See*
   **Marathons, injuries in; Running
   injuries; Triathlons, injuries in**
Distraction test, **3**:973, **4**:1587. *See also*
   Apley distraction test
Diuretics, 1:376–377, 2:685
defined, **4**:1587
in exercise, **3**:1082
for performance enhancement, **1**:377,
   1:382, **1**:388, **3**:1063
Diversity in sports, 1:377–382
benefits of, **1**:377–378
disability and, **1**:380–381
gender and, **1**:377, **1**:378, **2**:495,
   4:1488–1490
Dividing attention, **1**:124–125. *See also*
   Attention focus in sports
Diving
   atlantoaxial instability and, **1**:123
   body composition in, **1**:189
   catastrophic injuries in, **1**:252
   from cliffs, **2**:482
   ear injuries in, **2**:399
   headaches and, **2**:636
   neck injuries in, **3**:976
   seizure control in, **4**:1276
   spondylolysis in, **4**:1374
   wrist injuries in, **4**:1501
See also **SCUBA diving, injuries in**
DLCO (diffusing capacity of the lung for
   carbon monoxide) test, **1**:109
DM. *See* Diabetes mellitus
DNA testing, **1**:320. *See also* Genetic
   testing and screening
Doping, meaning of, **3**:1064, **3**:1065
**Doping and performance enhancement: a
   new definition, 1:382–386**
data analysis of doping test results,
   1:383
doping control in blood, **1**:383–384
gene doping, **1**:384–385
types of drug tests, **1**:382–383
UNESCO Convention, **1**:385
See also **Anabolic steroids; Blood
   doping; Narcotic analgesics;
   World Anti-Doping Agency**
**Doping and performance enhancement:
   historical overview, 1:386–389**
Olympic Games of 1886-1932,
   1:386–387
Olympic Games of 1936-1960, **1**:387
Olympic Games of 1968-1980,
   1:387–388
Olympic Games of 1978-2008,
   1:389 (table)
Olympic Games of 1984-2000, **1**:388
terminology of, **1**:386
WADA, founding of, **1**:388–389

Italy, preparticipation screening in, 3:1125–1126
Itchy skin, in allergic contact dermatitis, 1:28. *See also* **Jock itch**
Item-intensity specificity and arousal intensity, 1:95

Jammed finger, 1:141, 2:532–533, 3:1165. *See also* **Finger sprain; Proximal interphalangeal joint dislocation**
Japanese encephalitis, 4:1499
Jaundice, 2:812
Javelin (track-and-field event), 3:997, 3:1002, 3:1219, 3:1221, 4:1298, 4:1529
Jaw. *See* Mandible; Maxilla
Jaw thrust maneuver, 2:512
Jazzercise, 1:18
JCAHO (Joint Commission on Accreditation of Healthcare Organizations), 3:999
Jefferson fracture, 1:259
Jerk test, 2:585, 4:1311, 4:1591
Jersey finger, 2:625 (table), 2:729–731, 4:1404
 anatomy of, 2:729, 2:729 (figure)
 evaluation of, 2:730
 imaging of, 2:730
 mechanism of, 2:730
 return to sports, 2:730–731
 sports associated with, 2:554, 2:729
 surgery for, 2:629, 2:730–731
 treatment of, 2:730
Jervell and Lange-Neilson syndrome, 3:1129
Jet lag, 2:731–733
 chronobiology of, 2:731–733
 circadian rhythms and, 1:285, 1:286, 1:287–288, 2:731–732
 compared to travel fatigue, 2:731
 dealing with, 2:732–733, 4:1499–1500
 factors affecting, 2:732
 sleep deprivation and, 4:1348
 See also **Travel medicine and the international athlete**
Jet skiing, 2:482. *See also* Skiing; **Skiing, injuries in**
Jiujitsu, 3:874
Jobe, Frank, 1:137, 3:1005, 3:1238
Jobe empty can test, 2:585, 3:945–946, 3:946 (image), 4:1591. *See also* Empty can test
Jobe relocation test, 3:1112
Jock itch, 2:570, 2:733–734
 defined, 4:1601
 diagnosis of, 2:709
 pathophysiology of, 2:733
 physical examination and history for, 2:733
 prevention of, 2:734

 treatment of, 2:571, 2:709, 2:733–734
 in wrestlers, 4:1327
Jogger's nipples, 2:563, 2:734–735, 3:1136
Jogger's toe, 3:1135–1136
Jogging
 black nail in, 1:176
 seizure control in, 4:1276
 warming up for, 3:1138 (box)
 See also Running; **Running injuries**
John, Tommy, 1:137
Joint aspiration, defined, 4:1591
Joint Commission on Accreditation of Healthcare Organizations (JCAHO), 3:999
Joint Commission on Sports Medicine and Medical Science, 4:1642
Joint effusion, 3:926, 4:1591
Joint fluid, removal and analysis of, 1:98, 2:735
Joint injection, 2:735–737
 for diagnosis and treatment, 2:735
 follow-up for, 2:736
 injection sites for, 2:736
 risks and benefits of, 2:735–736
 types of medications injected, 2:736
 See also Injection of drugs
Joint integrity
 defined, 4:1591
 physical therapy for, 3:1150–1151
Joint line tenderness test, 3:929, 3:935–936, 3:936 (image)
Joint National Committee on the Detection, Evaluation and Treatment of High Blood Pressure, 2:683
Joint of Luschka, 1:266, 1:269 (figure), 1:270, 4:1591
Joint reduction techniques, 2:414–415
Joint stability and therapeutic exercise, 4:1472
Joints, magnetic resonance imaging of, 2:737–745
 arthroscopy and, 2:737
 for knees, 2:737–739
  ACL, 2:737, 2:737 (images), 2:739 (image)
  hyaline cartilage, 2:738, 2:740 (image)
  MCL, 2:737, 2:738 (image)
  menisci, 2:738, 2:738 (image)
  PCL, 2:739 (image)
  posterolateral corner, 2:738, 2:739 (image)
 for shoulders, 2:740–745
  glenoid labrum, 2:740, 2:742 (image)
  internal impingement, 2:742–743, 2:743 (images)
  paralabral cysts, 2:742, 2:743 (image)

  Parsonage-Turner syndrome, 2:744, 2:744 (images)
  quadrilateral space syndrome, 2:743–744, 2:744 (image)
  rotator cuff, 2:740, 2:741 (images)
 See also Magnetic resonance imaging
Jokl, Ernst, 2:668
Jones fracture, 1:130, 1:140, 2:543, 4:1591
Judo, 2:487, 2:523, 3:874
Jujitsu, 2:523
Jumper's knee, 3:1035, 3:1038–1039, 3:1195, 4:1533. *See also* **Patellar tendinitis; Quadriceps tendinitis**
Jumping, and incontinence, 2:583
Jumping, forces produced by, 2:477, 3:899
Jumping, injuries in
 Achilles tendon rupture, 1:11, 1:12
 ACL tear, 1:84
 ankle injuries, 1:61, 1:63, 1:67, 2:538, 2:539, 2:541, 4:1532
 apophysitis, 1:89, 1:90
 arch pain, 1:90
 avulsion fractures, 1:129
 foot injuries, 2:538, 2:541, 2:544
 foot stress fracture, 2:549, 2:550
 gluteal strain, 2:587
 hip, pelvis, and groin injuries, 2:596, 2:652, 2:656, 2:661, 3:1056
 knee injuries, 2:478, 2:771, 3:1011, 3:1035
 medial tibial stress syndrome, 3:851
 posterior tibial tendinitis, 3:1113
 quadriceps tendinitis, 3:1195
 Sever disease, 4:1287
 spinal injuries, 1:142
 stress fractures, 1:141, 2:549, 2:550, 3:851, 4:1485
 thigh injuries, 4:1474
 tibia and fibula stress fractures, 3:851, 4:1485
Juvenile osteochondritis dissecans of the knee, 2:745–747, 4:1575
 etiology of, 2:745
 imaging of, 2:746
 physical examination and history for, 2:745–746
 return to sports, 2:746, 2:747
 stages of, 2:746, 2:747
 surgery for, 2:746–747
 treatment of, 2:746–747
 See also **Knee, osteochondritis dissecans of the**

Karate, injuries in, 2:749–751, 3:874
 commotio cordis injuries, 1:228 (table)
 concussion, 2:750
 ear injuries, 2:750
 eye injuries, 2:750
 finger injuries, 2:523, 2:750
 lacerations, 2:750

biomechanics of, 2:764, 3:1107
epidemiology of, 3:1107
imaging of, 2:739 (image), 3:1108, 3:1109
mechanism of, 3:1108
in musculoskeletal tests, 3:934–935, 3:934 (images)
physical examination and history for, 3:1108
return to sports, 3:1109
sports associated with, 1:139, 3:1107
sprains, 1:139
surgery for, 3:1109
treatment of, 3:1108–1109
Posterior drawer test, 2:774–775, 2:783, 3:934–935, 3:934 (image), 3:1108, 4:1596. *See also* Drawer tests
Posterior impingement syndrome, 1:65, 1:66, **3:1110–1112**
anatomy of, 3:1110–1111
causes of, 3:1110, 3:1111
etiology of, 3:1111
imaging of, 3:1112
management of, 3:1112
physical examination and history for, 3:1111–1112
sports associated with, 3:1110, 3:1111
surgery for, 3:1112
See also **Ankle impingement**
Posterior Lachman test, 3:1108, 4:1596. *See also* Lachman test
Posterior oblique ligament, 2:782. *See also* Medial collateral ligament (MCL)
Posterior sag sign, 3:934, 3:934 (image)
Posterior sag test, 2:774–775, 3:1108, 4:1596
Posterior superior iliac spine, 3:915, 3:916, 3:958
Posterior talofibular ligament (PTFL), 1:68 (figure), 1:71, 1:77, 3:887, 4:1362
Posterior tibial tendinitis, 3:1113–1115
anatomy of, 3:1113, 3:1113 (figure)
causes of, 3:1113–1114
diagnosis of, 3:1114
imaging of, 3:1114
physical examination and history of, 3:1114
return to sports, 3:1115
sports associated with, 3:1113
surgery for, 3:1115
symptoms of, 3:1114
treatment of, 3:1114–1115
Posterior tibialis muscle, 3:1019, 3:1113
Posterior tibialis tendon, 3:1018, 3:1020, 3:1113, 3:1113 (figure), 3:1114, 3:1115
Posterior vertebral line, 3:974
Posterolateral corner (PLC)
ligament complex in, 2:783
MRI of, 2:738, 2:739 (images)

in musculoskeletal tests, 3:935, 3:935 (images)
PCL injuries and, 3:1108
Posterolateral drawer test, 3:935. *See also* Dial test; Drawer tests
Posterolateral rotatory instability, 3:1115–1117
anatomy of, 3:1116
causes of, 3:1115–1116
imaging of, 3:1116–1117
physical examination and history for, 3:1116
return to sports, 3:1117
stages of, 3:1115
surgery for, 3:1117
treatment of, 3:1117
Posterotalofibular ligament, 4:1362
Postgame meal, 3:1117–1121
carbohydrate loading in, 3:1120–1121
carbohydrate-protein mix in, 3:1120
carbohydrates in, 3:1118, 3:1120–1121
fat in, 3:1120
goals of, 3:1117–1118
hydration in, 3:1118, 3:1120
insulin from, 3:1118
liquid versus complex in, 3:1120
for marathon runners, 3:841
nitrogen balance in, 3:1120–1121
protein in, 1:226, 3:1118–1119, 3:1120
rest and, 3:1121
salt in, 3:1120
timing of, 3:1118
See also **Nutrition and hydration**
Posthypnotic suggestions, 2:687
Postpartum exercise, 2:455. *See also* **Exercise during pregnancy and postpartum**
Postseason conditioning, 1:316
Posture
in biking, 1:155, 1:156, 1:157, 1:158, 2:677, 2:720
in cervical nerve stretch syndrome, 1:273
in complementary treatment, 1:307, 1:308, 1:309
in costosternal syndrome, 1:328
defined, 4:1596
in disk degeneration, 1:267
evaluation of, 3:900–901, 3:913–915, 3:942, 3:955, 3:1150
in figure skating, 2:522
hyperlordotic, 2:522
kinesiology of, 2:755
in Scheuermann kyphosis, 1:263
types of, 2:755
See also Alignment
Potassium (in nutrition), 1:369, 3:993, 4:1384
Potassium hydroxide (KOH) test, 2:570, 2:733, 3:1136

Power
bioenergetics and, 1:160
defined, 4:1596
formula for, 3:1102
plyometrics and, 3:1102–1105
Power law of practice, 4:1323
Power lifting
atlantoaxial instability and, 1:123
disk disease and, 2:720
slipped disk in, 4:1354
See also Weight lifting; **Weight lifting, injuries in**
Power profile, 4:1365
Powerboat racing, 2:482
Practice
imagery for, 2:699
power law of, 4:1323
skill acquisition through, 4:1323
Practice statements, in sports medicine, 2:802. *See also* Recommendations and guidelines for
Prader-Willi syndrome, 2:608
Prague 2004 consensus guidelines, on concussion management, 2:553
Prayer, in mind-body medicine, 1:300. *See also* Meditation
Prayer position, 4:1564
Preconditioning, 1:317
Precordial catch syndrome, 1:328
Pregame meal, 3:988, 3:1121–1124
alcohol in, 3:1123
carbohydrate loading in, 3:1122
carbohydrates in, 3:1122–1123
for endurance events, 3:841, 3:1121
glycemic index and, 3:1121–1122, 3:1123
goals of, 3:1122
hydration in, 3:1122
insulin from, 3:1123
to prevent muscle cramps, 3:886, 3:1123
protein in, 3:1122
salt in, 3:1122, 3:1123
timing of, 3:1122
See also **Nutrition and hydration**
Pregnancy
carpal tunnel syndrome and, 1:239
exercise during, 2:453–455, 2:497, 2:580–581
osteoarthritis and, 1:97
sacroiliac joint during, 4:1252
See also Childbirth
Premature birth and childhood obesity, 3:1047, 3:1048
Premature ventricular contractions, 3:1133
Preparatory phase, in periodization, 3:1070, 3:1070 (table)
Preparticipation cardiovascular screening, 3:1124–1126
for athlete's heart syndrome, 1:114
for bleeding disorders, 1:179

Pyrogen, 2:506, 4:1597
Pyruvate
  as dietary supplement, 1:368–369
  in glycolysis, 2:793, 2:794 (figure)
  in Krebs cycle, 2:793, 2:795 (figure)

Q angle, 3:1191–1192, 3:1191 (figure)
  ACL injuries and, 3:1192
  in extensor mechanism injury, 2:477
  femoral anteversion and, 2:501,
      3:872–873, 3:928, 3:1191
  gender differences in, 2:496, 3:1191
  in knock-knees, 3:1144,
      3:1144 (figure), 3:1191
  measurement of, 3:1191
  in miserable malalignment syndrome,
      3:872–873
Qi (energy, life force), 1:301, 1:302,
    1:308
Qigong, 1:305, 1:307, 1:308
QT syndrome, long, 1:227, 3:1089,
    3:1124, 3:1129, 4:1419, 4:1420
Quadratus lumborum muscle, 1:44
Quadratus plantae muscle, 1:48
Quadriceps angle. *See* **Q angle**
Quadriceps contusion, 1:322, 2:694,
    4:1476 (table)
Quadriceps cramps, 3:885
Quadriceps inhibition test, 3:940,
    3:941 (image)
Quadriceps muscles, 2:477, 2:772
  anatomy of, 1:47, 4:1472, 4:1474
  patellar dislocation and, 3:1032–1033
  patellofemoral pain syndrome and,
      3:1037–1038
  quadriceps strain and, 3:1192
  strength differential ratio of, with
      hamstrings, 3:1247
  in thigh injuries, 4:1472–1474,
      4:1475
Quadriceps strain, 3:1192–1194
  anatomy and histology of,
      3:1192–1193, 3:1193 (figure)
  grading of, 3:1193
  imaging of, 3:1194
  physical examination and history for,
      3:1193
  return to sports, 3:1194
  sports associated with, 2:508, 3:1193
  treatment of, 3:1193–1194
  wrap for, 4:1622–1623,
      4:1622 (images), 4:1623 (image)
Quadriceps tendinitis, 3:1194–1197
  anatomy of, 3:1195, 3:1195 (figure)
  causes of, 3:1195
  diagnosis of, 3:1196
  imaging of, 3:1196
  physical examination and history for,
      3:1195–1196
  prevention of, 3:1197
  return to sports, 3:1197
  sports associated with, 1:157, 3:1195

surgery for, 3:1196–1197
  treatment of, 3:1196–1197
Quadriceps tendon, defined, 4:1597
Quadriceps tendon rupture, 3:1038
Quadrilateral space syndrome,
    2:743–744, 2:744 (image)
Quadriplegia, 1:262, 3:1084, 3:1226
Quads. *See* Quadriceps muscles;
    **Quadriceps strain; Quadriceps
    tendinitis**
Quarantine
  in impetigo, 4:1335
  in methicillin-resistant *Staphylococcus
      aureus* infections, 3:870, 3:872
QuickVue influenza test, 2:705

Rabies, 4:1499
Race, diversity of, in sports, 1:377,
    1:378–380
Race phase, in periodization,
    3:1070 (table)
Racquet wrist, 4:1464–1465
Racquetball and squash, cooling down
    in, 3:1139 (box)
**Racquetball and squash, injuries in,
    3:1199–1201**
  carpal tunnel syndrome, 1:239
  compared to other racquet sports,
      4:1462
  de Quervain tenosynovitis, 3:1200
  elbow and wrist sprains, 3:1200
  eye injuries, 2:569, 3:1199–1200
  facial injuries, 2:487
  foot and ankle injuries, 2:549, 3:1200
  knee injuries, 3:1200, 4:1462
  lower extremity injuries,
      3:1200–1201
  lumbar disk prolapse, 4:1462
  rib injuries, 3:1221
  shoulder separation, 3:1200
  SLAP lesions, 4:1428
  upper extremity injuries, 3:1200
  See also **Tennis and racquet sports,
      injuries in**
Radial artery, Allen test of, 3:898
Radial collateral ligament (RCL)
  anatomy of, 4:1257 (figure), 4:1480
  taping for, 4:1629, 4:1631
  in thumb sprain, 4:1533
Radial head, 2:416–417, 3:892
Radial nerve, 2:414, 2:556
Radial shock wave therapy, 2:479
Radial snuffbox, 4:1564. *See also*
    Snuffbox
Radiation, in body heat loss, 1:293,
    2:638, 4:1597. *See also* **Heat illness**
Radiation injury to the eye, 2:485. *See
    also* **Sunburn**
Radiation therapy, 4:1425
Radicular pain, 1:256, 1:269, 3:1201,
    4:1597. *See also* **Referred pain**
Radicular symptoms, 4:1355, 4:1597

Radiculopathy, 1:133, 3:980, 3:1203,
    4:1518, 4:1597
Radioallergoabsorbant testing (RAST),
    1:30
Radiocapitellar articulation, 3:1031,
    3:1116
Radiocarpal joint, 4:1563. *See also*
    Carpal bones; Radius
Radiocarpal ligaments, 4:1566
Radiographs. *See* X-rays and
    radiographs
Radiologic technologists, careers as,
    1:236
Radioulnar joint
  in triangular fibrocartilage complex,
      4:1501, 4:1502, 4:1504
  in wrist injuries, 4:1563, 4:1566
  See also Falls on the outstretched hand
      (FOOSH); Radius; Ulna
Radius
  anatomy of, 1:296, 2:402,
      2:405, 2:410, 2:416, 2:556,
      4:1257 (figure), 4:1501, 4:1502
  fractures of, 1:141, 1:296, 2:557,
      2:558, 2:558 (images), 2:610.
      See also **Forearm fracture; Wrist
      fracture**
  in Kienböck disease, 2:752, 2:753
  in posterolateral rotatory instability,
      3:1116
  scaphoid and, 4:1563
  in triangular fibrocartilage injuries,
      4:1501–1504
  See also entries beginning with Elbow
Range of motion (ROM) assessment
  of the ankle, 3:888
  of the elbow, 3:892–893,
      3:892 (images)
  of the foot, 3:902–903
  of the hand and wrist, 3:908
  of the hip, 3:917–918, 3:917 (images),
      3:918 (images)
  of the knee, 3:929, 3:929 (images)
  of the shoulder, 3:944–945,
      3:944 (images), 3:945 (images)
  of the spine, 3:955, 3:959,
      3:959 (images), 3:960 (images),
      3:973
  Staheli method for, 3:918,
      3:918 (images)
  See also the physical examination
      *subheading under names of
      specific injuries and conditions*
Range of motion (ROM) exercises,
    4:1411–1413, 4:1470–1471
Rapid strep test, 2:706
Rapid-eye-movement (REM) sleep,
    4:1345, 4:1346, 4:1348
Rashes
  athlete's foot as, 1:110–112
  from caterpillar contact,
      2:714–715

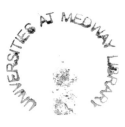